Operative Strategies in
Inflammatory Bowel Disease

Springer
New York
Berlin
Heidelberg
Barcelona
Hong Kong
London
Milan
Paris
Singapore
Tokyo

Fabrizio Michelassi, MD

Professor and Chief, Section of General Surgery, University of Chicago, Chicago, Illinois

Jeffrey W. Milsom, MD

Professor and Chief, Division of Colon and Rectal Surgery, Mount Sinai Medical Center, New York, New York

Editors

Operative Strategies in Inflammatory Bowel Disease

With 254 Illustrations, 36 in full color

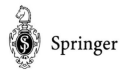 Springer

Fabrizio Michelassi, MD
Professor and Chief
Section of General Surgery
University of Chicago
Chicago, IL 60637, USA

Jeffrey W. Milsom, MD
Professor and Chief, Division of Colon
  and Rectal Surgery
Mount Sinai Medical Center
New York, NY 10029, USA

Library of Congress Cataloging-in-Publication Data
Operative strategies in inflammatory bowel disease / [edited by]
  Fabrizio Michelassi, Jeffrey W. Milsom
    p. cm.
    ISBN 0-387-94966-6 (hardcover : alk. paper)
    1. Inflammatory bowel diseases—Surgery. I. Michelassi,
  Fabrizio, 1950– . II. Milsom, Jeffrey W.
    [DNLM: 1. Inflammatory Bowel Diseases—surgery. 2. Inflammatory
  Bowel Diseases—complications. WI 420 061 1997]
  RD540.6.064 1997
  617.5'547—dc21   97-20702

Printed on acid-free paper.

Production coordinated by Chernow Editorial Services, Inc., and managed by Lesley
Poliner; manufacturing supervised by Joe Quatela.
Typeset by Agnew's, Inc., Grand Rapids, MI.
Printed and bound by Maple-Vail Book Manufacturing Group, York, PA.
Printed in the United States of America.

9 8 7 6 5 4 3 2 1

ISBN 0-387-94966-6 Springer-Verlag New York Berlin Heidelberg SPIN 10552790

Probably more than in most professions, the surgeon relies on the teaching and examples of others to master the clinical skills and the judgment necessary to care for patients. Therefore, this book is dedicated to the physicians and surgeons who have been instrumental in guiding me to this point in my professional life.

Fabrizio Michelassi

This book is dedicated to all patients with inflammatory bowel diseases and the determination to find a cure for their suffering.

Jeffrey W. Milsom

Preface

Inflammatory bowel disease (IBD) surgery has undergone major progress in the last twenty years, with strides in the care of both ulcerative colitis and Crohn's disease. There are now new operations available for most patients with IBD that alleviate suffering in Crohn's disease and offer curative therapy in ulcerative colitis, while permitting ever increasing chances of nearly normal intestinal, urologic, and sexual function.

Gastrointestinal surgeons have always been stimulated to treat the complexities of IBD. Patients are generally young, active, and highly motivated. Successful therapy is extremely gratifying to the patient and the medical team; there is reasonable hope after treatment for an active, long, and productive life.

The other alluring aspect of IBD surgery is its diversity. Pan intestinal, retroperitoneal, and pelvic anatomy must be understood in minute detail. Surgeons must be prepared to tackle unexpected problems in an extension of ileal Crohn's into the duodenum or a carcinoma of the rectum complicating ulcerative colitis—as a matter of course.

Not all surgeons are as fortunate as the authors of this book to be working in medical centers that have a long history of healing patients with IBD. In part, it was this responsibility that encouraged us to pursue the writing and editing of this book. Because IBD is very common in most Western countries (and is rising in incidence in many non-Western countries), we believe that assembling a single volume of expertise on the surgical aspects of IBD will be of great benefit to surgeons and patients alike. This book has been designed so that at a moment's notice, any surgeon may open it and consult an authority on a particular topic related to IBD surgery. In addition, consultants in related fields have written excellent summaries on major developments in the field outside of surgery, providing surgeons with important insights into the many nonsurgical aspects of IBD.

We hope this book will not only serve as a reference for surgeons, but also stir some controversies that will lead to further improvements in the care of IBD patients.

FABRIZIO MICHELASSI, MD
JEFFREY W. MILSOM, MD

Acknowledgments

We are greatly indebted to those who have contributed generously to producing this book. We want to thank the contributing authors who donated countless hours to enrich the book with their knowledge and expertise. We understand how difficult it can be to find those "extra" hours in busy schedules that are already stretched to the limit. We hope that gathering this extensive knowledge into one book will shed light on the surgical management of patients with inflammatory bowel disease and be of benefit to other surgeons and specialists in this increasingly complex field and to the patients who suffer with this condition.

We wish to thank Roberta Carden and Cynthia Scott for their professional secretarial assistance—the book would never have been completed without their help—and to Natalie Johnson and Joseph Pangrace for their many beautiful illustrations. We are also indebted to Laura Gillan and Jeffrey Sands from Springer-Verlag for their commitment to this project and for their ceaseless assistance, patience, and support in putting together a book about a complex subject discussed from many points of view. Barbara Chernow, our production editor, was also a steady hand in the final preparation of the book, and we owe many thanks to her and to her staff for their efforts in the final push to complete this project.

Our families also deserve our deeply felt gratitude for supporting us in our professional lives and for giving up those "extra" hours that we needed to complete this work. So to CH, RHM, and FEM, and to Susan, Alexandra, and Geoffrey, profound thanks as always for your support and generosity.

FABRIZIO MICHELASSI, MD
JEFFREY W. MILSOM, MD

Contents

Section III   Crohn's Disease
Part II   Surgical Treatment of Specific Complications

Section III   Crohn's Disease
Part III   Strategy According to Specific Anatomical Sites

Section III   Crohn's Disease
Part IV   Recurrent Disease

Section IV   Inflammatory Bowel Disease: Surgical Treatment
Part I   General Complications

Section IV   Inflammatory Bowel Disease: Surgical Treatment
Part II   Septic Complications Following Restorative Proctocolectomy

Contributors

MARK E. BAKER, MD
Head, Section of Abdominal Imaging, Department of Radiology, Cleveland Clinic Foundation, Cleveland, OH 44194, USA

DAVID C.C. BARTOLO, MD
Consultant, Colorectal Surgeon, Department of Surgery, Royal Infirmary of Edinburgh, Edinburgh EH3 9YW, UK

JAMES M. BECKER, MD
Surgeon-in-Chief, Department of General Surgery, Boston University School of Medicine, Boston Medical Center, Boston, MA 02215, USA

DIANE BRYANT, RN, MS, CETN
Clinical Nurse Specialist, Brigham and Women's Hospital, Boston, MA 02115, USA

AARON BRZEZINSKI, MD
Staff Gastroenterologist, Department of Gastroenterology, Cleveland Clinic Foundation, Cleveland, OH 44194, USA

DOMINICK J. CARBONE JR., M.D.
Fellow, Section of Male Infertility, Department of Urology, Cleveland Clinic Foundation, Cleveland, OH 44194, USA

SERGIO CASILLAS, MD
Research Resident, Department of Colon and Rectal Surgery, Cleveland Clinic Foundation, Cleveland, OH 44194, USA

ANTONINO CAVALLARI
Professor and Chairman, Clinica Chirurgica II dell' Università di Bologna, Ospedale S. Orsola, 40138 Bologna, Italy

ZANE COHEN, MD
Professor of Surgery, Department of Surgery, University of Toronto, Toronto, Ontario M5G 1X9, Canada

KEMAL I. DEEN, MD
Research Fellow, Department of Surgery, Division of Colon and Rectal Surgery, University of Minnesota Medical School, Minneapolis, MN 55405, USA

DAVID W. DIETZ, MD
Resident and Research Fellow, Department of Colon and Rectal Surgery, Cleveland Clinic Foundation, Cleveland, OH, 44194 USA

ROGER R. DOZOIS, MD
Professor of Surgery, Division of Colon and Rectal Surgery, Mayo Clinic and Mayo Foundation, Rochester, MN 55905, USA

DAVID M. EINSTEIN, MD
Head, Residency Program, Member, Section of Abdominal Imaging, Department of Radiology, Cleveland Clinic Foundation, Cleveland, OH 44194, USA

RIDZUAN FAROUK, MCH
Fellow, Division of Colon and Rectal Surgery, Mayo Clinic and Mayo Foundation, Rochester, MN 55905, USA

VICTOR W. FAZIO, MD
Chairman, Department of Colon and Rectal Surgery, Cleveland Clinic Foundation, Cleveland, OH 44194, USA

CLAUDIO FIOCCHI, MD
Professor of Medicine, School of Medicine, Division of Gastroenterology, Case Western Reserve University, Cleveland, OH 44106, USA

ERIC W. FONKALSRUD, MD
Professor of Surgery, Department of Surgery, UCLA Medical Center, Los Angeles, CA, 90024, USA

LAWRENCE J. GOTTLIEB, MD
Professor of Clinical Surgery, Section of Plastic and Reconstructive Surgery, University of Chicago, Chicago, IL 60637, USA

ADRIAN J. GREENSTEIN, MD
Professor of Surgery, Department of Surgery, Mount Sinai School of Medicine, New York, NY 10029, USA

STEPHEN B. HANAUER, MD
Professor of Medicine and Clinical Pharmacology, Department of Medicine, University of Chicago, Chicago, IL 60637, USA

BRUCE A. HARMS, MD
Professor of Surgery, Department of Surgery, University of Wisconsin Hospital and Clinics, Madison, WI 53715, USA

TOMAS M. HEIMANN, MD
Professor of Surgery, Department of Surgery, Mount Sinai School of Medicine, New York, NY 10029, USA

JACQUES HEPPELL, MD
Consultant, Department of Surgery, Mayo Medical School, Mayo Clinic, Scottsdale, AZ 85259, USA

TRACY L. HULL, MD
Staff Colorectal Surgeon, Department of Colon and Rectal Surgery, Cleveland Clinic Foundation, Cleveland, OH 44194, USA

ROGER HURST, MD
Assistant Professor of Surgery, Department of Surgery, University of Chicago, Chicago, IL 60637, USA

SANDEEP S. JEJURIKAR, MD
Fellow, Section of Plastic and Reconstructive Surgery, University of Chicago, Chicago, IL 60637, USA

JEFFREY A. KATZ, MD
Assistant Professor of Medicine, Division of Gastroenterology, University Hospitals of Cleveland, Cleveland, OH 44106, USA

M.R.B. KEIGHLEY, MD
Professor, Head of Surgery, Department of Surgery, Queen Elizabeth Hospital, Birmingham B15 2TH, UK

KEITH A. KELLY, MD
Professor of Surgery, Department of Surgery, Mayo Medical School, Mayo Clinic, Scottsdale, AZ 85259, USA

SEON-HAHN KIM, MD
Research Fellow, Department of Colon and Rectal Surgery, Cleveland Clinic Foundation, Cleveland, OH 44194, USA

JOSEPH B. KIRSNER, MD, PHD
Louis Block Distinguished Service Professor of Medicine, Department of Medicine, University of Chicago, Chicago, IL 60637, USA

S. KORSGEN, MD
Clinical Research Registrar, Department of Surgery, Queen Elizabeth Hospital, Birmingham BI5 2TH, UK

BRET A. LASHNER, MD MPH
Assistant Professor of Surgery, Department of Gastroenterology, Cleveland Clinic Foundation, Cleveland, OH 44194, USA

IAN C. LAVERY, MD
Professor of Surgery, Department of Colon and Rectal Surgery, Cleveland Clinic Foundation, Cleveland, OH 44194, USA

TOMAS LINDHAGEN, MD, PHD
Surgeon, Department of Surgery, University of Lund, Lund, Sweden

WALTER E. LONGO, MD
Associate Professor of Surgery, Department of Surgery, Saint Louis University Hospital, St. Louis, MO 63110, USA

ROBIN S. MCLEOD, MD, FRCSC, FACS
Head, Division of General Surgery, Professor, Department of Surgery, University of Toronto, Toronto M5G 1X5 Ontario, Canada

FABRIZIO MICHELASSI, MD
Professor and Chief, Section of General Surgery, University of Chicago, Chicago, IL 60637, USA

JEFFREY W. MILSOM, MD
Professor and Chief, Division of Colon and Rectal Surgery, Mount Sinai Medical Center, New York, NY 10029, USA

RONALD J. NICHOLLS, MD
Professor of Surgery, Department of Surgery, St. Marks Hospital, London EVIV 2PS, UK

BERNARD NORDLINGER, MD
Professor of Surgery and Chief, Hôpital Ambroise-Pazé, 92100 Boulogne, France

DENIS C.N.K. NYAM, MB
Department of Colorectal Surgery, Singapore General Hospital, Singapore 169608, The Republic of Singapore

ROLLAND PARC, MD
Professor of Surgery and Chief, Centre de Chirurgie Digestive, Hôpital Saint-Antoine, Paris 75571, France

JOHN H. PEMBERTON, MD
Professor of Surgery, Department of Colon and Rectal Surgery, Mayo Graduate School of Medicine, Rochester, MN 55905, USA

CHRISTOPHE PENNA, MD
Professor of Surgery, Centre de Chirurgie Digestive, Hôpital Saint-Antoine, Paris 75571, France

GILBERTO POGGIOLI, MD
Associate Professor, Clinica Chirurgica II dell' Università di Bologna, Ospedale S. Orsola, 40138 Bologna, Italy

ROBERT H. RIDDELL, MD
Professor of Pathology, Department of Pathology, McMaster University Medical Centre, Hamilton, Ontario L8N 3Z5, Canada

VIANNEY ROGER, MD
Professor of Surgery, Centre de Chirurgie Digestive, Hôpital Saint-Antoine Paris 75571, France

DAVID A. ROTHENBERGER, MD
Clinical Professor and Chief, Department of Surgery, Division of Colon and Rectal Surgery, University of Minnesota Medical School, Minneapolis, MN 55405, USA

OLIVIER SAINT-MARC, MD
Professor of Surgery, Centre de Chirugie Digestive, Hôpital Saint-Antoine, Paris 75571, France

DAVID J. SCHOETZ, MD
Colon and Rectal Surgeon, Chairman, Department of Colon and Rectal Surgery, Lahey Hitchcock Medical Center, Burlington, MA 01805, USA

JAMES R. STARLING, MD
Professor of Surgery, Department of Surgery, University of Wisconsin Hospital and Clinics, Madison, WI 53715, USA

ROBERT B. STEIN, MD
Fellow in Gastroenterology, Department of Medicine, University of Chicago, Chicago, IL 60637, USA

JAN STEWÉNIUS, MD, PHD
Attending Surgeon, Helsingborg Hospital, S-252 22 Helsingborg, Sweden

LUCA STOCCHI, MD
Clinica Chirurgica II dell' Università di Bologna, Ospedale S. Orsola, 40138 Bologna, Italy

DANNY TAKANISHI, MD
Assistant Professor of General Surgery, Department of Surgery, University of Chicago, Chicago, IL 60637, USA

H.T. TAN
Clinical Research Registrar, Department of Surgery, Queen Elizabeth Hospital, Birmingham B15 2TH, UK

ANTHONY J. THOMAS JR., MD
Head, Section of Male Infertility, Department of Urology, Cleveland Clinic Foundation, Cleveland, OH 44194, USA

JOE J. TJANDRA, MBBS, MD
Department of Colo-Rectal Surgery, Royal Melbourne Hospital, University of Melbourne, Royal Parade, Parkville, Victoria, 3050 Australia

ANTHONY M. VERNAVA, MD
Assistant Professor of Surgery, Department of Surgery, Section of Colon and Rectal Surgery, St. Louis University, School of Medicine, St. Louis, MO 63110, USA

CIARAN J. WALSH, MBBSC, MCH
Clinical Fellow, Department of Colon and Rectal Surgery, Cleveland Clinic Foundation, Cleveland, OH 44194, USA

BRUCE G. WOLFF, MD
Consultant, Division of Colon and Rectal Surgery, Professor of Surgery,
Department of Surgery, Mayo Clinic and Mayo Foundation, Rochester, MN
55905, USA

Section I
Inflammatory Bowel Disease: Overview

1 Etiologic Concepts of Inflammatory Bowel Diseases: Past, Present, and Future

Joseph B. Kirsner

All at present known in medicine is almost nothing in comparison with what remains to be discovered.
R. Descartes (1596–1650)

Ulcerative colitis and Crohn's disease represent a group of inflammatory and ulcerative disorders of the large and small intestine of unknown etiology and pathogenesis (1). They occur chiefly in developed countries (United States, Europe), affecting people of all ages, males and females approximately equally, and principally younger individuals. The common symptoms of ulcerative colitis are early constipation, rectal bleeding and urgency, abdominal discomfort, diarrhea, and weight loss. Laboratory data include iron deficiency anemia, lowered serum proteins, and the absence of conventional bacterial pathogens in the stool. The typical clinical manifestations of Crohn's disease are cramping lower abdominal pain, diarrhea, fever, anorexia, and weight loss. The laboratory data include normal or elevated leukocyte counts; increased erythrocyte sedimentation rate; iron, B_{12}, or folate deficiency; lowered serum proteins; and other indications of undernutrition. Their course is acute and chronic with remissions and exacerbations, intestinal and systemic complications, and variable responses to medical and surgical treatment.

The precise historical origins of ulcerative colitis and Crohn's disease are not known (2). Emerging as clinical entities early in the 20th century, ulcerative colitis dominated the first half and Crohn's disease the second half of the century; changing incidence trends are consistent with an environmental precipitating onset. Knowledge of inflammatory bowel disease (IBD) has increased in recent decades paralleling advances in the biomedical sciences, but many questions remain. This chapter examines current etiologic concepts of IBD, their source, their status, and their direction.

General Observations

Ulcerative Colitis

Based on the autopsy descriptions of pathologist Matthew Baillie (1761–1823) (Fig. 1.1), Morson (3) dates the first description of ulcerative colitis back at least two centuries. The first impact description of "ulcerative colitis" in 1859 (4) by Wilks (Figs. 1.2 and 1.3), was later changed to Crohn's disease, but a second paper in 1875 (5) described a young woman with a history of bloody mucoid diarrhea consistent with the diagnosis of ulcerative colitis. The 1909 London Symposium described the clinical features of more than 300 patients collected from seven London hospitals, including complications such as hemorrhage, perforation, and carcinoma of the colon and rectum, and a 50% mortality. Early speculation as to etiology, at a time of bacteriologic discovery, emphasized a "dysentery infection," prompting treatment with a "polyvalent antidysentery serum" (6). Bargen et al. (7) in 1924 implicated an intestinal diplostreptococcus and administered an autogenous vaccine of fecal bacteria. Additional reports from Great Britain, Europe, and the United States documented the unpredictable exacerbations and remissions and additional complications, including undernutrition and retardation of growth in children, vascular thromboses, erythema nodosum, and pyoderma gangrenosum. The early surgical approaches of appendicostomy, cecostomy, and "temporary" ileostomy, were based on the principle of "resting" the diseased bowel. Into the second quarter of the 20th century, possible causes included psychogenic mechanisms and gastrointestinal allergy to foods and pollens.

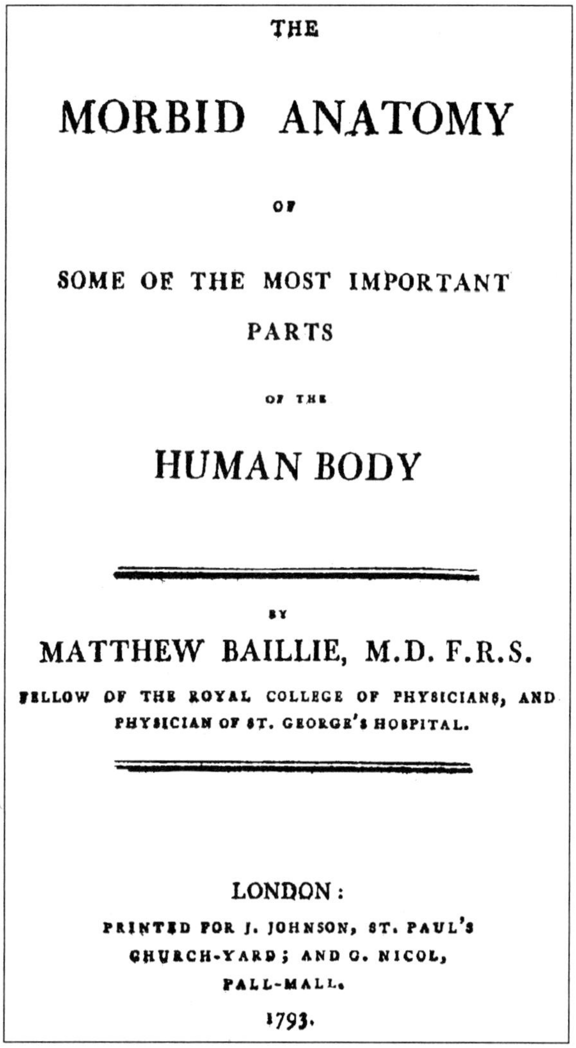

THE

MORBID ANATOMY

OF

SOME OF THE MOST IMPORTANT

PARTS

OF THE

HUMAN BODY

BY

MATTHEW BAILLIE, M.D. F.R.S.

FELLOW OF THE ROYAL COLLEGE OF PHYSICIANS, AND
PHYSICIAN OF ST. GEORGE'S HOSPITAL.

LONDON:

PRINTED FOR J. JOHNSON, ST. PAUL'S
CHURCH-YARD; AND G. NICOL,
PALL-MALL.
1793.

Fig. 1.1.   M. Baillie's hitherto unrecognized 1793 description of "ulcerative colitis."

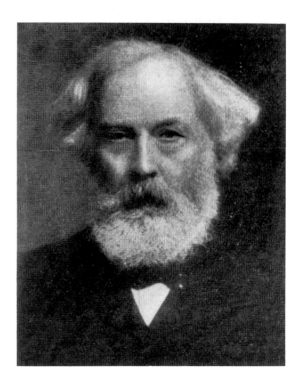

Fig. 1.2.   S. Wilks, first "impact" describer of ulcerative colitis (1859).

Pathologically, ulcerative colitis was identified as a diffuse inflammation characterized by an hyperemic, friable mucosa, numerous tiny superficial ulcers, and sanguinopurulent exudate, beginning in the rectum and progressing to involve the entire colon. The histologic features of intense vascular congestion of the mucosa and submucosa, pronounced cellular infiltration of the lamina propria with polymorphonuclear cells, lymphocytes, monocytes and other inflammatory cells, crypt abscesses, and architectural distortion, suggested the action of an injurious agent in the fecal stream but none has been identified thus far.

By mid 20th century, etiologic consideration continued to focus upon psychogenic problems, infection, and an injurious agent in the fecal stream, and extended to a "vascular disorder" (e.g., "thrombo-ulcerative ulcerative colitis" [8]) and

"nonspecific" damage to the colonic epithelium by multiple injurious agents. Therapy included nutritional and emotional supports and added sulfasalazine and other sulfonamides, antibiotics, ACTH, adrenal steroids, 6MP, and azathioprine, encouraging early speculation as to immunological mechanisms. Surgical approaches progressed to partial and total colectomy, with ileostomy, and abdominal-perineal resection. Experimental operative procedures such as pelvic autonomic neurectomy, distal vagotomy, and selective electrocoagulation of the prefrontal lobes reflected the preoccupation with unsubstantiated neurogenic and psychogenic hypotheses.

Beginning in the late 1920s many attempts to reproduce ulcerative colitis experimentally were based upon microbial, psychogenic, and vascular hypotheses. Although the bowel was readily injured, healing was rapid and human ulcerative colitis was not reproduced. However, reproduction of the classic Arthus and Shwartzman reactions and the Auer-Kirsner immune complex colitis in rabbits revealed the immunologic potential of the colon (9).

Crohn's Disease

Inflammatory bowel disease descriptively consistent with Crohn's disease may have been described

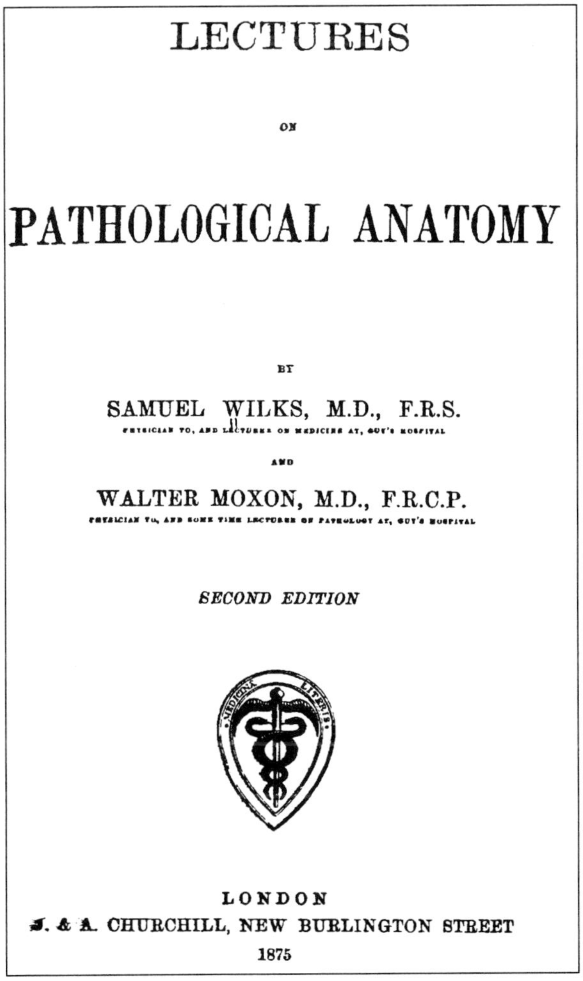

LECTURES

ON

PATHOLOGICAL ANATOMY

BY

SAMUEL WILKS, M.D., F.R.S.
PHYSICIAN TO, AND LECTURER ON MEDICINE AT, GUY'S HOSPITAL

AND

WALTER MOXON, M.D., F.R.C.P.
PHYSICIAN TO, AND SOME TIME LECTURER OF PATHOLOGY AT, GUY'S HOSPITAL

SECOND EDITION

LONDON
J. & A. CHURCHILL, NEW BURLINGTON STREET
1875

Fig. 1.3. Early "impact" description of pathology of ulcerative colitis (1875).

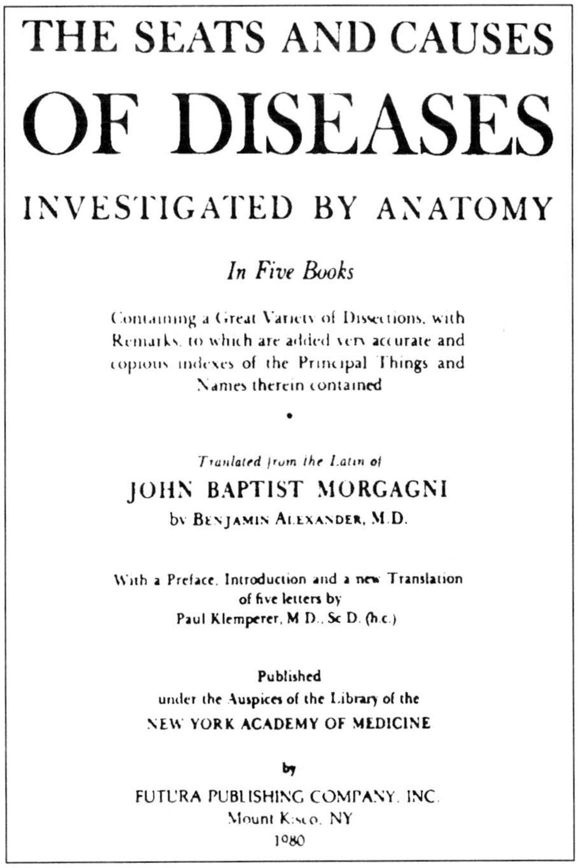

THE SEATS AND CAUSES

OF DISEASES

INVESTIGATED BY ANATOMY

In Five Books

Containing a Great Variety of Dissections, with
Remarks, to which are added very accurate and
copious indexes of the Principal Things and
Names therein contained

•

Translated from the Latin of
JOHN BAPTIST MORGAGNI
by BENJAMIN ALEXANDER, M.D.

With a Preface, Introduction and a new Translation
of five letters by
Paul Klemperer, M.D., Sc D. (h.c.)

Published
under the Auspices of the Library of the
NEW YORK ACADEMY OF MEDICINE

by
FUTURA PUBLISHING COMPANY, INC.
Mount Kisco, NY
1980

Fig. 1.4. Morgagni's 1761 description of "regional ileitis."

in 1612 by Fabry (10) in a teen-age boy who died after experiencing severe cramping abdominal pain. Autopsy revealed a contracted, ulcerated and fibrous cecum invaginating the ileum and causing complete bowel obstruction. Morgagni (Fig. 1.4) (11) in 1761 described ulceration and perforation of an inflamed distal ileum and enlarged mesenteric lymph nodes in a young man of 20 with a history of diarrhea and fever. Reports from Great Britain, Ireland, France, Germany, and the United States during the latter part of the 19th century and early in the 20th century documented the increasing frequency of a disease, often presenting with an abdominal mass, initially labeled as a "neoplasm" and, at a time of limited abdominal surgery, mistakenly dismissed as "untreatable." The 1913 paper by Dalziel (Fig. 1.5) (12) of Glasgow, comprising 13 patients included a physician who since 1901 had experienced recurrent intestinal obstruction and died. Autopsy demonstrated a

chronically inflamed and narrowed small intestine and enlarged mesenteric lymph nodes. Coffen's (13) patient, a 20 year old man, required three bowel resections in 1916 for recurrent intestinal obstruction. The 1932 report by Crohn, Ginzburg, and Oppenheimer (14) (Fig. 1.6) increased general awareness of regional ileitis and numerous case reports appeared during the 1930s, 1940s, and 1950s. In some instances patients had been operated upon for a suspected "acute appendicitis." In several countries (United States, England, Sweden), the disease appeared more common among Jewish people, an unexplained association. Etiologic possibilities included a bowel infection, a mesenteric endolymphangitis of the ileocecal region, "intestinal stagnation" proximal to the ileocecal valve and "intestinal allergy." Clinical observations extended the gastrointestinal involvement to the upper GI tract (esophagus, stomach, proximal small bowel). Surgery now included radical bowel resection and intestinal by-pass procedures. Although Crohn's disease of the colon had been observed earlier, not until

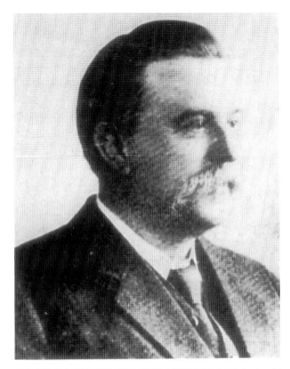

CHRONIC INTERSTITIAL ENTERITIS.
By T. K. DALZIEL, M.B., C.M., F.R.F.P.S.G.,
Surgeon, Western Infirmary, Glasgow.

Br Med J (Clin. Res.) 2:1068–1070, 1913

Fig. 1.5. Sir T. Kennedy Dalziel, author of the 1913 "classical" clinical and pathologic description of "Crohn's disease" (or "Dalziel-Crohn's disease").

the 1959 and 1960 reports of Lockhart-Mummery and Morson (15) was Crohn's disease of the colon fully recognized as a valid entity in the United States.

The intriguing predilection of Crohn's disease for the terminal ileum (40% of patients) and after intestinal resection and reanastomosis for the neo-terminal ileum implicated the fecal stream but remains unexplained. Early pathologic studies of Crohn's disease noted the focal distribution of an inflammatory reaction involving the entire thickness of the bowel wall, granulomas located deep within the bowel, and abscess and fistula formation. The cicatrizing tendency of Crohn's disease, initially attributed to an endolymphangitis presumably following the intralymphatic absorption of an "irritating lipid" (16), prompted unsuccessful attempts to reproduce regional enteritis via the intra-lymphatic injection of silica, talc, and sclerosing solutions (17). The dilated submucosal lymphatics and prominent lymphoid aggregates directed at-

tention to the intestinal lymphoid apparatus but the nature of this relationship remains obscure. The earliest and perhaps most intriguing histologic feature of Crohn's disease is the aphthoid ulcer located precisely over the M cell in the epithelium overlying lymphoid follicles in Peyer's patches, probably the site of entry of an etiologic agent(s).

Moschowitz and Wilkensky from New York's Mt. Sinai described four patients in 1923 with "nonspecific" granulomas of the intestine, reflecting the long-time interest of that institution in intestinal granulomas. Subsequent review of these cases demonstrated clinical and pathological features consistent with Crohn's disease. A fifth patient is included in the 1927 paper with the same "extraordinary association with acute appendicitis." Leon Ginzburg, associated with the surgeon A. A. Berg, who had operated on all patients, and Gordon Oppenheimer, then resident in surgical pathology, collected 12 patients dating back to 1920, characterized by a thickened and ulcerative stenosis of the distal two or three feet of terminal ileum, "ending rather abruptly at the ileocecal valve." In 1930 Burrill Crohn had under his care two young patients with a similar process. Crohn's first case was a 16-year-old boy with abdominal pain, diarrhea, fever, and a mass in the right lower abdominal quadrant, requiring ileocecal resection. The patient's sister also required an operation for regional ileitis several years later. Amebiasis, syphilis, actinomycosis, and intestinal tuberculosis were excluded. The two groups united at the suggestion of pathologist Paul Klemperer, providing the 14 cases published in the 1932 JAMA article as "regional ileitis" (Figs. 1.6 and 1.7) (14). The article was credited to the surgical service of Dr. A. A. Berg and had Berg accepted the invitation to join the alphabetically arranged authorship of the paper, we might be writing today about Berg's disease!

British reports of granulomatous inflammation of the small bowel in the 1930s occasionally designated the process as Crohn's disease. Cushway in 1934, Barbour and Stokes and Hurst and Lintott in 1937 also utilized this term. Other designations included "Crohn-Dalziel" and CGO disease to reflect in America the contributions of Ginsburg and Oppenheimer in addition to Crohn. "Whatever the labeling circumstances, the eponym Crohn's disease is now sanctioned by worldwide usage as a convenient designation for an unique (2) inflammatory process of the gastrointestinal tract."

Fig. 1.6. The "Crohn's disease" trio in 1932.

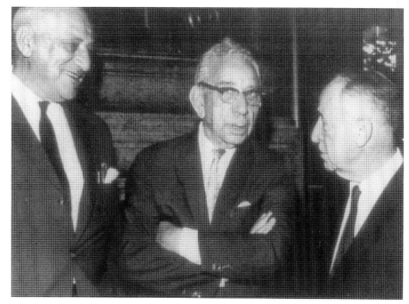

G. Oppenheimer
1900 - 1974

B. Crohn
1884 - 1983

L. Ginzburg
1898 - 1988

Author's Comment

The IBD literature during the early 20th century began with single case and small group reports, expanding into larger series and steadily expanded the geographic distribution and the clinical spectrum of ulcerative colitis and Crohn's disease. Population surveys from Denmark indicated many instances of mild to moderate illness, whereas reports from major medical centers tended to emphasize the more severe, complicated problems. Recurrences were associated with upper respiratory illness, the ingestion of salicylates, emotional stress and physical fatigue. Etiologic speculation on ulcerative colitis focused on bacterial infection, emotional disturbances, and gastrointestinal allergy. In Crohn's disease, etiologic interest centered on bacterial infection, an endolymphangitis of the ileoce-

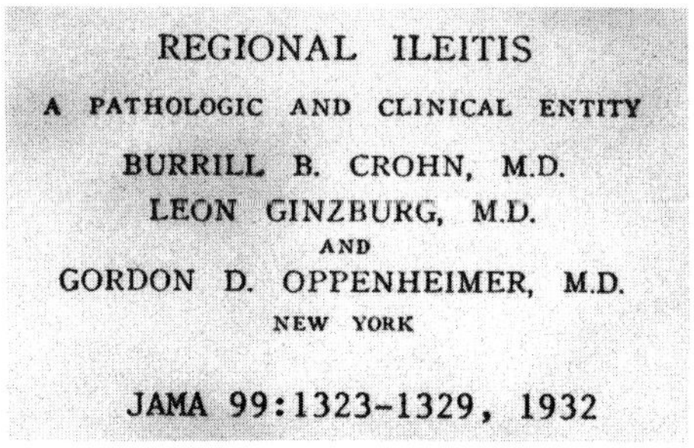

REGIONAL ILEITIS

A PATHOLOGIC AND CLINICAL ENTITY

BURRILL B. CROHN, M.D.
LEON GINZBURG, M.D.
AND
GORDON D. OPPENHEIMER, M.D.
NEW YORK

JAMA 99:1323-1329, 1932

Fig. 1.7. The 1932 "classical" report of intestinal inflammation, later recognized as Crohn's disease.

cal region, and "intestinal allergy." Beginning in the 1950s epidemiologic studies documented the occurrence of colorectal cancer and the increased familial occurrences. Etiologic speculation now advanced to immune mechanisms and genetic influences. The clinical and pathologic mimicry of ulcerative colitis and Crohn's disease by enterocolonic infections reflected not only the limited morphologic response of the bowel to injury but also implied multiple causes. Increased efforts to reproduce human IBD in animals, utilizing cholinergic stimulation, chemical irritants and immune mechanisms for ulcerative colitis, the introduction of bacteria (e.g., mycobacteria), and the attempted production of a mesenteric endolymphangitis for Crohn's disease all failed. Nevertheless, the experiments demonstrated the remarkable capacity of normal small bowel and colon to heal rapidly after injury and encouraged closer examination of the small and large bowel.

Etiology and Pathogenesis of IBD

Epidemiology

Epidemiological studies of inflammatory bowel disease were not feasible until the 1950s because of the small number of patients and the limited interest. A British study of 1425 patients with chronic ulcerative colitis in 1955 indicated an overall incidence of 11% (18). The rate of 6.9% for five Scottish towns in contrast to 15.5% for five London hospitals was early recognition of the urban-rural difference. A 1960 survey of U.S. veterans with the diagnosis of either ulcerative colitis or regional ileitis (19) revealed a bimodal incidence, a four-fold increase among Jewish patients, and a twenty-fold increase in the incidence of ankylosing spondylitis. Studies in the 1960s and 1970s indicated an overall incidence range of 4 to 6 per 100,000 population per year and a prevalence range of 40 to 100 for ulcerative colitis, probably under-estimates because of the omission of undiagnosed ulcerative proctitis and proctosigmoiditis. Lower figures were reported for Crohn's disease but a rising incidence trend already was apparent.

The Baltimore epidemiologic studies of Mendeloff et al. in the 1960s and 1970s (20,21) reported higher hospital incidence and prevalence rates for both ulcerative colitis and regional enteritis among whites than nonwhites, for Jews than nonJews, and for ulcerative colitis over Crohn's disease; a trend now reversed. A 1980 study (22) characterized the IBD population as including: (a) approximately equal numbers of males and females, (b) more "western" people than orientals, (c) more whites than blacks (now increasing), (d) higher figures among urban than rural residents, and (e) an increasing familial incidence, especially for Crohn's disease.

Incidence and prevalence figures for IBD from various geographic areas continue to vary and probably are higher than have been recorded; but recent epidemiologic surveys suggest an overall incidence for both ulcerative colitis and Crohn's disease approximating 20 per 100,000 population per year and a prevalence of approximately 300, equally divided between the two diseases (1). Incidence trends for both ulcerative colitis and Crohn's disease appear to have stabilized in some areas (Great Britain, United States) but in other areas ulcerative colitis (Scotland, Norway) and Crohn's disease (United States, Great Britain, Europe) continue to rise. In Israel IBD is more frequent among Ashkenazi (European Jews) than among Sephardic (North African) Jews. The genetic significance of these observations is obscured by the ethnic heterogeneity of the Jewish people. Today, ulcerative colitis and Crohn's disease are identifiable among most ethnic groups and are appearing in formerly low incidence countries (India, Japan).

The curious relationship between ulcerative colitis and nonsmoking, including former smokers, though observed clinically, was first reported from Upsala, Sweden in 1976 (23), expanded by Rhodes et al. (24) from Wales, confirmed from numerous geographic areas. The reverse occurs in Crohn's disease, namely excessive cigarette smoking and a higher rate of recurrence after surgery among smokers than nonsmokers. The negative association of cigarette smoking with ulcerative colitis and its positive association with Crohn's disease after 20 years remains unexplained. The nonsmoking association also has been observed in Parkinson's disease (25).

Epidemiologic studies have contributed important information on IBD (26), including the steadily rising incidence of Crohn's disease in industrialized, colder (northern) geographic areas (United States, Europe) in some areas exceeding the incidence of ulcerative colitis; the appearance of Crohn's disease among previously low risk individuals who move from rural to urban centers; the increased familial incidence; the higher risk of cancer of the colon and rectum in both ulcerative colitis and Crohn's disease of the colon; and the association of ulcerative colitis with immune disorders and of Crohn's disease with genetic diseases.

The clinical studies also have identified risk factors for recurrence, including upper respiratory infections, the use of aspirin and nonsteroidal compounds, and the early oral intake of penicillin-type antibiotics. The implication of food intolerance to refined sugars and margarine for Crohn's disease and to food additives remains unconfirmed except for lactose sensitivity. Seasonal relationships are reported by individual patients but ulcerative colitis and Crohn's disease are not seasonal disorders.

Author's Comment

Despite the considerable epidemiologic information, more definitive demographic studies are now necessary, including: (a) population based surveys to more completely characterize the clinical spectrum of IBD, (b) the identification of subsets of ulcerative colitis and Crohn's disease with common clinical features and complications, (c) more complete documentation of the association of genetic-immune disorders such as multiple sclerosis in ulcerative colitis and psoriasis in Crohn's disease, (d) longitudinal observations of IBD in children and teenagers with particular reference to significant early life events, (e) demographic and sociocultural features of IBD patients who had moved from rural to urban areas, and (f) more comprehensive epidemiologic investigations of the environment associated with high risk and low risk IBD occurrence, including the local agriculture, soil and water supply, the atmosphere (industrial pollutants), and socioculturally-determined dietary differences.

Psychogenic Aspects

The responsiveness of the gastrointestinal tract to emotional stress, known since the dawn of civilization, was documented scientifically 100 years ago in the studies of Pavlov (27) and Cannon (28). Additional scientific validity came in the 1940s and 1950s from the physiologic studies of Wolf and Wolff (29) and Almy et al. (30) who demonstrated the significant changes in gastrointestinal function associated with experimentally induced and spontaneous emotional stress. An etiologic role for emotionally significant life events in ulcerative colitis was suggested by Murray (31) in 1930 in a clinical study of 12 patients and was reemphasized by Sullivan (32) in 1932 in a review of 15 patients. Both observers noted the chronological relationship between emotional problems and the onset or recurrence of the colitis. Each described an "ulcerative colitis personality" characterized by emotional immaturity, dependence, rigidity, and inhibited interpersonal relationships. The observation of increased numbers of parasympathetic ganglion cells in the myenteric plexus of the ulcerative colitis colon appeared to provide an anatomic-physiologic basis for this hypothesis and a psychogenic causation for ulcerative colitis was widely accepted throughout the 1930s, 1940s, and 1950s, a time when psychiatric hypotheses dominated gastrointestinal pathogeneses. However, the absence of sustained control of the disease following psychotherapy and the prompt psychological improvement of patients with ulcerative colitis after curative total colectomy and ileostomy (33) seriously challenged psychiatric concepts. Karush (34) summarized the psychiatric position in 1977: "We do not claim that ulcerative colitis is 'caused' by unusual reactions of the mind alone. We claim only that these reactions almost always play a vital role in the interaction of the four etiological determinants: genetic endowment, constitutional vulnerability, intrapsychic processes, and the external environment. . . ." Subsequent analyses by Alpers and his colleagues confirmed significant methodological defects in the psychiatric studies in both ulcerative colitis and Crohn's disease (35,36), further weakening the validity of this concept. Beginning in the 1960s, the etiologic emphasis upon psychiatry in inflammatory bowel disease diminished and now has virtually disappeared.

Author's Comment

Mental illness (e.g., psychosis, schizophrenia) is not involved in the pathogenesis of IBD. Notwithstanding the variable clinical assessments of psychogenic disturbances in IBD, emotional stress, as in all human illnesses, contributes significantly to the severity of established disease and "everyday" emotional disturbances cannot be ignored in the management of IBD. The similar neurohumoral and neurotransmitter peptide-producing cells in the central nervous system (pituitary gland, sensory ganglia) and in the gastrointestinal tract (e.g., VIP, somatostatin, substance P), and the extensive neural innervation of the bowel wall provide important pathways for psycho-neuro-humoral-immunologic interactions between the brain and the gut and the intestinal expression of emotional stress. Continued investigation of the "stress system" (corticotropin-releasing hormone, the pituitary-adrenal axis and the limbs of the autonomic nervous system [37]), and its relationship to human illness via the neuroendocrine interactions involving such peptide hormones as galanin, CCK, and Substance P, located within enteric nerves, also should clarify the somatopsychic and psychosomatic aspects of inflammatory bowel disease.

Microbial Causes

Ulcerative Colitis

Infection ("dysentery") was suggested early in the 20th century, a time when microbial causes of many diseases were being identified (38). Numerous bacteria were implicated, including *Escherichia coli, Baccilus proteus, Baccilus morgagni,* histoplasma, *S. typhi,* the anaerobe *Spherophorus necrophorus,* mycobacteria, *Entameba histolytica,* cytomegalovirus and the intestinal diplostreptococcus, and subsequently discarded for lack of conclusive evidence. Interest in a microbial etiology for ulcerative colitis has been renewed by the identification of "new" bacterial and viral pathogens (39), including helicobacter pylori, *E. coli* 0157.H7, and hantavirus, the development of more sensitive methods of identification and the emergence of "new" pathogenetic roles for bacterial components in IBD.

Crohn's Disease

A microbial etiology always appeared more likely in Crohn's disease because of the increased gut microflora, the suppurative complications, and the favorable clinical response to antibiotics in some patients (1). Dalziel in 1913 suggested Johne's mycobacterial disease of cattle but could not pursue this possibility. Tuberculosis was a major differential consideration of Crohn et al. in 1932. Since then numerous organisms have been implicated, including anaerobes (40) (Eubacteria, Bacteroides, *Baccilus vulgatos*, peptostreptococcus, and coprococcus), Campylobacter, *Yersinia enterocolitica*, mycobacteria (Kansasii, paratuberculosis), and viruses (rotavirus). Recent interest has focused on *Listeria monocytogenes, Saccharomyces cerevisiae,* and paramyxovirus (measles [41]), on bacterial products, including lipopolysaccharides, toxins, and peptidoglycan-PS, and on abnormal bacterial constituents in the bowel content, including mucin-degrading enzymes and the ubiquitous nitric oxide.

Author's Comment

Ulcerative colitis and Crohn's disease are not conventional infectious diseases. The occasional delayed development of either ulcerative colitis or Crohn's disease in the initially healthy mate of an IBD patient suggests an "infectious agent" though neither ulcerative colitis nor Crohn's disease is increased among physicians (gastroenterologists) and nurses in frequent or prolonged contact with IBD patients. There is no evidence that an animal species is serving as a reservoir for putative infectious agents. Apart from ethnic groupings, time-space clustering of IBD patients implicating an external source of infection (e.g., contaminated water or food supply) has not been documented. There also is no serological evidence of unusual exposure of IBD patients to known viruses, including rotavirus, mumps, Epstein-Barr virus, and probably also the measles virus. The elevated serum titers of cytomegalovirus reflect the diminished immunocompetence of the chronically ill, undernourished IBD patient. A genetically-mediated antecedently increased intestinal permeability favoring the entry of microbial, viral, and other antigens has not been demonstrated. Other potential mechanisms such as stimulation of the gut mucosal immune system by bacterial products, activating cellular and cytokine mechanisms of inflammation, and perhaps down-regulating the gut mucosal response to intestinal antigens also have not been proven. An increased vulnerability of the gut mucosal immune system to "dysregulation" because of the lack of exposure to enteric pathogens early in life (especially in developed countries) is an interesting hypothesis requiring documentation.

Substantial gaps remain in our knowledge of the human gut microflora, including the vast anaerobic flora, and the commensal microflora, the role of the M cell in facilitating microbial or viral entry into the bowel wall, and the ecology of enterocolonic viruses. Nevertheless, a microbial agent (bacteria, viruses) remains a strong possibility in

the pathogenesis of both inflammatory bowel diseases, especially Crohn's disease. The newer techniques of bacterial identification, DNA hybridization and the search for extrachromosomal genetic elements (plasmids, phages), should aid in the identification of "new" pathogens and clarify microbial relationships in IBD.

Sartor (42) has suggested the following sequence of events: "Infection with common intestinal pathogens or exposure to microbial or environmental toxins induces tissue injury and increases mucosal permeability, leading to secondary invasion by endogenous luminal bacteria and enhanced uptake of ubiquitous bacterial components (PG-PS, LPS, FMLP). The subsequent inflammatory response is self-limited in the normal host as a result of appropriate down-regulation of the immune response, leading to resolution of inflammation and healing with no residual damage. However, in the genetically susceptible host there is an inappropriate amplification of the immune response that leads to chronic intestinal inflammation. Systemic uptake of luminal bacterial cell wall polymers leads to extraintestinal manifestations. Complications such as fibrosis depend on the cytokine and growth factor profile in the inflammatory response. Inflammation may continue unabated under the influence of specific immune events (to anaerobic bacteria in Crohn's disease and possible molecular mimicry-related autoimmunity in ulcerative colitis) or eventually may be controlled by intrinsic immunosuppression. Environmental triggers may reactivate disease at any time."

Immune Mechanisms

Immunology of the gut, a major consideration in the etiology and pathogenesis of the inflammatory bowel diseases, developed in part as an extension of the concept of hypersensitivity (allergy) of mucous membranes of the gastrointestinal tract. Andresen (43) and Rowe (44) in the 1920s had postulated an allergic basis for ulcerative colitis, implicating pollens (trees, grasses, weeds), house dust, as well as foods (milk, eggs, wheat, potato, orange, tomato, coffee, tea, and chocolate). Walzer and Gray et al. (45) later demonstrated an allergic reaction to specific protein in the passively sensitized ileal, colonic, and rectal mucosa of human subjects and the rhesus monkey. However, elimination diets based upon positive skin tests to various foods, during the 1930s, were ineffective and the lack of definitive evidence subsequently discredited the concept of food allergy in IBD.

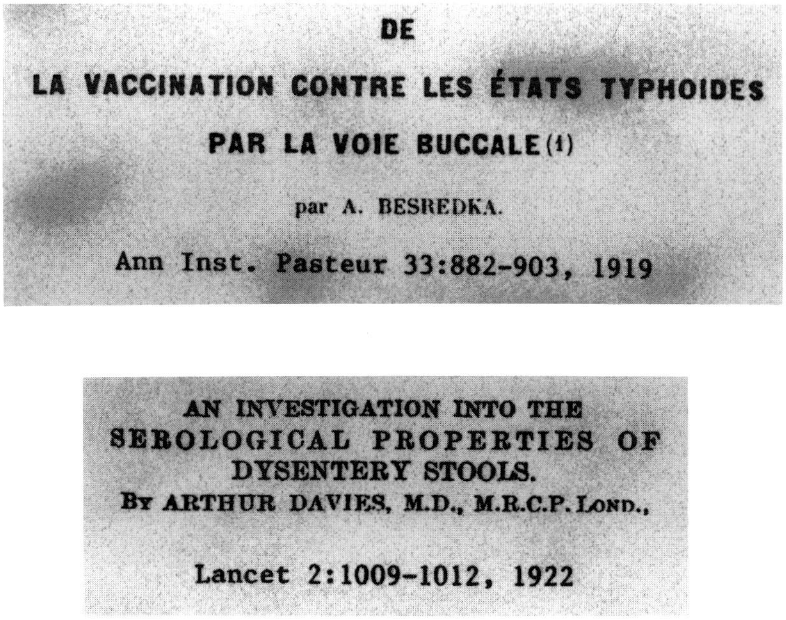

Fig. 1.8. Initial recognition of immunologic capacity of bowel (1919 and 1922).

DE
LA VACCINATION CONTRE LES ÉTATS TYPHOIDES
PAR LA VOIE BUCCALE (1)

par A. BESREDKA.

Ann Inst. Pasteur 33:882–903, 1919

AN INVESTIGATION INTO THE
SEROLOGICAL PROPERTIES OF
DYSENTERY STOOLS.
By ARTHUR DAVIES, M.D., M.R.C.P. Lond.,

Lancet 2:1009–1012, 1922

Immune mechanisms in the late 1940s and early 1950s were increasingly considered in the pathogenesis of diseases of unknown etiology (46). A series of clinical experiences between 1947 and 1952 suggested the possible involvement of immune processes in ulcerative colitis. These events included the abrupt onset of severe ulcerative colitis in several young patients following independent episodes of acute food poisoning and intestinal infection with *E. histolytica* (during the 1933 to 1934 Chicago epidemic), the association of ulcerative colitis with other immune diseases (e.g., autoimmune hemolytic anemia, systemic lupus erythematosus), the familial occurrences of inflammatory bowel disease and the beneficial therapeutic effects of ACTH and the adrenal corticosteroids.

Although the early hypothesis of IBD as "immune-mediated" disorders provided a sense of conceptual progress, the immunologic potential of the GI tract and just what "immune-mediated" inferred were not known. Besredka (47) in 1919 had demonstrated that oral "immunization of rabbits provided protection against otherwise fatal Shiga bacillus infection" and Davies (48) in 1922 had documented the presence of fecal antibody in the stools of patients with bacillary dysentery before serum antibody appeared (Fig. 1.8). Nevertheless, there was almost no awareness of the immunologic resources and responsiveness of the gastrointestinal tract until the 1950s. Kirsner and Palmer (49) in 1954 suggested sensitization of the bowel via an early microbial infection, "as in an antigen-antibody reaction occurring among hyperreactive persons . . ." Experiments by Kirsner and Goldgra-

ber (50) in 1959 demonstrated the positive response of the rabbit colon to the classic Arthus and Shwartzman reactions. In 1956, Kirsner and Elchlepp (51), utilizing the 1920 Auer (52) principle of local autosensitization to foreign protein as observed in the rabbit ear exposed to dilute xylol, produced immune complexes with crystalline egg albumin as the antigen in rabbits, localized to the distal bowel via the rectal instillation of a dilute formalin solution. An ulcerative colitis developed in precisely the areas of the rectum demonstrated immunologically to contain the immune complexes and nowhere else. The Auer-Kirsner colitis with modifications is utilized today as an immune model of human ulcerative colitis.

Further progress came when Heremans (53) in 1960 and Tomasi et al. (54) in 1965 identified the secretory IgA class of immunoglobulins and Bienenstock (55) and his colleagues described the components of the gastrointestinal immune apparatus and their interactions with the neuroendocrine network of the gastrointestinal tract. By the 1960s and 1970s the immunology of the gastrointestinal tract and the possible role of immune mechanisms in ulcerative colitis and Crohn's disease had become the most active area of IBD research. Early interest focused vaguely upon "autoimmunity," the identity of possible intestinal antigens, the search for anticolon antibodies, and for evidence of an immune abnormality (9). The methodology was crude: the "antigens" were poorly characterized, the relationship of the circulating "antibodies" to IBD was never established, and although "the colon was demonstrated as capable of generating immunologic reactions, an auto-immune colitis could not be reproduced experimentally."

Research on the immunology of the gastrointestinal tract and on inflammatory bowel disease subsequently expanded as improved methods of investigations were developed (56). Systemic immunity in IBD was found to be normal, IBD patients were not vulnerable to ordinary or "exotic" infections as indicated by normal antibody responses to standard bacterial immunizations, common viral agents, and enteropathogens. Although ulcerative colitis serum contained IgM antibodies, (cross-reactive with *E. Coli*), antibodies against surface antigens in mucus-secreting colonic epithelial cells, fetal colonic tissue, and against colonic epithelium from germ-free rats, these heterogeneous antibodies did not correlate with the age or sex of the patient, a family history of IBD, the extent, duration, or severity of IBD and were not pathogenic for colon epithelial cells. IBD serum also contained antibodies to a wide variety of antigens (cow's milk proteins, intestinal epithelial cells, bile ductule epithelium, and pancreatic homogenates), reflecting the secondarily increased permeability of the inflamed bowel wall. Shorter et al. (57) in 1972 suggested early "priming" of the gut-associated mucosal immune system via the more permeable intestinal epithelium during infancy as "preparing" the bowel for later development of an inflammatory bowel disease, similar to the concept implied in the patients with food poisoning and amebic dysentery mentioned earlier.

More recently, immunologic research (58) has focused on the responsiveness of the gut mucosal immune system, including the role of Peyer's patches and lymphoid follicles; the role of intraepithelial and lamina propria T and B lymphocytes; the immunologic and genetic significance of the antineutrophil cytoplasmic antibodies (different from those associated with vasculitis) in ulcerative colitis; the specific antigens involved in the elevated Ig1 (ulcerative colitis) and Ig2 (Crohn's disease); the possible immunological role of nitric oxide; and the nature of the immune mechanisms regulating gut-mediated oral tolerance. As indicated by Weiner (59): "Immunologically active lymphoid tissue in the gut is preferentially programmed to inhibit autoimmune reactions, a property that can be exploited by oral administration of self-antigen . . . but identifying the target autoantigens to use in oral preparations may not be necessary. The trigger for oral tolerization is antigen-specific but suppressive events in the target organ are nonspecific." Weiner also noted the two subclasses of helper T cells, "characterized by the cytokines they secrete." One subclass Th_1 is predominately involved in priming and sustaining cell-mediated immune responses; in autoimmune disease, these helper cells tend to be pathogenic. The other subclass "Th_2 tends to suppress Th_1 immune cells; these are the helper T cells needed to restore or maintain tolerance." Thus, an overreacting gut mucosal immune system in IBD may result from an overactivity of Th_1 cells or a decrease in Th_2 cells activity.

Author's Comment

After approximately forty years (1950s–1990s) of IBD-related research, no conclusive evidence of an antecedent immune abnormality preceding the onset of IBD (e.g., in initially healthy members of IBD families) has been obtained. Nor is there convincing evidence as yet for an autoimmune pathogenesis. Most, if not all, of the immunologic phenomena described thus far, including the varied antibodies, appearing and disappearing with the activity and the quiescence of ulcerative colitis or Crohn's disease, represent secondary events, reflections of a chronically activated gut mucosal immune system; events independent of the type, extent, severity, and duration of the disease. The infrequency of ANCA in healthy twin siblings to twins (60) with ulcerative colitis suggests that p-ANCA, whereas clinically useful in identifying ulcerative colitis (61), is not a subclinical marker of genetic susceptibility to ulcerative colitis. The most important immunologic finding thus far probably is the increased immune responsiveness (or decreased immune down-regulation) of the gastrointestinal mucosal immune system, a concept also requiring more extensive investigation.

Future immunologic studies should include: the normal immunophysiology of the gut, particularly the immunological regulation of epithelial function (62); the gut-associated mucosal immune system; mechanisms of oral tolerance and mucosal cytoprotective processes, including the inhibiting action of the intestinal intraepithelial lymphocytes; the nature of intestinal immune reactions to enteric bacteria and bacterial products, including the role of T and B cells (Th_1 and Th_2 cells); the role of immune cellular components (macrophages, neutrophils, and other cellular constituents (colonic epithelial cells, fibroblasts, muscle, and vascular endothelial cells) in the immune response; the interactions of the gut mucosal immune system with the enteric and central nervous systems; the immunologic basis of the intestinal granulomas of Crohn's disease; and gastrointestinal defenses against the complex mix of bacterial and dietary antigens, enzymes, and other biologically active molecules in the bowel content (63).

Inflammation, Lymphokines, Cytokines

Interest in the biology of inflammation and its involvement in immune reactions dates back to the observations on cellular immunity (phagocytosis) by Metchnikoff (64) in 1882, humoral immunity by Ehrlich (65), and in the 1930s and 1940s to the biochemistry of inflammation by Menkin (66).

The cellular and molecular nature of the inflammation in IBD and its tendency to persist or recur are incompletely understood. The increases in polymorphonuclear leukocytes, lymphocytes, monocytes, eosinophiles, and in macrophages, mast cells and Paneth cells also are observed in bowel infections of known etiology and also in various types of experimental intestinal injury and thus cannot be regarded as specific for IBD. Accordingly, the proinflammatory cytokines and anti-inflammatory products of the arachidonic acid cascade (originating in cell membranes) and other biologically active molecules such as nitric oxide have become a major research area in IBD.

During the 1950s and 1960s, the tissue reaction of ulcerative colitis was arbitrarily attributed to bacteria and to the action of enzymes such as trypsin, fibrinolytic mechanisms, mast cell products, and bradykinin. McCord and Fridovich (67) in 1969 were the first to discover the enzyme superoxide dismutase and to demonstrate the production of superoxide anion free radicals in mammalian systems. Babior et al. (68) in 1973 demonstrated that activated polymorphonuclear cells produce large quantities of the superoxide anion radical. Many investigators subsequently related inflammatory tissue injury to the action of superoxide anion radicals and other proinflammatory molecules. Granger and colleagues (69) in 1981 demonstrated their role in postischemic injury of the small bowel. In 1988 Grisham and Granger (70) identified the inhibitory effect of 5 amino salicylic acid on free oxygen radicals and the subsequent healing of experimental enterocolitis.

Interest in the role of cytokines (glycosylated proteins produced by all body cells) in the inflammatory reaction and as regulators of the immune response dates to the 1972 discovery (71) of a factor produced by macrophages stimulating T cell responses to antigens, later designated as interleukin-1 (IL-1) and to the discovery of interleukin-2

(IL-2) by Paetkau et al. (72) and by Chen and di Sabato (73) in 1976. In 1984 Sharon and Stenson (74) demonstrated a 50-fold increase in the proinflammatory leukotriene LTB4 in the colonic mucosa of ulcerative colitis. Increased LTB4 also characterized radiation proctitis and the ulcerative colitis of the captive cottontop tamarin. An increasing number and variety of cytokines and other biologically active molecules now have been identified in IBD, but not yet in patterns absolutely specific for IBD. Fiocchi (75), Podolsky (76), and Sartor (77) currently are endeavoring to clarify the complex cellular and molecular bases of intestinal inflammation.

Author's Comment

Many aspects are under investigation: cell trafficking and cellular-epithelial cell interactions, with particular emphasis upon the types of inflammatory cells recruited into the inflamed IBD intestine; the threefold actions of chemokines in the inflammatory reaction; the expression of adhesion molecules by endothelial cells permitting the transendothelial migration of monocytes and T cells; the proinflammatory cytokines (interleukin 1 and interleukin 1 receptor antagonist, interleukin 6, interleukin 8, and related cytokines); the immunomodulating cytokines (interleukin 2 and IL-2 receptor, interleukin 4, 5, 7, 9, 10, 11, 12, tumor necrosis factor α, interferon α, and epidermal, transforming, colony-stimulating growth factor). As to the future, Fiocchi and Podolsky (1) state: "There is much evidence to indicate that the complex network of cytokines and growth factors present within the intestinal mucosa plays a critical and multifaceted role in the pathogenesis of inflammatory bowel disease. The involvement of these mediators in most aspects of immune and inflammatory injury, as well as reparative processes, suggests that a comprehensive understanding of their properties may provide insights into disease pathogenesis and new approaches to therapy. However, their apparent extensive redundancy also indicates that such approaches will require a detailed understanding and precise manipulation of these regulatory peptides and their activities."

Genetic Aspects of IBD: Early Observations

The first published instances of "familial IBD" in the 1909 London symposium on ulcerative colitis (brother and sister, father and sibling, and father and sister of a third patient) were labeled as "coincidences," and this view prevailed until the publications of Sherlock and Almy (78), Kirsner et al. (79), and R. McConnell (80) during the 1960s. Reports of "familial" inflammatory bowel disease subsequently increased, clinically supporting a genetic relationship in IBD. Moltke (81) in 1936 had described five families with ulcerative colitis (mother and daughter, two; brother and sister, two; and father and daughter, one). Schlesinger and Platt (82) (1958) obtained a family history of ulcerative colitis in 17% of 60 children with ulcerative colitis; almost one fourth of the series were of Jewish origin, four-fold higher than the usual ethnic distribution of the hospital population.

Familial distributions of IBD involves first-degree relatives (parent, child, or siblings) more often than second-degree or third-degree relatives (aunts, uncles, nieces, and nephews) in accord with a polygenic inheritance. In the 1963 University of Chicago study (79) for ulcerative colitis, 50 of the 89 family members were brothers and sisters and cousins, approximately the same generation as that of the probands. For regional enteritis, 15 of the 22 family members involved brothers, sisters, and first cousins.

Multiple Family Occurrences

The occurrence of IBD in three or more members of the same family, a possibility estimated as only one in 12 billion, strongly supported a genetic relationship. In the 1963 Chicago study, triple or more familial occurrences of inflammatory bowel disease included: (a) mother, brother and sister with ulcerative colitis; (b) two sisters and a grandfather with ulcerative colitis; (c) three sisters with ulcerative colitis; and (d) three sisters and one brother with ulcerative colitis.

The eight members of the Morris family (83) (1965) represented three generations, all apparently with ulcerative colitis, four males and four females, a distribution compatible with the involvement of an autosomal dominant gene. Thayer's (84) (1972) unusual family included a 21-year-old male with ulcerative colitis since the age of 8 who developed a carcinoma of the descending colon. A maternal aunt developed ulcerative colitis at the same time. One year after the death of the index patient, his brother, 2 years younger, developed ulcerative colitis and required colectomy and ileostomy. Within a year after this operation, the boy's father developed ulcerative colitis and after 5 years of medical treatment, he also underwent a colectomy and ileostomy. In the Kuspira et al. (85) fam-

ily, six members were affected with Crohn's disease, spanning three generations.

Intermingling of Diseases: Twins and Genetic Associations

Ulcerative colitis was more likely to occur than Crohn's disease among the families of probands with ulcerative colitis and the same relationship held for probands with Crohn's disease, but disease incidence was mixed in approximately 25% of families. The seven affected members of the Ashkenazi Jewish family studied by Sherlock et al. (1963) included five with regional enteritis and two with ulcerative colitis. Seven unaffected relatives of the same family had varying degrees of genetically-related deafness. In the 1973 Chicago study, 31 of the 103 positive families included mixed inflammatory bowel disease (86).

Early surveys of monozygotic twins demonstrated moderate concordance for ulcerative colitis and strong concordance for Crohn's disease, powerful supporting evidence for a genetic influence in inflammatory bowel disease. Discordance was more common for ulcerative colitis than for Crohn's disease. Purrmann et al. (87) in 1986 reported monozygotic triplets with Crohn's disease of the colon developing within a period of 11 months; both parents were free of digestive disease. The association of ulcerative colitis and Crohn's disease with genetically-mediated conditions, such as for ulcerative colitis, primary sclerosing cholangitis, ankylosing spondylitis and Turner's syndrome, and for Crohn's disease, psoriasis, glycogan wastage disease, and the Hermansky-Pudlak syndrome, strengthened the genetic evidence. Two "controlled" studies of familial IBD, documenting a significantly increased incidence, provided additional support (88,89).

Genetic Possibilities

Genetic possibilities in IBD have included a polygenic mode of inheritance, "a specific form of somatic gene mutation in mesenchymal stem cells . . . (and) the growth of a 'forbidden clone' of cells whose 'mutant' humoral products attack the colonic mucosa," and a "rare additive major gene" (90). Kuster et al. (91) (1989), utilizing complex segregation analysis of data obtained in studying the pedigrees of 265 probands with Crohn's disease (5,387 relatives), suggested the presence of a recessive gene with incomplete penetrance for susceptibility to the disease. Approximately 30% of cases were related to the presence of this gene in the family. Rotter (92) has suggested that: "Early non-use of IBD predisposing genes with a later hyperimmune response of the mucosal immune system or (more likely) nonexposure to a potentially injurious agent" conceivably leaves the gut immunological system in a continually poised state and "thus sets up the system for subsequent dysregulation."

The gene clusters ordinarily involved in the expression of immune responses possibly relevant to IBD include HLA genes on chromosome 6, immunoglobulin heavy chain markers on chromosome 14, immunoglobulin light chain marker on chromosome 2, complement-controlling genes on chromosomes 6 and 19, and T-cell antigen receptor genes on chromosomes 14 (alpha chain) and 7 (beta chain) important in the pathogenesis of autoimmunity. The possible role of these gene patterns in IBD is under investigation (92).

Author's Comment

Ulcerative colitis and Crohn's disease are genetically heterogeneous disorders with complex genetic predispositions. Inheritable protein, enzymatic metabolic defects or chromosomal abnormalities have not been demonstrated. ABO blood groups and secretor status are distributed normally. Classic mendelian ratios are not observed in affected families. A generation often is skipped and consanguinity, an essential condition to a recessive gene is absent. The genetic abnormality probably involves the combined interaction of several genes, the polygenic or multifactorial type of inheritance, interacting with environmental influences to precipitate inflammatory bowel disease in susceptible individuals.

Current evidence strongly indicates a genetic influence in at least 15% of patients with ulcerative colitis and in 25% of patients with Crohn's disease. Sartor (42) has demonstrated a genetic vulnerability also in experimental intestinal inflammation, occurring in Lewis rats challenged by purified bacterial cell wall polymers or small bowel bacterial overgrowth (not in Fischer and Buffalo rats). The identity of the IBD genes remains to be determined but increasing knowledge of the HLA system and HLA linkages at the molecular level and new genetic techniques, including restriction fragment length polymorphism analysis of genomic DNA, recombinant DNA and monoclonal antibody methodology, the polymerase chain reaction and in situ hybridization methods for cellular localization of RNA transcripts, should help identify the complex molecular events involved in gene regulation of antigen processing within the IBD intestinal epithelium. Other areas for future investigation are the identification of specific biological markers of ulcerative colitis and Crohn's disease, the possible role of the complement system, and the T-cell receptor. The genetically-modified transgenic rat, the Jackson Laboratories heritable mouse enterocolitis (Elson), and the genetic "knockout" animal model (e.g., deletion of genes for IL2, IL-10, G protein [93]) are useful models for genetically-oriented study. Finally, the investigation of Class II antigens (HLA-DR, DP genes) associated with the clinical variability of certain diseases, such as rheumatoid arthritis and type I diabetes (94), should yield useful data applicable also to IBD.

Overview

The chronological events described for ulcerative colitis and for Crohn's disease, their emergence during the latter part of the 19th century, increasing early in the 20th century, the prominence of ulcerative colitis during the first half and of Crohn's disease during the second half of this century indicate slowly evolving, environmentally-influenced disorders characterized by the youthfulness of the patients, chronicity, recurrences, and numerous gastrointestinal and systemic complications. The early higher incidence of ulcerative colitis, exceeding Crohn's disease three or fourfold, appears to have stabilized and may be decreasing in several areas. Although affecting prevalently children and young adults, more IBD patients today are older (50–80 years). The clinical manifestations of ulcerative colitis have changed partially during the past half century. Ulcerative proctitis and proctosigmoiditis have increased in frequency or are diagnosed more often via flexible proctosigmoidoscopy. Improved supportive and anti-inflammatory therapy has decreased the previously high mortality of initially severe episodes. The major complications of massive hemorrhage, toxic dilatation of the colon, perforation, and severe malnutrition are less common now than 50 years ago because of improved nutritional and supportive care. The strong association between ulcerative colitis and primary sclerosing cholangitis (PSC) also represents an increased risk for colon cancer and further study of PSC may reveal pathogenetically important information. The severe hepatic disease in some IBD patients has necessitated liver transplantation. Cancer of the rectum and colon remains a problem but closer supervision of patients, frequent colonoscopic examination, biopsy recognition of dysplasia, together with earlier colectomy for patients not responding to medical treatment or requiring excessive amounts of steroids have reduced the magnitude of the problem. Population surveys in Denmark (95) have demonstrated a mild to moderate, medically controllable course in a substantial proportion of the ulcerative colitis population. The treatment of ulcerative colitis, though not curative, has improved significantly because of increased medical resources, better understanding of drug actions, clearer indications for operation, and improved surgical procedures.

Crohn's disease today also differs from its initial "tumor-like" presentation although inflammatory abdominal masses remain part of the clinical spectrum. The incidence of Crohn's disease continues to rise in many areas but may have stabilized in Sweden. The worldwide prevalence of Crohn's disease, especially in cooler, industrialized, urban areas, its infrequency in underdeveloped less sanitary geographic areas, and its emergence in "westernized" countries (e.g., Japan) pose intriguing environmental questions (e.g., the role of sanitation, pollution of water, food and air, microbial infection). Such initial features as limitation of Crohn's disease to the ileocecal valve and its presentation as "acute appendicitis" common during the 1930s have disappeared. Involvement of the colon has increased. The endoscopic demonstration of recurrent Crohn's disease of the small bowel postoperatively, immediately proximal to the surgical anastomosis, implicates the intestinal contents in the pathogenesis of the disease (role for bacteria, cytotoxin). An important aspect of Crohn's disease, increasingly evident in the 1990s, is the individuality of the clinical course and the repetitiveness of particular complications in the same patient; strictures, abscesses, fistulas, or bleeding, necessitating the identification of subsets of patients, in addition to acceptable guidelines of disease activity/severity in evaluating IBD. The tendency to cicatrization in Crohn's disease has been attributed to the proliferation of muscle cells in the muscularis mucosa. The uniquely aggressive nature of the inflammatory reaction, unlike the inflammatory response of ulcerative colitis, has not been explained. As with ulcerative colitis, the medical treatment of Crohn's disease has improved, including the restoration of normal nutrition (absence of anemia, normal serum proteins), the judicious use of broad-spectrum antibiotics, limited administration of steroids, and individually selective use of anti-inflammatory agents. Surgeons, once committed to extensive histologically influenced resections of small intestine, now limit bowel resection to grossly visible disease or perform stricturoplastics.

The intriguing relationship between ulcerative colitis and Crohn's disease, entities with similar clinical, epidemiologic, and demographic features and intermingling of both diseases in 25% of families, after 50 years, now appears closer to resolution as etiologically independent entities yet related perhaps via "similar perpetuating stimuli and common pathways of tissue injury." The Crohn's disease involvement of the entire gastrointestinal tract contrasts with the limitation of ulcerative colitis to the colon and rectum. Histologically, the diffuse mucosal-submucosal involvement of ulcerative colitis contrasts with the focal transmural inflammation of Crohn's disease but mucosal disease early in Crohn's disease has become more evident. The prominent lymphoid aggregates, dilated submucosal lymphatics and the granulomas distributed throughout the bowel wall in Crohn's disease, features not seen in ulcerative colitis, remain pathogenetically significant for Crohn' disease. The recurrence of Crohn's disease after surgery is in contrast to the "cure" of ulcerative colitis following total colectomy and ileostomy or ileoanal anastomosis, but pouchitis is an increasing problem and the observation of dysplasia in pouchitis is disquieting. The principal epidemiologic difference between Crohn's disease and ulcerative colitis is the infrequency of smokers among patients with ulcerative colitis and their excess among patients with Crohn's disease. The biologic basis of this difference is unknown. The genetic influence has become increasingly apparent in Crohn's disease.

Biologically, increased titers of serum antineutrophil cytoplasmic antibodies and antibodies against goblet cells are typical of patients with ulcerative colitis and their first degree relatives. Antibodies to a trypsin-sensitive antigen in pancreatic juice and the increased antiendothelial cell antibodies characterize Crohn's disease. Interleukin-2 messenger RNA is increased in the intestinal lesions of Crohn's disease but not ulcerative colitis and similar increases are reported for IL-8 and IL-10. Though much remains to be learned in this area, the differing genetic patterns now being disclosed (HLA-DR2 in ulcerative colitis and HLA-DR1/DQ5 in Crohn's disease) further separates the two illnesses. The more focused etiologic concepts of the 1990s revolve around microbial elements, gut mucosal immunologic mechanisms, cellular and cytokine mechanisms of inflammation, mechanisms of gut mucosal cytoprotection, and genetic influences.

In summary, ulcerative colitis and Crohn's disease are heterogeneous diseases with broadening and overlapping clinical features. Each results

Table 1.1. Inflammatory bowel diseases—possible pathogenetiic events.

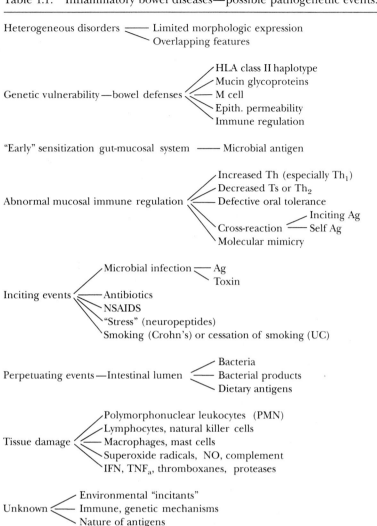

from the conjunction of multiple etiologic factors (genetic vulnerability, altered host intestinal defenses, abnormal gut mucosal immune system), priming the responsiveness of the gut immune system. (Table 1.1) Each involves the entry of an environmental agent into the GI tract or the generation of an etiologic agent within the alimentary canal. The immediate cytopathic agent appears to reside within the intestinal content, acting on the mucosa and submucosa in ulcerative colitis and on the postsurgical anastomosis in Crohn's disease. The focal tissue reaction of Crohn's disease suggests specific cellular-site attachments of a microbial or viral agent or constituent, subsequently entering the intestinal lymphatic network, accounting for the lymphatic dilatation, the lymphoid prominence, and the enlarged mesenteric lymph notes. Precipitating factors include environmental agents (bacteria, viruses, industrial, atmospheric,

and water pollutants, and chemicals) and "pathophysiological stress," and are not limited to any geographic area or to any ethnic group. The inflammatory reaction, possibly amplified by mucin-degrading enzymes (i.e., hyaluronidase), involves a series of nonspecific but complex proinflammatory events mediated by cytokines, and leukotrienes of the lipoxygenase pathway, insufficiently balanced by protective elements of the cyclo-oxygenase pathway (prostaglandins, other eicosanoids), with important contributions from activated macrophages and inflammatory cells (polymorphonuclear cells, lymphocytes, eosinophils, mast cells, and Paneth cells), as well as nitric oxide. Autoimmunity remains an unproven concept but immune reactions are an integral component of the tissue reaction.

Many issues remain to be investigated: the cytoprotective and immunologic integrity of the normal gastrointestinal tract continuously exposed to the vast array of bacterial, dietary, and environmental antigens; the mucosal cytoprotective effects of secretory IgA, heat-shock proteins, adhesion molecules, and other cytoprotective agents; the status of the vast aerobic and anaerobic flora of the gut; the biology of the IBD intestinal content; the mechanism and the significance of the hyperresponsive gut mucosal immune system; the molecular biology of inflammation; the nature of the genetic vulnerability; the tobacco enigma; the role of neurohumoral and neurotransmitter peptides acting via the autonomic and the enteric nervous systems in the immune and inflammatory responses, and genetic studies of programmed patterns of cell death (apoptosis) applied to the intestinal epithelial cell. These studies now are facilitated by the many genetically engineered animal models of intestinal inflammation.

Sartor's (42) working hypothesis of IBD pathogenesis, extending Shorter's earlier hypothesis, is relevant. Nonspecific intestinal inflammation induced, for example, by enteric infections, increases intestinal permeability with the increased absorption of anaerobic bacterial products (antigens) in Crohn's disease or aerobic bacterial products in ulcerative colitis, potentiating bowel injury. Normally these responses are down-regulated by the gut mucosal immune system, with rapid healing of the tissue injury. The genetically-vulnerable individual ("IBD patient") lacks the capacity (partially or completely) to fully suppress the inflammatory reaction, with consequent excessive amplification of the immune cascade, including the complex array of proinflammatory cytokines and other biologically active molecules. The result is "an unrestrained inflammatory response leading to tissue destruction, chronic inflammation, and fibrosis." The challenge for the future will be to determine the precise nature of these events and thereby establish the cause(s) of ulcerative colitis and Crohn's disease.

References

1. Kirsner JB, Shorter RG. Inflammatory Bowel Disease. 4th ed. Baltimore, MD: Williams & Wilkins, 1995.
2. Kirsner JB. The historical basis of the idiopathic inflammatory bowel diseases. J Inflamm Bowel Diseases 1995;1:2–26.
3. Morson BC. Current concepts of colitis. The 1970 Lettsomian Lectures, Trans Med Soc, London, 1970;86:159–76.
4. Wilks S. Morbid appearances in the intestine of Miss Bankes. London Medical Gazette 1859;2:264–5.
5. Wilks S., Moxon W. Lectures on Pathological Anatomy. London 2nd ed. 1875;408.
6. Hurst AF. Ulcerative colitis. Guy's Hosp Rep 1921; 71:26–41.
7. Bargen JA. Experimental studies on the etiology of chronic ulcerative colitis (Preliminary Report). JAMA 1924;83:332–6.
8. Bargen JA, Jackman RJ, Kerr JG. Studies on the life histories of patients with chronic ulcerative colitis (thrombo ulcerative colitis) with some suggestions for treatment. Ann Int Med 1938;12:339–52.
9. Kirsner JB, Goldgraber MB. Hypersensitivity, autoimmunity and the digestive tract. Gastroenterology 1960;38:536–62.
10. Fabry W. Cited by: Fielding JF. Crohn's disease and Dalziel's syndrome. J Clin Gastroenterol 1988;10: 279–85.
11. Morgagni GB. The seats and causes of disease investigated by anatomy. Five books containing a great variety of dissections with remarks (Translated from the Latin of John Baptist Morgagni by Benjamin Alexander.) 3 Vol. London: Millar A., Cadell T., 1769.
12. Dalziel TK. Chronic interstitial enteritis. Br Med J (Clin Res) 1913;2:1068–70.
13. Coffen TH. Nonspecific granuloma of the intestine causing intestinal obstruction. JAMA 1925;35: 1303–4.
14. Crohn BB, Ginzburg L, Oppenheimer GD. Regional ileitis: a pathologic and clinical entity. JAMA 1932; 99:1323–9.
15. Lockhart-Mummery HE, Morson BC. Crohn's disease (regional enteritis) of the large intestine and its distinction from ulcerative colitis. Gut 1960;1:87–105.
16. Warren S, Sommers SC. Cicatrizing enteritis (regional ileitis) as a pathologic entity: analysis of 120 cases. Am J Pathol 1948;24:475–501.
17. Reichert FL, Mathes ME. Experimental lymphoderma of the intestinal tract and its relation to regional cicatrizing enteritis. Ann Surg 1936;104:601–14.
18. Melrose AG. The geographic incidence of chronic ulcerative colitis in Britain. Gastroenterology 1955; 29:1055–60.
19. Acheson ED. The distribution of ulcerative colitis and regional enteritis in United States veterans with particular reference to the Jewish religion. Gut 1960;1:291–3.
20. Monk M, Mendeloff AI, Siegel CI, et al. An epidemiologic study of ulcerative colitis and regional enteritis among adults in Baltimore. I. Hospital incidence and prevalence 1960–1963. Gastroenterology 1967;53:198–210.
21. Mendeloff AI. The epidemiology of idiopathic inflammatory bowel disease. In: Kirnser JB, Shorter RG, eds. Inflammatory Bowel Disease, Philadelphia: Lea & Febiger, 1975;3–19.
22. Mendeloff AI. The epidemiology of inflammatory bowel disease. Clin Gastroenterol 1980;9:259–70.

23. Samuelsson SM. Ulceros colit och proktit. Thesis, University of Upsala 1976;1–182.

24. Harries AD, Baird A, Rhodes J. Nonsmoking: a feature of ulcerative colitis. Brit Med J 1982;284:706.

25. Kessler H, Diamond KI. Epidemiological studies of Parkinson's disease. I. Smoking and Parkinson's Disease. Am J Epidemiol 1971;94:16–25.

26. Calkins BM. Inflammatory bowel disease. In Digestive Diseases in the United States—Epidemiology and Impact. Everhart JK, National Digestive Disease Working Group. U. S. Department Health and Human Services. National Institutes of Health, Bethesda, MD 1994;509–50.

27. Pavlov I. Conditioned Reflexes (Anrep GV, trans.), New York: Oxford, 1927.

28. Cannon WB. Bodily Changes in Pain, Hunger, Fear and Rage. 2nd ed., New York: Appleton, 1929.

29. Grace WJ, Wolf S, Wolff HG. The Human Colon, New York: Hoeker, PB; 1951;225–7.

30. Almy TP, Tulin M. Alterations in colonic function in man under stress. I. Experimental production of changes simulating the irritable colon. Gastroenterology 1947;8:616–26.

31. Murray CD. Psychogenic factors in the etiology of ulcerative colitis. Am J Dig Dis 1930;180:239–48.

32. Sullivan AJ, Chandler CA. Ulcerative colitis of psychogenic origin: report of six cases. Yale J Biol Med 1932;4:779–86.

33. White BV. Effect of ileostomy and colectomy on personality adjustment of patients with ulcerative colitis. New Engl J Med 1951;244:537–40.

34. Karush A, Daniels GE, Flood C, et al. Psychotherapy in chronic ulcerative colitis. Philadelphia: W.B. Saunders, 1977.

35. North CS, Clouse RE, Spitznagel EL, et al. The relation of ulcerative colitis to psychiatric factors: a review of findings and methods. Am J Psychiatry 1990;147:974–81.

36. Helzer JE, Chammas S, Norland CC, et al. A study of the association between Crohn's disease and psychiatric illness. Gastroenterology 1984;86:324–30.

37. Sternberg EM, Chrousos GP, Wilder RL, et al. The stress response and the regulation of inflammatory disease. Ann Int Med 1992;117:854–66.

38. Kirsner JB. The Development of American Gastroenterology. New York: Raven Press, 1990.

39. Peterson EA, Mandel RM. Infectious diseases—old diseases return and new agents emerge (editorial). Arch Int Med 1995;155:1571–2.

40. Wensinck F. Cited by: Van de Merwe JP. A possible role of Eubacterium and Peptostreptococcus species in the aetiology of Crohn's disease. In Pena AS, Weterman IT, Booth CC, Strober W, eds. Recent Advances in Crohn's Disease. The Hague: Martinus Nijhoff 1981;201–206.

41. Ekbom J, Wakefield AJ, Zack M, et al. Perinatal measles infection and subsequent Crohn's disease. Lancet 1994;344:508–10.

42. Sartor RB. Current concepts of the etiology and pathogenesis of ulcerative colitis and Crohn's disease. Gastroenterol Clin of North Am 1995:24:475–507.

43. Andresen AFR. Ulcerative colitis—an allergic phenomenon. Am J Dig Dis 1942;9:91–8.

44. Rowe AH. Chronic ulcerative colitis: allergy in its etiology. Ann Int Med 1942;17:83–100.

45. Walzer M, Gray I, Straus HW, et al. Studies in experimental hypersensitiveness in the rhesus monkey: allergic reaction in passively locally sensitized abdominal organs. J Immunol 1938;34:91–5.

46. Kirsner JB, Shorter RG. Recent developments in "nonspecific" inflammatory bowel disease. New Engl J Med 1982;306:775–85, 837–48.

47. Besredka A. La vaccination contre les etats typhoides par la voie Buccale. Ann Inst Pasteur 1919;33:882–903.

48. Davies A. An investigation into the serological properties of dysentery stools. Lancet 1922;2:1009–12.

49. Kirsner JB, Palmer WL. Ulcerative colitis (considerations of its etiology and treatment). JAMA 1954;155:341–6.

50. Goldgraber MB, Kirsner JB. The arthus phenomenon in the colon of rabbits. AMA Arch Path 1959;67:556–71.

51. Kirsner JB, Elchlepp J. The production of an experimental colitis in rabbits. Trans Assoc American Physicians 1957;70:102–19.

52. Auer J. Local autoinoculation of the sensitized organism with foreign protein as a cause of abnormal reactions. J Exper Med 1920;32:427–44.

53. Heremans JF. Les Globulines Seriques du Systeme Gamma, leur Nature et leur Pathologie. Brussels: Arcia 1960.

54. Tomasi TB, Tan EM, Solomon A, et al. Characteristics of an immune system common to certain external secretions. J Exp Med 1965;121:101–24.

55. Bienenstock J. The physiology of the local immune response. In: Immunology of the Gastrointestinal Tract. Asquith P, ed. London: Churchill Livingstone 1979.

56. Kirsner JB. Inflammatory bowel disease—overview of etiology and pathogenesis. In: Berk JE, ed. Bockus Gastroenterology. Philadelphia: W.B. Saunders 1985.

57. Shorter RG, Huizenga KA, Spencer RJ. A working hypothesis for the etiology and pathogenesis of nonspecific inflammatory bowel disease. Digest Dis Sci 1972;17:1024–32.

58. Elson CO. The Immunology of Inflammatory Bowel Disease. In: Inflammatory Bowel Disease. 4th ed. Kirsner JB, Shorter RG, eds. Baltimore: Williams & Wilkins, 1994.

59. Weiner HL. Oral tolerance: mobilizing the gut. Hospital Practice (Sept) 1995;15:53–8.

60. Yang P, Jarnerot G, Danielsson D, et al. P-ANCA in monozygotic twins with inflammatory bowel disease. Gut 1995;36:887–90.

61. Hertervig E, Wieslander J, Johansson C, et al. Anti-neutrophil cytoplasmic antibodies in chronic inflammatory bowel disease. Scand J Gastroenterol 1995; 30:693–8.

62. Castro G. Immunological regulation of epithelial function. Am J Physiol 1982;243 (Gastrointestinal Liver Physiol. 6):G321–9.

63. Pulverer G, Ko HL, Berth J. Immunomodulating effect of antibiotics on intestinal microflora. Path Biol 1993;41:753–8.

64. Metchnikoff E. Untersuchungen uber die intracellularle verdauung bei wirbellosen thieren. Arbeit Zool Inst Univ Wien 1883;5:141–68. (See also Metschnikoff O. Life of Elie Metschnikoff. New York: Houghton Mifflin Co. 1921).

65. Ehrlich P. Experimental researches on specific therapy: on immunity with special reference to the relationship between distribution and action of antigens. In: Himmelwert F, ed. Collected Papers. Vol. 3. New York: Pergamon Press, 1960 (Originally Published 1908).

66. Menkin V. Studies on inflammation; mechanisms of fixation by inflammatory reaction. J Exper Med 1931;53:171–7.

67. McCord JM, Fridovich I. Superoxide dismutase. An enzymic function for erythrocuprein (hemocuprein). J Biol Chem 1969;244:6049–55.

68. Babior BM, Kipnes RS, Curnutte JT. Biological defense mechanisms, the production by leukocytes of superoxide—a potential bactericidal agent. J Clin Invest 1973;52:741–4.

69. Granger DN, Rutili G, McCord JM. Superoxide radicals in feline intestinal ischemia. Gastroenterology 1981;81:22–9.

70. Grisham MB, Granger DN. Neutrophil mediated mucosal injury—role of reactive oxygen metabolites. Dig Dis Sci 1988;33:6S–15S.

71. Gery I, Gersham RK, Waksman BH. Potentiates of the T-lymphocyte response to mitogens. I. The responding cell. J Exp Med 1972;136:128–42.

72. Paetkau V, Mills G, Gerhart S, et al. Proliferation of murine thymic lymphocytes in vitro is mediated by the concanavalin-α-induced release of a lymphokine (Costimulator). J Immunol 1976;117:1320–4.

73. Chen DM, di Sabato G. Further studies on the thymocyte stimulating factor. Cell Immunol 1976;22:211–24.

74. Sharon P, Stenson WK. Enhanced synthesis of leukotriene B4 by colonic mucosa in inflammatory bowel disease. Gastroenterology 1984;86:453–60.

75. Fiocchi C. Production of inflammatory cytokines in the intestinal lamina propria. Immunol Res 1991;10:239–46.

76. Podolsky DK. Inflammatory bowel disease. New Engl J Med 1991;325:928–37, 1008–16.

77. Sartor RB. Cytokines in intestinal inflammation. Pathophysiological and clinical considerations. Gastroenterology 1994;106:533–9.

78. Almy TP, Sherlock P. Genetic aspects of ulcerative colitis and regional enteritis. Gastroenterology 1966; 51:757–60.

79. Kirsner JB, Spencer JA. Family occurrences of ulcerative colitis, regional enteritis, and ileocolitis. Ann Int Med 1963;59:133–44.

80. McConnell RB. The genetics of gastrointestinal disorders. London: Oxford University Press, 1966; 128–42. Cited in: Genetics of gastrointestinal disorders. Clin Gastroenterol 1973;2:489–724.

81. Moltke O. Familial occurrence of non-specific ulcerative colitis. Acta Med Scand 1936;78(suppl 72):426–32.

82. Schlesinger B, Platt J. Ulcerative colitis in childhood and a follow-up study. Proc Royal Soc Med 1958;51:733–5.

83. Morris PJ. Familial ulcerative colitis. Gut 1965;6:176–8.

84. Thayer WR, Jr. Crohn's disease (regional enteritis). Scand J Gastroenterol 1970;6:165–85.

85. Kuspira J, Bhambhani R, Singh SM, et al. Familial occurrences of Crohn's disease. Human Heredity 1972;22:239–42.

86. Kirsner JB. Genetic aspects of inflammatory bowel disease. Clin Gastroenterol 1973;2:557–76.

87. Purrmann J, Bertrams J, Borchard F, et al. Monozygotic triplets with Crohn's disease of the colon. Gastroenterology 1986;91:1553–9.

88. Singer HC, Anderson JGD, Frischer H, et al. Familial aspects of inflammatory bowel disease. Gastroenterology 1971;61:423–30.

89. Kirsner JB. Inflammatory Bowel Disease. Part I. Nature and Pathogenesis. II. Clinical and Therapeutic Aspects. Disease-A-Month (Masters in Medicine) 1991;37:(10):610–66, 673–746.

90. Monsen U, Iselius L, Johansson C, et al. Evidence for a major additive gene in ulcerative colitis. Clin Gen 1989;36:411–4.

91. Kuster W, Pascoe L, Purrmann J, et al. The genetics of Crohn's disease—complex segregation analysis of a family study with 265 patients with Crohn's disease. Am J Med Gen 1989;32:105–8.

92. Yang H, Rotter JI. Genetics of inflammatory bowel disease. In Targan SR, Shanahan K, eds. Inflammatory Bowel Disease (From Bench to Bedside). Baltimore: Williams & Wilkins, 1994.

93. Elson CO, Sartor RB, Tennyson GS, et al. Experimental models of inflammatory bowel disease. Gastroenterology 1995;109:1344–67.

94. Nepom GT. Class II antigens and disease susceptibility. Ann Rev Med 1995;46:117–25.

95. Binder V, Park H, Hansen PK. et al. Incidence and prevalence of ulcerative colitis and Crohn's disease in the county of Copenhagen—1962 to 1978. Gastroenterology 1982;83:563–8.

2 Epidemiology

Jan Stewénius and Tomas Lindhagen

Epidemiology is the study of disease occurrence in a population in relation to "time, place, and person" (1). The intention is to generate hypotheses as to its cause and treatment by describing the geographical pattern of the disease, by following time trends of incidence and by describing the socio-demographic and clinical characteristics.

Epidemiological research concerning inflammatory bowel disease (IBD) began in the 1950s. Most of the early studies, however, included only hospital cases. The first population-based study, including both in- and out-patients, came from Oxford in 1965 (2) and for the first time in an epidemiological study, specific criteria were established for both ulcerative colitis and Crohn's disease. This was also the first study to discuss colitis of "mixed forms," which would probably have been labeled indeterminate colitis today. Many studies of both in- and out-patients have since then emanated from northwest Europe but also from the United States and Israel and, in later years, from an increasing number of countries all over the world.

This review presents the incidence trends in ulcerative colitis, Crohn's disease, and indeterminate colitis and the most common sources of errors in epidemiological studies in IBD. These errors are summed up in Table 2.1 and have been discussed in detail earlier by others (3).

Ulcerative Colitis

Most studies up to the 1980s showed an increase in incidence (Fig. 2.1). However, a recent study from Cardiff, Wales, between 1968 and 1987 showed a stable incidence over the whole period (4).

From Copenhagen, Denmark, an increase in the incidence has been reported for men but not for women (5). By contrast, some studies have shown a decrease in incidence for the first half of the 1980s (5,6,7). No studies have so far presented the incidence trend for the early years of the 1990s.

The incidence figures vary, however. A high annual incidence of more than 10 per 100,000 population have been reported from Scandinavia, Great Britain, and the United States, with the highest figure of 20.3 from the Faroe Islands (8). Medium high figures of two to seven have been found in central Europe and low ones from southern and eastern Europe. However, recent studies have shown a considerable increase in both Greece and Italy up to an incidence of about five (9,10), and thus it is doubtful if a north-south gradient in Europe exists. Such a north-south gradient has also been discussed in the United States (11). Medium high incidence rates are reported from New Zealand and Israel, whereas low figures have been reported in the few studies presented from other parts of the world.

Only one study has presented the incidence trends of all types of IBD including indeterminate colitis (Fig. 2.2) (12). In this study from Malmö, Sweden, from 1958 to 1982, with a follow-up study of at least seven years, almost all radiographs and histopathologic specimens were reexamined. Very few patients get a diagnosis of ulcerative colitis during the first decade of life. The peak incidence is between 20 and 29 years for both males and females; second incidence peak has been reported in the 60 to 70 age group in many but not in all studies. The onset of this disease at other ages is not common. Most earlier studies showed ulcerative colitis

Table 2.1.   Sources of error in epidemiological studies of IBD.

A. Within a study
  Population
    size
    mobility
    length of the study period
    length of the follow-up
  Medical care system
    changed access to medical care
    changed attitude to seeking medical attention
    introduction of new investigative techniques
  Case ascertainment
    children patients
    availability of registers of
      diagnosis for in- and outpatients
      radiology
      histo-pathology
      endoscopy
      gastroenterological clinics
      general practitioners' clinics

  Criteria
    uniformity during the whole study period
  Diagnosis
    exclusion of infectious and ischemic colitis
    indeterminate colitis separately registered
  Validity
    availability for re-examination of
      medical case history
        radiographs
      histopathological specimens
B. Comparing studies
  Population
    different lengths of the study period
    age-standardized incidence or not
  Criteria
    uniformity
    indeterminate colitis separately presented
    possible exclusion of patients with proctitis

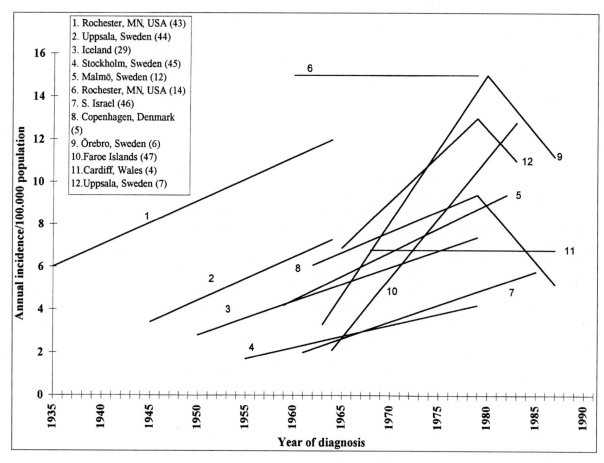

Fig. 2.1.   Incidence trend of ulcerative colitis in series with a study period of 20 years or more.

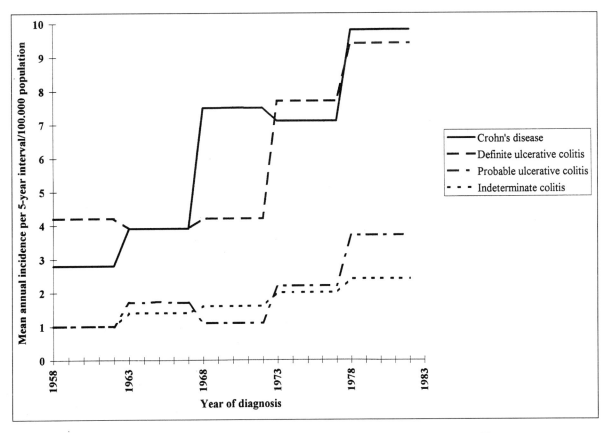

Fig. 2.2. Incidence of all patients wth IBD in Malmö, Sweden, 1958–82.

to be more common in women. Interestingly, several recent studies show that men are more commonly affected (6,9,10,12,13). Urban populations have in some but not all studies been found to have a higher incidence than rural ones. The earlier lower incidence of nonwhites versus whites has been found to be eliminated (14). Jews in the United States and other countries have been found to run a risk of developing IBD at least four times higher than other ethnic groups (15). South Asian immigrants in Leicestershire were found to develop ulcerative colitis significantly more often than the native population (16).

Mortality was high up until the 1970s, especially in severe attacks. Today mortality is hardly considered to be increased at all, or at least only among aged patients and in connection with severe attacks (17,18).

Indeterminate Colitis

In 1978, Price, from St. Mark's Hospital in London, reported on a surgical series of 330 patients where

30 cases were impossible to classify and the term *indeterminate colitis* was adopted (19). An update of the St. Mark's Hospital surgical series, now including 53 cases with indeterminate colitis out of 675 cases of colitis has been published (20).

Even in nonoperated cases, patients with indeterminate colitis have been delineated (21). In the incidence study of indeterminate colitis from Malmö, Sweden, the relative frequencies of IBD were 49% for ulcerative colitis, 41% for Crohn's disease and 10% for indeterminate colitis (Fig. 2.1) (12). The importance of this problem has been discussed in only very few other epidemiological studies. In one, 21 cases were excluded from a study of 373 patients with ulcerative colitis (6). In another, 11 out of 167 patients with ulcerative colitis and 79 with Crohn's disease were excluded (22). The highest frequency of indeterminate colitis so far reported is 24%, 127 cases out of 539 children with IBD, including small bowel disease (23). In other studies, if patients with indeterminate colitis are discussed at all, the number of these patients is usually not specified (Table 2.2).

Table 2.2.   Review of epidemiological studies on ulcerative colitis, grouped with special reference to indeterminate colitis.

Area	Year of publication	Study period
Cases of indeterminate colitis excluded		
Oxford, England[2]	1965	1951–60
Rochester, MN, USA[43]	1972	1935–64
Malmö, Sweden[49]	1975	1958–70
N Tees Health District, England[50]	1980	1971–77
Northeastern Scotland[51]	1983	1967–76
Israel[46]	1987	1961–85
Leiden, The Netherlands[52]	1987	1979–83
Örebro, Sweden[6]	1992	1963–87
Sweden (Children)[23]	1991	1984–85
Leicestershire, England[18]	1992	1972–89
Malmö, Sweden[12]	1995	1958–82
Cases of indeterminate colitis included either as ulcerative colitis or as Crohn's disease		
Rochester, MN, USA[14]	1987	1960–79
Uppsala, Sweden[7]	1991	1965–83
Indeterminate colitis not mentioned		
Uppsala, Sweden[44]	1976	1945–64
Stockholm, Sweden[45]	1985	1955–79
Faroe Islands[47]	1986	1964–83
Faroe Islands[8]	1989	1981–88
Iceland[29]	1989	1950–79
Copenhagen, Denmark[5]	1991	1962–87
Cardiff, Wales[4]	1992	1968–87

Crohn's Disease

Crohn's disease is most common in central and northern Europe, especially in Great Britain and Scandinavia, and in North America. The incidence in eastern and southern Europe is low. (9,10,24,25) A low incidence has been reported from Australia (26). The disease is seldom seen in Asia, South America, or Japan. The incidence of Crohn's disease in Africa is practically unknown since there are very few reports from this continent and then only concerning the white population in South Africa (27,28). Interestingly, the incidence in Iceland, a Nordic country, is low and has not increased since 1960 (29).

In high incidence areas an increasing rate of Crohn's disease is a typical finding. The increase started in the early 1960s and continued through the 1970s. High incidence rates are reported from Cardiff, Wales (30) and in Malmö, Sweden, the incidence was 11.3 per 100,000 inhabitants in 1980. During the 1980s there are some reports showing a decreasing incidence (7,31), whereas in Örebro (Sweden), Copenhagen (Denmark), and Israel there is still a rise (32,33,34) (Fig. 2.3).

An interesting finding is that people from countries with a low or practically no incidence of

Crohn's disease who move to countries with a high incidence seem to suffer the same risk of getting Crohn's disease as the native population in the area to which they have moved (35). However, this is not applicable to Hindus moving to and living in England (35). Jews born and living outside Israel, especially in central European countries and in northeast America, are more prone to develop Crohn's disease than those born and living in Israel (34). They also have a higher risk than the non-jewish population in these areas (36). Among Arabs living in Israel the disease is more or less unknown (36).

In many studies a distinct difference in the incidence in urban and rural areas is reported, the urban one being higher (7,37,38). There is an age-specific incidence peak in patients 15 to 30 years of age. In some studies a bimodal curve has been demonstrated with a second peak in elderly patients (30,39). In most studies women are slightly more affected than men by the disease. In Iceland, however, there are twice as many males as females (29).

The mortality rate of Crohn's disease is probably not higher than the one expected for different age-matched groups. In a large study of the mortality among 610 patients with Crohn's disease diag-

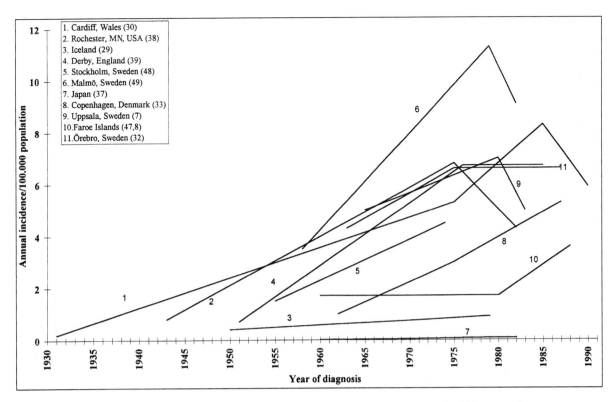

Fig. 2.3. Incidence trend of Crohn's disease in series with a study period of 20 years of more.

nosed in Leicershire during the years 1972 through 1989 the mortality rate did not differ from that of the background population (40). Similar findings are reported from Copenhagen (41). From Leiden (The Netherlands), however, an excess mortality among 670 patients with Crohn's disease diagnosed between 1934 and 1984 was found (42).

Summary

Most studies of both ulcerative colitis and Crohn's disease have shown an increased incidence from the 1950s to the beginning of the 1980s. Thereafter, however, several studies have shown a decrease, a finding supported by clinical observations (Figs. 2.1 and 2.3).

High and low incidence areas have been described, the same for both diseases. Such high incidence areas are northwestern Europe and North America whereas rather low incidence areas are to be found in southern and eastern Europe and Israel. Low incidence areas are probably Africa, Asia, and South America but very few studies or only studies with a low number of patients have so far been presented.

In many studies the male to female ratio has been reported to have changed to a male predominance. The earlier high mortality in patients with IBD is today eliminated.

It is uncertain whether indeterminate colitis is a condition of its own. A subclassification of IBD with indeterminate colitis as a special group might avoid misclassification and might also be used as a therapeutic guideline (19).

The different incidence figures in Figures 2.1 and 2.3 even from places that are geographically close probably only mirror the problems in IBD epidemiological studies summed up in Table 2.1. These problems and the different criteria used in at least studies concerning ulcerative colitis, make comparisons uncertain or even impossible. The most important information is probably to be found in trend analysis of well defined studies extending over long periods of time.

References

1. Roht LH, Selwyn BJ, Holguin AH Jr, et al. Principles of epidemiology. A self-teaching guide. New York: Academic Press.

2. Evans JG, Acheson ED. An epidemiological study of ulcerative colitis and regional enteritis in the Oxford area. Gut 1965;6:311–24.

3. Mendeloff AI, Calkins BM. The epidemiology of idiopathic inflammatory bowel disease. Inflammatory Bowel Disease 3rd ed. 1988:3–34.

4. Srivastava ED, Mayberry JF, Morris TJ, et al. Inci-

dence of ulcerative colitis in Cardiff over 20 years: 1968–1987. Gut 1992;33:256–8.

5. Langholz E, Munkholm P, Haager Nielsen H, et al. Incidence and prevalence of ulcerative colitis in Copenhagen county from 1962 to 1987. Scand J Gastroenterol 1991;26:1247–56.

6. Tysk C, Järnerot G. Ulcerative proctocolitis in Örebro, Sweden. A retrospective epidemiologic study, 1963–1987. Scand J Gastroenterol 1992;27:945–50.

7. Ekbom A, Helmick C, Zack M, et al. The epidemiology of inflammatory bowel disease: a large, population-based study in Sweden. Gastroenterology 1991;100:350–8.

8. Róin F, Róin J. Inflammatory bowel disease of the Faroe Islands, 1981–1988. Scand J Gastroenterology 1989;24(suppl 170):44–6.

9. Tsianos EV, Masalas CN, Merkouropoulos M, et al. Incidence of inflammatory bowel disease in northwest Greece: rarity of Crohn's disease in an area where ulcerative colitis is common. Gut 1994;35:369–72.

10. Tragnone A, Hanau C, Bazzocchi G, et al. Epidemiological characteristics of inflammatory bowel disease in Bologna, Italy—Incidence and risk factors. Dig 1993;54:183–8.

11. Sonnenberg A, Wasserman IH. Epidemiology of inflammatory bowel disease among U.S. military veterans. Gastroenterology 1991;101:122–30.

12. Stewénius J, Adnerhill I, Ekelund G, et al. Ulcerative colitis and indeterminate colitis in the city of Malmö, Sweden, 1958 to 1982. A 25-year incidence study. Scand J Gastroenterol 1995;30:38–43

13. Gower-Rousseau C, Salomez J-L, Dupas J-L, et al. Incidence of inflammatory bowel disease in northern France (1988–1990). Gut 1994;35:1433–8.

14. Calkins BM, Lilienfeld AM, Garland CF, et al. Trends in incidence rates of ulcerative colitis and Crohn's disease. Dig Dis Sci 1984;29:913–20.

15. Calkins BM, Mendeloff AI. Epidemiology of inflammatory bowel disease. Epidemiol Rev 1986;8:60–91.

16. Probert CSJ, Jayanthi V, Pinder D, et al. Epidemiological study of ulcerative proctocolitis in Indian migrant and the indigenous population of Leicestershire. Gut 1992;33:687–93.

17. Stonnington CM, Phillips SF, Melton LJ III, et al. Chronic ulcerative colitis: incidence and prevalence in a community. Gut 1987;28:402–9.

18. Probert CSJ, Jayanthi V, Wicks AC, et al. Mortality in patients with ulcerative colitis in Leicestershire. Dig Dis Sci 1993;38:538–41.

19. Price AB. Overlap in the spectrum of non-specific inflammatory bowel disease—"colitis indeterminate." J Clin Path 1978;31:567–77.

20. Wells AD, McMillan I, Price AB, et al. Natural history of indeterminate colitis. Br J Surg 1991;78:179–81.

21. Margulis AR, Goldberg HI, Lawson TL, et al. The overlapping spectrum of ulcerative and granu-

lomatous colitis: a roentgenographic-pathologic study. Am J Roentgenol Radiat Therapy Nucl Med 1971;113:325–34.

22. Martínez-Salmeron JF, Rodrigo M, de Teresa J, et al. Epidemiology of inflammatory bowel disease in the province of Granada, Spain: a retrospective study from 1979 to 1988. Gut 1993;34:1207–9.

23. Hildebrand H, Fredrikzon B, Holmquist L, et al. Chronic inflammatory bowel disease in children and adolescents in Sweden. J Ped Gastroenterol Nutr 1991;13:293–7.

24. Vucelic B, Korac B, Sentic M, et al. Epidemiology of Crohn's disease in Zagreb, Yugoslavia: a ten-year prospective study. Int J Epiderm 1991;20:216–20.

25. Maté-Jimenez J, Munoz S, Vicent D, et al. Incidence and prevalence of ulcerative colitis and Crohn's disease in urban and rural areas of Spain from 1981 to 1988. J Clin Gastroenterol 1994;18(1):27–31.

26. Anseline PF. Crohn's disease in the Hunter Valley region of Australia. Aust NZ J Surg 1995;65(8):564–9.

27. Novis BH, Marks IN, Bank S, et al. Incidence of Crohn's disease at Groote Schuw Hospital during 1970–1974. S Afr Med J 1975;49:693–7.

28. Wright JP, Marks IN, Jameson C, et al. The Cape Town experience of CD. In: Lee ECG, ed. Crohn's Workshop. London: Heyden 1981:95–100.

29. Björnsson S. Inflammatory bowel disease in Iceland during a 30-year period, 1950–1979. Scand J Gastroenterrol 1989;24(suppl 170):47–9.

30. Rose JDR, Roberts GM, Williams G, et al. Cardiff Crohn's disease jubilee: the incidence over 50 years. Gut 1988;29:346–51.

31. Thomas GA, Millar-Jones D, Rhodes J, et al. Incidence of Crohn's disease in Cardiff over 60 years: 1968–1990 an update. Eur J Gastroenterol Hepatol 1995;7(5):401–5.

32. Lindberg E, Jarnerot G. The incidence of Crohn's disease is not decreasing in Sweden. Scand J Gastroenterol 1991;26:495–500.

33. Munkholm P, Langholz E, Nielsen OH, et al. Incidence and prevalence of Crohn's disease in the county of Copenhagen, 1962–1987: a sixfold increase in incidence. Scand J Gastroenterology 1992;27:609–14.

34. Odes HS, Fraser D, Hollander L. Epidemiological data of Crohn's disease in Israel: etiological implications. Public Health Reviews 1989/90;17:321–35.

35. Jayanthi V, Probert CS, Pinder D, et al. Epidemiology of Crohn's disease in indian migrants and the indigenous population in Leicestershire. Q J Med 1992;82(298):125–38.

36. Odes HS, Fraser D, Krugliak P, et al. Inflammatory bowel disease in the bedouin Arabs of southern Israel: rarity of diagnosis and clinical features. Gut 1991;32:1024–6.

37. Yoshida Y, Murata Y. Inflammatory bowel disease in Japan: studies of epidemiology and etiopathogenesis. Med Clin North Am 1990;74:67–90.

38. Gollop JH, Phillips SF, Melton LJ, et al. Epidemiologic aspects of Crohn's disease: a population based study in Olmsted County, Minnesota, 1943–1982. Gut 1988;29:49–56.

39. Fellows IW, Freeman JG, Holmes GTK. Crohn's disease in the city of Derby, 1951–1985. Gut 1990; 31:1262–65.

40. Probert CSJ, Jayanthi V, Wicks ACB, et al. Mortality from Crohn's disease in Leicestershire 1972–1989: an epidemiological community based study. Gut 1992;33:1226–8.

41. Munkholm P, Langholz E, Davidsen M, et al. Intestinal cancer risk and mortality in patients with Crohn's disease. Gastroenterology 1993;105:1716–23.

42. Weterman IT, Biemond I, Pena AS. Mortality and causes of death in Crohn's disease. Review of 50 years' experience in Leiden University Hospital. Gut 1990;31:1387–90.

43. Sedlack RE, Nobrega FT, Kurland LT, et al. Inflammatory colon disease in Rochester, Minnesota, 1935–1964. Gastroenterology 1972;62:935–41.

44. Samuelsson S-M. Ulcerative colitis in the county of Uppsala. Clinical, epidemiological and sociomedical aspects (thesis). University of Uppsala, Sweden, 1976. ISBN 91–554–0421–9.

45. Nordenvall B, Broström O, Berglund M, et al. Incidence of ulcerative colitis in Stockholm county 1955–1979. Scand J Gastroenterol 1985;20:783–90.

46. Odes HS, Fraser D, Krawiec J. Ulcerative colitis in the Jewish population of southern Israel 1961–1985: epidemiological and clinical study. Gut 1987;28:1630–6.

47. Berner J, Klaer T. Ulcerative colitis and Crohn's disease on the Faroe Islands 1964–1983. Scand J Gastroenterol 1986;21:188–92.

48. Hellers. Crohn's disease in Stockholm County, 1955–1974. Acta Chir Scand 1979;490(suppl):1–84.

49. Brahme F, Lindstrom C, Wenckert A. Crohn's disease in a defined population. An epidemiological study of incidence, prevalence, mortality and secular trends in the city of Malmo, Sweden. Gastroenterology 1975;69:342–51.

50. Devlin HB, Datta D, Dellipiani AW. The incidence and prevalence of inflammatory bowel disease in North Tees health district. World J Surg 1980;4:183–93.

51. Sinclair TS, Brunt PW, Mowat NAG. Nonspecific proctocolitis in northeastern Scotland: a community study. Gastroenterology 1983;85:1–11.

52. Shivananda S, Peña AS, Mayberry JF, et al. Epidemiology of proctocolitis in the region of Leiden, the Netherlands. A population study from 1979 to 1983. Scand J Gastroenterol 1987;22:993–1002.

3 Pathogenesis

Jeffrey A. Katz and Claudio Fiocchi

Despite intensive investigation over the past several decades, the cause and mechanism of inflammatory bowel disease (IBD) remain unknown. The pathogenesis of IBD is certainly more complex than a simple single cause-and-effect relationship, and probably results from the interaction of predisposing genetic factors, exogenous and endogenous triggers, and host modifying factors (1–3). The outcome of these multiple interactions is the chronic remitting and relapsing inflammatory process recognized clinically as ulcerative colitis or Crohn's disease. Although we, as yet, do not fully understand the intimate mechanisms of the complicated host-environment relationship which result in IBD, research in the areas of genetics, intestinal microbiology and ecology, immunology, and experimental animal models have greatly increased our understanding of the individual components of the disease process and how they may interrelate. This chapter will synthetically review the state-of-the-art knowledge on the possible causes and mechanisms of ulcerative colitis and Crohn's disease.

Genetics

Though clearly not governed by simple Mendelian genetics, there is ample evidence that Crohn's disease and ulcerative colitis are in part the result of genetic predisposition. Several lines of evidence support this concept, including familial aggregation, ethnic differences in disease prevalence, genetic syndromes associated with IBD, and linkage of genetic markers with IBD. It is reasonable to assume that there are specific genes that put a person at risk for the potential development of IBD,

and indeed, a few candidate genes have been identified. Some have suggested that as many as 10 to 15 genes may be involved in the pathogenesis of IBD (4). Alternatively, others have hypothesized that IBD is a genetically heterogeneous disease, and that various individual genes are associated with distinct clinical subsets of IBD (5). Regardless of whether one or several genes are involved in the pathogenesis of IBD, acknowledging the importance of a genetic risk holds the promise that one day culprit genes can be identified. This, in turn, should allow the identification of persons at risk and permit the development of possible preventive approaches.

Familial Aggregation

Familial aggregation of IBD is common, though the inheritance patterns fit no simple Mendelian systems (5). There is an approximately ten-fold increase in the prevalence of IBD among siblings compared to the general population (6). Between 10% to 20% of IBD patients report a positive family history of IBD (6–8). In general, ulcerative colitis is increased among relatives with ulcerative colitis and Crohn's disease is increased among relatives with Crohn's disease (9,10). However, the two illnesses may exist in the same family at a frequency higher than expected by chance alone, suggesting that Crohn's disease and ulcerative colitis are etiologically related. In patients with a family history of IBD, the disease onset appears to be earlier. Several studies have shown that a positive family history is more common in Crohn's disease, and that the relatives of Crohn's disease patients have a greater likelihood of having IBD than the relatives of ulcerative colitis patients (5). This suggests that there may be a stronger component of genetic predisposition for Crohn's disease than for ulcerative colitis.

Several recent studies have looked closely to determine whether a family history of IBD correlates with age of onset of disease, site of initial disease, type of disease (i.e., inflammatory, stricturing, or perforating), or course of the disease (11–15). Up to 86% of families were concordant for the site of Crohn's disease, and 82% were concordant for the clinical type (12,15). Younger age at diagnosis was associated with a family history of IBD, and predicted a more complicated course in some studies, (11,14), but not others (13). Intriguingly, there appeared to be a trend towards symptomatic disease at progressively younger ages in successive generations (12,13).

The concordance rate for IBD among monozygotic twins is greater than the concordance rate among dizygotic twins (16). Because monozygotic twins share 100% and dizygotic twins only 50% of their genes, the higher concordance rate for monozygotic twins supports the argument that genetic factors are important for the development of IBD. Nevertheless, the concordance rate for monozygotic twins is not 100% and nongenetic factors are probably operating to reduce penetrance of the IBD phenotype. The concordance rate among both monozygotic and dizygotic twins with Crohn's disease is greater than in twins with ulcerative colitis (5). This finding mirrors the results of family studies, and supports the concept that heredity may play a greater role in Crohn's disease than in ulcerative colitis.

Ethnicity

The incidence of IBD is highest among whites, lower in blacks, and lowest in Asians (5). For Caucasians, an increase in the frequency of IBD has been consistently observed among people of Jewish descent, and is estimated to be three to four times higher than for non-Jews (10,17). Importantly, this increase has been reported from multiple observations, in several different countries, and in various time periods, strongly suggesting that this is a true ethnic phenomenon and not an environmentally conditioned one. Even the incidence of IBD varies between the different historical subpopulations of the Jewish religion. Studies from Israel show that the prevalence of IBD is greater among the Ashkenazi Jews of European descent than among the Sephardic Jews of North African and Asian origin (17,18).

Genetic Syndromes Associated with IBD

A number of well defined genetic syndromes are clearly associated with IBD, lending further support to the concept of a strong genetic background for ulcerative colitis and Crohn's disease. The three syndromes most closely linked to the development of IBD are Turner's syndrome (19,20), Hermansky-Pudlak syndrome (21,22), and glycogen storage disease type Ib (23). In addition, IBD has been reported in individuals and families with various inherited immunodeficiencies (5). Although none of these illnesses precisely mimics Crohn's disease or ulcerative colitis, the association of rare immunodeficiencies, congenital syndromes and IBD suggests that genetic studies of shared immune pathways may help to understand IBD immunopathogenesis.

Genetic Markers

The complex genetics of IBD, involving incomplete penetrance and genetic heterogeneity, make identification of candidate genes difficult. The availability of subclinical markers to distinguish clinically unaffected individuals with a susceptibility genotype, and markers to stratify IBD into genetically more homogeneous subsets would greatly simplify the search for IBD-predisposing genes. Among the most interesting studies of subclinical markers reported are those of perinuclear antineutrophil cytoplasmic antibodies (p-ANCA) and intestinal permeability. p-ANCA is a highly specific and moderately sensitive marker of ulcerative colitis when compared to other forms of colitis (24,25), and it can be present in up to 85% of patients with sclerosing cholangitis (26). p-ANCA has been proposed as a marker of genetic heterogeneity in ulcerative colitis. In a study from Los Angeles, California, and Calgary, Alberta, p-ANCA was found more frequently in relatives of patients with ulcerative colitis than in the relatives of healthy controls (27). More specifically, p-ANCA was identified in 21.4% of healthy relatives of p-ANCA positive ulcerative colitis patients, but in only 7% in p-ANCA negative ulcerative colitis patients (27). Other studies from Germany, England, and France, however, have found no significant increase in p-ANCA frequency among the healthy relatives of subjects with ulcerative colitis (28–30). Although found in some patients with colonic Crohn's disease, the existence of p-ANCA is not significantly more common in Crohn's disease than in other colitides. Thus, the actual role of p-ANCA as a potential marker of genetic heterogeneity in IBD remains to be clarified.

Increased intestinal permeability is another potential subclinical marker of genetic susceptibility to IBD that has received considerable attention. Several studies have shown that intestinal permeability is greater in patients with Crohn's disease than in patients with ulcerative colitis or normal controls (31–34). Unexpectedly, however, Hollander and colleagues found increased intestinal permeability in a number of healthy relatives of patients with Crohn's disease, suggesting that the absorptive defect might be primary and perhaps genetically determined (33). Other studies have yielded conflicting results (35,36), but analysis of the available data suggests that a small percent of the healthy relatives of patients with Crohn's disease does have an increase in intestinal permeability (37). This may be a marker of low-level, subclinical intestinal inflammation and identify a population of genetically similar individuals at risk for Crohn's disease.

Candidate Genes

Human Leukocyte Antigen (HLA) Associations

Given the central role of the immune system in the pathogenesis of IBD, most of the genetic marker studies in IBD have focused on genes involved in the development and regulation of immune function. Many studies have examined the association between IBD and HLA class I and II alleles (for complete review see reference 5). The results from these studies have been largely inconclusive, but some interesting points emerge from review of the existing knowledge. HLA class I association studies have shown a consistent increased frequency of HLA-B5 or HLA-B52 in Japanese patients with ulcerative colitis (38). Several HLA class II association studies document a relationship between HLA-DR2 and ulcerative colitis in the Japanese population (38–40). In contrast, the investigation of HLA class II associations in non-Japanese subjects with ulcerative colitis yields conflicting results. Some studies show a significant increase in HLA-DR2 in ulcerative colitis (41), whereas others do not (42). However, the HLA-DRB1*1502 allele, which is responsible for the association between HLA-DR2 and Japanese ulcerative colitis but is rare in whites in the United States, has been found in a few ulcerative colitis patients, but none of the controls, in a recent study from the United States (42). Though the data remain conflicted, there does appear to be a real association between HLA-DR2 and at least a subset of patients with ulcerative colitis.

Fewer data are available on Crohn's disease and HLA associations. Several HLA class I association studies have shown a significantly increased frequency of HLA-B44 in CD (43,44). HLA class II associations have been found for HLA-DR7 (44,45), HLA-DR4 (46,47), and the combination of HLA-DR1 and HLA-DQB1*0501 (41).

Cytokine Genes

Genes outside the HLA system have recently come under scrutiny in the search for IBD genes. A number of investigators have looked for mutations or genetic polymorphisms in cytokine genes. Considering the intestinal inflammation observed in some cytokine knock-out models of IBD (see Cytokines below), the central role of cytokines in modulating intestinal inflammation, and the clinical benefit derived from anti-cytokine therapy, it is logical to investigate genetic variation in cytokine genes. The interleukin-1 (IL-1) receptor antagonist (IL-1ra) is a naturally occurring inhibitor of IL-1. An insufficient production of IL-1ra to counterbalance the well known increased IL-1 production in IBD has been suggested to lead to inadequate anti-inflammatory activity (48,49). Several recent studies have shown that allele 2 of the IL-1ra gene is associated with ulcerative colitis (50,51). Other investigators have looked at the tumor necrosis factor-α (TNF-α) gene. Plevy and colleagues have shown a strong association between a specific TNF microsatellite haplotype and Crohn's disease (52). Interestingly, the specific TNF microsatellite haplotype was associated with HLA DR1/DQ5, one of the HLA loci found more frequently in some patients with Crohn's disease.

Other Genes

Ultimately, the most direct approach to the identification of the IBD susceptibility genes is to collect large family kindreds with several affected individuals and perform a genome-wide search for susceptibility loci. A French group recently performed a genome-wide search in 53 Caucasian families with at least two members affected with Crohn's disease and reported a susceptibility locus on chromosome 16. Within this region of chromosome 16 are genes involved in cell adhesion (CD11 integrin cluster, CD19, sialophorin), as well as the interleukin-4 (IL-4) receptor (53). Further investigation of this genetic site might lead to new clues on the pathogenesis of Crohn's disease.

Intestinal Microbiology and Ecology

Only a single layer of epithelial cells separates the intestinal mucosa, rich in immunologically responsive cells, from the massive antigenic challenge of the intestinal lumen. Thus, it is little wonder that, ever since the recognition of ulcerative colitis and Crohn's disease as distinct disease entities, investigators have searched the luminal contents for etiologic factors. Clinical observations, such as the improvement of Crohn's disease with fecal diversion (54), elemental diets (55), and anti-bacterial agents (56), as well as laboratory observations, such as amelioration of gut inflammation in the IL-10 "knock-out" mice kept in specific pathogen-free conditions (57), highlight the key importance of the intestinal milieu in IBD pathogenesis. Despite acknowledging this, we are far from fully understanding the complex world of the intestinal microenvironment, and how it may impact on the initiation or perpetuation of intestinal inflammation. This section will review the potential roles of microorganisms and their products, dietary factors, and intestinal defenses in the pathogenesis of ulcerative colitis and Crohn's disease.

Infectious Agents

Bacteria

The list of bacteria, viruses, and fungi implicated as potential etiologic agents for IBD is astonishingly long (Table 3.1). Given the volume and variety of bacteria in the intestinal lumen it is not surprising that researchers have long searched for a bacterial etiology for Crohn's disease and ulcerative colitis. Although no single microorganism has been identified, several abnormalities of the enteric flora have been documented. Cultures of obligate anaerobic flora have demonstrated greater numbers of gram-positive coccoid rods and gram-negative rods in patients with Crohn's disease compared to healthy controls (58). Although cultures from ulcerative colitis patients have found fecal flora similar to that of control subjects, *Escherichia coli* isolated from ulcerative colitis show substantially greater adherence to colonocytes than similar organisms isolated from control subjects (59). No single unique bacterial pathogen has been isolated from either Crohn's disease or ulcerative colitis intestines, but mucosal cultures have identified unusual cell wall-deficient bacterial L-forms in some patients with IBD (60–62). Revertants to parental forms have revealed *Pseudomonas*-like species, *E. coli*, and *Staphlococcus faecalis*. Although IBD patients have increased serum antibody titers to a wide array of bacterial pathogens (63), this is likely secondary to an inflamed or damaged epithelium, rather than being of primary pathogenic importance. Even though no specific bacterial pathogen

Table 3.1. Bacteria, viruses, and fungi investigated in the etiology of inflammatory bowel disease.

Bacteroides	Listeria
Brucella	Measles virus
Citrobacter	Mycobacterium avium
Coprococcus	Mycobacterium kansasii
Candida albicans	Mycobacterium paratuberculosis
C. Colinum	Paramyxovirus
Campylobacter fetus	Peptostreptococcus
C. jejuni	Pseudomonas sp
C. Sputorum	Rotavirus
Chlamydia psittaci	Saccharomyces cerevisiae
C. trachomatis	Streptococcus faecalis
Eubacterium	Yersinia enterocolitica
Escherichia coli	Y. paratuberculosis

has been identified in either Crohn's disease or ulcerative colitis, it is worth remembering that until the discovery of *Helicobacter pylori* ulcer disease was not felt to have an infectious cause.

Mycobacteria

In 1913, Dalziel commented on the pathologic similarity between Crohn's disease and Johne's disease, a chronic mycobacterial enteritis of ruminants due to infection with *Mycobacterium paratuberculosis* (64). Seventy years later Chiodini and colleagues cultured *M. paratuberculosis* from a few patients with Crohn's disease (65,66). The growth conditions of this organism are very fastidious, and most laboratories have had very limited success in attempting to culture *M. paratuberculosis* from Crohn's disease tissue (67,68). In the past few years, sophisticated molecular biology techniques have been used to try to more closely link *M. paratuberculosis* to Crohn's disease. A specific mycobacterial DNA insertion sequence, IS900, found in multiple copies of the genome of *M. paratuberculosis,* has been cloned and used in highly sensitive polymerase chain reactions to probe Crohn's disease intestinal specimens (69). IS900 has been found in as many as 65% of Crohn's disease specimens (70) and as few as 3% (71). Whether *M. paratuberculosis* is a real etiologic agent in a small subset of patients with Crohn's disease or simply represents an irrelevant organism remains uncertain. Attempts to treat Crohn's disease patients with antimycobacterial therapy has been generally unrewarding (72–74).

Viruses

There is epidemiological evidence showing that perinatal viral infections are a risk factor for the future development of IBD (75). However, although transmissible agents suggestive of a RNA virus were identified in Crohn's disease patients in the 1970s (76–78), a definite viral cause for Crohn's disease has yet to be identified. Increased serum antibody titers to cytomegalovirus have been detected in ulcerative colitis patients, but this is considered a phenomenon secondary to mucosal inflammation (79).

Recently, Wakefield and colleagues have published a series of reports arguing that Crohn's disease may be due to a latent measles virus (paramyxovirus) infection (80,81). These authors first proposed that Crohn's disease was the result of multifocal gastrointestinal infarctions caused by chronic mesenteric vasculitis (82). In a series of elegant anatomic and histologic investigations, they gathered evidence of a microvascular vasculitis based on careful microinjection studies using surgical specimens (82,83). Electron micrograph studies of these lesions then identified viral-like inclusions resembling paramyxoviruses (80). Subsequent immunohistochemical staining and *in situ* hybridization for measles virus lended support to this conclusion. Some epidemiologic data also support the association of Crohn's disease and measles virus infection (84). This hypothesis of Wakefield and colleagues is certainly provocative, but additional work by other independent investigators must be performed to prove or disprove such a hypothesis.

Yeasts

Although a classical fungal infection has never been considered a primary etiologic possibility, it has recently been proposed that *Saccharomyces cerevisiae* (baker's and brewer's yeast) may be important in Crohn's disease (85,86). On the basis of an increased peripheral lymphocyte response to *S. cerevisiae* in Crohn's disease patients, yeast cell-wall material may selectively activate the local and systemic immune system. Others have suggested that this immune response is characteristic of, but not specific for Crohn's disease, as it has also been found in celiac disease (87).

Bacterial Products

Although few convincing data exist that any one particular microorganism causes ulcerative colitis or Crohn's disease, there is increasing evidence that the bacterial flora as a whole as well as its products play an important role in the pathogenesis of IBD. This theory has been recently bolstered by reports of several experimental models of IBD, in which animals kept in specific pathogen-free or germ-free environment develop little or no intestinal inflammation (57,88,89). Various products of

bacterial cell wall origin can reproduce the histological and immunological inflammatory responses caused by the intact organism. These products include peptidoglycan-polysaccharide complex (PG-PS), lipopolysaccharide (LPS), N-formylmethionyl-leucyl-phenylalanine (FMLP), and muramyl peptides (90). These bacterial products can activate macrophages to release cytokines, induce cell adhesion molecule expression, modulate T- and B-cell responses, and trigger the kinin and complement cascades (91). Therefore, these combined actions could potentially explain many of the pathophysiologic processes ongoing in IBD.

Mucus

The mucus layer covering the intestinal epithelium is the first line of defense for the host against the immunologic challenge of luminal dietary and bacterial antigens. Occupying such a strategic location, it has been hypothesized that some abnormality in mucin composition may contribute to the pathogenesis of IBD. This concept has been most intensively studied in ulcerative colitis, and early studies suggested depletion of specific mucin subclasses (92). Subsequent analyses, however, failed to identify differences between the mucin composition of ulcerative colitis, Crohn's disease, and normal controls (93). No specific defect in mucin composition may be present in IBD, but altered lectin binding has been documented in both ulcerative colitis and Crohn's disease, indicating that the attachment of bacteria and other substances to epithelial cells may be altered in IBD (94). This could represent a breakdown in mucosal defenses relevant to the pathophysiology of IBD, but more likely represents a secondary nonspecific phenomenon.

Dietary Factors

Since IBD is an inflammatory condition affecting the whole digestive system, it is logical to consider diet as a possible etiologic factor. Dietary antigens represent the major nonbacterial, non-self antigens present in the gut. The existence of antibodies to dietary wheat, corn, and milk protein have been well documented in both ulcerative colitis and Crohn's disease (95,96). Epidemiological studies have evaluated refined sugar (97), fruit and vegetable consumption (98), and coffee and alcohol intake (99) as possible etiologic determinants of IBD. At present no particular dietary product has been convincingly shown to be closely linked to the development or IBD, nevertheless, evidence from clinical trials clearly still suggests a role for food-derived components in perpetuating inflammation. Dietary manipulations including total parenteral nutrition (100), elimination diets (101), elemental diets (55), and polymeric diets (102) have all been shown to help improve symptoms in patients with ulcerative colitis and Crohn's disease. However, it remains unclear how these various dietary manipulations act to improve disease activity. Some investigators argue that the low fat content of these diets reduce the availability of precursors for arachidonate derived eicosanoid synthesis (103). Others believe these dietary manipulations decrease the antigenic burden on an already injured gut. Finally, it is possible that these specialized diets provide some missing key nutrient necessary to heal the damaged intestine. Given the benefit of the above diets in symptomatic improvement and the success of more refined and subtle manipulations, such as the administration of ω-3 fatty acids in Crohn's disease (104), it is likely that continued investigation will focus on the role of food antigens in the pathogenesis of IBD.

Results of recent investigations have helped sustain a steady interest in the role of diet in IBD, particularly after the identification of glutamine as the primary fuel for the enterocyte (105), and short chain fatty acids (SCFA) as the preferred energy source of the colonocyte (106). There is some evidence indicating that ulcerative colitis patients are deficient in SCFA (107) and treatment of distal ulcerative colitis with SCFA enemas improves inflammation (106). Furthermore, both pouchitis and diversion colitis appear to be, at least in part, due to a deficiency of SCFA as both may improve with SCFA supplementation (108,109). Glutamine can also be helpful in pouchitis (109,110). Whether these observations represent a primary etiologic defect, or are secondary to chronic inflammation is uncertain, but the use of specific supplements will likely continue to be an area of active investigation.

Immune Factors

Alterations of the immune system are frequently involved in diseases manifested by chronic inflammation. This is certainly the case for IBD where overwhelming evidence points to immune abnormalities as an intrinsic component of the mechanism of inflammation and tissue injury. An in depth review of all the immunologic factors potentially implicated in the pathogenesis of IBD is beyond the scope of this chapter and the interested reader can take advantage of several reviews on the subject (3,111,112). This section will discuss selected humoral, cellular, and other immune components potentially important to IBD.

Humoral Immunity

Serum Antibodies

Early evidence that IBD could be an immune-mediated process came from the demonstration of serum antibodies against colonic epithelial cells in patients with ulcerative colitis (113). Later work showed that such antibodies cross react with *E. coli*, suggesting that sensitization to a common bacteria could result in autoreactivity leading to gut injury (114). More studies have uncovered a number of different antibodies that may play a role in the pathogenesis of IBD. Circulating antibodies to *E. coli* and a number of other bacterial pathogens have been found in both ulcerative colitis and Crohn's disease (63,115). Antibodies to cow's milk protein have been described in IBD patients (116), as have lymphocytotoxic antibodies (117). However, most of these studies have been unable to show a specific correlation between the level or type of antibodies and specific clinical disease activity. Thus, the presence of these antibodies likely represents an epiphenomenon of inflammation rather than a primary pathogenic event.

Intestinal Antibodies

The presence of circulating antibodies in IBD is interesting, but the identification of abnormalities in mucosal antibodies is potentially more pathogenetically important. Several investigators have reported abnormalities of antibody production by mucosal plasma cells. Alterations of IgA, IgG, and IgM have been reported in both ulcerative colitis and Crohn's disease, and a specific increase in IgG1 is found in ulcerative colitis (118–120). One group has been able to purify a specific IgG antibody from ulcerative colitis mucosa (121). This antibody recognizes a 40 kD peptide shared by cells in the colon, bile ducts, skin, joints, and eyes (122–124). The 40 kD protein has been tentatively characterized as a cytoskeletal protein member of the tropomyosin family (125). Most patients with ulcerative colitis have antibodies against this protein which are localized on epithelial cells (126), and spontaneous production of tropomyosin IgG and IgG1 antibodies by lamina propria mononuclear cells has been recently reported (127). Thus, this series of investigations have characterized a potential autoantigen in ulcerative colitis, identified a consistent antibody response to it, and localized the antigenic epitope(s) to precisely the tissues most commonly involved in this disease.

Such studies are arguments in favor of an autoimmune pathogenesis for IBD. However, other investigators have been unable to detect autoantibodies in the mucosa of patients with IBD (128), and the existence of true autoimmunity in patients with ulcerative colitis and Crohn's disease remains unresolved.

Cell-Mediated Immunity

Extensive investigation over several decades supports the concept that some abnormality of cell-mediated immunity is present in patients with IBD, though the data remain contradictory (129–133). None of these studies, however, has provided direct evidence of a primary T-cell defect, and all systemic abnormalities of immune cell function in Crohn's disease and ulcerative colitis must presently be considered secondary to the underlying inflammatory disease process.

In contrast to circulating immune cells, there are subtle, but reproducible, abnormalities in immune cells at the level of the intestinal mucosa in IBD. Normally, intraepithelial T-cells are CD8-positive (suppressor/cytotoxic), whereas most lamina propria T-cells are CD4-positive (helper/inducer). Both epithelial and lamina propria T-cells preferentially express the αβ T-cell receptor (TCRαβ), whereas cells expressing the γδ T-cell receptor (TCR γδ) are less common. In IBD, the distribution of CD4- and CD8-positive T-cells is maintained (134), but there is an overall decrease in the number of TCRγδ cells (135). Additionally, there is a selective change in the TCR Vβ chain utilization of CD4- but not CD8-positive lymphocytes in Crohn's disease (136). The significance of these subtle changes in the mucosal T-cell repertoire remains to be determined.

Compared to the peripheral blood, mucosal immune cells are an activated cell population (137). In IBD lamina propria mononuclear cells display increased expression of lymphocyte activation antigens and immune activation gene products (138,139). Interestingly, there appears to be a differential response to activating stimuli between lamina propria mononuclear cells from patients with Crohn's disease compared to ulcerative colitis. In an assay measuring lymphokine activated killer cell activity, mononuclear cells from the mucosa of patients with Crohn's disease show enhanced cytotoxicity, whereas cells from the mucosa of patients with ulcerative colitis become less cytotoxic when stimulated with equal amounts of IL-2 (140). In summary, the immune function of mucosal immune cells is altered in IBD, and different between

Crohn's disease and ulcerative colitis: in Crohn's disease T-cell dependent functions are normal or increased, whereas in ulcerative colitis they are suppressed.

Nonimmune Cells: Epithelial Cells, Endothelial Cells, Mesenchymal Cells

It is being increasingly recognized that a variety of "nonimmune" cells in intestinal mucosa can function as antigen presenting cells, serve accessory cell functions, secrete and respond to cytokines and perform a variety of other functions previously thought to be exclusive for T-cells, B-cells, and monocytes/macrophages. Human epithelial cells can express HLA-DR molecules and function as antigen presenting cells (141), respond to typical T-cell cytokines (142), and produce cytokines (143). Evidence suggests that the intestinal epithelial cell immune response may be abnormal in IBD. Although epithelial cells from normal mucosa normally stimulate CD8-positive T-cells, epithelial cells from IBD mucosa preferentially stimulate CD4-positive T-cells (144). This suggests that in the nondiseased intestine epithelial cells may induce or maintain suppressive tolerance, but in the mucosa of patients with IBD these same cells may amplify and perpetuate a state of chronic inflammation. In addition to intestinal epithelial cells, studies show that both endothelial cells and mesenchymal cells may also be important in controlling inflammation in the intestine and may be abnormal in IBD (145–147).

Cytokines

Cytokines are secreted molecules that affect the behavior of neighboring cells. The shear number of cytokines available for study and their multiple and varied actions on immune cells and immunologic function have generated an enormous amount of information on the role of cytokines in IBD. Reviews on the role of cytokines in IBD are available (148), and this section will focus on selected aspects of cytokine biology felt most relevant to the pathogenesis of Crohn's disease and ulcerative colitis. It is important to keep in mind that assessing the relative importance of an individual cytokine measurement in IBD depends critically on the patient population (Crohn's disease vs. ulcerative colitis), the source of the specimen (serum vs. mucosal), and the type of assay (protein measurement vs. DNA/RNA measurement). Cytokines can generally be divided into immunoregulatory cytokines and pro-inflammatory cytokines.

Immunoregulatory Cytokines

The immunoregulatory cytokines are the primary products of T-cells and function to modulate the activity of other immune cells. IL-2, IL-4, IL-10, and interferon-γ (IFN-γ) are the main immunoregulatory cytokines. Although the overall status of immunoregulatory cytokines in IBD is not entirely defined, abnormal production of and response to these potent immunologic mediators has been described in Crohn's disease and ulcerative colitis.

IL-2 is central to T-cell function and has been intensely studied in IBD with controversial results. Protein levels of IL-2 by intestinal mononuclear cells have been found to be decreased (149), whereas mRNA levels have been reported to be increased in active Crohn's disease (150). There is also evidence for a differential response of the intestinal mucosa to IL-2 between Crohn's disease and ulcerative colitis. Compared to control cells, the response of Crohn's disease mucosal lymphocytes to IL-2 is enhanced, whereas in ulcerative colitis this response is decreased (140). The finding of elevated serum and intestinal IL-2 receptor, especially in Crohn's disease provides additional evidence of an important role for IL-2 in IBD (151).

Like IL-2, IFN-γ production by lamina propria mononuclear cells appears to be greater in Crohn's disease than in ulcerative colitis or control mucosa (152). Fewer data are available for the other immunoregulatory cytokines, IL-4 and IL-10. IL-4 has potent anti-inflammatory activity, and its mucosal production has been reported to be decreased at both the protein and mRNA levels (153). Additionally, the response of IBD mucosa to the immunomodulatory effects of IL-4 and IL-10 may be impaired (154,155). No differential response to these two cytokines between Crohn's disease and ulcerative colitis has been reported. Recent reports of enterocolitis in IL-10 deficient mice (57) and clinical improvement in Crohn's disease activity in patients treated with intravenous IL-10 (156) argue that a deficiency of this potent immunomodulatory molecule may be relevant to the pathogenesis of IBD.

Proinflammatory Cytokines

The proinflammatory cytokines IL-1, IL-6, IL-8, and TNF-α are primarily the products of monocytes and macrophages. These molecules are central to the pathophysiology of the body's acute inflammatory response. In general, there is a detectable increase in the levels of these inflammatory molecules during active inflammation.

As expected, the production of IL-1 is very much increased in actively involved IBD mucosa (157). However, it may not be the absolute level of this cytokine, but rather the level of its naturally occurring receptor antagonist (IL-1ra) that is important in IBD pathogenesis, since there is a mucosal imbalance between IL-1 and IL-1ra (48). This imbalance may create a relative deficiency of anti-inflammatory activity and contribute to chronic inflammation.

IL-6 is elevated in the circulation of Crohn's disease, but not ulcerative colitis patients (158), and has been suggested as a possible marker of disease activity. Mucosal levels of IL-6 are also elevated (159). A similar situation exists for IL-8 and monocyte chemoattractant protein-1 (MCP-1), potent neutrophil and monocyte chemoattractants respectively, both of which are elevated in IBD (160,161).

TNF-α is a potent proinflammatory cytokine with extensive tissue destructive properties. One would expect constantly elevated TNF-α levels in active IBD, but surprisingly, this cytokine has been inconsistently detected (159). Some studies in children with Crohn's disease, however, do report a correlation between TNF-α levels in the stool and disease activity (162). Reports of marked improvement in refractory Crohn's disease treated TNF-α monoclonal antibodies argue, that, despite difficulties in detection, TNF-α likely plays some role in the intestinal inflammation (163).

Lipid Mediators

In addition to cytokines produced by immune cells, the metabolites of arachidonic acid also mediate intestinal inflammation in IBD. The main products of arachidonic acid metabolism are the prostaglandins and leukotrienes, both of which play a role in inflammatory events including increased vascular permeability, vasodilatation, platelet aggregation, muscle contraction, neutrophil chemotaxis, and electrolyte secretion (164). Studies have shown that the inflamed mucosa in IBD produces increased levels of eicosanoids, with production localized to infiltrating leukocytes and the epithelium (165,166). Although elevation of arachidonic acid metabolites is probably a nonspecific event associated with gut inflammation, there appears to be distinct eicosanoid profiles in ulcerative colitis compared to Crohn's disease. In ulcerative colitis, but not Crohn's disease, prostaglandin E_2 and thromboxane B_2 are greatly elevated (167). Clinical studies have shown that treating Crohn's disease patients with fish oils, which modulate eicosanoid production, may reduce the rate of disease relapse, suggesting that selective down-regulation of some arachidonic acid metabolites may be beneficial to IBD patients (104).

Growth Factors

In addition to cytokines, growth factors, including transforming growth factor (TGF)-α and -β, insulin-like growth factor (IGF), fibroblast growth factor (FGF), and trefoil factor also play a role in mucosal damage in human IBD. These peptides, through actions on intestinal epithelial cells and mucosal mononuclear cells, help maintain intestinal integrity by stimulating epithelial cell proliferation, a process central to wound healing and repair (168). Several experimental models of intestinal injury in IBD exist in which mucosal protection is mediated by growth factors such as keratinocyte growth factor (KGF) (169). Trefoil peptide, FGF, and KGF are all abundantly expressed in IBD tissue (170,171). In IBD tissues, TGF-α and TGF-β have been reported to be differentially expressed, implying a role for TGF-α in epithelial hyperproliferation and for TGF-β in epithelial cell restitution after injury (172). This data point out that, in addition to forces injurious to the intestinal lining, we must also consider the counterbalancing restorative properties of growth factors when investigating the pathophysiology of IBD.

Adhesion Molecules

Adhesion molecules represent a large class of cell surface proteins that allow for attachment and direct communication between cells. The potential importance of adhesion molecules in IBD is considerable, given the complex interactions between immune and non immune cells in the intestinal mucosa. Multiple abnormalities of adhesion molecules have been reported in IBD patients. Increased expression of E-selectin has been observed in actively inflamed mucosa (173), as has the expression of the leukocyte adhesion molecule ICAM-1 by mucosal mononuclear phagocytes (174). The profile of integrin expression has also been found to be distinct between Crohn's disease and ulcerative colitis (175). The importance of these observations is that they represent the cellular and molecular events responsible for the recruitment of circulating leukocytes into the inflamed bowel wall. Understanding these events may allow the development of novel therapies for IBD, as suggested by animal studies showing attenuation of intestinal inflammation by the administration of antibodies to the integrins LFA-1 or VLA-4 (176,177).

Reactive Oxygen and Nitrogen Metabolites

Neutrophil and macrophage infiltration of the intestinal mucosa is a characteristic feature of active IBD. In addition to releasing proteolytic enzymes, these cells produce reactive oxygen metabolites (ROM) and nitrogen oxides (NO), both extremely potent mediators of inflammation. Actively inflamed mucosa of ulcerative colitis and Crohn's disease show an increased production of ROMs (178), and increased NO synthesis in the mucosa of ulcerative colitis, but not Crohn's disease, has been reported (179). Several studies also show that, not only is there an increase in the production of oxidative products in IBD mucosa, but a concomitant decrease in antioxidant defenses may be present as well. In both Crohn's disease and ulcerative colitis the levels of antioxidants such as peroxyl radical scavengers, glutathione, and ubiquinol-10 are significantly diminished (180). It is likely that both increased ROM and NO production and decreased antioxidant defenses are secondary, nonspecific reactions to the presence of intestinal inflammation, rather than primary pathogenetic events. Still, these processes are part of the spectrum of forces damaging the mucosa and interfering in these processes may help improve inflammatory disease activity (181).

Neuropeptides

Many patients with IBD will note a correlation between life stressors and disease activity. Although definitive proof is lacking, there is good evidence that the nervous system influences the immune system (182) and that the nervous, endocrine, and immune systems communicate with one another via neuropeptides, hormones, and cytokines (183). Although anatomic abnormalities of the enteric nervous system have been described in IBD, it is unclear how these alterations effect neuroimmune interactions. Studies have shown a decrease in vasoactive intestinal peptide (VIP) containing nerve fibers in both ulcerative colitis and Crohn's disease closely associated with inflammation (184). By contrast, substance P tends to be elevated in IBD mucosa (185). Although much remains to be learned about the role of neuropeptides in IBD, some preliminary studies using the topical anesthetic lidocaine in ulcerative colitis suggest that neuromodulation may be a future therapeutic option (186).

Table 3.2. Animal models of inflammatory bowel
disease: exogenous induction.

Irritants	Acetic acid
Drugs	Indomethacin
Immunologic	Immune complex/formalin, trinitrobenzene sulfonic acid/ethanol
Infectious	Lymphogranuloma venereum
Bacterial products	Peptidoglycan-polysaccharide complexes
Feeding	Dextran sulfate sodium, carrageenan (poligeenan)
Surgery	Infarction, ileopouchitis

Table 3.3. Animal models of inflammatory bowel
disease: endogenous induction.

Spontaneous	Cotton-top tamarin, C3H/HeJ Bir mouse
Clonal deletion	Cyclosporin A in neonatal mice
Cell reconstitution	CD45RB^{high}, CD4-positive T cells in SCID mice
Transgenic	HLA-B27 rats, dominant negative N-cadherin mutant mice
Gene targeting	IL-2, IL-10, TGF-β, TCRαβ, Gα$_{i2}$, keratin 8 "knock out" mice

Animal Models

The complexity of IBD and the inherent limitations of human studies make it difficult to perform the detailed investigations necessary to understand the intimate mechanisms of inflammation and tissue damage in this disease. Experimental animal models allow study of early initiating events, evaluation of the interactions among different components of the inflammatory response, and analysis of different immunologic factors and genes that determine susceptibility, in ways that are impossible in humans. The study of animal models of IBD helps stimulate new ideas to test in patients; they complement and expand studies in humans, but do not replace them. An ideal animal model would be identical to human IBD, with the same causal factors, pathology, pathophysiology, and clinical findings (187). No such model is available, and for many years only a few rudimentary animal models of IBD were at hand. During the last decade, however, a larger number of animal models have been developed (Tables 3.2 and 3.3), greatly advancing our knowledge of the pathophysiology of bowel inflammation (111,188,189). The most useful models of IBD are easily induced and consistently reproducible, inexpensive, and use animals with a defined genetic background and an immune system comparable to that of humans. It is critical to bear in mind, however, that the appropriateness of an animal model for a given study depends entirely on the experimental question being asked. The details of some of the animal models most relevant to understanding ulcerative colitis and Crohn's disease are discussed below.

Exogenous Induction

Among the exogenously induced animal models several have been widely used. Perhaps the simplest animal model is the acute inflammatory response generated by the luminal instillation of diluted acetic acid (190). The initial contact injury is bland necrosis of the epithelial cells, followed by acute mucosal and submucosal inflammation. This nonspecific acute inflammation can be inhibited through a number of different anti-inflammatory pathways including leukotriene blockade, prostaglandin analogues, phospholipase A$_2$ inhibitors, prevention of neutrophil recruitment, IL-1ra, somatostatin analogues, mast cell stabilizers, and scavengers of reactive oxygen metabolites (111). The secondary inflammatory phase also involves luminal bacterial products and inflammation can be potentiated by luminal PG-PS (191). This model of acute intestinal inflammation can been used in a variety of animals, is easy to reproduce, and cheap. The beneficial therapeutic effect of sulfasalazine and corticosteroids in this model and the profile of inflammatory mediators make this model useful for the study of new therapeutics and the evaluation of the role of luminal factors in the perpetuation of chronic inflammation. However, the nonspecific nature of the initial mucosal injury and lack of chronicity limit its ultimate relevance to human IBD.

Colitis can also be induced in rats and mice by the administration of an enema containing trinitrobenzene sulfonic acid (TNBS) in ethanol (192). There are strong patterns of susceptibility and resistance among different strains of mice (193). TNBS-colitis seems to be a classic delayed-type hypersensitivity reaction to the contact substance. This type of immune response is T-cell mediated, though under the regulation of other immune cells. Researchers can study the immune control of a localized delayed-type hypersensitivity reaction in the intestine and the effect of various therapies on the intestinal inflammation. The variability in response to the TNBS among strains allows for investigation of susceptibility factors and for the definition of genes involved in the inflammatory response. The model is also simple, inexpensive, and reproducible.

Another type of acute colonic inflammation of the mucosal layer can be induced in mice, rats, and hamsters by continuous oral administration of dextran sulfate sodium (DSS) (194,195). By giving DSS in a cyclic fashion, a chronic colitis develops that is characterized by inflammatory cells, patchy distribution, and fissuring ulcers. Dysplastic changes and colonic adenocarcinoma can also develop in the DSS-induced chronic colitis model (196). The development of dysplasia and colon cancer makes this model more relevant to ulcerative colitis, but prominent lymphoid aggregates, fissuring ulcerations, and discontinuous inflammation are reminiscent of Crohn's disease. This model is most useful for studying genetic susceptibility in inbred mice, oral tolerance, drug screening studies, and for understanding mechanisms of dysplasia and carcinoma associated with colonic inflammation.

Sartor and colleagues have developed a fascinating model of spontaneously relapsing acute and chronic granulomatous enterocolitis in rats by injecting purified streptococcal bacterial cell wall products (PG-PS) into the bowel wall of rats (197). Marked strain susceptibility is evident, highlighting the influence of genetic susceptibility to intestinal inflammation: Lewis rats develop a severe systemic illness with enterocolitis, arthritis, hepatitis, anemia, and leukocytosis, whereas Sprague-Dawley rats develop a persistent enterocolitis, but without arthritis or hepatitis (198). Similar to human IBD, the IL-1ra/IL-1 ratio seems to be genetically determined and is lower in the more susceptible species (199). These studies help show that the products of normal bacterial flora can induce granulomatous intestinal inflammation and extraintestinal symptoms in the proper genetically susceptible host, a picture reminiscent of Crohn's disease.

Endogenous Induction

Cotton-top tamarins, nonhuman primates normally living in the tropical forest of Columbia, spontaneously develop a pancolitis when held in captive breeding colonies in temperate climates (200). The colitis in this South American monkey is age-related, flares and relapses spontaneously, responds to therapy with anti-inflammatory medications, and is associated with adenocarcinoma of the colon in older animals (111). Another fascinating feature of this model is that animals in the wild do not develop colitis, raising questions about the psychological or other stress factors of captivity and the pathogenic role of neuroendocrine factors in colitis (201). All of these features make cotton-top tamarins an excellent model of human ulcerative colitis. However, the small number of these animals in captivity, their endangered species classification, and the difficulties of working with them limit their widespread use. Another type of spontaneous colitis has been created by the continuous inbreeding of C3H/HeJ mice (202). These animals are cheaper to obtain and easier to work with than the cotton-top tamarins and work with this new model is under development.

Advances in molecular biology allow the genetic manipulation of animals and have resulted in a number of new animal models of IBD. The joint transfection of the HLA-B27 and β_2-microglobulin molecules in rats induces a generalized inflammation in multiple organs including the small and large bowel (203). This model represents primarily a systemic illness with secondary bowel involvement. Animal models of IBD have also been generated from the specific manipulation of distinctive immune cell subpopulations. Mice mutant for the TCR α, β, and $\beta x\delta$ chains, as well as class II major histocompatibility all develop chronic colitis (204), strongly highlighting the central role of T-cells in the modulation of intestinal inflammation. Still other models have been developed through the selective deletion or inactivation of cytokine genes. Interleukin-2 deficient mice develop a colitis resembling human ulcerative colitis, while IL-10-deficient mice develop a colitis and enterocolitis reminiscent of Crohn's disease (57,89). Other more recent models of experimental inflammation include the $G\alpha_{i2}$- and keratin 8-deficient mice (205,206), and the dominant negative N-cadherin transfected mice (207). All of the above models develop intestinal inflammation despite having diverse and seemingly unrelated genetic alterations, demonstrating how completely different immune and non-immune mechanisms ultimately result in some form of IBD.

Conclusion

The progress achieved in understanding the pathogenesis of IBD during the last decade is unquestionably greater than all previous progress since modern scientific investigation has been applied to the study of Crohn's disease and ulcerative colitis. Precise knowledge of the exact cause and specific mechanisms of gut inflammation continues to escape us, but some recently acquired concepts are clearly fundamental and almost certainly dominant. First, a contribution of immunogenetics to the predisposition, initiation, modulation, and/or perpetuation of IBD is essentially established. How many genes might be involved and the relative balance of genes vs. environment in determining disease variability will be determined by ongoing and future studies. Second, the role of the intestinal milieu, and the enteric flora in particular, appears to have a much more dominant role than previously anticipated. Lack of experimental IBD in germ-free animals, reconstitution experiments with whole or partial flora, and the effect of antibiotics in altering disease severity, all point to the microorganisms normally living in the lumen as major modulators of IBD. This concept might be modified some day by the unexpected isolation of unique infectious agents directly causing Crohn's disease or ulcerative colitis. Third, the mucosal immune system is the central effector of intestinal inflammation and injury. The mechanisms of its abnormal and persistent activation leading to a chronic, tissue damaging response are certainly multiple and complex, but the key controlling steps must be finite; once they are clearly identified, these immune factors will ultimately be subject to pharmacologic control. Finally, the advent of several good and reproducible animal models with defined molecular defects, or induced by known effector cells or controlled environmental changes, has revolutionized the approach to the study of IBD pathogenesis. It is likely that most of the progress in the immediate future will come from detailed studies of such models. Once knowledge from these different areas is integrated, a clear understanding of IBD pathogenesis will emerge. Until then, current clinical and surgical approaches will help in bridging the gap between the present and the future management of patients suffering from IBD.

References

1. Shanahan F. Pathogenesis of ulcerative colitis. Lancet 1993;342:407–11.
2. Fiocchi C. Overview of inflammatory bowel disease pathogenesis. Can J Gastroenterol 1990;4:309–16.
3. Fiocchi C. New concepts of pathogenesis in inflammatory bowel disease. In: Collins SM, Martin F, McLeod RS, Targan SR, Wallace JL, Williams CN, eds. Inflammatory Bowel Disease. Basic Research, Clinical Implications and Trends in Therapy. Lancaster: Kluwer Academic 1994:243–61.
4. McConnell R, Vadheim C. Inflammatory bowel disease. In: King R, Rotter J, Motulsky A, eds. The Genetic Basis of Common Diseases. New York: Oxford University Press, 1992:326–48.
5. Yang H, Rotter J. Genetics of inflammatory bowel disease. In: Targan S, Shanahan F, eds. Inflamma-

tory Bowel Disease: From Bench to Bedside. Baltimore: Williams & Wilkins, 1994:32–64.
6. Orholm M, Munkholm P, Langholz E, et al. Familial occurence of inflammatory bowel disease. N Engl J Med 1991;324:84–8.
7. Singer H, Anderson J, Frischer H, et al. Familial aspects of inflammatory bowel disease. Gastroenterology 1971;61:423–30.
8. Lashner B, Evans A, Kirsner J, et al. Prevalence and incidence of inflammatory bowel disease in family members. Gastroenterology 1986;91:1396–400.
9. Meucci G, Vecchi M, Torgano G, et al. Familial aggregation of inflammatory bowel disease in northern Italy: a multicenter study. Gastroenterology 1992;103:514–9.
10. Yang H, McElree C, Roth M-P, et al. Familial empirical risks for inflammatory bowel disease: differences between Jews and non-Jews. Gut 1993;34:517–24.
11. Polito J, Childs B, Mellits E, et al. Crohn's disease: influence of age at diagnosis on site and clinical type of disease. Gastroenterology 1996;111:580–6.
12. Peeters M, Nevens H, Baert F, et al. Familial aggregation in Crohn's disease: increased age adjusted risk and concordance in clinical characteristics. Gastroenterology 1996;111:597–603.
13. Lee J, Lennard-Jones J. Inflammatory bowel disease in 67 families each with three or more affected first-degree relatives. Gastroenterology 1996;111:587–96.
14. Colombel J, Grandbastien B, Gower-Rousseau C, et al. Clinical characterisitics of Crohn's disease in 72 families. Gastroenterology 1996;111:604–7.
15. Bayless T, Tokayer A, Polito J, et al. Crohn's disease: concordance for site and clinical type in affected family members-potential heriditary influences. Gastroenterology 1996;111:573–9.
16. Tysk C, Lindberg E, Jarnerot G, et al. Ulcerative colitis and Crohn's disease in an unselected population of monozygotic and dizygotic twins: a study of heritability and the influence. Gut 1988;29:990–6.
17. Gilat T, Grossman A, Fireman Z, et al. Inflammatory bowel disease in Jews. In: McConnell R, Rozen P, Langman M, Gilat T, eds. The Genetics and Epidemiology of Inflammatory Bowel Disease. New York: Krager, 1986:135–40.
18. Krawiec J, Odes H, Lasry Y, et al. Aspects of the epidemiology of Crohn's disease in the Jewish population of Beer Sheva, Israel. Isr J Med Sci 1984;20:16–21.
19. Weinreb I, Fineman R, Spiro H. Turner's syndrome and inflammatory bowel disease. N Engl J Med 1976;294:1221, 1222.
20. Kohler J, Grant D. Crohn's disease in Turner's syndrome. Br Med J 1981;282:950.
21. Schinella R, Greco A, Cobert B, et al. Hermansky-Pudlak syndrome with granulomatous colitis. Ann Intern Med 1980;92:20–3.

22. Mahadeo R, Markowitz J, Fisher S, et al. Hemansky-Pudlak syndrome with granulomatous colitis in children. J Pediatr 1991;118:904–6.

23. Roe T, Schonfeld N, Thomas D, et al. Regional enteritis and glycogen storage disease type Ib. Lancet 1984;1:1077.

24. Duerr RH, Targan SR, Landers CJ, et al. Anti-neutrophil cytoplasmic antibodies in ulcerative colitis. Comparison with other colitides/diarrheal diseases. Gastroenterology 1991;100:1590–6.

25. Saxon A, Shanahan F, Landers C, et al. A distinct subset of anti-neutrophil cytoplasmic antibodies is associated with inflammatory bowel disease. J Allergy Clin Immunol 1990;86:202–10.

26. Duerr R, Targan S, Landers C, et al. Neutrophil cytoplasmic antibodies: a link between primary sclerosing cholangitis and ulcerative colitis. Gastroenterology 1991;100:1385–91.

27. Shanahan F, Duerr RH, Rotter JI, et al. Neutrophil autoantibodies in ulcerative colitis: familial aggregation and genetic heterogeneity. Gastroenterology 1992;103:456–61.

28. Reumaux D, Colombel J, Delecourt L, et al. Antineutrophil cytoplasmic anitbodies (ANCA) in patients with ulcerative colitis (UC): influence of disease activity and family study. Adv Exp Med Biol 1993;336:515–8.

29. Siebold F, Weber P, Klein R, et al. Clinical significance of antibodies against neutrophils in patients with inflammatory bowel disease and primary sclerosing cholangitis. Gut 1992;33:657–62.

30. Lee J, Lennard-Jones J, Cambridge G. Anti-neutrophil antibodies in familial inflammatory bowel disease. Gastroenterology 1995;108:428–33.

31. Bjarnason I, O'Morain C, Levi AJ, et al. Absorption of 51-chromium-labelled ethylenediaminetetracetate in inflammatory bowel disease. Gastroenterology 1983;85:318–22.

32. Adenis A, Colombel J, Lecouffe P, et al. Increased pulmonary and intestinal permeability in Crohn's disease. Gut 1992;33:678–82.

33. Hollander D, Vadheim C, Brettholz E, et al. Increased intestinal permeability in patients with Crohn's disease and their relatives. Ann Int Med 1986;105:883–5.

34. Pearson AD, Eastman EJ, Laker MF, et al. Intestinal permeability in children with Crohn's disease and coeliac disease. Br Med J 1982;285:20–1.

35. Katz K, Hollander D, Vadheim C, et al. Intestinal permeability in patients with Crohn's disease and their healthy relatives. Gatroenterology 1989;97:927–31.

36. Teahon K, Smethurst P, Levi A, et al. Intestinal permeability in patients with Crohn's disease and their first degree relatives. Gut 1992;33:320–3.

37. May G, Sutherland L, Meddings J. Is small intestinal permeability really increased in relatives of patients with Crohn's disease? Gastroenterology 1993;104:1627–32.

38. Sugimura K, Asakura H, Mizuki N, et al. Analysis of genes within the HLA region affecting susceptibility to inflammatory bowel disease. Hum Immunol 1993;36:112–8.

39. Futami S, Aoyama N, Honsako Y, et al. HLA-DRB1*1502 allele, subtype of DR15, is associated with susceptibility to ulcerative colitis and its progression. Dig Dis Sci 1995;40:814–8.

40. Asakura H, Tsuchiya M, Aiso S, et al. Association of the human lymphocyte-DR2 antigen with japanese ulcerative colitis. Gastroenterology 1982;82:413–8.

41. Toyoda H, Wang SJ, Yang HJ, et al. Distinct associations of HLA class II genes with inflammatory bowel disease. Gastroenterology 1993;104:741–8.

42. Duerr R, Neigut D. Molecularly defined HLA-DR2 alleles in ulcerative colitis and an antineutrophil cytoplasmic antibody-positive subgroup. Gastroenterology 1995;108:423–7.

43. Purrmann J, Bertrams J, Knapp M, et al. Gene and haplotype frequencies of HLA antigens in 269 patients with Crohn's disease. Scand J Gastroenterol 1990;25:981–5.

44. Smolen J, Gangl A, Polterauer P, et al. HLA antigens in inflammatory bowel disease. Gastroenterology 1982;82:413–8.

45. Boehm B, Reinshagen M, Loeliger C, et al. HLA class II genes in Crohn's disease: a population based analysis (abstract). Gasteoenterology 1994;106:A654.

46. Matake H, Okabe N, Naito S, et al. An HLA study on 149 Japanese patients with Crohn's disease. Gastroenterol Jpn 1992;27:496–501.

47. Fujita K, Naito S, Okabe N, et al. Immunological studies in Crohn's disease. I. Assocaition with HLA systems in the Japanese. J Clin Lab Immunol 1984;14:99–102.

48. Casini-Raggi V, Kam L, Chong YJT, et al. Mucosal imbalance of interleukin-1 and interleukin-1 receptor antagonist in inflammatory bowel disease: a novel mechanism of chronic inflammation. J Immunol 1995;154:2434–40.

49. Isaacs KL, Sartor RB, Haskill S. Cytokine messenger RNA profiles in inflammatory bowel disease mucosa detected by polymerase chain reaction amplification. Gastroenterology 1992;103:1587–95.

50. Duerr R, Tran T. Association between ulcerative colitis and a polymorphism in intron 2 of the interleukin-1 receptor antagonist gene (abstract). Gastroenterology 1995;108:A812.

51. Mansfield JC, Holden H, Tarlow JK, et al. Novel genetic association between ulcerative colitis and the anti-inflammatory cytokine interleukin-1 receptor antagonist. Gastroenterology 1994;106:637–42.

52. Plevy S, Targan S, Yang H, et al. Tumor necrosis factor microsatellites define a Crohn's disease-

associated haplotype on chromosome 6. Gastroenterology 1996;110:1053–60.

53. Hugot J, Laurent-Puig P, Gower-Rousseau C, et al. Mapping of a susceptibility locus for Crohn's disease on chromosome 16. Nature 1996;379:821–3.

54. Rutgeerts P, Goboes K, Peeters M, et al. Effect of faecal stream diversion on recurrence of Crohn's disease in the neoterminal ileum. Lancet 1991;2: 771–4.

55. O'Morain C, Segal A, Levi A. Elemental diet as primary treatment of acute Crohn's disease: a controlled study. Br Med J 1984;288:1859–62.

56. Ursing B, Alm T, Barany F, et al. A comparative study of metronidazole and sulfasalazine for active Crohn's disease: the Cooperative Crohn's Disease Study in Sweeden. Gastroenterology 1982;83:550–62.

57. Kuhn R, Lohler J, Rennick D, et al. Interleukin-10-deficient mice develop chronic enterocolitis. Cell 1993;75:263–74.

58. Wensinck R. The fecal flora in patients with Crohn's disease. Antonie van Leeuwenhoek 1975;41:214–5.

59. Burke D, Axon A. Hydrophobic adhesion of E. coli in ulcerative colitis. Gut 1988;29:41–3.

60. Belsheim MR, Darwish RZ, Watson WC, et al. Bacterial L-form isolation from inflammatory bowel disease patients. Gastroenterology 1983;85:364–9.

61. Ibbotson JP, Pease PE, Allan RN. Cell-wall deficient bacteria in inflammatory bowel disease. Eur J Clin Microbiol 1987;6:429–31.

62. Parent K, Mitchell PD. Bacterial variants: etiologic agents in Crohn's disease? Gastroenterology 1976; 71:365–8.

63. Blaser M, Miller R, Lacher J, et al. Patients with active Crohn's disease have elevated serum antibodies to antigens of seven enteric bacterial pathogens. Gastroenterology 1984;87:888–94.

64. Dalziel TK. Chronic interstitial enteritis. Br Med J 1913;2:1068–70.

65. Chiodini R, van Kruiningen H, Thayer W, et al. Possible role of mycobacteria in inflammatory bowel disease: I. An unclassified Mycobacterium species isolated from patients with Crohn's disease. Dig Dis Sci 1984;29:1073–9.

66. Chiodini R, van Kruiningen H, Merkal R, et al. Characteristics of an unclassified Mycobacterium species isolated from patients with Crohn's disease. J Clin Microbiol 1984;20:966–71.

67. Gitnick G, Collins J, Beaman B, et al. Preliminary report on isolation of Mycobacteria from patients with Crohn's disease. Dig Dis Sci 1989;34:925–32.

68. Graham DY, Markesich DC, Yoshimura HH. Mycobateria and inflammatory bowel disease. Results of culture. Gastroenterology 1987;92:436–42.

69. McFadden JJ, Thompson J, Hull E, et al. The use of cloned DNA probes to examine organisms isolated from Crohn's disease tissue. In: MacDermott RP, ed. Inflammatory Bowel Disease: Current Status and Future Applications. Amsterdam: Elsevier, 1988:515–20.

70. Sanderson J, Moss M, Tizard M, et al. *Mycobacterium paratuberculosis* DNA in Crohn's disease tissue. Gut 1992;33:890–6.

71. McFadden JJ, Seechurn P. Mycobacteria and Crohn's disease. A molecular approach. In: MacDermott RP, Stenson WF, eds. Inflammatory Bowel Disease. New York: Elsevier, 1992:259–71.

72. Afdhal NH, Long A, Lennon J, et al. Controlled trial of antimycobacterial therapy in Crohn's disease: clofazimine versus placebo. Dig Dis Sci 1991;36:449–53.

73. Shaffer JL, Hughes S, Linaker BD, et al. Controlled trial of rifampicine and ethambutol in Crohn's disease. Gut 1984;25:203–5.

74. Swift GL, Srivastava ED, Stone R, et al. A controlled trial of 2 years' antituberculous chemotherapy in Crohn's disease (abstract). Gastroenterology 1993; 104:A787.

75. Ekbom A, Adami HO, Hernick CG, et al. Perinatal risk factors of inflammatory bowel disease: a case control study. Am J Epidemiol 1990;132:1111–9.

76. Gitnick GL, Arthur MH, Shibata I. Cultivation of viral agents from Crohn's disease. Lancet 1976;2: 215–7.

77. Mitchell D, Rees R. Agent transmissible from Crohn's disease tissue. Lancet 1970;2:168–71.

78. Aronson M, Phillips C, Beeken W, et al. Isolation and characterization of a viral agent from intestinal tissue of patients with Crohn's disease and other intestinal disorders. Prog Med Virol 1975;21:165–76.

79. Farmer GW, Vincent MM, Fuccillo DA, et al. Viral investigations in ulcerative colitis and regional enteritis. Gastroenterology 1973;65:8–18.

80. Wakefield A, Pittilo R, Sim R, et al. Evidence of persistent measles virus infection in Crohn's disease. J Med Virol 1993;39:345–53.

81. Wakefield AJ, Ekbom A, Dhillon AP, et al. Crohn's disease: pathogenesis and persistent measles virus infection. Gastroenterology 1995;108:911–6.

82. Wakefield AJ, Dhillon AP, Rowles PM, et al. Pathogenesis of Crohn's disease: multifocal gastrointestinal infarction. Lancet 1989;2:1057–62.

83. Wakefield A, Sankey E, Dhillon AP, et al. Granulomatous vasculitis in Crohn's disease. Gastroenterology 1991;100:1279–87.

84. Ekbom A, Wakefiled A, Zack M, et al. The role of perinatal measles infection in the aetiology of Crohn's disease: a population based epidemiological study. Lancet 1994;344:508–10.

85. Lindberg E, Magnusson KE, Tysk C, et al. Antibody (IgG, IgA, and IgM) to baker's yeast (Saccharomyces cerevisiae), yeast mannan, gliadin, ovalbumin and betalactoglobulin in monozygotic twins

with inflammatory bowel disease. Gut 1992;33:909–13.

86. McKenzie H, Main J, Pennington CR, et al. Antibody to selected strains of Saccharomyces cerevisiae (baker's and brewer' yeast) and Candida albicans in Crohn's disease. Gut 1990;31:536–8.

87. Giaffer MH, Clark A, Holdsworth CD. Antibodies to *Saccharomyce cerevisiae* in patients with Crohn's disease and their possible pathogenic importance. Gut 1992;33:1071–5.

88. Onderdonk AB, Franklin ML, Cisneros RL. Production of experimental ulcerative colitis in gnotobiotic guinea pigs with simplified microflora. Infect Immun 1981;32:225–31.

89. Sadlack B, Mertz H, Schorle H, et al. Ulcerative colitis-like disease in mice with a disrupted interleukin-2 gene. Cell 1993;75:253–61.

90. Chadwick VS, Anderson RP. Microorganisms and their products in inflammatory bowel disease. In: MacDermott RP, Stenson WF, eds. Inflammatory Bowel Disease. New York: Elsevier, 1992:241–58.

91. Sartor R. Role of intestinal microflora in initiation and perpetuation of inflammatory bowel disease. Can J Gastroenterol 1990;4:271–7.

92. Podolsky DK, Isselbacher KJ. Glycoprotein composition of colonic mucosa. Specific alterations in ulcerative colitis. Gastroenterology 1984;87:991–8.

93. Raouf A, Parker N, Ryder S, et al. Ion exchange chromatography of purified colonic glycoproteins in inflammatory bowel disease: absence of a selective subclass defect. Gut 1991;32:1139–45.

94. Rhodes JM, Black RR, Savage A. Altered lectin binding by colonic epithelial glycoconjugates in ulcerative colitis and Crohn's disease. Dig Dis Sci 1988;33:1359–63.

95. Glassman M, Newman L, Berezin S, et al. Cow's milk protein sensitivity during infancy in patients with inflammatory bowel disease. Am J Gastroenterol 1990;85:838–40.

96. Elson C. The immunology of inflammatory bowel disease. In: Kirsner J, Shorter R, eds. Inflammatory Bowel Disease. 3rd ed. Philadelphia: Lea & Febiger, 1988:97–164.

97. Mayberry J, Rhodes J, Newcombe R. Increased sugar consumption in Crohn's disease. Digestion 1980;20:323–6.

98. Thornton J, Emmett P, Heaton K. Diet and Crohn's disease: characteristics of the pre-illness habit. Br Med J 1979;2:762–4.

99. Boyko E, Perera D, Koepsell T, et al. Coffee and alcohol use and the risk of ulcerative colitis. Am J Gastroenterol 1989;84:530–4.

100. Strobel C, Byrne W, Ament M. Home parenteral nutrition in children with Crohn's disease: an effective management alternative. Gastroenterology 1979;77:272–9.

101. Riordan AM, Hunter JO, Cowan RE, et al. Treatment of active Crohn's disease by exclusion diet: East Anglian multicentre controlled trial. Lancet 1993;342:1131–4.

102. Rigaud D, Cosnes J, LeQuintrec Y, et al. Controlled trial comparing two types of enteral nutrition in treatment of active Crohn's disease: elemental *v* polymeric diet. Gut 1991;32:1492–7.

103. Royall D, Jeejeebhoy KN, Baker JP, et al. Comparison of amino acid vs peptide based enteral diets in active Crohn's disease: clinical and nurtitional outcome. Gut 1994;35:783–7.

104. Belluzzi A, Brignola C, Campieri M, et al. Effect of an enteric-coated fish-oil preparation on relapses in Crohn's disease. N Engl J Med 1996;334:1557–60.

105. Scheppach W, Loges C, Bartram P, et al. Effect of free glutamine and alanyl glutamine dipeptide on mucosal proliferation of the human ileum and colon. Gastroenterology 1994;107:429–34.

106. Scheppach W, Sommer H, Kirchner T, et al. Effect of butyrate enemas on the colonic mucosa in distal ulcerative colitis. Gastroenterology 1992;103:51–6.

107. Roediger WEW. Bacterial short-chain fatty acids and mucosal diseases of the colon. Br J Surg 1988;75:346–8.

108. Harig J, Soergel K, Komorowski R, et al. Treatment of diversion colitis with short-chain fatty acid irrigation. N Engl J Med 1989;320:23–8.

109. Wischmeyer P, Pemberton J, Phillips S. Chronic pouchitis after ileal pouch-anal anastamosis: responses to butyrate and glutamine suppositories in a pilot study. Mayo Clin Proc 1993;68:978–81.

110. Winter HS, Crum PM, King NW, et al. Expression of immune sensitization to epithelial cell-associated components in the cotton-top tamarin: a model of chronic ulcerative colitis. Gastroenterology 1989;97:1057–82.

111. Elson C, Sartor R, Tennyson G, et al. Experimental models of inflammatory bowel disease. Gastroenterology 1995;109:1344–67.

112. Mayer L. Mucosal immune system in inflammatory bowel disease. In: MacDermott RP, Stenson WF, eds. Inflammatory Bowel Disease. New York: Elsevier, 1992:53–75.

113. Broberger O, Perlmann P. Autoantibodies in human ulcerative colitis. J Exp Med 1959;110:657–74.

114. Perlmann P, Hammarstrom S, Lagercrantz R, et al. Autoantibodies to colon in rats and human ulcerative colitis: cross reactivity with Escherichia coli 0:14. Proc Soc Biol Med 1967;125:975–80.

115. Tabaqchali S, O'Donaghue DP, Bettelheim KA. *Esherichia coli* antibodies in patients with inflammatory bowel disease. Gut 1978;19:108–13.

116. Knoflach P, Park B, Cunningham R, et al. Serum antibodies to cow's milk proteins in ulcerative colitis and Crohn's disease. Gastroenterology 1987;92:479–85.

117. Korsmeyer S, Strickland RG, Wilson ID, et al. Serum lymphocytotoxic and lymphocytophilic antibody

activity in inflammatory bowel disease. Gastroenterology 1974;67:578–83.

118. MacDermott RP, Nash GS, Bertovich MJ, et al. Alterations of IgM, IgG, and IgA synthesis and secretion by peripheral blood and intestinal mononuclear cells from patients with ulcerative colitis and Crohn's disease. Gastroenterology 1981;81:844–52.

119. Scott MG, Nahm MH, Macke K, et al. Spontaneous secretion of IgG subclasses by intestinal mononuclear cells: differences between ulcerative colitis, Crohn's disease, and controls. Clin Exp Immunol 1986;66:209–15.

120. Kett K, Rognum TO, Brandtzaeg P. Mucosal subclass distribution of immunoglobulin G-producing cells is different in ulcerative colitis and Crohn's disease of the colon. Gastroenterology 1987;93:919–24.

121. Das KM, Dubin R, Nagai T. Isolation and characterization of colonic tissue-bound antibodies from patients with idiopathic ulcerative colitis. Proc Natl Acad Sci USA 1978;75:4528–32.

122. Bhagat S, Das K. A shared and unique epitope in the human colon, eye, and joint detected by a monoclonal antibody. Gastroenterology 1994;107:103–8.

123. Das KM, Vecchi M, Sakamaki S. A shared and unique epitope(s) on human colon, skin, and biliary epithelium detected by a monoclonal antibody. Gastroenterology 1990;98:464–9.

124. Takahashi F, Das KM. Isolation and characterization of a colonic autoantigen specifically recognized by colon tissue-bound immunoglobulin G from idiopathic ulcerative colitis. J Clin Invest 1985;76:311–8.

125. Das KM, Dasgupta A, Mandal A, et al. Autoimmunity to cytoskeletal protein tropomyosin. A clue to the pathogenetic mechanisms for ulcerative colitis. J Immunol 1993;150:2487–93.

126. Halstensen TS, Das KM, Brandtzaeg P. Epithelial deposits of immunoglobulin G1 and activated complement colocalise with the Mr 40kD putative autoantigen in ulcerative colitis. Gut 1993;34:650–7.

127. Biancone L, Mandal A, Yang H, et al. Production of immunoglobulin G and G1 antibodies to cytoskeletal protein by lamina propria cells in ulcerative colitis. Gastroenterology 1995;109:3–12.

128. Cantrell M, Prindiville T, Gershwin ME. Autoantibodies to colonic cells and subcellular fractions in inflammatory bowel disease: do they exist? J Autoimmunity 1990;3:307–20.

129. Hodgson H, Wands J, Isselbacher K. Decreased suppressor cell activity in inflammatory bowel disease. Clin Exp Immunol 1978;32:451–8.

130. Holdstock G, Chastenay B, Kravitt E. Increased suppressor cell activity in inflammatory bowel disease. Gut 1981;22:1025–30.

131. Ginsburg C, Falchuk Z. Defective autologous mixed-lymphocyte reaction and suppressor cell generation in patients with inflammatory bowel disease. Gastroenterology 1982;83:1–9.

132. MacDermott RP, Bragdon MJ, Kodner IJ, et al. Deficient cell-mediated cytotoxicity and hyporesponsivenss to interferon and mitogen lectin by inflammatory bowel disease peripheral blood and intestinal mononuclear cells. Gastroenterology 1986;90:6–11.

133. Shanahan F, Leman B, Deem R, et al. Enhanced peripheral blood T-cell cytotoxicity in inflammatory bowel disease. J Clin Immunol 1989;9:55–64.

134. Selby WS, Janossy G, Bofill M, et al. Intestinal lymphocyte subpopulations in inflammatory bowel disease: an analysis by immunohistological and cell isolation technique. Gut 1984;25:32–40.

135. Fukushima K, Masuda T, Ohtani H, et al. Immunohistochemical characterization, distribution, and ultrastructure of lymphocytes bearing T-cell receptor gd in inflammatory bowel disease. Gastroenterology 1991;101:670–8.

136. Gulwani-Akolkar B, Akolkar P, McKinley M, et al. Crohn's disease is accompanied by changes in the CD4+, but not CD8+, T cell receptor Vβ repertoire of lamina propria lymphocytes. Clin Immunol Immunopathol 1995;77:95–106.

137. Fiocchi C, Battisto JR, Farmer RG. Studies on isolated gut mucosal lymphocytes in inflammatory bowel disease. Detection of activated T cells and enhanced proliferation to Staphylococcus areus and lipolysaccharides. Dig Dis Sci 1981;26:728–36.

138. Matsuura T, West GA, Youngman KR, et al. Immune activation genes in inflammatory bowel disease. Gastroenterology 1993;104:448–58.

139. Schreiber S, MacDermott RP, Raedler A, et al. Increased activation of isolated intestinal lamina propria mononuclear cells in inflammatory bowel disease. Gastroenterology 1991;101:1020–30.

140. Kusugami K, Youngman KR, West GA, et al. Intestinal immune reactivity to interleukin 2 differs among Crohn's disease, ulcerative colitis and control. Gastroenterology 1989;97:1–9.

141. Mayer L, Shlien R. Evidence for function of Ia molecules on gut epithelial cells in man. J Exp Med 1987;166:1471–83.

142. Watanabe M, Ueno Y, Yajima T, et al. Interleukin-7 is produced by human intestinal epithelial cells and regulates the proliferation of intestinal mucosal lymphocytes. J Clin Invest 1995;95:2945–53.

143. Jung H, Eckmann L, Yang S-K, et al. A distinct array of proinflammatory cytokines is expressed in human colonic epithelial cells in response to bacterial invasion. J Clin Invest 1995;95:55–65.

144. Mayer L, Eisenhardt D. Lack of induction of suppressor T cells by intestinal epithelial cells from patients with inflammatory bowel disease. J Clin Invest 1990;86:1255–60.

145. Musso A, Ina K, Fiocchi C. Extracellular matrix (ECM) from inflammatory bowel disease (IBD) displays enhanced adhesiveness for T-cells (abstract). Gastroenterology 1996;110:A977.

146. Ina K, Binion D, West G, et al. Secretion of soluble factors and phagocytosis by intestinal fibroblasts regulate T-cell apoptosis (abstract). Gastroenterology 1995;108:A841.

147. Binion D, West G, Ina K, et al. Analysis of human intestinal microvascular endothelial cell activation: enhanced leukocyte binding capacity in inflammatory bowel disease, submitted.

148. Fiocchi C. Cytokines in Inflammatory Bowel Disease. Austin, Texas: R.G. Landes Company, 1996.

149. Fiocchi C, Hilfiker ML, Youngman KR, et al. Interleukin 2 activity of human intestinal mucosal mononuclear cells. Decreased levels in inflammatory bowel disease. Gastroenterology 1984;86:734–42.

150. Mullin GE, Lazenby AJ, Harris ML, et al. Increased interleukin-2 messenger RNA in the intestinal mucosal lesions of Crohn's disease but not ulcerative colitis. Gastroenterology 1992;102:1620–7.

151. Matsuura T, West GA, Klein JS, et al. Soluble interleukin 2, CD8 and CD4 receptors in inflammatory bowel disease. A comparative study of peripheral blood and intestinal mucosal levels. Gastroenterology 1992;102:2006–4.

152. Fuss I, Neurath M, Boirivant M, et al. Disparate CD4+ lamina propria (LP) lymphokine secretion profiles in inflammatory bowel disease. Crohn's disease LP manifest increased secretion of IFN-γ, whereas ulerative colitis LP cells manifest increased secretion of IL-5. J Immunol 1996;157:1261–70.

153. West G, Matsuura T, Levine A, et al. Interleukin-4 in inflammatory bowel disease and mucosal immune reactivity. Gastroenterology 1996;110:1683–95.

154. Schreiber S, Heinig T, Thiele HG, et al. Immunoregulatory role of interleukin 10 in patients with inflammatory bowel disease. Gastroenterology 1995;108:1434–44.

155. Schreiber S, Heinig T, Panzer U, et al. Impaired response of activated mononuclear phagocytes to interleukin 4 in inflammatory bowel disease. Gastroenterology 1995;108:21–33.

156. Van Deventer S, Elson C, Fedorak R, and the IL-10 cooperative study group. Safety, tolerance, pharmacokinetics, and pharmacodynamics of recombinant interleukin-10 (SCH 5200) in patients with steroid refractory Crohn's disease (abstract). Gastroenterology 1996;110:A1034.

157. Ligumsky M, Simon PL, Karmeli F, et al. Role of interleukin 1 in inflammatory bowel disease-enhanced production during active disease. Gut 1990;31:686–9.

158. Mahida YR, Kurlak L, Gallagher A, et al. High circulating levels of interleukin 6 in active Crohn's disease but not ulcerative colitis. Gut 1991;32:1531–4.

159. Stevens C, Walz G, Singaram C, et al. Tumor necrosis factor-α, interleukin-1β, and interleukin-6 expression in inflammatory bowel disease. Dig Dis Sci 1992;37:818–26.

160. Reinecker HC, Loh EY, Ringler DJ, et al. Monocyte-chemoattractant protein 1 gene expression in intestinal epithelial cells and inflammatory bowel disease mucosa. Gastroenterology 1995;108:40–50.

161. Izutani R, Loh EY, Reinecker HC, et al. Increased expression of interleukin-8 mRNA in ulcerative colitis and Crohn's disease mucosa and epithelial cells. Inflammatory Bowel Diseases 1995;1:37–47.

162. Braegger CP, Nicholls S, Murch SH, et al. Tumour necrosis factor alpha in stool as a marker of intestinal inflammation. Lancet 1992;339:89–91.

163. Van Dulleman H, Van Deventer S, Hommes D, et al. Treatment of Crohn's disease with anti-tumor necrosis factor chimeric monoclonal antibody (cA2). Gastroenterology 1995;109:129–35.

164. Stenson W. Arachidonic acid metabolites in inflammatory bowel disease. In: Fiocchi C, ed. Cytokines in Inflammatory Bowel Disease. Austin: R.G. Landes, 1996:157–76.

165. Sharon P, Stenson WF. Enhanced synthesis of leukotriene B4 by colonic mucosa in inflammatory bowel disease. Gastroenterology 1984;86:453–60.

166. Shannon VR, Stenson WF, Holtzman MJ. Induction of epithelial arachidonate 12-lipoxygenase at active sites of inflammatory bowel disease. Am J Physiol 1993;264:G104–11.

167. Lauritsen K, Laursen LS, Bukhave K, et al. In vivo profiles of eicosanoids in ulcerative colitis, Crohn's colitis, and Clostridium difficile colitis. Gastroenterology 1988;95:11–7.

168. Dignass A, Podolsky D. Peptide growth factors in inflammatory bowel disease. In: Fiocchi C, ed. Cytokines in Inflammatory Bowel Disease. Austin: R.G. Landes, 1996:137–55.

169. Zeeh J, Procaccino F, Hoffman P, et al. Keratinocyte growth factor ameliorates mucosal injury in an experimental model of colitis in rats. Gastroenterology 1996;110:1077–83.

170. Finch P, Pricolo V, Wu A, et al. Increased expression of keratinocyte growth factor messenger RNA associated with inflammatory bowel disease. Gastroenterology 1996;110:441–51.

171. Wright NA, Poulsom R, Stamp G, et al. Trefoil peptide gene expression in gastrointestinal epithelial cells in inflammatory bowel disease. Gastroenterology 1993;194:12–20.

172. Babyatsky M, Rossiter G, Podolsky D. Expression of transforming growth factor α and β in colonic mucosa in inflammatory bowel disease. Gastroenterology 1996;110:975–84.

173. Koizumi M, King N, Lobb R, et al. Expression of vascular adhesion molecules in inflammatory bowel disease. Gastroenterology 1992;103:840–7.

174. Malizia G, Calabrese A, Cottone M, et al. Expression of leukocyte adhesion molecules by mucosal mononuclear phagocytes in inflammatory bowel disease. Gastroenterology 1991;100:150–9.

175. Yacyshyn BR, Lazarovits A, Tsai V, et al. Crohn's disease, ulcerative colitis, and normal intestinal lymphocytes express integrins in dissimilar patterns. Gastroenterology 1994;107:1364–71.

176. Palmen M, Dijkstra C, VanderEnde M, et al. Anti-CD11b/CD18 antibodies reduce inflammation in acute colitis in rats. Clin Exp Immunol 1995;101:351–6.

177. Podolsky DK, Lobb R, King N, Benjamin CD, Pepinsky B, Seghal P, et al. Attenuation of colitis in the cotton-top tamarin by anti-alpha4 integrin monoclonal antibody. J Clin Invest 1993;92:372–80.

178. Simmonds NJ, Allen RE, Stevens TRJ, Niall R, Someren MV, et al. Chemiluminescence assay of mucosal reactive oxygen metabolites in inflammatory bowel disease. Gastroenterology 1992;103:186–96.

179. Boughton-Smith NK, Evans SM, Hawkey CJ, Cole AT, Balsitis M, et al. Nitric oxide synthase activity in ulcerative colitis and Crohn's disease. Lancet 1993;342:338–40.

180. Buffington G, Doe W. Depleted mucosal antioxidant defenses in inflammatory bowel disease. Free Radical Biol Med 1995;19:911–8.

181. Yamada T, Grisham M. Pathogenesis of tissue injury: role of reactive metabolites of oxygen and nitrogen. In: Targan S, Shanahan F, eds. Inflammatory Bowel Disease: from Bench to Bedside. Baltimore: Williams & Wilkins, 1994:133–50.

182. Stanisz A. Neuronal factors modulating immunity. Neuroimmunomodulation 1994;1:217–30.

183. Reichlin S. Neuroendocrine-immune interactions. N Engl J Med 1993;329:1245–53.

184. Kubota Y, Petras RE, Ottaway CA, et al. Colonic vasoactive intestinal peptide nerves in inflammatory bowel disease. A digitized morphometric immunohistochemical study. Gastroenterology 1992;102:1242–51.

185. Mazumdar S, Das KM. Immunohistochemical localization of vasoactive intestinal peptide and substance P in the colon from normal subjects and patients with inflammatory bowel disease. Am J Gastroenterol 1992;87:176–81.

186. Bjorck S, Dahlstrom A, Ahlman H. Topical treatment of ulcerative proctitis with lidocaine. Scand J Gastroenterol 1989;24:1061–72.

187. Strober W. Animal models of inflammatory bowel disease-an overview. Dig Dis Sci 1985;30:3S-10S.

188. Stenson WF. Animal models of inflammatory bowel disease. In: Targan SR, Shanahan F, eds. Inflammatory Bowel Disease. From Bench to Bedside. Baltimore: Williams & Wilkins, 1994:180–92.

189. Sartor RB. Insights into the pathogenesis of inflammatory bowel diseases provided by new rodent models of spontaneous colitis. Inflammatory Bowel Diseases 1995;1:64–75.

190. Yamada T, Grisham M. Role of neutrophil-derived oxidants in the pathogenesis of intestinal inflammation. Klin Wochenschr 1991;69:988–94.

191. Sartor RB, Bond TM, Schwab JH. Systemic uptake and intestinal inflammatory effects of luminal bacterial cell wall polymers in rats with acute colonic injury. Infect Immun 1988;56:2101–8.

192. Morris G, Beck P, Herridge M, et al. Hapten-induced model of chronic inflammation and ulceration in the rat colon. Gastroenterology 1989;96:795–803.

193. Beagley K, Black C, Elson C. Strain differences in susceptibility to TNBS-induced colitis (abstract). Gastroenterology 1991;100:A560.

194. Cooper H, Murthy S, Shah R, et al. Clinico-pathologic study of dextran sulfate sodium experimental murine colitis. Lab Invest 1993;69:238–49.

195. Okayasu I, Hatakeyama S, Yamada M, et al. A novel method in the induction of reliable experimental acute and chronic ulcerative colitis in mice. Gastroenterology 1990;98:694–702.

196. Yamada M, Ohkusa T, Okayasu I. Occurrence of dysplasia and adenocarcinoma after experimental chronic ulcerative colitis in hamsters induced by dextran sulphate sodium. Gut 1992;33:1521–7.

197. Sartor RB, Cromartie WJ, Powell DW, et al. Granulomatous enterocolitis induced in rats by purified bacterial cell wall fragments. Gastroenterology 1985;89:587–95.

198. Sartor R. Animal models of intestinal inflammation: Relevance to inflammatory bowel disease. In: MacDermott R, Stenson W, eds. Inflammatory Bowel Disease. New York: Elsevier, 1992:337–53.

199. McCall RD, Haskill S, Zimmermann EM, et al. Tissue interleukin-1 and interleukin-1 receptor antagonist expression in enterocolitis in resistant and susceptible rats. Gastroenterology 1994;106:960–72.

200. Chalifoux L, Bronson R. Colonic adenocarcinoma associated with chronic colitis in cotton top marmosets, *Sanguinis oedipus*. Gastroenterology 1981;80:942–6.

201. Wood J, Peck O, Sharma H, et al. Captivity promotes colitis in the cotton-top tamarin (*Sanguinis oedipus*) (abstract). Gastroenterology 1990;98:A480.

202. Sundberg JP, Elson CO, Bedigian H, et al. Spontaneous, heritable colitis in a new substrain of C3H/HeJ mice. Gastroenterology 1994;107:1726–35.

203. Hammer RE, Maika SD, Richardson JA, et al. Spontaneous inflammatory disease in transgenic rats expressing HLA-B27 and human β2m: an animal model of HLA-B27-associated human disorders. Cell 1990;63:1099–112.

204. Mombaerts P, Mizoguchi E, Grusby MG, et al. Spontaneous development of inflammatory bowel disease in T cell receptor mutant mice. Cell 1993;75: 275–82.

205. Rudolph U, Finegold M, Rich S, et al. Ulcerative colitis and adenocarcinoma of the colon in Gαi2-deficient mice. Nature Genetics 1995;10:143–50.

206. Hermiston M, Gordon J. Inflammatory bowel disease and adenomas in mice expressing a dominant negative N-cadherin. Science 1995;270: 1203–7.

207. Baribault H, Penner L, Iozzo R. Colorectal hyperplasia and inflammation in keratin 8-deficient FVB/N mice. Genes & Dev 1994;8:2964–73.

4 Surgical Pathology

Robert H. Riddell

Idiopathic inflammatory bowel disease (IBD) is used in this chapter for primary chronic inflammatory diseases of unknown etiology, which specifically include ulcerative colitis and Crohn's disease; these are part of a much wider spectrum of diseases as shown in Table 4.1. It will also include their complications including fulminant disease, dysplasia and carcinoma, diversion disease and pouchitis. Increasingly it is necessary to be aware of the effects of drugs and medications both in causing diseases and modifying their usual pathology.

Histological Diagnosis: Fact, Fiction, and Oral Tradition

Number of Biopsies: Theory versus Practice

Morphological studies of IBD have largely been directed at the value of specific criteria by one or few pathologists based almost entirely on rectal biopsies in untreated patients in their first attack, and rarely on more than one biopsy or site. In practice, pathologists have also been using the distribution of disease as well on multiple biopsies around the large bowel, as well as specific histological features to both diagnose IBD as well as distinguish its subtypes. Thus active right sided colitis with absolutely normal left sided biopsies is very unlikely to be ulcerative colitis.

Interobserver variability studies have not used biopsies obtained at colonoscopy which can demonstrate not only the distribution of disease within the terminal ileum and large bowel, but also such major criteria as focality of disease within the same segment of bowel and whether, if erosions or ulcers are present they occur on a background of normal or inflamed mucosa. This implies that colonoscopists need to deliberately target biopsies to demonstrate the presence of these features. Data from the literature therefore provide poor indices of features that may be of value in IBD, and only a few of these stand up reproducibly to critical inter and intraobserver variability studies. None have specifically asked colonoscopists to demonstrate the distribution and focality of disease throughout the large bowel in their biopsies.

Interpretation of biopsies from patients with inflammatory bowel disease is the result of examining patterns of inflammation and architecture in multiple biopsies and the distribution of the disease in the terminal ileum and large bowel, and sometimes the upper gastrointestinal tract in addition. The standard of practice is such that diagnostic criteria, and those used in practice in differential diagnosis on colonoscopic biopsies have been taught primarily as an oral tradition. This likely results in considerable variation of biopsy diagnoses from hospital to hospital depending on one's mentors. Most colonoscopists have little notion of the criteria used by pathologists and therefore do not take the biopsies required to establish a diagnosis or refute a differential diagnosis (discussed subsequently). Much of what follows is therefore based on the limited literature, personal experience and practices, some of which have never been formally tested (an attempt to design such a study will rapidly allow the reader to see why this is the case—the variables are numerous).

Oral Tradition

Personal experience also translates into what we were taught, what of that we have personally found

Table 4.1. Classification of inflammatory bowel diseases.

Idiopathic	Ulcerative colitis/proctitis, Crohn's disease
Infective	Viral, chlamydia, bacteria, spirochetes, fungi, protozoa, nematodes, trematodes
Inflammation	Diverticular disease, Solitary rectal ulcer syndrome, Systemic disease (e.g., Behcet's), Iatrogenic—diversion, ostomies, reservoirs, GVH
Ischemia	Low/no flow, mechanical, trauma, stercoral, drug-related, radiation, vasculitis
Descriptive colitides	Pseudomembranous, hemorrhagic, collagenous, follicular, eosinophilic, granulomatous, microscopic/lymphocytic etc.
Drugs, chemicals and foodstuffs	NSAID's, Gold, penicillamine, sulfasalazine, Me-DOPA, antibiotics, antifungal, Cytotoxics, kayexalate Oral contraceptives, metals, enemas/laxatives, food allergens

useful, and which of this we teach our peers and residents. This is the foundation of oral tradition, and the unlikely hope that this is the same for all pathologists. However, such individual variation also extends to clinical practice; at a workshop at which this author participated along with numerous distinguished gastroenterologists consisting of many of the leaders in the field of IBD, fully 1/3 accepted typical granulomas as part of the spectrum of ulcerative colitis, and a different 1/3 aphthoid ulcers as part of the typical endoscopic appearances of ulcerative colitis. As both of these need alternative explanations, one presumes that for most of the time the distinction between ulcerative and Crohn's colitis tends to be of little clinical significance.

Initial Diagnosis

The original surgical pathology of IBD was described in surgical resections, which were then used as a primary therapy. Now resections are carried out almost entirely for complications of the disease. The intimal diagnosis of IBD may therefore be made in those few patients initially presenting with surgical complications such as obstruction—whether from primary disease such as Crohn's disease or from complications such as carcinoma, from fulminant disease or bleeding, or from an erroneous diagnosis of appendicitis, or from a fistula. The primary diagnosis is therefore

made radiologically or endoscopically usually including biopsies taken in patients to answer a specific question. For example, in patients with diarrhea the main questions arising include:

1. Am I in the right organ?
   a. If an endoscopic lesion is present what kind of colitis/proctitis does the patient have?
   b. If no endoscopic abnormality is present could the patient have microscopic disease causing symptoms?
2. In a patient with established inflammatory bowel disease
   a. If the patient is not responding to therapy—why not? Have I underestimated the extent of the disease
   b. Do I have the wrong diagnosis?
   c. Is anything present histologically that might change the patient's management e.g., dysplasia or carcinoma?

In all of these situations, unless the endoscopist appreciates the features used by the pathologist to make the diagnosis, it is unlikely that appropriate biopsies will be taken. The role of the endoscopist is to ascertain whether an endoscopic abnormality is present, and to obtain histologic confirmation of the endoscopic impression, even if normal, to exclude diseases such as microscopic (lymphocytic) colitis. If an endoscopic lesion is present, what kind of colitis/proctitis does the patient have? In patients with bloody diarrhea the endoscopic appearance may vary from relatively nonspecific findings such as mild focal erythema and possible erosions, or be more severe, sometimes with ulceration superimposed on mucosa that may be normal or focally or diffusely abnormal, or be diffuse and extend to the anus. The objective for the endoscopist is therefore to define histologically as well as endoscopically the nature and extent of the disease particularly those that might indicate chronic inflammatory bowel disease. A knowledge of the histological criteria used to make specific diagnoses is therefore required so that appropriate biopsies can be taken.

Guide to Colonoscopic Biopsy Requirements in Patients with Potential IBD

Technical Points

There are no absolutes about taking biopsies other than ensuring that: a) sufficient tissue is taken to answer the question at hand, and b) the question for which the biopsies have been taken, together with relevant history and any therapy that the patient is on is made known to the pathologist.

The day of deliberately sending little or no history is long past, and encourages the use of descriptive diagnosis (e.g., nonspecific acute and chronic inflammation) that are without value. Rubbish in—rubbish out. Increasingly in a cost efficient method of practice, costs can be kept to a minimum by ensuring that biopsies are utilized to obtain full value. In many institutions multiple biopsies from the same site may be put directly into a histology cassette on a piece of filter paper or similar mounting medium to ensure good orientation as far as possible. Although this can be helped to some extent during embedding in the laboratory, a twisted biopsy cannot be readily oriented. Particularly when dealing with IBD it is essential to see the deep mucosa in the region of the muscularis mucosae, as the type of inflammation in this region such as an excess of plasma cells, is found in long-standing disease, and particularly ulcerative colitis, Crohn's disease, collagenous and microscopic colitis.

Diffuse Disease

This usually means disease extending in continuity down to the anorectal junction. The endoscopist should demonstrate in multiple biopsies that this is the case. If an upper limit is visualized, biopsies should be taken not only of the involved area, but also from the apparently normal mucosa 5 to 10 cms above this demarcation. The lower biopsies will in most instances allow the ready distinction between acute ulcerative colitis and an acute infection, by far the two most common diseases that cause this endoscopic appearance. If the disease proves to be ulcerative colitis it will also be apparent in the proximal biopsies whether the disease is limited to the rectum or rectosigmoid, or if the patient has at least left sided ulcerative colitis. The presence of the latter, or failure to visualize an upper limit will, in a patient with ulcerative colitis, necessitate a further investigation at some point to determine the extent of the disease. Ultimately, this may determine whether the patient will require to be entered into a surveillance program. Conversely, limitation of the disease to the rectum is associated with a good longterm prognosis.

Focal or Patchy Disease, Including Aphthoid Ulcers

The question regarding whether an upper and/or lower border is present remains and should be demonstrated in biopsies to confirm that microscopic disease is not present. An attempt should also be made to determine whether normal and abnormal mucosa coexists side by side. If obvious ulcers are present these should clearly be biopsied, if possible *at their edges;* these are also particularly useful for demonstrating pseudomembranes or aphthoid ulcers in Crohn's disease when the immediately adjacent apparently normal mucosa may be almost spared histologically. Biopsies should also be taken of endoscopically normal, or relatively normal bowel at the same level as the focal lesion and can be included in the same specimen container. If clearly visible upper or lower limits are present these should also be sampled in separate containers. These biopsies determined whether endoscopic focality is also reflected microscopically; in some infections and ulcerative colitis undergoing remission endoscopic patchiness is frequently much more diffuse histologically (1). Features of idiopathic inflammatory bowel disease, specifically architectural distortion and an inflammatory infiltrate down to the muscularis mucosa on the background of a normal mucosa virtually excludes infection but are highly suggestive of Crohn's disease.

Microscopic Disease and Collagenous Colitis

If no endoscopic abnormality is present could the patient have microscopic disease causing symptoms? If endoscopy is normal biopsies are required to exclude entities characterized by only a histologic abnormality including, particularly collagenous colitis, microscopic/lymphocytic colitis, some infections and non-specific inflammation that may still be the cause of the patient's symptoms (see Table 4.2). Biopsies should be taken from a minimum of three sites. The first should be taken as proximally as possible, even during flexible sigmoidoscopy, by extending the forcep well beyond the tip of the endoscope. The main purpose is to exclude collagenous colitis that spares the rectosigmoid. The other two biopsies should be taken from the sigmoid and the rectum to exclude other proctitides and abnormalities that may be focal, or ensure that enema induced artifacts are minimized where Fleets or similar enemas known to cause superficial mucosal damage are used. If colonoscopy is being done as the first approach or because biopsies at flexible sigmoidoscopy were normal then biopsies should sample the terminal ileum and the landmark areas of the colon (i.e., cecum ascending colon, proximal and distal transverse colon, and the three sites mentioned above for flexible sigmoidoscopy). In patients with diarrhea, but normal endoscopy, histologic abnormalities will be

Table 4.2.   Possible causes of microscopically abnormal biopsies from endoscopically normal patients.

Descriptive colitides
   Collagenous colitis
   Microscopic colitis
     Lymphocytic colitis
   Granulomatous colitis
Specific infections (detectable on examination or culture)
   Cryptosporidiosis
   (Spirochetosis)
Nonspecific inflammation or granuloma
   Possible infection
   Possible Crohn's disease
   Possible quiescent ulcerative colitis
   Iatrogenic disease
   Medications e.g., NSAIDs
Miscellaneous conditions
   Melanosis coli (Ingested anthraquinones)
   Amyloid
   (Diabetes—electron microscopic)

found on biopsy in 15% to 20% of patients (2,3). Under these circumstances microscopic and collagenous colitis are particularly being sought, but patients with quiescent ulcerative colitis may have normal biopsies (4).

Does the Patient Have IBD?

The histological criteria for the diagnosis are well established. Their main problem is that they are not always all present, particularly in the very early and the resolved phases of the disease. Features that are most useful are (Fig. 4.1):

a.   Crypt atrophy.
b.   Crypt distortion is present.
c.   Plasmacytosis (especially immediately above the muscularis mucosae where they are not normally present other than in the cecum) with severe chronic inflammation.
d.   Distal Paneth cell metaplasia (5).

Some studies add features such as excess of polymorphonuclear leucocytes polymorphonuclear cryptitis, crypt abscesses, basal lymphoid aggregates (6,7). However, neutrophils crypt abscesses are found whenever an acute inflammatory process is present, suggesting that these studies were inadequately controlled. A surface villiform pattern is highly suggestive of ulcerative colitis, and is therefore of value in the small proportion of patients in whom it is present. Similarly, granulomas always raise the question of Crohn's disease whenever they occur in the gastrointestinal tract. Interestingly, on multiple biopsies a formula can be used to de-

termine the likelihood of IBD being present derived from regression analysis (5).

Does the Patient Have Ulcerative Colitis or Crohn's Disease?

Once the criteria for IBD have been fulfilled, other than granulomas, the features that really suggest underlying Crohn's disease in multiple colonoscopic biopsies are (5) (Fig. 4.2):

a.   The presence of segmental crypt architectural abnormalities.
b.   Segmental mucin depletion.
c.   Mucin preservation with surrounding neutrophils or adjacent ulcer edge.
d.   focal chronic inflammation

In IBD patients the fewer of these criteria that are filled or presence of the converse features—diffuse crypt architectural abnormalities: diffuse mucin depletion, mucin depletion with surrounding neutrophils or adjacent ulceration, diffuse chronic inflammation—strongly suggest that the underlying disease is ulcerative colitis (5). In many studies additional criteria for ulcerative colitis include: an irregular or villous surface and polymorphonuclear cryptitis (8). In the differential diagnosis, neutrophils that are diffusely cryptophilic (Fig. 4.3) also highly suggest ulcerative colitis, while lamina propria neutrophils that remain in the lamina propria strongly suggest Crohn's disease, or, in the absence of features of IBD, acute infectious colitis.

Ulcerative Colitis

Definition and Terminology

Ulcerative colitis is a chronic inflammatory disease of unknown cause affecting primarily the mucosa of the large bowel and characterized by exacerbations and remissions of bloody diarrhea. Histologically, exacerbations are characterized by a predominantly acute inflammatory process associated with destruction of mucosal elements, primarily epithelial. Loss of crypts (atrophy) and/or distortion of crypt architecture can be seen in all stages of the disease. The rectum is invariably involved. The disease may extend proximally in a symmetric manner, and in some patients involves the entire large bowel and occasionally the distal terminal ileum in continuity. In some patients, the entire large bowel appears involved from the beginning. There is an increased risk of developing colorectal cancer that is related to the extent of disease. Because the proximal extent of disease is variable and depends

Fig. 4.1. (A) Normal large bowel biopsy with regularly spaced test tube-like crypts and few cells immediately above the muscularis mucosae (bottom and right) taken above the proximal margin of disease. (B) Distal biopsy from the same patient. There is marked architectural distortion and a transmucosal inflammatory infiltrate. (C) Detail of (b) showing basal plasma cells. This combination of features indicates that the patient has IBD of some kind.

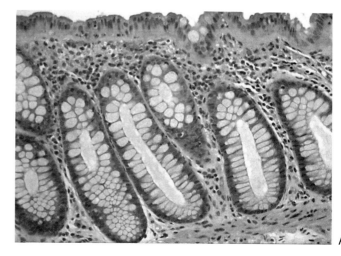

A

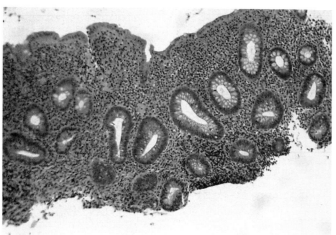

B

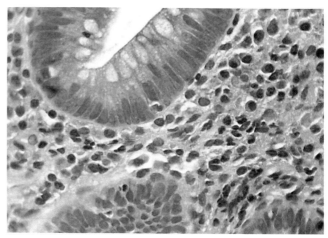

C

on the method of demonstration, the following clinical terms are often used:

1. ***Ulcerative proctitis*** Ulcerative proctitis is identical to ulcerative colitis in many ways, but disease remains confined to the rectum, i.e., the distal 10 to 12 cm of large bowel. It comprises about a quarter of the cases of ulcerative colitis depending on the series examined and their selection biases (9,10). Because most of the colon is intact, these patients do not usually have diarrhea. Instead, they have recurrent bouts of rectal bleeding, characterized by the passage of stool coated on the outside by bright red blood or by the passage of small amounts of bright red blood without stool. In a proportion of patients the disease involves the sigmoid colon as well as the rectum; some prefer the term ulcerative proctosigmoiditis or left sided colitis for this group (11,12) Unfortunately some clinicians use the term ulcerative proctitis to include proctosigmoiditis. This is potentially confusing in terms of outlining

prognosis to patients. Ulcerative proctitis limited to the distal 10 to 12 cm rarely spreads proximally; conversely, involvement of the sigmoid colon, even if only for 10 to 15 cm beyond the rectum portends the possibility that one may be dealing with ulcerative colitis at the outset.

The histology of ulcerative proctitis is very similar to that of ulcerative colitis; however, in one study there appeared to be more intense inflammation, particularly in plasma cells, in the affected mucosa (13). Therapy involves corticosteroids and sometimes maintenance sulfasalazine, to which there is a good response in about three-quarters of the patients. The remainder have a less satisfactory response. Some of the newer agents based on local anesthetics show promise. Overall, about 15% to 50% of patients have a relatively intractable disease which responds poorly to therapy but which nevertheless fails to extend. Considering the few centimeters of bowel involved, the disease can be surprisingly incapacitating. The only re-

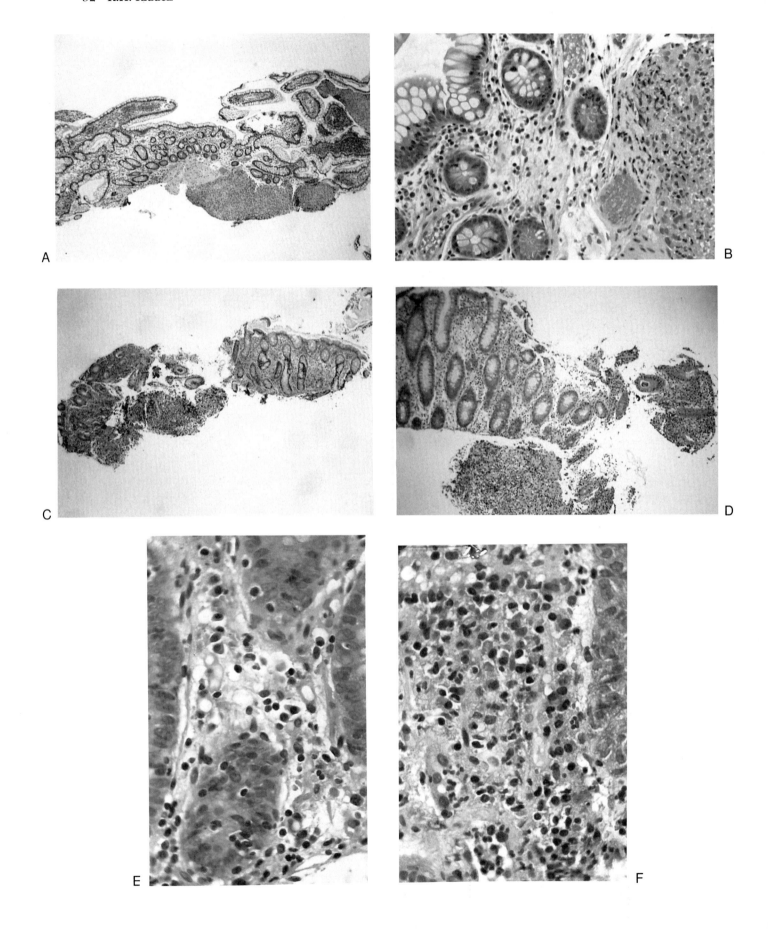

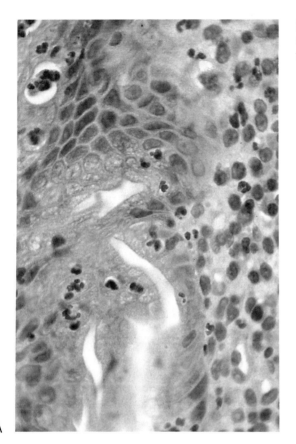

A

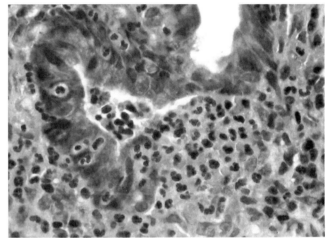

B

Fig. 4.3. Ulcerative colitis. (A) Crypt with occasional neutrophils (cryptitis) primarily in the crypt. (B) Cryptitis with crypt abscess.

assurance that can be given is that the condition is not serious, rarely requires operation, involves no additional risk of carcinoma, and virtually all problems occur in the first 5 years. More than 90% of these patients never have proximal extension of their disease to produce typical ulcerative colitis (12,14,15). Those in whom the disease does extend may have had more than limited disease at the outset. However, one study found that in 13/96 patients (13.6%), ulcerative proctitis was the initial manifestation of Crohn's disease, evidence of which usually appeared within the first 3 years (16).

Currently, it is impossible to predict accurately which patients will have disease that extends proximally, but the risk is highest in patients whose disease remains active with spontaneous bleeding at proctoscopy, and those who present before age 21; in this group, one study suggested that 38% develop proximal extension despite distal localization of the disease. Virtually all patients who experience extension do so within 5 years, and in most cases within 2 years. These patients are also more likely to have diarrhea, anemia, and systemic symptoms. In one group, operation was ultimately required in 16% for bleeding, fulminant colitis or toxic dilatation (17).

2. *Left-sided colitis* Although literally "disease confined to the large bowel distal to the mid-transverse colon," this term is most frequently used for disease extending proximally as far as the splenic flexure. When the disease is limited to the rectum and sigmoid colon, some use the term "proctosigmoiditis." There is no standard terminology for disease extending proximal to the splenic flexure; the following is therefore suggested.

Fig. 4.2. Crohn's disease. (A) Terminal ileal biopsy with normal villi but focal necrotic exudate bottom and right. (B) Detail showing the focal exudate (right) and relatively normal mucosa (left). (C) Colonic biopsy with two halves of the same biopsy showing very different quantities of inflammation in the inflamed part left compared to the normal part right. (D) Biopsy from the same patient showing normal mucosa left and an inflamed portion right. (E) and (F) are details of (D) showing the relatively normal mucosa and the inflamed part with numerous neutrophils in the lamina propria, a combination that is highly suggestive of Crohn's disease.

3. *Extensive colitis* Although this is clearly a subjective term, and is used as a synonym for any condition from proctosigmoiditis to disease extending proximally to the hepatic flexure; I arbitrarily use it for disease extending in continuity proximal to any point in the transverse colon as defined by endoscopy and biopsy. At some centers these patients are entered into surveillance programs.

4. *Pancolitis (synonyms: total colitis/"universal" colitis/pan proctocolitis):* This literally means disease involving the entire colon, but is used occasionally and loosely for disease extending proximal to the hepatic flexure (we accept the last definition).

Terminology

Much of the terminology applied to inflammatory bowel disease is ambiguous in that terms such as "active" and "inactive," and "acute" and "chronic," may be used by clinicians either to describe the patients' symptoms or as an attempt at clinicopathological correlation, or to define the duration of the disease. The same terms may be used by pathologists to describe the presence or absence of acute inflammatory cells (neutrophils), again inferring a degree of clinicopathological correlation. The correlation between symptoms and histology is far from absolute, generally reasonable but with numerous exceptions. Multiple biopsies from a patient in clinical remission may show occasional neutrophils or crypt abscesses, and occasionally endoscopy suggests disease that is far more intense than that seen histologically. Whatever the preferences of both the pathologist and clinician regarding terminology, it is essential that they communicate to leave little room for mutual misunderstanding. In this respect, endoscopists can help by using simple literate descriptions of what was seen rather than attempting histological interpretations

Clinical Features and Implications for Pathology

Ulcerative colitis is a disease which waxes and wanes and is characterized by acute exacerbations of bloody diarrhea which resolve either spontaneously or following treatment. Conventional wisdom has always been that ulcerative colitis inevitably involves the rectum and tapers as it goes proximally (Table 4.3). Recent data in a prospective study and some earlier anecdotal reports suggest that there may be considerable patchiness and some rectal sparing in up to a third of patients who are on treatment (1,18), while rectal biopsies may also revert to normal following successful therapy (4,19). The implication is that a normal rectal biopsy never excludes ulcerative colitis.

Extent is gauged differently in different centres and may be the upper limit of disease visualized by proctoscopy, colonoscopy or radiology; the last may be either single or air contrast, and may be inaccurate unless the disease is total. The addition of biopsy, ideally in active disease, is required to carry out this study on a representative patient population. Depending on the series, between 20% and 60% of patients have disease limited to the rectum or rectum and sigmoid colon, about 30% to 40% have left sided colitis, and about 20% have extensive or total disease. Patients with extensive or total large bowel disease are prone to develop colorectal cancer and also a variety of extraintestinal manifestations.

Table 4.3.   Gross pathology of idiopathic inflammatory bowel disease in resected specimens.

Macroscopic	Active UC	Toxic megacolon	Crohn's disease
Distribution	Diffuse, rectum usually involved	Diffuse, proximal and distal colon often spared	Segmental, variable rectal disease
Inflammatory masses	None	Only if Crohn's	Frequent
Cobblestoning	No	Only if Crohn's	Yes
Aphthoid ulcers	No	Only if Crohn's	Yes
Extensive small bowel disease	No	Only if Crohn's	May occur
Creeping fat	No	Only if Crohn's	May occur
Perianal disease	Uncommon	Uncommon	Common
Mesenteric adenopathy	Occasional	Occasional	Frequent
Inflammatory polyps	Frequent	Residual mucosal islands may resemble polyps, especially on x-ray	Less frequent
Fissures	None	Only if Crohn's	Frequent
Serositis	Absent	Peritonitis common	Usually present

Gross Pathology and Endoscopic Appearances

The macroscopic appearances in ulcerative colitis vary, depending primarily on the clinical activity of the disease, its severity, and the presence of complications. The major characteristic of untreated ulcerative colitis is that, with few exceptions, it is a diffuse disease which involves the rectum and may extend proximally to varying degrees, always in continuity with the rectal disease.

Macroscopic examination of the colon is now most frequently a function of the endoscopist. Except for the risk or presence of carcinoma, elective resection in disease that is quiescent or only mildly active is now uncommon. In active ulcerative colitis the mucosa endoscopically is typically red, friable, and granular with contact bleeding, the "skinned knee" appearance (Fig. 4.4; see color plate).

Endoscopic Appearances

In long-standing disease, erythema, loss of vascular pattern, and friability are present. In milder cases, friability may be evident only because pressure of the endoscope against the colonic wall elicits oozing of blood or petechiae. Surface ulceration, if present, is usually relatively superficial (erosions) and may be obscured by an overlying mucopurulent exudate. The finding of ulcers indicates severe disease or some other form of inflammatory bowel disease, even if the intervening mucosa is extremely friable. Importantly, with rare exception, epithelial destruction occurs on the background of an inflamed mucosa, in contrast to Crohn's disease, where sudden transitions from ulcers to normal mucosa may be found.

The transition from diseased to normal mucosa is usually gradual, but occasionally abrupt. Proximal spread is in continuity, without intervening areas of uninvolved mucosa. This is an important feature of ulcerative colitis which contrasts with the discontinuous pattern of involvement often seen in Crohn's colitis. It remains even in patients in whom active disease affects only the distal bowel, when the patient is known to have had much more extensive disease proximally. Bowel that has been quiescent for long periods of time may regain a normal haustral pattern.

Patchiness of disease can be seen at the proximal margin of active disease and in response to therapy. The rectum may occasionally be spared in patients with fulminant colitis, particularly in the first attack, and sometimes relatively spared following the use of steroid enemas. The endoscopic and histologic sparing seen in up to one third of patients with treated mild or moderate disease (1,18,19) sometimes raises the disturbing spectre of Crohn's disease. This becomes an important issue if total proctocolectomy is contemplated.

Resected Specimens

Unless fulminant disease is present, the serosa is normal. The creeping fat that is so characteristic of Crohn's disease is distinctly uncommon and should cause the diagnosis to be questioned. If there has been previous active disease the bowel may be markedly shortened, with loss of the haustral pattern, so that the colon is converted into a tube-like structure (Fig. 4.4) which is usually most apparent distally and may be severe. Such shortening in ulcerative colitis is attributed to muscular contraction and thickening; fibrosis, if present, tends to be limited to the submucosa histologically. Strictures are usually a reflection of prior severe disease or malignancy. Undermining mucosal in-

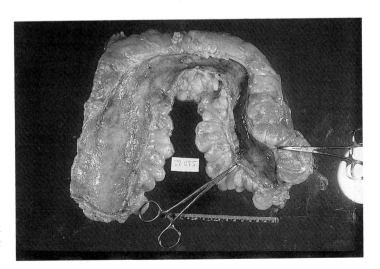

Fig. 4.4. Ulcerative colitis with quiescent disease proximally but with blood oozing from the mucosa distally. (See color plate.)

flammation may result in inflammatory polyps that may be numerous or mucosal bridges. If the disease is severe and involves the entire large bowel, "backwash ileitis" may be present in continuity The appendix is also frequently affected, usually in continuity, but occasionally with intervening normal disease (20).

Histology of Ulcerative Colitis

The distinction of IBD from other inflammatory diseases and ulcerative colitis from Crohn's disease has been considered above. The inflammatory infiltrate in the lamina propria consists primarily of plasma cells; however, in the vicinity of the muscularis mucosae lymphocytes may predominate often associated with histiocytes and eosinophils, either in aggregates or as a more diffuse band. A deep plasmacytic infiltrate with readily identifiable plasma cells immediately above the muscularis mucosae is virtually pathognomonic of longstanding chronic inflammation particularly ulcerative colitis (Fig. 4.1), Crohn's disease, collagenous, microscopic and lymphocytic colitis and is rarely found in acute infectious type colitis (7,21). In IBD, its presence correlated with the duration of symptoms prior to biopsy, in one study being present in only 38% of those undergoing biopsy in the first 2 weeks, but in 89% of those with symptoms for more than 4 months (22).

Histological activity traditionally depends quantitatively on the additional presence of neutrophils. *Neutrophilic infiltration* begins as small accumulations of neutrophils in the capillaries and lamina propria but appear immediately attracted to adjacent crypt epithelium, which they invade (cryptitis—Fig. 4.3). This crypt invasion by neutrophils in ulcerative colitis is characteristically diffuse, involving most crypts in a biopsy. Diffuse crypt abscesses are uncommon in Crohn's disease but may be present in acute infections. However, in infection there is often a surprising reproducibility of the level of crypt abscesses from crypt to crypt, with a tendency to occur in the middle or upper crypt zone. In contrast, the crypt bases are most involved in ulcerative colitis but they occur throughout the mucosa. Ultimately, epithelial destruction occurs (crypt ulcers) which can result in crypt abscesses. These can enlarge, completely destroy the crypt epithelium, and extend into the lamina propria or submucosa, particularly distally. I prefer to amalgamate cryptitis, crypt abscess, and crypt ulcer into "crypt abscesses." Although not all stages may be present at the same time, all seem to occur under the same pathological circumstances.

The use of "crypt abscess" will include any or all of these situations. When activity is severe it may result in erosions or full thickness ulceration (Fig. 4.5).

It is important to realize that crypt abscesses are also a feature of acute colitis of numerous other causes; they indicate the activity of the acute inflammatory process rather than the underlying etiology. In contrast to other diseases, in ulcerative colitis the tendency for neutrophils to invade crypt or surface epithelium is so great that, if not present, the possibility that the disease under review is not ulcerative colitis should be strongly considered. Further, the presence of cryptitis and crypt abscesses in the face of architectural distortion and numerous basal lymphoid aggregates or a band is virtually pathognomonic, and a confident diagnosis of ulcerative colitis can be made. This picture is so rarely seen in Crohn's disease that, in view of its specificity, the term "nonspecific ulcerative colitis" should be abandoned.

Biopsy Reporting in Ulcerative Colitis

Large bowel biopsies in ulcerative colitis fall into distinctive categories, depending largely on the activity of the underlying disease; the way the results are reported varies with the reason the biopsies were taken (see preceding diagnostic criteria and the cases at the end of this chapter). No morphologic feature is specific for ulcerative colitis, but the certainty that ulcerative colitis is the underlying disease grows as the number of features increases.

Exceptions apply only to the inflammatory component as follows:

1. Distal biopsies may be less inflamed if the patient has been taking intensive steroid enemas. This information needs to be available for interpretation; relative rectal sparing does not therefore exclude the diagnosis (18) particularly in those with quiescent or treated disease.
2. Conversely, if the most proximal large bowel biopsy is from the vicinity of the ileocecal valve, it may be heavily inflamed in a patient with no other evidence of inflammation until much further distally (23). We have no idea why the 'kick' in inflammation occurs, but it should not by itself detract from the diagnosis.
3. Biopsies from inflammatory polyps, particularly if they consist only of a nubbin or granulation tissue, may give a false impression of focality (see Case 6 at the end of this chapter). This information should also be available.

Response to Therapy (Resolution)

When patients respond to treatment following an exacerbation of ulcerative colitis, the signs of clini-

Fig. 4.5. Ulceration of the rectum. Mucosa is completely destroyed with no visible epithelium.

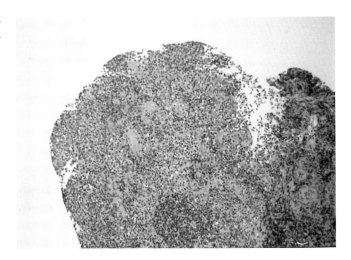

cal resolution often precede those of histologic resolution. In biopsies, the number of neutrophils begins to decrease, regenerative features become prominent, and epithelial continuity is restored. Goblet cells again became apparent and Paneth cells may (re)appear. Nuclei may remain enlarged but slowly return to their normal size. Architectural distortion is apparent but may completely resolve (4).

Change in Extent of Disease and Endoscopic/Histologic Correlation

Few studies have examined, by endoscopy and biopsy, the extent of disease and whether, or how, this changes with time. The problems of being certain exactly where one is to within a few centimeters between colonoscopies are almost impossible to solve. Despite these reservations, in one such study of 31 patients, 12 (39%) appeared to show an increase in the extent of disease, in 12 it appeared reduced, and in the remaining 7 it remained the same. In 61% of colonoscopies there was agreement between endoscopic and histologic extent of disease; the histologic extent exceeded the endoscopic extent in 28%; and the endoscopic extent was greater in the remaining 11% (24).

Unusual Histological Appearances in Ulcerative Colitis

It should be appreciated that while the patterns described above are classical, exceptions occur. Further, these exceptions have clinical significance and should be appreciated. These are as follows:

Lack of Atrophic or Regenerative Changes

The finding of an atrophic mucosa with typical regenerative features in patients with longstanding ulcerative colitis is always reassuring when review-

ing their histology, as it tends to confirm the correctness of the diagnosis. Nevertheless, such changes are not always present in patients with known ulcerative colitis, particularly under the following well-defined clinical circumstances:

1. Proximal biopsies, for example, from the right colon of patients with known extensive or total disease; in these patients, only the distal biopsies may show typical changes of atrophy. Similarly, patients with diffuse atrophic changes may only show evidence of active disease distally.
2. In patients with long-standing disease or at risk of developing carcinoma, not only may there be no evidence of atrophic changes, but crypts may be packed tightly together. Persistent Paneth cell metaplasia and a thickened muscularis mucosae may be the only markers of previous disease, but even these may be absent, particularly in biopsies.
3. There has been a suggestion that even in the first attack it may be impossible to readily distinguish between infection and inflammatory bowel disease because biopsies may not always show all of the expected abnormalities (4,25). This requires confirmation.

Granulomas and Giant Cells in Ulcerative Colitis

A recurring question is whether one is allowed granulomas in ulcerative colitis. Well-formed, sarcoid-like granulomas are not part of the spectrum of ulcerative colitis and if these are present, an alternative explanation must be sought. Isolated giant cells may, however, occur in ulcerative colitis close to ulcers, adjacent to crypts, or, rarely, isolated in the lamina propria (Fig. 4.6) (7,26), although the last always raises the question of Crohn's disease. Occasionally crypt abscesses may rupture,

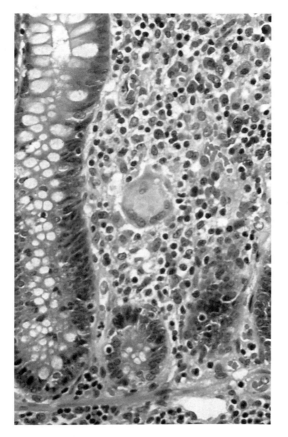

Fig. 4.6.   Ulcerative colitis with giant cells in the lamina propria (center).

causing extravasation of mucin into the lamina propria; this can stimulate the production of histiocytes, foreign body giant cells, and granulomas (27) immediately adjacent to ruptured crypts. They are usually not numerous and are acceptable in a patient with typical ulcerative colitis. A mucin stain may confirm this etiology, but may also be negative, in which case we accept them only if located adjacent to an ulcerated crypt. Lamina propria mac-

rophages frequently also stain positively in the absence of granulomas. It should be remembered that apart from Crohn's disease, there are numerous other causes of granulomas

Rectal Sparing and Irregular Transition to Active Disease in Fulminant Colitis

In patients with severe active disease, relative rectal sparing may be present (Fig. 4.7; see color plate). This may be marked in a first attack of what by all other criteria appears to be ulcerative colitis, with a very irregular and patchy transition to active ulcerating disease which may suggest that the underlying disease is Crohn's disease. Further, multiple biopsies may confirm this patchy tendency. Nevertheless, if these colons are resected, similar changes are often found at the proximal limit of disease. In most patients, there is nothing else to indicate that the underlying disease is anything but ulcerative colitis. However, some may prefer to call this pattern of involvement in a first attack "indeterminate colitis" (28,29). It is also possible that steroid enemas may result in a less severely affected rectal mucosa compared to that of the more proximal colon. Long-term studies to determine the natural history of this group of patients has not yet been carried out.

Backwash Ileitis

Backwash ileitis is a diffuse mucosal inflammation of the terminal ileum in continuity with active ulcerative colitis in the large bowel. It is observed in 10% to 20% of patients with total ulcerative colitis and usually extends only a few centimeters into the ileum, although it may sometimes extend up to 40 cm proximal to the ileocecal valve (30). Backwash ileitis may represent a reaction to regurgitation of colonic content into the terminal ileum, primary ileal involvement, or both. Interestingly, it

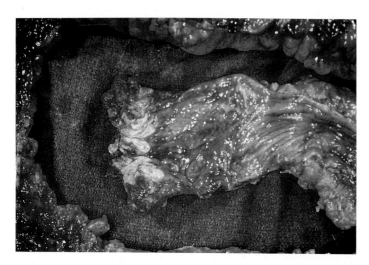

Fig. 4.7.   Active ulcerative colitis but with relative rectal sparing at resection ascribed to cecal steroid enemas. (See color plate.)

invariably resolves following colectomy. Although it is usually associated with a dilated, patulous ileocecal valve, it may occur when the cecum and ileocecal valve are not inflamed (31).

In backwash ileitis, the mucosa is macroscopically, diffusely abnormal and looks almost identical to the contiguous area of colonic disease; the calibre of the bowel is not greatly increased. In contrast, in terminal ileitis in Crohn's disease, the ileum may be strictured and contains aphthoid ulcers, as well as discontinuous or serpiginous ulceration, a cobblestone appearance, and fistulas (32).

Histologically, while backwash ileitis is very similar to colonic ulcerative colitis(32) although with less architectural distortion and fewer crypt abscesses, in some patients the redness is due to marked congestion rather than inflammation. However, studies in backwash ileitis have largely been carried out on resected specimens with its selection biases, so that the biopsy appearance is virtually undocumented. Acute terminal ileitis in Crohn's disease has many or all of the stigmata of that disease, including aphthoid ulcers, sarcoid-like granulomas, fissures, and transmural inflammation. Pyloric metaplasia may also be present.

The shallow ulceration in backwash ileitis rarely perforates (33), is rarely the site of carcinoma, and may be associated with the production of colonic-type sulfomucins (34). In addition, backwash ileitis does not seem to predispose the patient to the development of ileal pouchitis after ileal pouch-anal anastomosis (35). Nevertheless, pouches following colectomy for ulcerative colitis are at increased risk of developing pouchitis, in contrast to those in patients undergoing proctocolectomy for familial adenomatosis (see the next section). However, there is no contraindication to using the inflamed terminal ileum for construction of the ileal pouch or ileorectal anastomosis.

Crohn's Disease
Definition
Crohn's disease is a disease of unknown etiology that can affect any part of the gastrointestinal tract and occasionally other organs in addition. It is characterized in its active phase by aphthoid ulceration, often with adjacent cobblestoning, by a chronic inflammatory process that is usually transmural and composed of lymphoid aggregates and sometimes by granulomas, by fissures, abscesses and fistula tracts, and in the resolving phase by fibrosis that may result in strictures. It is characteristically a focal or multifocal disease radiologically, endoscopically, and pathologically, and has a remarkable capacity to recur following resections.

Like ulcerative colitis, there may be a variety of accompanying extra-intestinal manifestations that occasionally precede symptoms of the disease, but unlike ulcerative colitis there is some evidence that Crohn's disease, as manifest by granulomatous disease, may sometimes affect other organs such as bone as a metastatic process as well as by direct extension of local disease occasionally producing such conditions as granulomatous salpingitis.

Clinical Features
Ileocolic, small intestinal and upper gastrointestinal Crohn's disease occur in approximately 30% to 55%, 25% to 35%, and 5% to 10% of all cases respectively, whereas disease limited to the colon accounts for 15% to 25% (36–41). Anal lesions such as fistulae and ulceration are common. Symptoms are related to the location of the disease, its phase (active, resolving, fibrosed), or complications. Enterovaginal, enterovesical, and enterocutaneous fistulae may also occur resulting in passage of pus, gas, urine, or fecal material through the fistula. Perianal disease is common with a variety of features up to and including that described by the "watering-can," which is the result of numerous fistula.

Unusual Presentations
Fulminant colitis progressing to toxic dilatation is now rare but patients coming to colectomy following an unsatisfactory response to medical therapy is more common. Free perforation is rare and is seen particularly in the cecum or ascending colon (42) and may also occur through a carcinoma (43). Hemorrhage, which may be severe and sometimes catastrophic originates from aphthoid ulcers but is a further rare mode of presentation (44), although many of these are "indeterminate" colitis. Gastroduodenal disease may present as dyspepsia and multiple aphthoid ulcers may present in the oral cavity. Rarely, symptoms associated with carcinoma may occur in a by-passed small bowel, a rectal stump, and sometimes as a stricture with obstructive symptoms indistinguishable from that of the underlying disease. Ulcerative proctitis may be a presenting feature (16).

Gross and Endoscopic Appearances
Endoscopists are very familiar with the aphthoid ulcer/cobblestone phase of the disease (Fig. 4.8; see color plate), but pathologists are less familiar with this phase as resections are uncommon; it is particularly associated with new disease or its earliest recurrence clinically, and is also associated

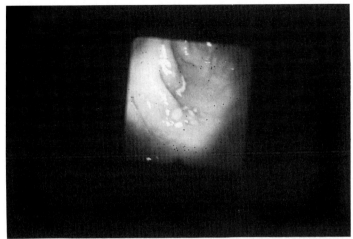

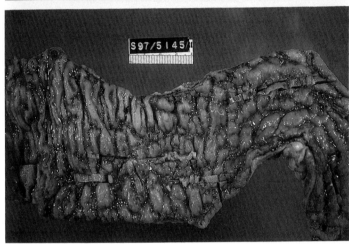

Fig. 4.8. (A) Crohn's disease with aphthoid ulcers forming snail tracks. (B) Resected colon showing cobblestoning and aphthoid ulcers some of which have linked up to form transverse and longitudinal ulcers. (See color plate.)

with focal acute inflammation histologically as discussed previously. Further, histological evidence suggests that fissures, and therefore fistulae, also have their origin in aphthoid or larger ulcers. If all of these are considered to be features of active disease, then the later phase is their sequelae, which can include abscesses, strictures, sometimes toxic dilatation and rarely carcinoma. Conceptually, it is both convenient, and reasonably correct to think of Crohn's disease in this manner.

Aphthoid Ulcer/Cobblestone Phase

The earlier macroscopic lesion of Crohn's disease seems to be the *aphthoid ulcer or erosion*. This is a pinpoint white based lesion surrounded by a halo with intervening normal mucosa; it is characteristic but not specific for the disease (45). In resected specimens aphthoid ulcers appear as red spots or focal mucosal depressions. When many aphthoid ulcers are present they may enlarge, become stellate and fuse with adjoining stellate (bear claw) ulcers (Fig. 4.8B). These may then enlarge to form ulcers that run primarily longitudinally (train track

ulcers) and usually overlay the tenia coli of the large bowel. Less obviously ulcers run transversely in the mucosa (Fig. 4.8B). The intervening mucosa and particularly the submucosa become very edematous and project into the lumen, the appearance resembling cobblestones. The cobblestoned mucosa may be surprisingly normal macroscopically. Ulcers may be the site of hemorrhage; although this usually occurs from large ulcers, occasionally a localized crop of small aphthoid ulcers may bleed profoundly. Some patients present with disease discretely affecting more than one region of the bowel; because the disease is discontinuous, ulcerative colitis should not be entertained.

Thickening of the Wall and Stricture Formation

This seems to follow the stage of aphthoid ulcers and cobblestoning. The wall is considerably thickened but the mucosa may retain the cobblestoned appearance often with longitudinal ulceration. The thickest areas are those in which transmural disease is usually found histologically (Fig. 4.9).

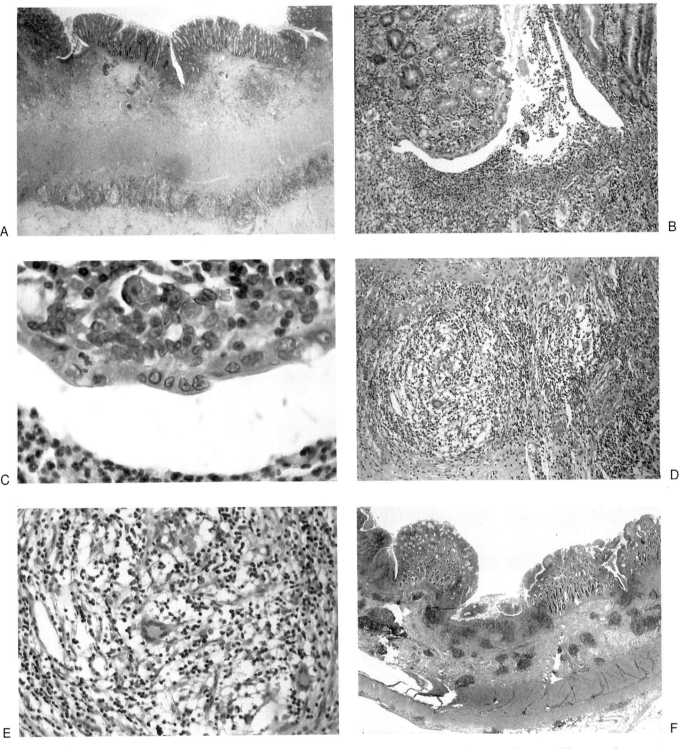

Fig. 4.9. Crohn's disease in which numerous aphthoid ulcers can be seen in the mucosa the details of one of which (top left) can be seen in (B) and (C). Note that transmural inflammation is already present with a row of lymphoid nodules and granulomas on the serosal aspect. The granulomas are shown in (D) and (E). However, the lymphoid tissue may not contain granulomas and be located primarily in the submucosa (F).

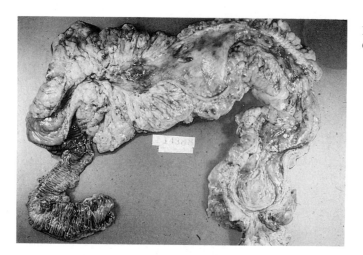

Fig. 4.10. Multiple large bowel strictures in Crohn's disease. (See color plate.)

The mechanism of narrowing seems to be a combination of development of a chronic inflammatory infiltrate, usually in the form of numerous submucosal and subserosal lymphoid aggregates that may also be admixed with granulomas. In addition, areas of ulceration heal by submucosal fibrosis that may be potentiated by duplication of the muscularis mucosae and thickening of the muscularis propria. The submucosal edema and lymphangiectasia that cause the cobblestoning may partly be reabsorbed but also has a distinct tendency to resolve by fibrosis contributing to the luminal narrowing. Tight and obstructing hosepipe strictures presumably are caused by fibrous contraction of thickened bowel and result in the typical "string sign" radiologically, or multiple strictures pathologically (Fig. 4.10; see color plate). The lumen within these strictures is frequently ulcerated. A further characteristic feature of strictures is the presence of a large irregular ulcer a few centimeters proximal. Obstructing strictures limited to a few cm of bowel are frequently treated with stricturoplasty rather than resection with subsequent resolution of most of the inflammation.

Fissures, Fistulae, and Abscesses

Sinuses and fissures both end blindly (sinuses are said to penetrate the muscularis propria) (46); in contrast fistula tracts have an origin and an exit. The smallest fissures seen microscopically are usually incidental findings arising directly from the edge of an aphthoid ulcer (Fig. 4.11). The origin of tracts is sometimes behind a sentinel inflammatory polyp. If an area of narrowing or stenosis is present, an ulcer immediately proximal is a common source, whereas if a previous anastomosis site is included in the resection, that should also be carefully probed.

Exit sites of fistula tracts are usually readily identified in adjacent loops of bowel because the mucosa in the immediately surrounding bowel appears completely uninvolved by the disease, although there is invariably an inflammatory polyp to identify the site. The course of tracts is often directly towards the muscularis propria, but they sometimes turn abruptly and run in the submucosa, often for a considerable distance, before

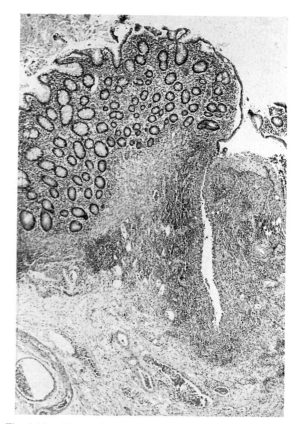

Fig. 4.11. Fissure beginning at the edge of an aphthoid ulcer.

Fig. 4.12. Crohn's disease with multiple fistulas. (See color plate.)

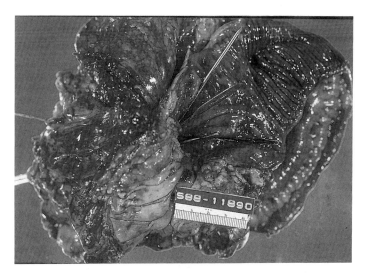

returning to the bowel, ending blindly, or turning into the muscularis propria; at this point it may again end blindly, run into an abscess cavity or continue as a fistula into another loop of bowel or organ (Fig. 4.12; see color plate).

Abscesses occur in about 10% to 25% of patients requiring surgery (47) and seem particularly associated with ileocecal and perianal disease. They can form at the end of a fissure, frequently in the mesentery but sometimes in the submucosa. Occasionally, large inflammatory masses are encountered that are the result of adherent loops of bowel with fistula and abscesses between. If a second tract opens into the same abscess the effect is to produce a fistula tract. They can also form in the postoperative period, particularly in patients with preoperative abscesses. Culture reveals the expected mixture of enteric flora, particularly *Escherichia coli*, Bacteroides, enterococci and *Streptococcus viridans* (48). Occasionally, unusual secondary organisms such as Actinomyces may be present (49).

Fissures are invariably lined by neutrophils with a surrounding infiltrate of histiocytes, other mononuclear cells beyond, and rarely granulomas. Yet, with time it is not uncommon to observe attempts to reepithelialize these tracts, at least in part (Fig. 4.13). The process of reepithelialization may extend not only into the submucosa and muscularis propria, sometimes causing colitis cystica profunda, but occasionally through the muscle into the pericolic tissues forming acquired diverticula. This has important clinical connotations, for while it is not unreasonable to suppose that if the driving force causing tracts to form is removed, whether by diversion of intestinal contents, parenteral nutrition, antibiotics, or combinations of

these, that these might undergo some degree of healing. Yet, if these were to become completely epithelialized, it is almost inconceivable that they could close down permanently any more than a loop of defunctioned bowel might become resorbed.

Other Unusual Appearances

A small proportion of patients present with more unusual macroscopic or clinical presentations including:

1. *Diffuse Disease.* Some patients have a relatively diffuse disease affecting what is usually most of the large bowel, and may bear a strong resemblance to ulcerative colitis (Fig. 4.14; see color plate). Areas of sparing are the major indicators that the underlying disease is likely not to be ulcerative colitis. Typically this may involve the rectum.

2. A *single longitudinal ulcer* limited to the mesenteric border of the small bowel. This presentation is seen particularly in parts of the world where Crohn's disease is relatively uncommon, and in those countries makes up quite a sizeable proportion of diagnosed cases.

3. *Single or multiple large punched out ulcers* arc occasionally the presenting feature of Crohn's disease; it is imperative to ensure that these patients are not on nonsteroidal antiinflammatory drugs (NSAIDs), which are the most frequent cause of solitary ulcers, particularly in the terminal ileum and right colon.

4. *Free perforation* may occur, usually in the right colon.

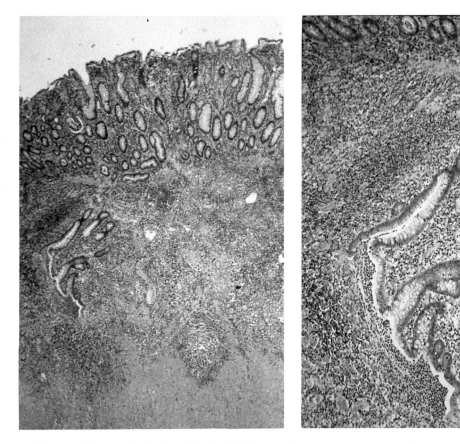

Fig. 4.13.   Partially reepithelialized fistula. (A) Mucosa is present at the top and a second group of crypts in the submucosa mid-left. (B) Detail shows the crypts to be part of a fistula which remains ulcerated on the left side.

5. *Miliary disease* is involvement of the bowel, usually the jejunum, in a granulomatous reaction visible on the outside of the bowel as numerous white specks and nodules resembling carcinomatosis peritonei or tuberculosis, often associated with free fluid. Histologically, they consist of a noncaseating granulomatous reaction (50–52).

In patients undergoing resection of the rectal stump, the gross and microscopic appearances may be particularly confusing. Diffuse disease may be

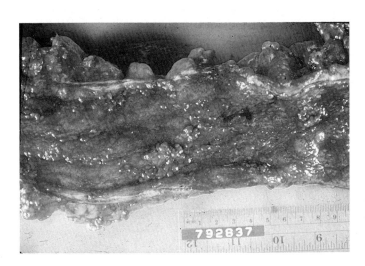

Fig. 4.14.   Crohn's disease masquerading as ulcerative colitis. Despite the diffuse colitis there were transmural granulomas histologically. (See color plate.)

part of the spectrum described above, or it may be part of diversion proctitis (see subsequent discussion).

Histology

The histological feature of Crohn's disease that can be found in resected specimens are (53,54):

1. *Ulcers*—initially aphthoid (Fig. 4.9A–C); that is, the ulcer often starts initially in a crypt base, or over a lymphoid nodule, an area which is known to contain cells designed for continuous sampling of luminal contents, the M-cells. Neutrophils migrate through this region with a stream of neutrophils emerging from it; it then forms a volcano-like lesion, and ultimately a nonspecific ulcer which may penetrate into or rarely through all layers of the bowel wall. Ulcers may have or develop an underlying zone of histiocytes, lymphocytes, and occasionally giant cells or granulomas (Fig. 4.9D,E).

   All changes tend to take place on a background of an uninflamed or relatively uninflamed mucosa.
2. *Fissures* may penetrate for a varying distance of direction into or through the bowel wall, may end blindly, or return to the lumen (Fig. 4.11).
3. *Abscesses* may form within or outside the bowel.
4. *Fistula tracts* may develop from fissures or abscesses.
5. *Lymphoid aggregates,* usually without germinal centres (Fig. 4.9F) are present focally in the most severely affected regions, arranged randomly or in a rosary bead array in the submucosa. A second row also resembling a rosary bead may be present in the subserosa with variable involvement of the muscularis propria or beyond.
6. *Granulomas* may be present in all layers of the bowel, nodes, or beyond.

One can also look at this in terms of the layer of the bowel affected as follows:

1. Epithelium
   a. Direct involvement in aphthoid ulcers.
   b. Crypts are not usually mucin depleted unless acutely inflamed.
   c. Features of previous healed ulcers.
   d. Intact epithelium may show architectural distortion.
   e. Pyloric metaplasia, mainly in the small bowel.
   f. Active regeneration may be present over ulcers.
   g. Adaptive changes, primarily in the terminal ileum (see text).
   h. Pyloric metaplasia, primarily in the terminal ileum.
2. Lamina propria
   a. Inflammation varies from normal, through an increase in all inflammatory cells in which plasma cells predominate; most importantly plasma cells may reach the muscularis mucosae, a feature of chronic disease and rarely seen in acute infections.
   b. If neutrophils are present they tend not to invade crypts, which for the most part are uninvolved, unlike active ulcerative colitis; a markedly focal acute cryptitis with surrounding focus of chronic inflammation may be present.
3. Muscularis mucosae
   a. Duplicated or markedly thickened and fibrotic at sites of present or previous ulceration.
4. Submucosa
   a. Marked edema and lymphangiectasia in cobblestoning.
   b. Fibrosis with proliferation of smooth muscle cells as cobblestoning resolves and strictures form.
   c. Neuronal hyperplasia may be present.
5. Muscularis propria
   a. Thickened, fibrotic, neuronal hyperplasia, pseudodiverticula.
6. Vascular
   a. Focal endothelial damage.
   b. Intimal proliferation and sometimes obliteration or thrombosis.
   c. Involvement in adjacent acute and chronic inflammation.
   d. Focal necrosis of the vessel wall.
   e. Granulomatous vasculitis (rare) (Fig. 4.15).
   f. Acute necrotizing vasculitis (rare).

Appearances in Biopsies
Although the diagnosis of IBD from other forms of colitis, and the distinction of Crohn's disease from ulcerative colitis have been discussed above, the criteria on which the diagnosis of Crohn's disease are made can be summarized as follows:

1. Large bowel, terminal ileal or gastroduodenal biopsies.
   a. Granulomas.
   b. Aphthoid ulcers (focal ulceration) (Fig. 4.2A,B).
   c. Markedly focal cryptitis.

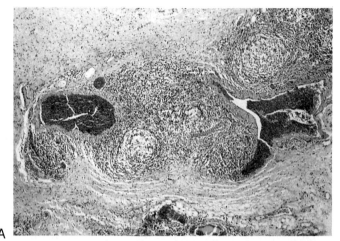

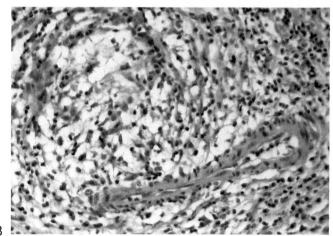

Fig. 4.15. Granulomatous involvement of vessels. (A) numerous veins filled with blood are surrounded by nodular granulomas. (B) Small venule towards the bottom and right apparently compressed by granulomas. Changes such as these give credence to a vascular component in some cases of Crohn's disease.

   d. Markedly focal chronic infiltration (Fig. 4.2C–F).
   e. Disproportionate submucosal inflammation.
2. Ileal biopsy.
   f. Pyloric metaplasia.
   g. Acute terminal ileitis especially in the absence of similar disease in the proximal colon.
   h. Jejunalization of ileal villi.
3. Gastroduodenal biopsies.
   i. Focal acute gastritis in *H. pylori* negative individuals not on NSAIDs.
   j. Focal acute duodenitis in *H. pylori* negative individuals not on NSAIDs.
4. Multiple large bowel biopsies.
   k. Proximal or focal distribution of ulceration.
   l. Evidence of prior focal or proximal ulceration.
      i. Proximal biopsies with architectural distortion together with distal biopsies showing architectural preservation.
      ii. Random architectural distortion in some biopsies but not others.
5. A false impression of focal disease can be obtained from.
   i. Biopsies of inflammatory polyps.
   ii. Biopsies of granulation tissue at anastomotic lines.
   iii. Chronic inflammation in cecal biopsies—(normal).
   iv. Lymphoid aggregates in terminal ileal biopsies (normal).

Aphthoid ulceration tends to occur over a lymphoid follicle but may occur in all epithelia in the gastrointestinal tract. However, larger ulcers appear to be surrounded by a zone of lymphoid tissue that could just as easily be reactive rather than primary.

Histological Sequence of Changes

Re-resections for a variety of reasons were examined histologically in patients who had undergone resection of all known Crohn's disease and in whom the margins were apparently free of disease.

This study suggested that the earliest lesions were small ulcers and granulomas, but that features associated with healing such as regeneration and pyloric-type metaplasia followed. Pyloric-type metaplasia may be accompanied by surface metaplasia also resembling gastric foveolar cells; both cell types are strongly immunoreactive for epidermal growth factor (urogastrone). Formation of this type of gland may be required for healing particularly in the small intestine (55). Lymphoid aggregates, whether submucosal or transmural, were a later phenomenon but were also closely related to each other. Large ulcers, sinuses, and strictures were in that order the final features that appeared, and required the longest time to develop (56). Fissures and fistula developed primarily proximal to sites of obstruction, which also supports the conclusion that they are a late feature of the disease (46,57).

Lack of Transmural Inflammation
Transmural inflammation may not be present in resections carried out for the following:

a. The acute or active phase of Crohn's disease, namely when fulminant disease (toxic dilatation) is present.
b. Uncontrollable bleeding during the cobblestone/aphthoid ulcer phase of the disease (58).
c. Rectal stumps that are excised for persistent anorectal disease.
d. Unremarkable Crohn's disease. A considerable search is sometimes required to find transmural disease emphasizing its focality. These findings suggest that lymphoid aggregates develop in longstanding disease and are a marker of chronicity.
e. Nonspecific ulcers that are sometimes the earliest feature of Crohn's disease.

Granulomas
In resected specimens granulomas have been present in 50% to 60% of cases (37,59,60) and in regional lymph nodes in 20% to 38% of cases (37,59,61,62). The reported frequency of granulomas in biopsies varies from 15% to 36% of cases (37,60,63,64), but depends on the definition used, and the number of biopsy specimens and sections examined (60). Microgranulomas can easily be overlooked due to their small size (less than about 200 μm) (65) and may require serial sections to demonstrate them. However, in clinical situations when a positive diagnosis of Crohn's disease will affect management, this may be essen-

tial. Careful examination of two large rectal biopsies may reveal granulomas in over 25% of patients if carefully sought (60). This significant chance of finding granulomas probably justifies taking multiple sections of a few biopsies.

Pathology of Recurrence Following Resection
The prevalence of recurrence varies with the means used to detect it. By far the highest prevalence occurs in those in whom recurrence is detected endoscopically, followed by symptomatic recurrence, and finally that proportion of patients requiring recurrent surgery. One endoscopic study examined 50 consecutive patients 6 weeks to 6 months after surgical resection of the terminal ileum and found that 70% had lesions in the neoterminal ileum. All had aphthoid ulcers and some larger or multiple ulcers. Half of the anastomotic lines were also ulcerated, and a third of these had large ulcers involving at least half of the circumference of the bowel (66). A similar study found a 73% recurrence rate in those undergoing endoscopy within a year of surgery although only 20% had symptoms; at 3 years these figures had increased to 85% and 34% respectively (67). It is possible that the recurrence rate can be reduced by longterm antibiotics (68) or immunosuppressive therapy. The pathology in resections is similar to that of typical disease, and can be considered as:

a. Persistent ulceration at an anastomosis line— this has the appearance of ulceration and granulation tissue.
b. Inflammatory polyps—these are usually larger portions of granulation tissue that may ultimately become reepithelialized.
c. Fistulas—these are only detected in resected specimens.
d. Strictures, often with ulceration within them. This is the only lesion in which transmural disease can be found if resection rather than stricturoplasty is carried out. The disease is usually immediately proximal to the anastomosis line reaching up to, and often a few millimeters or more beyond it.

Crohn's Disease in Sites Other Than the Small and Large Intestine

Crohn's disease may affect sites both within the gastrointestinal site and at a variety of sites beyond it, and should be considered separately from extraintestinal manifestations of inflammatory bowel, which are paraphenomena rather than direct involvement. Involvement may be by direct extension from disease within the gastrointestinal tract, but others seem to be examples of metastatic disease. Disease involving the mouth, pharynx, esophagus, stomach, or duodenum rarely represent as primary involvement and is invariably found in patients with disease elsewhere in the small or large intestine.

Oral Cavity

The mouth can be affected by granulomas, particularly within the minor salivary glands, but also by nodular granulomatous masses (69,70)

Esophageal Disease

This is rare and we are sceptical of cases with only esophageal disease, although we have seen large otherwise nonspecific esophageal ulcers precede other evidence of Crohn's disease. Esophageal disease can be transient and heal but others may persist despite steroids, or have multiple relapses in the esophagus (71,72). Usually it is found in patients with severe and extensive disease in other parts of the gastrointestinal tract (73) and ranges from longitudinal serpiginous ulcers and cobblestoning with stricture formation to nonspecific inflammation and superficial ulceration that can be impossible to distinguish from reflux disease. Granulomas are rare on biopsy.

Gastroduodenal Disease

There has also been a suggestion that in Crohn's disease there may be increased numbers of histiocytes in the duodenum (74).

At least 2% to 3% of patients have symptoms ascribable to gastroduodenal disease, and endoscopic or histologic changes may be present in up to 70% of patients if searched for and can affect oxyntic, antral, or duodenum (75) although granulomas are relatively infrequent (76).

Gastric disease is usually focal and antral (5,77), and in our population Crohn's gastritis is the most common cause of focal chronic and acute gastritis in *H. pylori* negative patients; NSAIDs tend not to have such intense focal chronic inflammation accompanying the acute inflammation. Rarely, giant gastric ulcers may be present (78).

Duodenal involvement is easiest to diagnose when it does not involve the first and second parts of the duodenum where *H. pylori* disease is most prevalent and with NSAIDs is probably the most common cause of *Helicobacter* negative duodenitis in our biased patient population. In patients with suspected but not definitively proven Crohn's disease on conventional gastroduodenoscopy, it is sometimes useful to examine the upper gastrointestinal tract with a long endoscope.

Endoscopic features are similar to those elsewhere in the intestinal tract; histologically typically focal disease is the rule in the absence of granulomas. *H. pylori* infection is relatively uncommon in patients with Crohn's disease, possibly because of the relatively young age of this population, or the large numbers of antibiotics taken by patients with Crohn's disease. The morphologic differential diagnosis is primarily with other causes of focal inflammation and ulceration, primarily nonsteroidal anti-inflammatory drugs (NSAIDs). Localized ulcer disease associated with NSAIDs can produce a virtually identical biopsy appearance to that seen in Crohn's disease. The endoscopic finding of cobblestoning in association with aphthoid ulcers, particularly when in the distal duodenum, markedly increased the likelihood that the underlying disease is due to Crohn's disease. Because upper gastrointestinal disease usually occurs in patients with documented disease elsewhere, caution should be exercised about making a primary diagnosis of Crohn's disease in the upper part of the gastrointestinal tract. Nevertheless the appearances are sometimes so characteristic that they can allow a "highly suggestive" diagnosis in the absence of other features clinically. Rare cases have been described presenting as Meckel's diverticulitis (79).

Appendiceal Disease

The appendix can be involved as an isolated finding, or in patients with Crohn's disease either contiguous or remote from other disease. As an isolated finding it rarely portends the development of Crohn's disease (80,81); investigation for Crohn's disease elsewhere is not justified. Only rarely is Crohn's disease of the appendix found with remote disease (82) although in about a quarter of terminal ileal resections that include the appendix, appendiceal inflammation is present often with little or no mucosal ulceration, but with a transmural infiltrate of lymphoid aggregates otherwise similar or identical to those seen in Crohn's disease. It is not known if this really is Crohn's disease localized to the appendix only. First, there appears to be no increased incidence of fistula formation after the resection of such an appendix. Second, unless Crohn's disease is also present in the adjoining colon or terminal ileum, there seems to be little evidence of an increased risk of subsequent Crohn's disease, and this seems at most to be no more than 10% (83,84). In patients with concurrent or prior Crohn's disease, symptoms may be more longstanding and other features of chronic disease may be present (85). Virtually all appendices in resections for Crohn's disease are abnormal, but more specific features are seen in about half (86)

Sometimes an appendix is removed that has features of Crohn's disease. This may be in the form of granulomas either affecting any or all layers of the appendix (80–84). Under these circumstances the most likely diagnosis is Yersinia, particularly if some of the granulomas have neutrophils at their center. However, other causes of granulomas including worms have to be considered. Granulomatous appendicitis seems rarely to progress to Crohn's disease unless there is other evidence of Crohn's disease at the time of resection.

Pathological Evaluation of Resected Margins

The main question here is whether the presence of Crohn's disease at the resected margin increased the likelihood of recurrence, or decreases the time interval to recurrence, and whether these parameters can be influenced by ensuring that where possible resection and therefore anastomoses are carried out through normal bowel. In one study with an 18 year follow-up, 31% of patients undergoing "radical" resection (not well defined) had "recurrence" compared with 83% undergoing "nonradical" resections (87). However, numerous biases are present, the most obvious being a lack of standardization of margins, patients with extensive disease invariable but not surprisingly having less normal bowel resected at the margins (88).

Inflammation likely extends well beyond any resected margins as judged by histologic inflammation including granulomas in apparently normal mucosa (65,89) and magnifying colonoscopy (90).

There is modest literature on whether microscopic involvement of resected margins is associated with an increased rate of recurrence. The definition of what constitutes disease at the margin is not standardized. The majority of papers suggest that microscopic disease at a resected margin is not associated with an increased rate of recurrence, but the trend is that microscopic disease usually has an increased clinical or suture line recurrence rate of about 5% to 35% more than those without disease over the time of study, and particularly if recurrence is in the form of aphthous ulceration, but that this never reaches clinical significance (91–96). One study utilizing frozen sections did not find these to be of value in predicting recurrence (97). However, one study found a very high "recurrence" rate of 90% at 8 years in what may be highly selected patients with unexpected microscopic

disease (98), whereas another found that as well as an age under 20 being a high risk for recurrence, that patients with a 10 cm margin of histopathologically normal bowel (not further defined) had a 21% chance of recurrence versus 50% of this was less (99). By multivariate analysis, microscopic involvement of the resected margin was second only to the number of resections carried out in predicting recurrence (100). Despite this, there has been little enthusiasm for carrying out frozen sections on margins, because it is recognized that this may be focal and also difficult to be certain about on suboptimal frozen sections.

Fulminant Colitis and Toxic Megacolon

Fulminant colitis results in hemorrhage or perforation and usually correlates with ulceration into the muscularis propria; if this progresses to involve the entire thickness of the muscularis propria, perforation is a distinct possibility. Cyclosporin appears to be playing a dramatic role in reducing the need for surgery in patients with fulminant disease. Overall mortality is said to be about 15%, but now seems to be considerably less. Perforation is the single most important determinant of the prognosis, with a mortality of about 50% (101,102). Although no definite explanation is yet available for toxic megacolon, of the specific factors studied, the extent and depth of ulceration have the strongest correlation with the area of dilatation (101,103). Life-threatening hemorrhage, which may be one of the manifestations of fulminant colitis, may also occur.

Toxic megacolon is reported to occur in 2% to 4% of all patients with ulcerative colitis (104,105). It may develop at any time but is most commonly seen early in the course of inflammatory bowel disease; it may be the presenting manifestation. The onset of fulminant disease is usually acute and severe, and there may be no previous symptoms of inflammatory bowel disease before the illness; most patients require urgent operation or surgery following a short period of unsuccessful medical management (29,105–108). Dilatation is usually greatest in the transverse colon (Fig. 4.16; see color plate) on the flexures or cecum but may involve other parts of the colon; occasionally it involves almost the entire colon.

Although tempting to want to divide all fulminant colitis into ulcerative colitis or Crohn's disease, life is never so simple. There are numerous causes of fulminant colitis including virtually every infection known. It should also be recalled that in

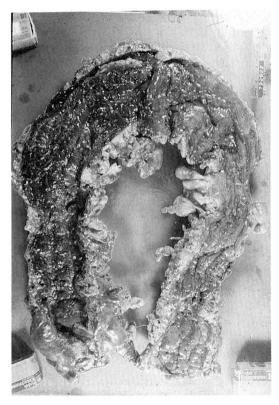

Fig. 4.16.   Fulminant ulcerative colitis with disease that is most severe on the left side and with dilatation in the transverse colon. (See color plate.)

Table 4.4.   Feature of indeterminate colitis of any cause.

Macroscopic features
    Rectal sparing.
    A patchy and often marked focal junction with active
       disease which can resemble aphthoid ulcers.
    Deep fissuring or broad ulcers with relatively little
       inflammation of variable death from the submucosa, into
       or through the muscularis propria, sometimes with
       perforation.
    Intervening mucosa may resemble cobblestoning and
       inflammation including longitudinal but not aphthoid
       ulcers, although histologic features.
    Ulcerated areas are frequently hemorrhagic with marked
       vasodilatation and little inflammation.
    Ulcers may be fissuring or broad extending into or through
       the muscularis propria.
    Residual mucosa may have architectural distortion
       indicating prior mucosal disease
       (if diffuse and worse distally this strongly suggests
       ulcerative colitis)
    Mucosal inflammation varies from none to intense, is
       usually sparse even in areas of ulceration.
    No granulomas unless containing foreign material.
    No well-formed lymphoid aggregates.
Additional features suggesting Crohn's or other disease/
    unlikely to be ulcerative colitis:
    Skip areas grossly.
    Granulomas unrelated to ulcers or lamina propria mucin.
    Lymphoid aggregates in submucosa or subserosa, especially
       if unrelated to adjacent ulceration.

acute infectious colitis a pathogen cannot be grown in up to 50% of patients; a similar proportion of culture-negative infections could therefore also occur in fulminant colitis. Further, even in patients with known ulcerative colitis or Crohn's disease some fulminant colitides may be infection-mediated. It is therefore perhaps not surprising that some cases do not fit conveniently into either ulcerative colitis or Crohn's disease. In patients with a clear history of ulcerative colitis, who have diffuse disease and additional features only of fulminant colitis, can remain classified as ulcerative colitis rather than as indeterminate colitis. The term "fulminant colitis of uncertain etiology" seems a preferable term in those in whom the diagnosis is not clearly ulcerative colitis or Crohn's disease, although it is these patients who are usually classified as indeterminate colitis (see subsequent section). A comparison of ulcerative colitis, Crohn's disease, and toxic megacolon is shown in Table 4.4.

There is a developing trend at some hospitals to construct a pouch at the same time as the colonic resection in patients with no evidence of Crohn's disease. Although histological examination to ensure that no features of Crohn's disease are present is ideal, this obviously cannot be carried out in a one stage procedure so that the validity of this approach must await the results of well performed prospective studies (see subsequent section and that on pouchitis).

Gross Appearances

In fulminant colitis without dilatation, external examination usually shows only minimal external changes, as might be expected in a disease predominantly affecting the mucosa and submucosa. However, the muscularis propria may be involved, and perforation may occur in the absence of toxic dilatation; in this case, serosal changes are again present. In the affected area mucosal ulceration is severe, with frequent ulceration extending into the muscularis propria, which may be completely penetrated and accompanied by extensive myocytolysis. The most severely involved mucosa is dark red or purple, hemorrhagic, and friable, with extensive ulceration that may bleed profusely, and may dominate the clinical picture. The mucosa is covered by a mixture of blood, mucus, pus, necrotic debris, and liquid stool. Extensive and deep ulceration, commonly exposes the underlying submucosa or muscularis propria. Because the circular muscle is the first exposed, numerous circumferential or partially circumferential, discrete ridges may be apparent. The more usual haustral pattern is not present at this stage of the disease. Confluence of ulcers may produce longitudinal furrows and often leaves isolated polypoid islands of mucosa. Deep fissuring, which in nonfulminant disease is more characteristic of Crohn's disease, can also be seen in fulminant colitis.

Some patients have rectal sparing usually attributed to local steroids (but sometimes seen in those receiving systemic steroids or immunosuppressives, and a transition zone consisting of aphthoid ulcers that continue into tram track ulcers or more diffuse disease. These features can be seen in fulminant colitis of any cause; it is when there is no prior documented colitis that these cases tend to be classified as indeterminate colitis (see subsequent section).

Histology

Irrespective of the underlying disease, the residual mucosa shows marked variation in the amount of architectural distortion, mucin depletion, inflammation, and congestion. It is frequently very congested and hemorrhagic, with large, dilated, vascular channels (Fig. 4.17A,B) and variable penetration into or through the submucosa and muscularis propria (Fig. 4.17C,D). The epithelium may show virtually no architectural distortion, particularly if this is part of the first attack either for the patient or in that part of the bowel. If there has been previous involvement, distortion is usual. The adjacent ulcers usually extend variably into the

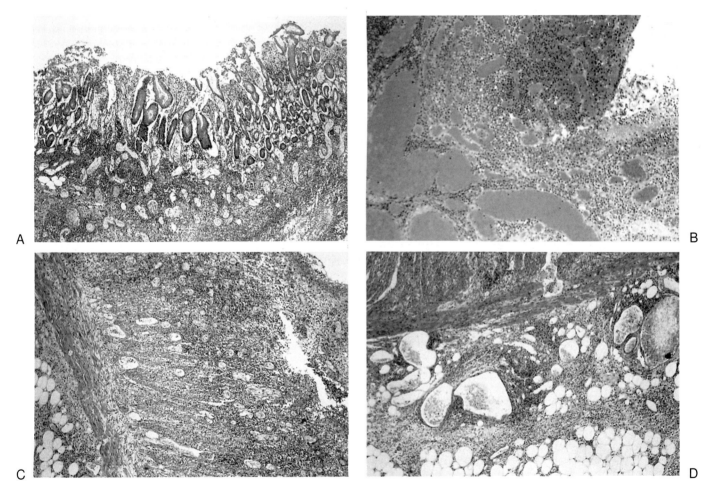

Fig. 4.17. Fulminant colitis. (A) Relatively unaffected mucosa with numerous dilated capillaries in the mucosa and submucosa. (B) Edge of true pseudopolyp left with adjacent ulceration into the submucosa (right). Note the marked vasodilatation (C) Vasodilatation with relatively mild inflammation can extend into and destroy the muscularis propria (myocytolysis)—the serosa is on the left (D) Detail of residual muscularis propria (top) with only a few remaining strands and inflammation well into the subserosa.

submucosa or muscularis propria, and knife-like fissures may develop and perforate in the absence of dilatation. Myocytolysis is marked, and the muscularis propria almost seems to have been melted away by ectatic vascular channels (Fig. 4.17C,D). Ultimately, this process may be complete, with the serosal tissue and peritoneum alone separating the lumen from the peritoneal cavity; perforation may therefore follow. Some patients have associated cytomegalovirus infection, which may well increase the severity of the disease (109). Rarely, subserosal fibrosis may be present, indicating a previous peritoneal reaction.

In patients treated medically the ulcerated surfaces may reepithelialize, so that new mucosa forms directly over or in the muscularis propria, presumably representing reepithelialization of prior deep ulcers; it may also result in numerous localized inflammatory polyps (Fig. 4.18; see color plate) or diffuse colitis cystica profunda.

Indeterminate Colitis (Colitis of Uncertain Etiology)

Originally, the term *indeterminate colitis* was proposed for unclassifiable cases (not overtly ulcerative colitis or Crohn's disease) of fulminant disease (28,110). However, this is now commonly used for any patient in whom the diagnosis of IBD has been made but in whom the underlying disease process is unclear, particularly regarding the presence of ulcerative colitis or Crohn's disease. For example, a Norwegian study examining new cases of IBD had a total of 525 cases of UC and 93 cases of indeterminate colitis yielding a mean annual incidence of 13.6/10(5) and 2.4/10(5), respectively (111). In another study indeterminate colitis had a worse long term prognosis than definite ulcerative colitis (112). Nevertheless the primary use of this term is in patients with fulminant colitis; its major implication the subsequent behavior. The major features of indeterminate colitis are shown in Table 4.4. In this setting the key data are why some patients apparently defy classification and the implications of this observation, in particular:

a.   Data regarding the proportion of these patients who subsequently develop Crohn's disease, hopefully before an ileoanal pouch anastomosis is carried out in whom Crohn's was found in the resected colon, and whether this is related to subsequent pouchitis or the need to remove the pouch.

b.   In those patients undergoing a ileoanal pouch anastomosis, the prevalence of pouchitis in patients clearly developing subsequent Crohn's disease and in those who do not.

c.   The frequency and reasons why pouches need to be removed.

In patients with a known history of ulcerative colitis or Crohn's disease, it is reasonable to assume that fulminant disease is occurring in that condition unless there is good evidence to the contrary. A more difficult problem arises in patients presenting for the first time with fulminant colitis, or in those in whom a firm clinical diagnosis was never established prior to colectomy. These are the 5% to 10% of patients in whom when all clinical and pathologic features have been reviewed, a firm diagnosis either of ulcerative colitis or of Crohn's disease is difficult or impossible.

Reasons that a firm diagnosis may be difficult or impossible include:

a.   Patients with fulminant colitis but with rectal sparing (histologically as well as clinically, suggesting that this is not ulcerative colitis). There is a distinct transition zone from normal to abnormal in which aphthoid ulceration may be present, and then longitudinal ulceration often in a tram-track manner that together strongly suggest Crohn's disease. In some patients the longitudinal ulcers are partially masked by relatively diffuse disease (Fig. 4.19; see color plate). Further, biopsies may show typical features of aphthoid ulcers as described above. It is these patients that if resected rarely have other supporting evidence of Crohn's disease such as transmural lymphoid aggregates or granulomas that would support a diagnosis of Crohn's disease). In many patients the focal transition is also present proximally (Fig. 4.19).

b.   Genuine overlapping histologic features—although this sounds reasonable, transmural inflammation is usually diffuse as any hint of lymphoid aggregates immediately raises the suggestion of Crohn's disease. Aggregates of inflammation in the subserosa are plasma cells rather than lymphoid as seen in Crohn's disease.

c.   Because the underlying disease is the result of another cause such as an infection or possibly a drug effect.

What is the likelihood of Crohn's disease occurring in patients with indeterminate colitis? In one report, a confident diagnosis of Crohn's disease was made in 9 of 23 "unclassified" cases utilizing

Fig. 4.18. Fulminant colitis (A) Residual mucosal islands and ulceration down to the visible circular muscle. (B) Inflammatory polyps with adjacent mucosa that has become re-epithelialized. Note that the submucosa is pink and fibrosed with direct continuity with the muscularis propria, indicating previous ulceration at this site. (See color plate.)

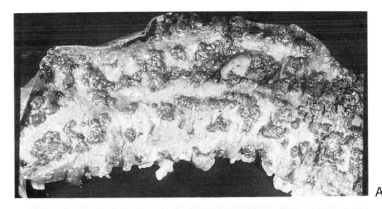

A

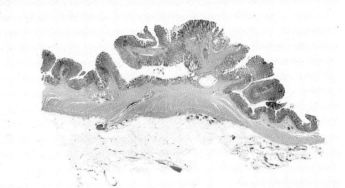

B

preoperative biopsy specimens and/or follow-up materials available. However, another report stated that none of the patients examined was subsequently reclassified as having Crohn's disease (28). Some patients with apparent ulcerative colitis who undergo resection for fulminant disease subsequently develop features of Crohn's disease. It is unclear whether these patients had Crohn's disease all along or whether they originally had ulcerative colitis or another form of colitis and subsequently developed Crohn's disease.

The implications of the diagnosis of indeterminate colitis for ileoanal pouch anastomoses is discussed in the following section under "failure."

Pouchitis

Although colectomy and ileostomy are suitable for both patients with ulcerative colitis and Crohn's disease with universal colitis, ileal anal pouch anastomosis appears to be an excellent alternative for most patients. However there are some drawbacks,

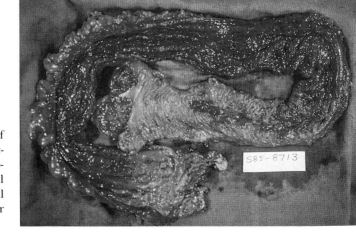

Fig. 4.19. Indeterminate colitis (colitis of unknown etiology), here resulting from rectal sparing (lower right), a transition to apparently diffuse disease but with longitudinal ulcers more proximally, and at the proximal limit of disease multifocal ulcers. (See color plate.)

primarily different forms of pouch dysfunction. This includes early problems associated with healing of anastomosis lines or transient ischemia to longterm complications such as pouchitis, pelvic sepsis, intestinal obstruction, and fistulas. Pouches are said to be contraindicated in those with Crohn's disease because of the problem of postoperative recurrence in the pouch. Interestingly pouchitis appears to develop almost entirely in those patients with IBD, the prevalence in patients with familial polyposis is rare—less than 5%. This has clear implications regarding the etiology of the disease and its implications. Other occasional complications include small bowel obstruction, and anal strictures, the latter being primarily seen in males.

Pouchitis is mucosal and submucosal inflammation in an ileal pouch used for continent ileostomy or ileal pouch-anal anastomosis. The reported frequency varies from 10% to almost 50% (35,113–118). In a series from the Mayo clinic the prevalence was 15% at 1 year, 36% at 5 years, and 46% at 10 years (119). Similar figures were obtained from Sweden where the cumulative risk of developing mild pouchitis was 21, 26, and 39% at 6, 12, and 48 months, respectively; the corresponding cumulative risk of developing severe pouchitis was 9, 11, and 14%, respectively. The overall risk was 51% at 48 months. The occurrence of pouchitis, calculated at six-month intervals after closure of the loop ileostomy, was highest (23.1 percent) during the first six months; during the next six-month period it was 11.4% and only 3.1% thereafter. Thirty-two patients (21.5%) had chronic continuous symptoms requiring long-term metronidazole treatment, and 14 (9.4%) of those had chronic severe pouchitis (120). Pouchitis can manifest at any time after construction of the pouch, but the first episode usually occurs in the first year postoperatively (121).

There is modest correlation between symptoms, endoscopic appearances, and pathology. Whereas some patients with severe symptoms have a severely inflamed and ulcerated pouch, in others both the endoscopic and biopsy findings are far less marked than might be expected from the symptoms. Pouchitis does not include the duskiness and even ulceration that may be present in the first days or weeks after construction of the pouch, and which likely has an ischemic component, and seems unrelated to subsequent pouchitis which occurs following the reanastomosis of the pouch in continuity with the rest of the intestinal tract.

The etiology of pouchitis is complex, and this subject is thoroughly discussed in Chapter 41.

Failure of Pouches—Risk from Indeterminate Colitis and Crohn's Disease

Poor functional results, pelvic sepsis, and unsuspected Crohn's disease are the major causes of pouch failure, while pouchitis was not (122,123). In one study, 8/158 patients with ulcerative colitis required removal of their pouches, and 3 of 16 patients with indeterminate colitis (124). Another study found that indeterminate colitis predisposed particularly to perianal complications (125). In a third study, of 18 patients with indeterminate colitis, 9 patients experienced complications (50%) vs. 8 of 235 patients with chronic ulcerative colitis (3%).

The risk of eventual ileostomy increased dramatically in some studies with the diagnosis of indeterminate colitis or Crohn's disease rather than ulcerative colitis following colectomy, often because of perineal complications. In one study this was 0.4% in patients with chronic ulcerative colitis vs. 28% in patients with indeterminate colitis (126). In a second study of 543 patients, the results were:

1. *Preoperative diagnosis*—UC-499, indeterminate colitis(IC)—42, CD in 2. *Postoperatively,* the diagnosis changed in 20 with UC (13 to IC, 7 to CD). Another 2 with IC showed evidence of CD in the resected rectal specimen.
2. *On follow up,* an additional 13 were found to have CD (5 from IC, 8 from UC). Thus the final diagnosis was:

	Perineal complications	Pouch failure
UC	23%	2%
IC	44%	12%
CD	63%	37%

Only 3% of patients with ulcerative colitis compared with 13% of patients with indeterminate colitis had a change in diagnosis to Crohn's disease (127).

Failure always raises the question of undiagnosed Crohn's disease. This occurs in about 5% of pouches, but tends to result in pelvic sepsis (127). Refractory pouchitis does not usually indicate Crohn's disease, but severe disease may be associated with extraintestinal manifestations such as arthritis. Failure also seems particularly to be associated with indeterminate colitis; in patients with indeterminate colitis coming to resection, there is increasing evidence that compared to patients with ulcerative colitis, those undergoing restorative proctocolectomy with indeterminate colitis have a greater number of complications including the need to remove the pouch (124,125,128–130).

Complications are more common in patients with possible Crohn's disease, whether called indeterminate colitis or outright Crohn's disease (130).

Histologic Findings

Histologic findings can mimic both ulcerative colitis, infection, and Crohn's disease. It includes a nonspecific increase in chronic inflammatory cells in the lamina propria with villous blunting, patchy intraepithelial and lamina propria neutrophils, and plasma cell infiltration. There is usually expansion of inflammatory cells into the villi, giving an impression of villous atrophy, with mucin changes more reflecting a large bowel rather than small bowel pattern, although with preservation of small bowel enzymes suggesting that this metaplasia is partial (131,132). Early changes (6 weeks) are characterized by neutrophilic and eosinophilic inflammation, mild villus atrophy, Paneth cell hyperplasia, a partial transition to colonic mucin phenotype, and an increased proliferation index. These features remained relatively stable after 6 months, except for a greater degree of mononuclear infiltration, a progressive increase in the degree of eosinophilic inflammation and a new higher steady state level of crypt epithelial kinetics (132). If the changes are severe, cryptitis, crypt abscesses, and ulceration may occur, but neutrophils may remain largely in the lamina propria with relatively little epithelial infiltration, thereby mimicking infection. Acute inflammation appears after chronic inflammation and is related to the severity of pouchitis. The histology can be very focal (Fig. 4.20). In one study of biopsies from 60 patients undergoing repeated pouch biopsies, patients could be divided into three groups based on the severity and fluctuation of histological inflammation: a) In 45% chronic changes were minor and acute inflammation was never seen, b) in 42% chronic changes were more severe and there were transient episodes of acute inflammation, c) in 13% severe chronic and severe acute inflammation were constantly present.

Differentiation of the three groups had clearly occurred within six months from closure of the ileostomy. Patients in the third group could be identified on histological criteria within weeks of closure of the ileostomy and were those exclusively at risk of developing chronic pouchitis. Chronic pouchitis never occurred in patients from the first two groups. Histological assessment of the reservoir mucosa within a few months after closure of the ileostomy therefore seemed to define patients who will and who will not subsequently develop pouchitis (133). One could therefore advocate pouch biopsy to determine which patients are most likely to encounter severe problems, but begs the question of longterm management.

If pouches are taken down, the question remains of whether the features present would support a diagnosis of Crohn's disease. Because fissuring ulcers, granulomas, and transmural lymphoid aggregates, are usually absent (114,134,135), the question is always whether to interpret their presence as evidence of Crohn's disease, but follow-up has not been long enough to confirm that this is correct. Pyloric metaplasia is a feature of ulceration irrespective of the underlying cause. It can therefore be expected nonspecifically and helps little in the differential diagnosis. Care must be taken particularly with granulomas to ensure that they do not contain foreign material.

Neoplastic Complications of Pouches

There are anecdotal reports of patients who have developed aneuploidy (136), adenomas, and even carcinoma associated with pouches, but these cases are currently rare (135,137,138). Similar rare cases are documented following conventional ileostomy (34), it is unclear whether pouches are at any additional risk.

Neoplasia in the Remaining Rectal Mucosa

In ulcerative colitis although theoretically all of the rectal mucosa down to the anoderm is excised, in practice this may not be carried out because anal function is better preserved if a centimeter or two of lower rectal mucosa is deliberately not removed. In both ulcerative colitis and familial adenomatous polyposis this mucosa remains at risk of development of carcinoma. In patients with ulcerative colitis undergoing a pouch procedure who already have rectal dysplasia this is particularly likely to be a problem (135,137,138). There is therefore little alternative to regular inspection of this cuff of mucosa in the same way that would be carried out had the initial operation carried out been an ileorectal anastomosis, with regular destruction of new polyps in familial adenomatous polyposis or biopsy for dysplasia in patients with ulcerative colitis. The question is whether the additional effort would justify the return. (This is discussed in more detail in Chapters 11 and 13).

Benign Strictures

Benign strictures are local sequelae of severe ulcerative colitis but part of the usual spectrum of Crohn's disease (Fig. 4.10). In ulcerative colitis strictures are usually of little consequence to the patient and are not an indication for colectomy

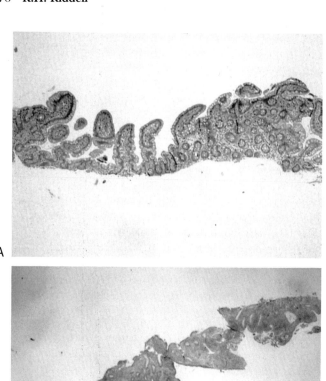

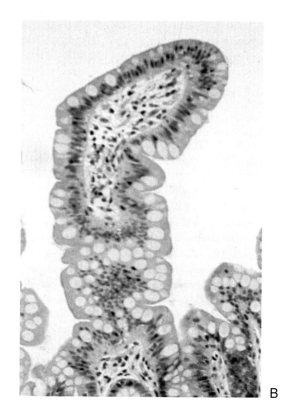

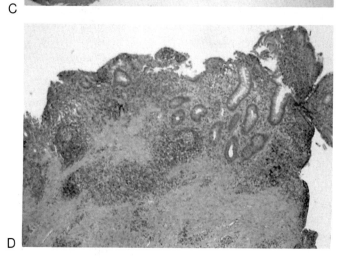

Fig. 4.20.   Pouchitis. (A) Biopsy in which the left half is largely normal (detail in B), but with inflammation on the right side. (C and D) Biopsy from a different part of the pouch at the same time. There is very heavy inflammation.

unless they are suspected of being malignant. However, colectomy is sometimes considered if there is doubt as to their underlying pathology or, in total colitis, if they prevent the colonoscopist from traversing the narrowest part of the stricture to biopsy the remainder of the colon. Strictures are usually smooth, may be multiple, and are sometimes reversible, either spontaneously or with glucagon (suggesting that they are primarily muscular). They are rarely sufficiently narrow to cause obstruction. Benign strictures have been attributed to hypertrophy of the muscularis mucosae (139), but they may also include fibrosis of the submucosa and often of the muscularis propria, presumably as a result of previous severe ulcerative disease as seen in benign strictures most commonly seen in patients with long-standing disease, although they are occasionally observed at presentation (140–142). The key question, particularly in ulcerative colitis, is the frequency with which apparently benign strictures may harbor an unsuspected carcinoma.

Diversion Proctocolitis

Diversion of the fecal stream is carried out either to bypass or protect diseased bowel, for example in Crohn's disease, and sometimes collagenous colitis, when it has beneficial effects on the distal diseased bowel. It can also be used to protect bowel, for example when an anal pouch is protected prior to reanastomosis with ileum. It may also be incidental when diseased bowel is resected proximally and a portion of bowel remains distally, usually the rectum. The latter occurs in patients with inflammatory bowel disease, diverticular disease and carcinoma. Its main problem is in patients who have undergone resection for colitis, in whom this may be misinterpreted as recurrence of the colitis, for which it may be resected, rather than diversion disease that will resolve following restoration of the fecal stream. Under these circumstances it is always useful to examine the distal margin of the colectomy specimen, which is frequently uninflamed.

Diversion proctocolitis and enteritis are inflammatory changes that can occur in the rectum and distal colon or small bowel after surgical diversion has been performed. In the large bowel it results in a bloody and mucoid discharge and is almost universal endoscopically and histologically if looked for, tends to cause a bloody discharge or abdominal pain, may be an incidental endoscopic finding, and resolves following reanastomosis (143,144). The etiology of diversion colitis is not yet clear. Because it resolves following reestablishment of the fecal stream, there is something in the fecal stream or resulting from its loss that potentiates this disease. It may be an inflammatory state resulting from a nutritional deficiency, especially short-chain fatty acids, in the lumen of the colonic epithelium (145). Although initial reports suggested a deficiency disease, prospective double blind trials have not demonstrated an advantage although anecdotal patients may respond (146).

The endoscopic appearances in diversion proctitis of the rectum may resemble those of ulcerative colitis, Crohn's disease, or infectious colitis in having a granular, nodular, erythematous and friable mucosa. Mucosal nodules or inflammatory polyps may be present; sometimes a patchy distribution and even aphthous ulcers are found (143–145, 147,148).

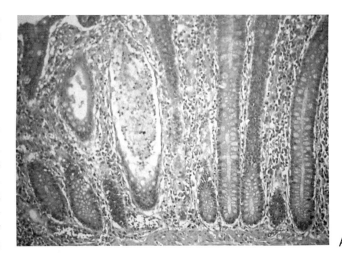

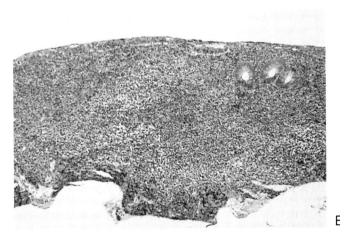

Fig. 4.21. Diversion colitis. (A) Chronic inflammation in the lamina propria reaching down to the muscularis mucosae and with a dilated crypt containing mucus and neutrophils (B) Follicular proctitis with numerous lymphoid nodules containing germinal centers.

Histologic findings can also mimic many of those found in ulcerative colitis, Crohn's disease, or infection and there are no specific pattern or features. Inflammation can be diffuse or focal and follicular inflammation is relatively common. Crypt abscesses, mucin depletion, epithelial cell regeneration, acute and chronic inflammation in the lamina propria, and architectural changes in the crypts may all be present (Fig. 4.21A). The last, in particular, may represent residual presurgical disease, especially in ulcerative colitis; as far as is known granulomas and fissures are absent (147). Additionally, some reports have suggested that ulceration may be so severe as to be pseudomembranous, fissuring may be present as may a transmural lymphoid infiltrate in a typical Crohn's like manner; this may therefore actually represent diversion disease rather than Crohn's disease and is therefore without clinical significance (149). However, unless one is aware of this it may easily be misinterpreted as being Crohn's proctitis. It is interesting that these changes appear to be limited to diversions for inflammatory bowel disease and are not apparently found in diversion for other diseases (150,151). The tipoff is the pronounced follicular proctitis in the mucosa (Fig. 4.21B). Although diversion disease can occur in Crohn's disease, amelioration of symptoms is the rule once reanastomosis is achieved. If the diverted rectum is removed in a patient with ulcerative colitis, there may be transmural lymphoid nodules in a pattern indistinguishable from Crohn's disease and fat wrapping (149). However, this does not appear to represent Crohn's disease. Well formed mucosal granulomas in the absence of crypt rupture clearly suggest recurrent Crohn's disease (148).

Diversion Pouchitis

Pouchitis sometimes develops after construction of the pouch but before continuation is restored with the fecal stream, a condition sometimes called pre-closure pouchitis (149). Although the histology is usually similar to that of typical pouchitis, case reports indicate that this can also have the typical features of diversion complete with apparent diffuse follicular hyperplasia (149), although care needs to be taken with this interpretation as the normal terminal ileum has numerous lymphoid follicles so that the distinction from hyperplasia may be problematic. However, it should be recalled that lymphoid tissue is prominent in the terminal ileum normally.

Neoplasia in Defunctioned Bowel

Occasional instances of carcinomas occurring in diverted bowel have been seen. Some have endocrine like features although microcarcinoidosis has also been seen (152).

Carcinoma in IBD

Carcinoma complicating ulcerative colitis accounts for about 1% of all large bowel cancers. It occurs in patients with extensive ulcerative colitis or pancolitis at a far greater rate than that observed in the general population, the risk starting after about 10 years of disease. In North America it is currently estimated that about 3% to 5% of the population will develop colorectal carcinoma, so that the in-

creased risk of total ulcerative colitis is probably on the order of 10 to 25 times, and even greater in young patients, partly because colorectal carcinoma is rare at this age. There is, however, wide geographical variation of this risk. For no apparent reason, some countries, such as Israel, have a low prevalence of dysplasia or carcinoma (135,153,154). In parts of Scandinavia, where surgery is performed relatively frequently for severe disease, the population at risk is small and these complications are correspondingly uncommon. One large study suggests a cumulative 25 year probability of only 9% (155).

The age at presentation of carcinoma is markedly less than that seen in the noncolitic population, the mean age of symptomatic presentation being between 40 and 45. When compared stage for stage with age-matched controls, the prognosis of cancer in ulcerative colitis is no worse in control patients, primarily because a large proportion of young patients present and die with advanced disease and aggressive tumors irrespective of the underlying predisposing cause. Most series including a reasonable proportion of young patients show high mortality rates. However, other series have a high proportion of Dukes' A carcinomas and correspondingly good overall prognosis (155–158).

Risk Factors
Practically, the risk factors for colorectal carcinoma complicating ulcerative colitis that really matter are the extent of disease (extensive tends to mean proximal to the splenic flexure) and the length of the history. The presence of sclerosing cholangitis may also predispose to dysplasia (159), while long-term therapy with sulfas may be protective, therapy for at least 3 months apparently being associated with a 60% reduction in the expected incidence of colorectal cancer in one study (160); the latter is surprising in view of the apparent lack of correlation between disease activity and cancer found in most studies. Immunosuppressives such as azathioprine do not appear to increase the risk (161), but folate loading might prevent it (162).

Extent of Disease
This is the single most important factor in predisposing patients with ulcerative colitis to carcinoma. Patients with disease, extending into the right side of the colon, can be considered at high risk (157). Perhaps as high as 15 times overall, 2.8 times that expected for left sided disease and 1.7 times for ulcerative proctitis (163). However, relative risks have to be treated with caution in the younger population as any cancer causes a huge

increase in relative risk because of the infrequency of the colorectal cancer in this age group. Extent of disease probably varies depending on how it was assessed. Radiologic assessment even with air-contrast barium enema is less sensitive than endoscopy with biopsy in assessing the extent of the disease. Biopsies performed proximal to the endoscopically visible limit of disease sometimes reveal clear evidence of quiescent and sometimes active disease. Some patients with left-sided disease have an inflamed mucosa in the vicinity of the ileocecal valve, that is also seen in normals and is likely without significance (23). It makes sense to use endoscopy and biopsy to determine the extent of colitis, possibly soon after an exacerbation to preclude extensive disease being missed should the vascular pattern and biopsies return to largely normal. In one study patients developing colitic cancers were not under surveillance because the extent of their disease was underestimated (164).

Duration of Disease and Age of Onset
Few patients develop clinically apparent carcinoma before 10 years duration of disease. However, in most studies, the curve starts to rise at this point. Others are less comfortable with the fact that cancers may present clinically after 10 years of disease and assume that there is a lead time for the dysplasia–carcinoma sequence to be effected; thus, they start screening after 7 years of disease. The actual risk is on the order of 0.5% to 2% per year after the first 10 years of disease (153,157, 165). Age of onset of disease is thought to be important, but almost certainly because patients developing ulcerative colitis early in life have a long time in which to develop carcinoma (166). Some data suggests that the risk after a given period of time is similar in all age groups (153), but others suggest a distinct risk related to age of onset of the

disease (163,167); in those with pancolitis for 35 years it has been suggested that the risk may be as high as 30%, reaching 40% in those in whom the age of onset was less than 15 years old (163).

Site of Tumors
In contrast to noncolitic carcinomas, three-quarters of which are in the rectosigmoid, colitic cancers may have a more diffuse distribution. However, more recent data suggest that at least 80% of cancers still occur within reach of a flexible sigmoidoscope (168,169); however, the possibility that some of these patients may be the result of referral bias because dysplasia was found at flexible sigmoidoscopy or on rectal biopsies cannot be entirely discounted.

Multiple Tumors
The multiplicity of tumors in patients with colitic cancer is well established, and it has been determined that about 25% of patients with one carcinoma will have a second (170–172). Nevertheless, these figures were obtained in patients presenting with symptoms of carcinoma. In our experience, the incidence of multiple tumors seems to be much less in patients in whom carcinomas are detected incidentally during surveillance.

Gross and Endoscopic Appearance
Large colitic carcinomas that present with clinical symptoms usually are circumferential, stenosing, and may obstruct, with dilatation of the proximal bowel and may be multiple (Fig. 4.22). Occasionally a linitis plastica appearance is seen, with long, tubular, neoplastic strictures. Some abnormalities seen endoscopically are dysplastic (high or low grade) when biopsied, but on subsequent resection some are found to contain invasive adenocar-

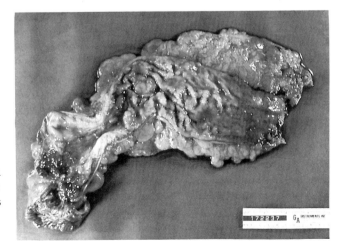

Fig. 4.22. Colitic carcinoma that presented with a palpable mass in the right iliac fossa. Apart from the large tumor, there are multiple smaller nodules that are independent carcinomas.

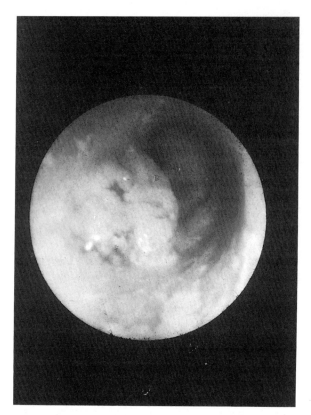

Fig. 4.23. Endoscopic nodular irregularity that was dysplastic on biopsy but proved to be an invasive carcinoma when resected—a so-called dysplasia-associated mass. (See color plate.)

cinoma, so-called dysplasia-associated lesions or masses (DALMs) (Fig. 4.23; see color plate) (170,171).

Smaller colitic carcinomas are unlike small non-colitic carcinomas and are easily missed. Rather than being polyps or polypoid they are much more likely to be irregular nodules, but the smallest carcinomas are often only plaques, which may be slightly raised, at the same level of the adjacent mucosa or a slight mucosal irregularity (Fig. 4.24; see color plate). These small, asymptomatic carcinomas are much more likely to be discovered incidentally in colectomy specimens or at colonoscopy. Rarely, nothing is seen endoscopically, and the diagnosis of carcinoma is made on random biopsy or histologic section (Fig. 4.24). Conversely, a proportion of carcinomas present as large polypoid masses resembling giant inflammatory polyps; surprisingly, infiltration in many of these polyps remains limited to the submucosa or internal muscularis propria.

Microscopic Appearance

The usual microscopic variation of tumors is seen in the large bowel but two major differences are

apparent. First, perhaps 50% of the tumors are colloid and arise in a villous-like mucosa (Fig. 4.25); these are notoriously difficult to diagnose on biopsy, because even in those patients in whom biopsy is deep enough to detect invasion, rather than the overlying dysplastic mucosa, only mucin or very well differentiated epithelium, often without desmoplasia, is present on biopsy. Hence, the concept of endoscopic dysplasia-associated lesions and masses (DALMs) (125,173) which may prove to be invasive carcinomas endoscopically (see below).

The second difference is that a variety of unusual morphological subtypes of carcinoma are encountered, some of which may not be immediately recognized as carcinoma because of the bland appearance of the nuclei but which can be seen to infiltrate into the lamina propria or submucosa on biopsy, or beyond (minimal deviation carcinomas) (Fig. 4.26). Endocrine carcinomas, and other unusual variants such as squamous cell carcinoma (174) can arise in areas of squamous metaplasia within the large bowel (175) or as part of an adenosquamous carcinoma can occur (176). Some of the more unusual variants of adenocarcinoma include choriocarcinoma and spindle cell variants.

Dysplasia in IBD

Dysplasia is defined as an unequivocally neoplastic proliferation essentially equivalent to an adenoma (177); it usually occurs on the background of a longstanding inflammatory disease. It excludes all equivocal or regenerative lesions but may also be the superficial part of an invasive carcinoma (Fig. 4.21) (177). All regenerative or doubtful epithelial proliferation should be excluded from this definition of dysplasia.

Use of Dysplasia in Surveillance of Ulcerative Colitis and Its Implications

Surveillance in ulcerative colitis is based on the concept that the mortality from colorectal cancer can be reduced, whether by detecting dysplasia and carrying out prophylactic colectomy, or detecting invasive cancer but curing it by resection at an early pathological stage. But no controlled study shows this to be the case, however asymptomatic cancers found incidentally at colonoscopy or in resections have a much lower mortality than cancers presenting symptomatically. The 5-year survival in 4 series were 15%, 33.5%, 36.5%, 55% for known cancers, compared with a 5-year survival of 77.2%, 88.2%, 87% in cancers detected as a result of a surveillance

Fig. 4.24. Flat colitis carcinoma that is infiltrating into and expanding the submucosa, and which was an incidental finding in a resection for dysplasia. (See color plate.)

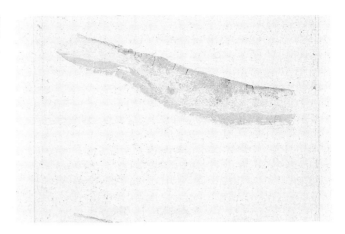

Fig. 4.25. Colitic carcinoma with a villous dysplastic mucosa superficially but with mucin pools of colloid carcinoma beneath.

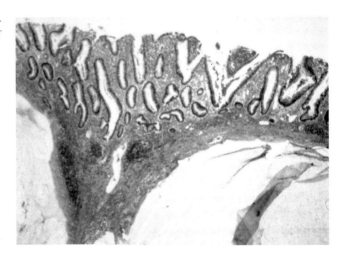

Fig. 4.26. Colitic carcinoma with overlying dysplastic mucosa and regular glands infiltrating into the muscularis mucosae into the submucosa.

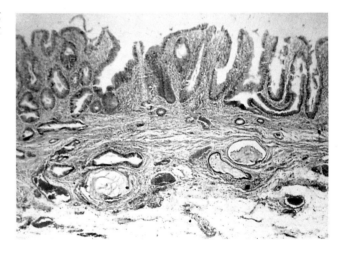

program (168,178–180). Such data is compelling and relates to the earlier pathological stage in asymptomatic cancers. Clearly if colonoscopy (surveillance) is not carried out the detection rate inevitably falls.

A second major tenet of surveillance is that if cancers are actually detected by surveillance that this occurs before they become lethal or that a marker such as the presence of dysplasia precedes all carcinomas for a long enough period to be detectable. Also, if dysplasia is present, it must be both endoscopically detectable and morphologically and reliably identifiable. The corollary of persistently negative surveillance colonoscopies is that patients with quiescent disease and no dysplasia are at extremely low risk of developing carcinoma (probably about 2% [181]), and can be successfully followed and not subjected to unnecessary colectomy.

The large step from the theoretical concept of dysplasia to its applications in patient management implies three major points. First, prophylactic proctocolectomy in all patients in the high-risk clinical group is unacceptable. Second, a laissez-faire attitude is similarly rejected. Third, there is no good method of anticipating easily which patients in the clinical high-risk group will develop carcinoma. Dysplasia is therefore best regarded as an aid to predicting which patients are at greater risk of developing carcinoma, so that prophylactic surgery would be offered only to this subgroup.

Classification and Grading of Dysplasia

In practice, there are major divisions within the spectrum from negative to high-grade dysplasia that need to be made because they are important clinically (see Table 4.5). Thus, biopsies can be divided into those that are unequivocally neoplastic (positive for dysplasia) and those that are unequivocally negative for dysplasia; the latter group comprises typical quiescent, active, or resolving colitis, including typical reparative changes. The midpart of the spectrum, namely, those not falling into either of these two categories, are indefinite for dysplasia. Some prefer three grades of dysplasia (mild, moderate, severe), but this rapidly turns into five with the addition of mild-moderate (effectively low-grade) and moderate-severe (effectively high-grade). Further data are few and it is now largely obsolete.

Gross Appearance of Dysplasia

Areas of dysplasia may be raised above the adjacent mucosa and may be evident as obvious nodules or polyps, but also as plaques or irregular areas of nodularity, which may be minimally or obviously raised; sometimes an entire segment of mucosa is affected. The mucosa may also appear finely villous and brushlike, resembling the pile of a carpet, or may be indistinguishable from adjacent nondysplastic mucosa. It may vary in size from a patch several millimeters or centimeters in maximum length or may involve extensive areas of mucosa.

Histologic Appearances

By far the most frequent type of dysplasia is that resembling typical adenomas (Fig. 4.27). A much less common type consists of large, hyperchromatic nuclei, each of which occupies as much as one-half of each cell usually the basal half (177).

Dysplasia in the Presence of Active Inflammation

The basic guidelines here are that dysplastic epithelium is only occasionally the seat of acute inflammation and that when the latter is present, no or very focal epithelial involvement or an occasional crypt abscess is observed (Fig. 4.28). In the same way that an adenoma that is ulcerated but biopsied is still an ulcerated adenoma, a biopsy specimen consisting of tall epithelium with little or no evidence of regeneration is still dysplastic. In the presence of active inflammation affecting most of the crypts present and/or in the presence of much actively regenerating epithelium, it is unwise to call a biopsy specimen dysplastic because it will usually improve gradually with therapy, thereby disproving the diagnosis of dysplasia.

Aids in the Diagnosis of Dysplasia

A variety of techniques have been used to assist the diagnosis of dysplasia, including carcinoembryonic antigen (182), mucins (183–185), or lectin binding (186,187). The lectin sialosyl-Tn frequently reflects and may precede areas of dysplasia but its clinical usefulness has not been established (188,189). A variety of monoclonal and polyclonal antibodies have been unrewarding, showing only trends (182,190–193), and nothing that looks likely to replace histology as an alternative gold standard.

The measurement of DNA content using flow cytometry is now well established as correlating with and preceding detectable dysplasia in many patients (194–196) even if the latter is not aneuploid. However, no prospective studies have yet been carried out using aneuploidy as a surveillance tool in place of the histological detection of dysplasia, possibly because it is already known that occasional tumors that are highly invasive are not accompanied by aneuploidy (197).

Table 4.5.   Classification of dysplasia.

Diagnosis	Suggested management
Negative for dysplasia	Regular surveillance
Indefinite for dysplasia (probably negative) unknown probably positive	Increased surveillance
Positive for dysplasia (any grade)	Seriously consider colectomy

Fig. 4.27. Dysplasia in ulcerative colitis. On the left is low grade dysplasia in which the nuclei are limited to the bases of the crypts, while in high grade dysplasia (right) the nuclei regularly reach the luminal portion of the cell.

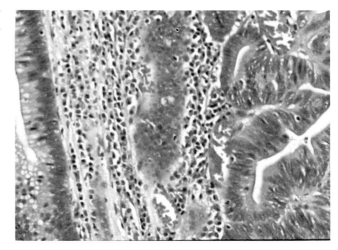

Work has been carried out on oncogenes and their products that might be expressed preferentially in adenomas and carcinomas. To date, the little work done suggests that colitic carcinomas may express different mutations to noncolitic carcinomas (198). K-ras and p53 are found but the former at a much lower rate than in sporadic large bowel cancer and the latter almost entirely in aneuploid mucosa; abnormalities on chromosome 8p and in *Rb, mcc, apc* genes are also found, but as yet none in a manner that may be of clinical usefulness (199–204). Their potential as markers in dysplasia remains uncertain (205).

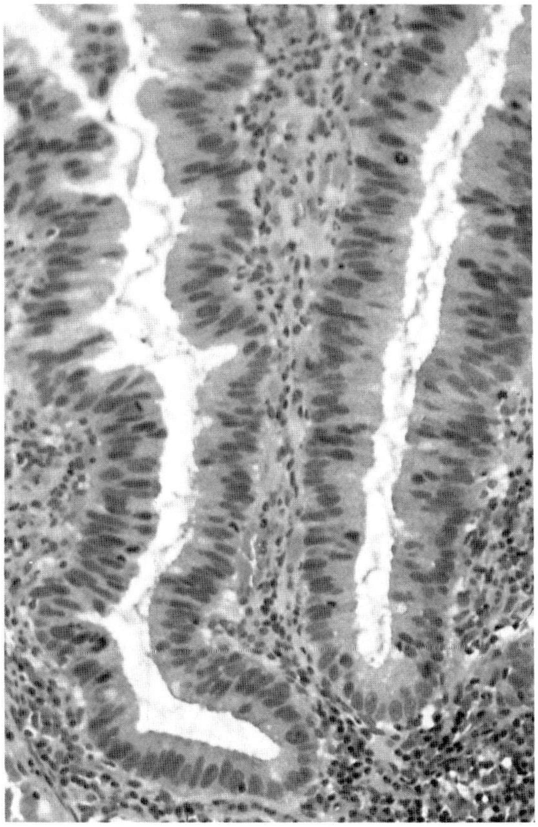

Dysplasia-Associated Lesions and Masses (DALMs)

This is an important concept in adenocarcinomas anywhere in the gastrointestinal tract. It means that if biopsies from an endoscopic abnormality with plaques, nodules, or polypoid masses is dysplastic, then an underlying carcinoma cannot be excluded unless that lesion is resected and examined histologically (Figs. 4.23, 4.25). The reason is that the underlying carcinoma may not be accessible to biopsy forceps, so that without resection, the diagnosis of carcinoma cannot be made. It is therefore imperative that endoscopists be aware of these lesions and their potential significance in patient management (171).

Differences Between Adenomas, Dysplasia, and Dysplasia Associated Lesions and Masses (DALMs)

In ulcerative colitis, pedunculated adenomas are uncommon but do occur. However, endoscopic excision of these lesions as if they were simple adenomas appears safe and is not apparently associated with an excess of carcinoma. It must be shown that the lesion has been completely excised locally by demonstrating nondysplastic mucosa in the stalk or lateral margin and by taking multiple biopsy specimens of the adjacent mucosa to ensure that the adenoma is not part of a more widespread area of nodular dysplasia. If it is, local excision is not curative and colectomy needs to be considered. The distinction of adenomas from DALMs can be

Fig. 4.28. Crypt abscess with focal epithelial involvement.

difficult or impossible. One study used primarily architectural distortion as the major diagnostic criterion for dysplasia, and the typical architectural characteristics of adenomas. Adenomas were associated with a much older mean age of 66 versus 43 for dysplasia, a shorter history (7 vs. 12 years), and were less frequently multiple or multifocal (35% vs. 73% for dysplasia) (206).

How Much Sampling Is Required?

Although in patients presenting with symptomatic cancer dysplasia may be widespread, in asymptomatic cancers this (as well as multiple tumors) is much less frequent, and mapping studies have demonstrated the focal nature of both dysplasia, as well as the aneuploid mucosa in which many of them develop (194,196,200,207). It has been estimated that 30 to 35 biopsies are required to give a 90% chance of detecting dysplasia if present (194), which amounts to 3 to 4/10 cm or anatomic segment. Even more disconcerting is a simple calculation to determine the number of biopsies required to detect a 2 cm patch of dysplasia, which of course has an area of exactly 3.14 cm². The increasingly uncommon shortened haustra-less gut with a circumference of 10 cm (a diameter of only 3.2 cm), each 10 cm length of bowel would have an area of 100 cm². In this segment of bowel it would require 100/3.14, or 32 biopsies to detect the 2 cm patch of dysplasia. In a colon 100 cm in length (short), it would therefore require 320 evenly spaced biopsies to reasonably guarantee detection of a 2 cm diameter patch of dysplasia, a completely daunting prospect. Yet the objectives of surveillance colonoscopy are to ensure as far as is possible that dysplasia or cancer is not present. In the absence of an endoscopic abnormality the detection of dysplasia is indeed dependent entirely on the number of biopsies taken. One can argue in addition that, as seems increasingly to be the case, that about 80% of colitic cancers occur in the left colon, that most of the sampling should be carried out here. Taking 2 to 4 biopsies every 10 cm appears reasonable.

Management of Dysplasia

The management of dysplasia involves balancing the risks and benefits of one particular form of therapy, such as colectomy, and any ensuing problems against the risks and benefits of continued follow-up in any particular patient. Major problems include the lack of objective data on which to base these judgments, failure of gastroenterologists to appreciate the cancer risk associated with dysplasia, and problems of interobserver variability of diagnosis amongst pathologists. The notion that all patients must be managed "individually" continues to guarantee that data will remain difficult to obtain. The problem is potentiated because many physicians are unclear about whether they are practicing cancer prevention (prophylaxis), its early detection, or a fortuitous combination of both. The presence of dysplasia does not mean that the patient will inevitably have or develop carcinoma, indeed many may never do so. However, a small proportion may already have an invasive carcinoma. This creates further tension in trying to prevent the patient developing a potentially lethal carcinoma on the one hand (an early curable cancer may be acceptable), and carrying out an unnecessary colectomy on the other.

Confirmation of Dysplasia

Confirmation of dysplasia was recommended to ensure that colectomy is not carried out unnecessarily for false positive diagnosis of dysplasia (177). Confirmation can be carried out by:

a. Sending the slides to a second pathologist
b. Repeating the colonoscopy to obtain further biopsies.

Confirmation by a second pathologist clearly depends on the competence of both pathologists and the gastroenterologist's confidence in that pathologist. Most of the time the diagnosis of dysplasia is straightforward, so that confirmation by a second pathologist is usually necessary only if either party is insecure. Unless dysplasia is wide-spread or an area of dysplasia can be visualized endoscopically, confirmation of dysplasia by repeated endoscopy and biopsy is usually doomed to failure because it has repeatedly been shown that dysplasia is patchy (157,170–172). This results in statements such as "dysplasia comes and goes," dysplasia regressed," and so on, that likely reflect sampling problems.

Decision for Colectomy and Timing for Dysplasia

Once dysplasia is diagnosed the options are: continue regular surveillance, increase surveillance, or resection. To make this decision data of risk of actually having or subsequently developing carcinoma is required. These are few and overall of modest quality, but have been combined to provide an index of risk as follows (Table 4.6), in which immediate colectomy usually applies to dysplasia being found on the first (diagnostic) colonoscopy, and subsequent to surveillance colonoscopy (208).

The implications are fairly obvious and in some ways surprising. The most obvious is that DALMs and high-grade dysplasia have a sufficiently high

Table 4.6. Risk of cancer in patients with dysplasia.

	Probability of carcinoma	
Diagnosis	Immediate colectomy	Subsequent colectomy
DALM	43% (17/40)	NA
High grade dysplasia	42% (10/24)	32% (15/47)
Low grade dysplasia	19% (3/16)	8% (17/204)
Indefinite for dysplasia	NA	9% (9/95)
No dysplasia	NA	2% (11/595)

risk of concurrent carcinoma to justify immediate colectomy. The data also suggest that the same is true for low grade dysplasia, particularly as about half of these patients continue to develop high grade dysplasia or carcinoma. The real surprise is that the longterm prognosis for indefinite dysplasia seems to be identical to low grade dysplasia. However, there are currently no recommendations to carry out colectomy at this stage. Nevertheless, this mucosa is frequently aneuploid, which may be part of the reason for the enlarged nuclei, and offer at least a partial explanation for the increased risk. Evidence increasingly supports colectomy when dysplasia of any grade is found (168,208,209).

What Can Be Achieved If Appropriate Surveillance Is Carried Out?

Since 1990, four other European studies have been published, three from Scandinavia and one from the UK (164,210–212). These reported a total of 423 patients at risk followed from 12 to 15 years. Eight cancers were reported, two of whom died— one before starting surveillance, the other after leaving the program, two were found at the screening colonoscopy (one Dukes' B and one C); none of these can be attributed to the programs. Four patients developed cancer while on surveillance. One had a Dukes' B cancer after refusing colectomy for dysplasia, resection being carried out for active disease. The worst possible interpretation of this is that the patient had a Dukes' B cancer when colectomy was initially recommended. Three other cancers were found under surveillance, an asymptomatic Dukes' A at colonoscopy, and two Dukes' A cancers found incidentally in resections carried out for dysplasia. Eleven other patients had resections for dysplasia, but were found to be cancer free. There was no mortality. No cancer deaths occurred. Although some of the authors were disappointed with their study as potentially poor use of resources, it is tough to imagine better results.

Why Is the Proportion of Cancer with Adenomas or Dysplasia in Ulcerative Colitis Less Than 100%?

Only about 75% of resected clinical carcinomas are accompanied by dysplasia (213,214). These may be summarized as follows, and apply to both usual carcinomas and those associated with inflammatory conditions.

1. As carcinomas enlarge, they destroy any associated adenomatous or dysplastic component.
2. As carcinomas enlarge, the pathologist is unlikely to increase the number of blocks taken commensurate with the size of the tumor, so that the dysplastic component may be missed.
3. The histologic appearances of mucosal and submucosal tumor may be identical so that distinction is similarly impossible.
4. Some poorly differentiated carcinomas prove to be poorly differentiated carcinoid tumors (215–217). These do not appear to arise from classical dysplasia.

It is also well known that classical dysplasia is relatively uncommon in gastric carcinomas unassociated with intestinal metaplasia (diffuse carcinomas including some signet ring carcinomas). Some colitic carcinomas are similar morphologically to these tumors, and a similar lack of conventional dysplasia may be expected in these tumors also.

Carcinoma and Dysplasia in Crohn's Disease

The risk of carcinoma of the small and large bowels in these patients has been estimated at 3 to 20 times greater than that of the general population (218). The characteristics of Crohn's cancers are very similar to those seen in patients presenting with symptomatic cancers in ulcerative colitis (219). Predisposing factors are patients with extensive large bowel disease (218) especially those relatively young (<30) when the diagnosis was made (220), possibly treatment with 6 mercaptopurine (221), and increasing duration of Crohn's disease (222–224). The average age at the time of diagnosis of carcinoma is approximately 48 years for the small bowel and 50 years for the large bowel, in contrast to a decade older for carcinoma of these sites in patients without Crohn's disease (222,223,245).

The distribution of gastrointestinal cancers in Crohn's disease is roughly 25% in the small bowel (30% in the jejunum and 70% in the ileum), 70% in the large bowel, and 5% in the remaining sites (222–224,226–228). Although the proportion of gastrointestinal cancers that arise in macroscopically normal bowels is greater in Crohn's disease than in ulcerative colitis (33% vs. 4%) (222), most cancers occur in inflamed segments of bowel, particularly in strictures and long-standing fistulas (223–225,227). Bypassed loops of small bowel and excluded colorectum are also liable to cancer (223,225,228–230). Multifocal carcinomas are commonly observed in Crohn's disease (225,228,231).

The preoperative diagnosis of carcinomas in Crohn's disease is even more difficult than in ulcerative colitis, due to the difficulty of examining the small bowel and of distinguishing neoplastic from inflammatory stricture (232); some carcinomas may be undetectable early, especially if they occur in fistulas or are also of the flat plaque-like type found in ulcerative colitis. Patients with Crohn's carcinoma therefore tend to have a very poor prognosis; mortality is about 80% (222,224,227,232), and likely worse in small bowel rather than large bowel tumors (233). Grossly and histologically, these carcinomas resemble other advanced small and large bowel and colitic cancers, except for the additional presence of Crohn's disease.

Carcinoma in Fistula Tracts

A small proportion of carcinomas in Crohn's disease occur in what appears to be a fistula tract. Most of them are incidental findings in resection specimens. Surprisingly, this is the only group of patients with a good prognosis, presumably because the tumor is largely confined to the bowel wall (234,235).

Dysplasia in Crohn's Disease

Dysplasia adjacent to small bowel carcinomas, as well as those in the large bowel, is well described and similar to that seen in ulcerative colitis. There is therefore no reason why surveillance should not be carried out in Crohn's colitis. However, because of the technical difficulty, cost and low yield, there is currently little interest in doing so. The other difficult problem is what to resect if dysplasia is found—the local area of bowel, the whole large bowel, all obvious disease. Dysplasia may be found adjacent to and/or distant from an infiltrating carcinoma and extend variably, ranging from widespread to multifocal and focal dysplasia (177,223,230,236,237). Several authors support a dysplasia-carcinoma sequence, especially when high-grade dysplasia is recognized as a precursor of cancer in Crohn's disease (236–239), but the sensitivity and positive predictive accuracy of dysplasia

for adjacent or remote carcinoma are unknown. Although aneuploidy has been looked for in small patient cohorts, it seems to be much less frequent than in ulcerative colitis, and is likely of little value in predicting dysplasia or cancer (240,241).

References

1. Bernstein CN, Shanahan F, Anton PA, et al. Patchiness of mucosal inflammation in treated ulcerative colitis: a prospective study. Gastroint Endosc 1995, in press.
2. Sanderson IR, Boyle S, Williams CB, et al. Histological abnormalities in biopsies from macroscopically normal colonoscopies. Arch Dis Child. 1986;61:274–7.
3. Prior A, Lessels AM, Whorwell PJ. Is biopsy necessary if colonoscopy is normal? Dig Dis Sci. 1987;32:673–6.
4. Odze R, Antonioli D, Peppercorn M, et al. Effects of topical 5-aminosalicylic acid (5-ASA) therapy on rectal mucosal biopsy morphology in chronic ulcerative colitis. Am J Surg Pathol 1993;17:869–75.
5. Wright C, Riddell RH. Gastroduodenal involvement in Crohn's disease. Am J Surg Pathol 1997; in press.
6. Winter HS, Madara JL, Stafford RJ, et al. Intraepithelial eosinophils: a new diagnostic criterion for reflux esophagitis. Gastroenterology 1982;83:818–23.
7. Surawicz CM, Haggitt RC, Husseman M, et al. Mucosal biopsy diagnosis of colitis: acute self-limited colitis and idiopathic inflammatory bowel disease. Gastroenterology 1994;107:755–63.
8. Le Berre N, Heresbach D, Kerbaol M, et al. Histological discrimination of idiopathic inflammatory bowel disease from other types of colitis. J Clin Pathol 1995;48:749–53.
9. Ritchie JK, Powell-Tuck J, Lennard-Jones JE. Clinical outcome of the first ten years of ulcerative colitis and proctitis. Lancet 1978;1:1140–3.
10. Nordenvall B, Brostrom O, Berglund M, et al. Incidence of ulcerative colitis in Stockholm county 1955–1979. Scand J Gastroenterol 1985;7:783–90.
11. Nugent FW, Veidenheimer MC, Zuberi S, et al. Clinical course of ulcerative proctosigmoiditis. Am J Dig Dis 1970;15:321–6.
12. Farmer RG. Longterm prognosis for patients with ulcerative proctosigmoiditis (ulcerative colitis confined to the rectum and sigmoid colon). J Clin Gastroenterol 1979;1:47–50.
13. Jenkins D, Goodall A, Scott BB. Ulcerative colitis: one disease or two? (Quantitative histological differences between distal and extensive disease). Gut 1990;31:426–30.
14. Sparberg M, Fennessy MB, Kirsner JB. Ulcerative proctitis and mild ulcerative colitis: a study of 220 patients. Medicine 1966;45:391–412.

15. Farmer RG. Ulcerative proctitis: tractable or intractable. In: Barkin JS, Rogers AL, eds. Difficult Decisions in Digestive Disease. Chicago: YearBook Medical Publishers, 1989:368–79.

16. Langevin S, Menard DB, Haddad H, et al. Idiopathic ulcerative proctitis may be the initial manifestation of Crohn's disease. J Clin Gastroenterol 1992;15:199–204.

17. Mir-Madjlessi SH, Michener WM, Farmer RG. Course and prognosis of idiopathic ulcerative proctosigmoiditis in young patients. J Pediatr Gastroenterol Nutr 1986;5:570–5.

18. Holmquist L, Ahren C, Fallstrom SP. Clinical disease activity and inflammatory activity in the rectum in relation to mucosal inflammation assessed by colonoscopy. A study of children and adolescents with chronic inflammatory bowel disease. Acta Paediatr Scand 1990;79:527–34.

19. Levine TS, Tzardi M, Mitchell S, et al. Diagnostic difficulty arising from rectal recovery in ulcerative colitis. J Clin Pathol 1996;49:319–23.

20. Davison AM, Dixon MR. The appendix as a skip organ in ulcerative colitis. Histopathology 1990;16:93–5.

21. Schumacher G, Sandstedt B, Mollby R, et al. Clinical and histologic features differentiating non-relapsing colitis from first attacks of inflammatory bowel disease. Scand J Gastroenterol 1991;26:151–61.

22. Schumacher G. First attack of inflammatory bowel disease and infectious colitis. A clinical, histological and microbiological study with special reference to early diagnosis. Scand J Gastroenterol Suppl 1993;198:1–24.

23. Ang ST, Bernstein CN, Robert ME, et al. Cecal inflammation occurs in health and may result in false diagnoses of pancolitis: a prospective study. (Abstract). Gastroenterology 1993;104:A1028.

24. Niv Y, Bat L, Ron E, et al. Change in the extent of colonic involvement in ulcerative colitis: a colonoscopic study. Am J Gastroenterol 1987;82:1046–51.

25. Therkildsen MH, Jensen BN, Teglbjaerg PS, et al. The final outcome of patients presenting with their first episode of acute diarrhoea and an inflamed rectal mucosa with preserved crypt architecture. A clinicopathological study. Scand J Gastroenterol 1989;24:158–64.

26. Theodossi A, Spiegelhalter DJ, Jass J, et al. Observer variation and discriminatory value of biopsy features in inflammatory bowel disease. Gut 1994;35:961–8.

27. Haggitt RC. The differential diagnosis of inflammatory bowel disease. In: Norris HT, ed. Pathology of the Colon, Small Intestine and Anus. New York: Churchill-Livingstone, 1983:21–60.

28. Lee KS, Medline A, Shockey S. Indeterminate colitis in the spectrum of inflammatory bowel disease. Arch Pathol Lab Med 1979;103:173–6.

29. Price AB. Overlap in the spectrum of non-specific inflammatory bowel disease: colitis indeterminate. J Clin Pathol 1978;31:567–77.

30. Thayer WR, Spiro HM. Ileitis after ileostomy: prestromal ileitis. Gastroenterology 1962;42:547–54.

31. Lumb G, Protheroe RHB. Ulcerative colitis: a pathologic study of 152 surgical specimens. Gastroenterology 1958;34:381–407.

32. Saltzstein SI, Rosenberg BF. Ulcerative colitis of the ileum and regional enteritis of the colon, a comparative histologic study. Amer J Clin Path 1963;40:610–23.

33. Markowitz AM. The less common perforations of the small bowel. Ann Surg 1960;152:240–57.

34. Berman JJ, Ullah A. Colonic metaplasia of ileostomies. Biological significance for ulcerative colitis patients following total colectomy. Am J Surg Pathol 1989;13:955–60.

35. Gustavsson S, Weiland LH, Kelly KA. Relationship of backwash ileitis to ileal pouchitis after ileal pouch-anal anastomosis. Dis Colon Rectum 1987;30:25–8.

36. Lockhart-Mummery HE, Morson BC. Crohn's disease of the large intestine. Gut 1964;5:493–509.

37. Price AB, Morson BC. Inflammatory bowel disease: the surgical pathology of Crohn's disease and ulcerative colitis. Hum Pathol 1975;6:7–29.

38. Farmer RG, Hawk WA, Turnbull RB. Clinical patterns in Crohn's disease: a statistical study of 615 cases. Gastroenterology 1975;68:627–35.

39. Truelove SC, Pea AS. Course and prognosis of Crohn's disease. Gut 1976;17:192–201.

40. Higgens CS, Allan RN. Crohn's disease of the distal ileum. Gut 1980;21:933–40.

41. Okada M, Yao T, Fuchigami T, et al. Anatomical involvement and clinical features in 91 Japanese patients with Crohn's disease. J Clin Gastroenterol 1987;9:165–71.

42. Katz S, Schulman N, Levin L. Free perforation in Crohn's disease: a report of 33 cases and review of the literature. Am J Gastroenterol 1986;81:38–43.

43. Greenstein AJ, Gennuso R, Sachar DB, et al. Free perforation due to cancer in Crohn's disease. Int J Colorectal Dis 1987;2:201–2.

44. Mellor JA, Chandler GN, Chapman AH, et al. Massive gastrointestinal bleeding in Crohn's disease: successful control by intra-arterial vasopressin infusion. Gut 1982;23:872–4.

45. Pera A, Bellando P, Caldera D, et al. Colonoscopy in inflammatory bowel disease. Diagnostic accuracy and proposal of an endoscopic score. Gastroenterology 1987;92:181–5.

46. Kelly JK, Siu TO. The strictures, sinuses, and fissures of Crohn's disease. J Clin Gastroenterol 1986;8:594–8.

88 **R.H. Riddell**

47. Dourmashkin RR, Davies H, Wells C, et al. Epithelial patchy necrosis in Crohn's disease. Human Pathol 1983;14:643–8.

48. Keighley MRB, Eastwood D, Ambrose ND, et al. Incidence and microbiology of abdominal and pelivc abscess in Crohn's disease. Gastroenterol 1982;83:1271–5.

49. Manley PN, Dhru R. Actinomycosis complicating Crohn's disease. Gastroentcrol 1980;79:934–7.

50. Heaton KW, McCarthy CF, Horton RE, et al. Miliary Crohn's disease. Gut 1967;8:4–7.

51. Otto HF, Gebbers JO, Kàgler S. Miliarer morbus. Crohn Dtsch Med Wschr 1975;100:505–7.

52. Scapa E, Marcus EL, Kaufman S, et al. Miliary Crohn's disease: early or different? J Clin Gastroenterol 1993;16:222–6.

53. Tanaka M, Riddell RH. The pathological diagnosis and differential diagnosis of Crohn's disease. Hepato-gastroenterol 1990;37:18–31.

54. Lewin KJ, Riddell RH, Weinstein WM. Gastrointestinal Pathology and its Clinical Implications. New York: Igaku-Shoin, 1992.

55. Wright NA, Pike C, Elia G. Induction of a novel epidermal growth factor-secretory cell lineage by mucosal ulceration in human gastrointestinal stem cells. Nature 1990;343:82–6.

56. Kelly JK, Sutherland LR. The chronological sequence in the pathology of Crohn's disease. J Clin Gastroenterol 1988;10:28–33.

57. Kelly JK, Preshaw RM. Origin of fistulas in Crohn's disease. J Clin Gastroenterol 1989;11:193–6.

58. McQuillan AC, Appelman HD. Superficial Crohn's disease—a study of 10 patients. Surg Pathol 1989;2:231–9.

59. Cook MG. The size and histological appearances of mesenteric lymph nodes in Crohn's disease. Gut 1972;13:970–2.

60. Surawicz CM, Meisel JL, Ylvisaker T, et al. Rectal biopsy in the diagnosis of Crohn's disease: value of multiple biopsies and serial sectioning. Gastroenterology 1981;81:66–71.

61. Warren S, Sommers SC. Cicatrizing enteritis (regional enteritis) as a pathological entity. Am J Pathol 1948;24:475–501.

62. Williams WJ. Histology of Crohn's syndrome. Gut 1964;5:510–6.

63. Chong SKF, Blackshaw AJ, Boyle S, et al. Histological diagnosis of chronic inflammatory bowel disease in childhood. Gut 1985;26:55–9.

64. De Dombal FT, Watts JMK, Watkinson G, et al. Incidence and management of anorectal abscess, fistula, and fissure in patients with ulcerative colitis. Dis. Colon Rectum 1966;9:201–6.

65. Rotterdam H, Korelitz BI, Sommers SC. Microgranulomas in grossly normal rectal mucosa in Crohn's disease. Amer J Clin Path 1977;67:550–4.

66. Tytgat GNJ, Muider CJJ, Brummelkamp WH. Endoscopic lesions in Crohn's disease early after ileocecal resection. Endoscopy 1988;20:260–2.

67. Rutgeerts P, Geboes K, Vantrappen G, et al. Predictability of the postoperative course of Crohn's disease. Gastroenterology 1990;99:956–63.

68. Rutgeerts P. Recurrence of Crohn's disease in the neoterminal ileum after ileal resection: is prevention therapy possible? Neth J Med 1994;45:60–4.

69. Basu MK, Asquith P. Oral manifestations of inflammatory bowel disease. Clin Gastroenterol 1980;9:307–21.

70. Scully C, Cochran KM, Russell RI, et al. Crohn's disease of the mouth: an indicator of intestinal involvement. Gut 1982;23:198–201.

71. D'Haens G, Rutgeerts P, Geboes K, et al. The natural history of esophageal Crohn's disease: three patterns of evolution. Gastrointest Endosc 1994;40:296–300.

72. Schmidt-Sommerfeld E, Kirschner BS, Stephens JK. Endoscopic and histologic findings in the upper gastrointestinal tract of children with Crohn's disease. J Pediatr Gastroenterol Nutr 1990;11:448–54.

73. Geboes K, Janssens J, Rutgeerts P, et al. Crohn's disease of the esophagus. J Clin Gastroenterol 1986;8:31–7.

74. Yao K, Iwashita A, Yao T, et al. Increased numbers of macrophages in noninflamed gastroduodenal mucosa of patients with Crohn's disease. Dig Dis Sci 1996;41:2260–7.

75. Cameron DJ. Upper and lower gastrointestinal endoscopy in children and adolescents with Crohn's disease: a prospective study. J Gastroenterol Hepatol 1991;6:355–8.

76. West AB, Isaac CA, Carboni JM, et al. Localization of villus, a cytoskeletal protein specific to microvilli, in human ileum and colon and in colonic neoplasms. Gastroenterology 1988;94:343–52.

77. Oberhuber G, Püspök A, Oesterreicher C, et al. Focally enhanced gastritis: a frequent type of gastritis in patients with Crohn's disease. Gastroenterology 1997;112:698–706.

78. Moonka D, Lichtenstein GR, Levine MS, et al. Giant gastric ulcers: an unusual manifestation of Crohn's disease. Am J Gastroenterol 1993;88:297–9.

79. Quint KM. Primary Crohn's disease of a Meckel's diverticulum. J Clin Gastroenterol 1986;8:187–8.

80. Mayerding E, Bertram HF. Non-specific granulomatous inflammation (Crohn's disease) of the appendix. Surgery 1953;34:891–4.

81. Ewen SWB, Anderson J, Galloway JMD, et al. Crohn's disease initially confined to the appendix. Gastroenterology 1971;60:853–7.

82. Hollings RM. Crohn's disease of the appendix. Med J Austr 1964;639–41.

83. Allen DC, Biggart JD. Granulomatous disease of the vermiform appendix. J Clin Pathol 1983;36:632–8.

84. Ariel I, Vinograd I, Hershlag A, et al. Crohn's disease isolated to the appendix. Truths and fallacies. Hum Pathol 1986;17:1116–21.

85. Oren R, Rachmilewitz D. Preoperative clues to Crohn's disease in suspected, acute appendicitis. Report of 12 cases and review of the literature. J Clin Gastroenterol 1992;15:306–10.

86. Kahn E, Markowitz J, Daum F. The appendix in inflammatory bowel disease in children. Mod Pathol 1992;5:380–3.

87. Krause U, Ejerblad S, Bergman L. Crohn's disease. A long-term study of the clinical course in 186 patients. Scand J Gastroenterol 1985;20:516–24.

88. McLeod RS. Resection margins and recurrent Crohn's disease. Hepato-gastroenterol 1990;37: 63–6.

89. Korelitz BI, Sommers SC. Rectal biopsy in patients with Crohn's disease: normal mucosa on sigmoidoscopic examination. J Amer Med Assoc 1977;237:2742–4.

90. Makiyama K, Bennett MK, Jewell DP. Endoscopic appearances of the rectal mucosa of patients with Crohn's disease visualised with a magnifying colonoscope. Gut 1984;25:337–40.

91. Pennington L, Hamilton SR, Bayless TM, et al. Surgical management of Crohn's disease. Influence of disease at the margin of resection. Ann Surg 1980;192:311–8.

92. Heuman R, Boeryd B, Bolin T, et al. The influence of disease at the margin of resection on the outcome of Crohn's disease. Br J Surg 1983;70:519–20.

93. Lindhagen T, Ekelund G, Leandoer L, et al. Recurrence rate after surgical treatment of Crohn's disease. Scand J Gastroenterol 1983;18:1037–44.

94. Cooper JC, Williams NS. The influence of microscopic disease at the margin of resections on recurrence rates in Crohn's disease. Ann Roy Coll Surg Eng 1986;68:23–6.

95. Adloff M, Arnaud J-P, Ollier J-C. Does the histologic appearance at the margin of resection affect the postoperative recurrence rate in Crohn's disease? Amer Surg 1987;53:543–6.

96. Kotanagi H, Kramer K, Fazio VW, et al. Do microscopic abnormalities at resection margins correlate with increased anastomotic recurrence in Crohn's disease? Retrospective analysis of 100 cases. Dis Colon Rectum 1991;34:909–16.

97. Hamilton SR, Reese J, Pennington L, et al. The surgical management of Crohn's disease: an appraisal of frozen section examination of resection margins for selecting an anastomotic site. Surg Gynecol Obstet 1985;160:57–62.

98. Wolff BG, Beart RJ, Jr, Frydenberg HB, et al. The importance of disease-free margins in resections for Crohn's disease. Dis Colon Rect 1983;26:239–43.

99. Softley A, Myren J, Clamp SE, et al. Factors affecting recurrence after surgery for Crohn's disease. Scand J Gastroenterol 1988;23(Supp 144):31–4.

100. Heimann TM, Greenstein AJ, Lewis B, et al. Prediction of early symptomatic recurrence after intestinal resection in Crohn's disease. Ann Surg 1993;218:294–9.

101. Norland CC, Kirsner JB. Toxic dilatation of colon (toxic megacolon): etiology, treatment and prognosis in 42 patients. Medicine 1969;48:229–50.

102. Greenstein AJ, Sachar DB, Gibas A, et al. Outcome of toxic dilatation in ulcerative and Crohn's colitis. J Clin Gastroenterol 1985;7:137–43.

103. Buckell NA, Williams GT, Bartram CI, et al. Depth of ulceration in acute ulcerative colitis. Gastroenterology 1980;79:19–25.

104. Jalan KN, Walker RJ, Sircus W, et al. Pseudopolyposis in ulcerative colitis. Lancet 1969;2: 555–9.

105. Edwards FC, Truelove SC. The course and prognosis of ulcerative colitis. Gut 1964;5:1–22.

106. Chandratre S, Bramble MG, Cooke WM, et al. Simultaneous occurrence of collagenous colitis and Crohn's disease. Digestion 1987;36:55–60.

107. Heppell J, Farkouh E, Dube S, et al. Toxic megacolon. An analysis of 70 cases. Dis Colon Rectum 1986;29:789–92.

108. Danovitch SH. Fulminant colitis and toxic megacolon. Gastroenterology Clin N Amer 1989;18:73–82.

109. Cooper HS, Raffensperger EC, Jonas L, et al. Cytomegalovirus inclusions in patients with ulcerative colitis and toxic dilatation requiring colonic resection. Gastroenterology 1977;72:1253–6.

110. Katz S, Schulman N, Levin L. Free perforation in Crohn's disease: a report of 33 cases and review of literature. Am J Gastroenterol 1986;81:38–43.

111. Moum B, Vatn MH, Ekbom A, et al. Incidence of ulcerative colitis and indeterminate colitis in four counties of southeastern Norway, 1990–93—A prospective population-based study. Scand J Gastroenterol 1996;31:362–6.

112. Lu ES, Lin TS, Harms BL, et al. A severe case of diversion colitis with large ulcerations. Am J Gastroenterol 1995;90:1508–10.

113. Flake WK, Altman MS, Cartmill AM, et al. Problems encountered with the Kock ileostomy. Am J Surg 1979;138:851–5.

114. Bonello JC, Thow GB, Manson RR. Mucosal enteritis: a complication of the continent ileostomy. Dis Colon Rectum 1981;24:37–41.

115. Kelly DG, Phillips SF, Kelley KA, et al. Dysfunction of the continent ileostomy: clinical features and bacteriology. Gut 1983;24:193–201.

116. Taylor BM, Cranley B, Kelly KA, et al. A clinicophysiological comparison of ileal pouch-anal and straight ileoanal anastomoses. Ann Surg 1983;198: 462–8.

117. Metcalf AM, Dozois RR, Kelly KA, et al. Ileal "J" pouch-anal anastomosis: clinical outcome. Ann Surg 1985;202:735–9.

118. Svaninger G, Nordgren S, Oresland T, et al. Incidence and characteristics of pouchitis in the Kock continent ileostomy and the pelvic pouch. Scand J Gastroenterol 1993;28:695–700.

119. Sandborn WJ. Pouchitis following ileal pouch-anal anastomosis: definition, pathogenesis, and treatment. Gastroenterology 1994;107:1856–60.

120. Ståhlberg D, Gullberg K, Liljeqvist L, et al. Pouchitis following pelvic pouch operation for ulcerative colitis—Incidence, cumulative risk, and risk factors. Dis Colon Rectum 1996;39:1012–8.

121. Phillips SF. Pathophysiology of symptoms and clinical features of inflammatory bowel disease. In: Kirsner JB, Shorter RG, eds. Inflammatory Bowel Disease. Philadelphia: Lea & Febiger, 1988:239–58.

122. Gemlo BT, Wong WD, Rothenberger DA, et al. Ileal pouch-anal anastomosis. Patterns of failure. Arch Surg 1992;127:784–6.

123. MacRae HM, McLeod RS, Cohen Z, et al. Risk factors for pelvic pouch failure. Dis Colon Rectum 1997;40:257–62.

124. Atkinson KG, Owen DA, Wankling G. Restorative proctocolectomy and indeterminate colitis. Am J Surg 1994;167:516–8.

125. Koltun WA, Schoetz DJ Jr, Roberts PL, et al. Indeterminate colitis predisposes to perineal complications after ileal pouch-anal anastomosis. Dis Colon Rectum 1991;34:857–60.

126. Koltun WA, Schoetz DJ Jr, Roberts PL, et al. Indeterminate colitis predisposes to perineal complications after ileal pouch-anal anastomosis. Dis Colon Rectum 1991;34:857–60.

127. Marcello PW, Schoetz DJ Jr, Roberts PL, et al. Evolutionary changes in the pathologic diagnosis after the ileoanal pouch procedure. Dis Colon Rectum 1997;40:263–9.

128. McIntyre PB, Pemberton JH, Wolff BG, et al. Indeterminate colitis: long-term outcome in patients after ileal pouch-anal anastomosis. Dis Colon Rectum 1995;38:51–4.

129. Luukkonen P, Jarvinen H, Tanskanen M, et al. Pouchitis—recurrence of the inflammatory bowel disease? Gut 1994;35:243–6.

130. Grobler SP, Hosie KB, Affie E, et al. Outcome of restorative proctocolectomy when the diagnosis is suggestive of Crohn's disease. Gut 1993;34:1384–8.

131. de Silva HJ, Millard PR, Kettlewell M, et al. Mucosal characteristics of pelvic ileal pouches. Gut 1991;32:61–5.

132. Apel R, Cohen Z, Andrews CW Jr, et al. Prospective evaluation of early morphological changes in pelvic ileal pouches. Gastroenterology 1994;107:435–43.

133. Carraro PS, Talbot IC, Nicholls RJ. Longterm appraisal of the histological appearances of the ileal reservoir mucosa after restorative proctocolectomy for ulcerative colitis. Gut 1994;35:1721–7.

134. Petras RE, Bona SJ, McGonagle B, et al. "Pouchitis" in patients with continent ileostomy: a histologic study. In: MacDermott RP, ed. Inflammatory bowel disease: current status and future approach. Elsevier Science Publishers BV (Biomedical Division), 1988:699–704.

135. Stern H, Walfisch S, Mullen B, et al. Cancer in an ileoanal reservoir: a new late complication? Gut 1990;31:473–5.

136. Lofberg R, Liljeqvist L, Lindquist K, et al. Dysplasia and DNA aneuploidy in a pelvic pouch. Report of a case. Dis Colon Rectum 1991;34:280–4.

137. Puthu D, Rajan N, Rao R, et al. Carcinoma of the rectal pouch following restorative proctocolectomy. Report of a case. Dis Colon Rectum 1992;35:257–60.

138. Wiltz O, Hashmi HF, Schoetz DJ Jr, et al. Carcinoma and the ileal pouch-anal anastomosis. Dis Colon Rectum 1991;34:805–9.

139. Goulston SJM, McGovern VJ. The nature of benign strictures in ulcerative colitis. N Eng J Med 1969;281:3290–5.

140. Sarin SK, Malhotra V, Sen Gupta S, et al. Significance of eosinophil and mast cell counts in rectal mucosa in ulcerative colitis. Dig Dis Sci 1987;32:363–7.

141. De Dombal FT, Watts JM, Watkinson G, et al. Local complications of ulcerative colitis: stricture pseudopolyposis and carcinoma of the colon and rectum. Brit Med J 1966;1:1442–7.

142. Gumaste V, Sachar DB, Greenstein AJ. Benign and malignant colorectal strictures in ulcerative colitis. Gut 1992;33:938–41.

143. Glotzer DJ, Glick ME, Goldman H. Proctitis and colitis following diversion of the fecal stream. Gastroenterology 1981;80:438–41.

144. Korelitz BI, Cheskin LJ, Sohn N, et al. Proctitis after diversion in Crohn's disease and its elimination with reanastomosis: implications for surgical management. Gastroenterology 1984;87:710–3.

145. Harig JM, Soergel KH, Komorowski RA, et al. Treatment of diversion colitis with short chain fatty acid irrigation. N Eng J Med 1989;320:23–8.

146. Guillemot F, Colombel JF, Neut C, et al. Treatment of diversion colitis by short-chain fatty acids. Prospective and double-blind study [see comments]. Dis Colon Rectum 1991;34:861–4.

147. Lusk LB, Reichen J, Levine JS. Aphthous ulceration in diversion colitis: clinical implications. Gastroenterology 1984;87:1171–3.

148. Ma CK, Gottlieb C, Haas PA. Diversion colitis: a clinicopathological study of 21 cases. Hum Pathol 1990;21:429–36.

149. Warren BF, Shepherd NA, Bartolo DC, et al. Pathology of the defunctioned rectum in ulcerative colitis. Gut 1993;34:514–6.

150. Geraghty JM, Charles AK. Aphthoid ulceration in diversion colitis. Histopathology 1994;24:395–7.

151. Haque S, Eisen RN, West AB. The morphologic features of diversion colitis: studies of a pediatric pop-

ulation with no other disease of the intestinal mucosa [see comments]. Hum Pathol 1993;24: 211–9.

152. Griffiths AP, Dixon MF. Microcarcinoids and diversion colitis in a colon defunctioned for 18 years. Report of a case. Dis Colon Rectum 1992;35:685–8.

153. Devroede G. Risk of cancer in inflammatory bowel disease. In: Winwer SJ, Schottenfield D, Sherlock P, eds. Colorectal cancer: prevention, epidemiology and screening. New York: Raven Press, 1980:325–6.

154. Gilat T, Fireman Z, Grossman A, et al. Colorectal cancer in patients with ulcerative colitis. A population study in central Israel. Gastroenterology 1988; 94:870–87.

155. Hughes RG, Hall TJ, Block GE, et al. The prognosis of carcinoma of the colon complicating ulcerative colitis. Surg Gynecol Obstet 1978;146:46–8.

156. Riddell RH. Why the variation in colitic cancer rates from different centers? In: Tytgat GNJ, van Blankenstein M, eds. Current Topics in Gastroenterology and Hepatology. Stuttgart: Georg Thieme Verlag, 1990:494–9.

157. Lennard-Jones JE, Melville DM, Morson BC, et al. Precancer and cancer in extensive ulcerative colitis: findings among 401 patients over 22 years. Gut 1990;31:800–6.

158. Lennard-Jones OR, Ritchie JK, Hawley PR, et al. Prognosis of carcinoma in ulcerative colitis. Gut 1981;22:752–5.

159. Broome U, Lindberg G, Lofberg R. Primary sclerosing cholangitis in ulcerative colitis—a risk factor for the development of dysplasia and DNA aneuploidy? [see comments]. Gastroenterology 1992;102:1877–80.

160. Pinczowski D, Ekbom A, Baron J, et al. Risk factors for colorectal cancer in patients with ulcerative colitis: a case-control study. Gastroenterology 1994; 107:117–20.

161. Connell WR, Kamm MA, Dickson M, et al. Long-term neoplasia risk after azathioprine treatment in inflammatory bowel disease. Lancet 1994;343: 1249–52.

162. Lashner BA, Provencher KS, Seidner DL, et al. The effect of folic acid supplementation on the risk for cancer or dysplasia in ulcerative colitis. Gastroenterology 1997;112:29–32.

163. Ekbom A, Helmick C, Zack M, et al. Ulcerative colitis and colorectal cancer. A population-based study. N Engl J Med 1990;323:1228–33.

164. Lynch DA, Lobo AJ, Sobala GM, et al. Failure of colonoscopic surveillance in ulcerative colitis [see comments]. Gut 1993;34:1075–80.

165. Greenstein AJ, Sachar DB, Smith H, et al. Cancer in universal and left-sided colitis: factors determining risk. Gastroenterology 1979;77:290–4.

166. Thirlby RC. Colonoscopic surveillance for cancer in patients with chronic ulcerative colitis: is it working? Gastroenterology 1991;100:570–2.

167. Sugita A, Sachar DB, Bodian C, et al. Colorectal cancer in ulcerative colitis. Influence of anatomical extent and age at onset on colitis-cancer interval. Gut 1991;32:167–9.

168. Connell WR, Talbot IC, Harpaz N, et al. Clinicopathological characteristics of colorectal carcinoma complicating ulcerative colitis. Gut 1994;35:1419–23.

169. Schneider A, Stolte M. Clinical and pathomorphological findings in patients with colorectal carcinoma complicating ulcerative colitis. Z Gastroenterol 1993;31:192–7.

170. Blackstone MO, Riddell RH, Rogers BHG, et al. Dysplasia-associated lesion or mass (DALM) detected by colonoscopy in long-standing ulcerative colitis: an indication for colectomy. Gastroenterology 1981;80:366–74.

171. Rosenstock E, Farmer RG, Petras R, et al. Surveillance for colonic carcinoma in ulcerative colitis. Gastroenterology 1985;89:1342–6.

172. Butt JH, Konoshi F, Morsom BC, et al. Macroscopic lesions in dysplasia and carcinoma complicating ulcerative colitis. Dig Dis Sci 1983;28:18–26.

173. Brostrom O, Lofberg R, Ost A, et al. Cancer surveillance of patients with longstanding ulcerative colitis: a clinical, endoscopical and histological study. Gut 1986;27:1408–13.

174. Mir-Madjlessi SH, Farmer RS. Squamous cell carcinoma of the rectal stump in a patient with ulcerative colitis. Cleveland Clinic Q 1985;52:257–61.

175. Adamsen S, Ostberg G, Norryd C. Squamous-cell metacarcinoma with severe dysplasia of the colonic mucosa in ulcerative colitis. Dis Colon Rectum 1988;31:558–62.

176. Patterson FK. Adenocanthoma and ulcerative colitis. Case report and review of the literature. South Med J 1973;66:681–90.

177. Riddell RH, Goldman H, Ransohoff DF, et al. Dysplasia in inflammatory bowel disease: standardized classification with provisional clinical applications. Human Pathol 1983;14:931–68.

178. Gyde SN, Prior P, Thompson H, et al. Survival of patients with colorectal cancer complicating ulcerative colitis. Gut 1984;25:228–31.

179. Choi PM, Nugent FW, Schoetz DJ Jr, et al. Colonoscopic surveillance reduces mortality from colorectal cancer in ulcerative colitis [see comments]. Gastroenterology 1993;105:418–24.

180. Giardiello FM, Gurbuz AK, Bayless TM, et al. Colorectal cancer in ulcerative colitis. effect of a cancer prevention strategy on survival. Gastroenterology 1993;104:705A.

181. Connell WR, Lennard-Jones JE, Williams CB, et al. Factors affecting the outcome of endoscopic surveillance for cancer in ulcerative colitis [see comments]. Gastroenterology 1994;107:934–44.

182. Allen DC, Biggart JD, Orchin JC, et al. An immunoperoxidase study of epithelial marker antigens in

ulcerative colitis with dysplasia and carcinoma. J Clin Path 1985;38:18–29.

183. Ehsanullah M, Naunton Morgan M, Filipe MI, et al. Sialomucins in the assessment of dysplasia and cancer-risk patients with ulcerative colitis treated with colectomy and ileorectal anastomosis. Histopathology 1985;9:223–35.

184. Jass ER, England J, Miller K. Value of mucin histochemistry in follow-up surveillance of patients with longstanding ulcerative colitis. J Clin Path 1986; 39:393–8.

185. Allen DC, Connolly NS, Biggart JD. Mucin profiles in ulcerative colitis with dysplasia and carcinoma. Histopathol 1988;13:413–24.

186. Boland CR, Lane P, Levin B, et al. Abnormal goblet cell glycoconjugates in rectal biopsies associated with an increased risk of neoplasia in patients with ulcerative colitis: early results of a prospective study. Gut 1984;25:1364–71.

187. Ahnen DJ, Warren GH, Greene LJ, et al. Search for a specific marker of mucosal dysplasia in chronic ulcerative colitis. Gastroenterology 1987;93:1346–55.

188. Chao CC, Sandor M, Dailey MO. Expression and regulation of adhesion molecules by gamma delta T cells from lymphoid tissues and intestinal epithelium. Eur J Immunol 1994;24:3180–7.

189. Nogueira AM, Barbosa AJ. Immunocytochemical study of intestinal endocrine cells in germ-free mice. Eur J Histochem 1994;38:213–8.

190. Olding LB, Ahren C, Thurin J, et al. Gastrointestinal carcinoma-associated antigen detected by a monoclonal antibody in dysplasia and adenocarcinoma associated with chronic ulcerative colitis. Int J Cancer 1985;36:131–6.

191. Cooper HS, Steplewski Z. Immunohistologic study with monoclonal antibodies against tumor-associated and/or differentiation antibodies. Gastroenterology 1988;95:686–93.

192. Filipe MI, Sandey A, Ma J. Intestinal mucin antigens in ulcerative colitis and their relationship with malignancy. Hum Pathol 1988;19:671–81.

193. Thor A, Itzhowitz SH, Schlom J, et al. Tumor-association glycoprotein (Tag-72) expression in ulcerative colitis. Int J Cancer 1989;43:810–5.

194. Rubin CE, Haggitt RC, Burmer GC, et al. DNA aneuploidy in colonic biopsies predicts future development of dysplasia in ulcerative colitis. Gastroenterology 1992;103:1611–20.

195. Befrits R, Hammarberg C, Rubio C, et al. DNA aneuploidy and histologic dysplasia in longstanding ulcerative colitis. A 10-year follow-up study. Dis Colon Rectum 1994;37:313–20.

196. Lofberg R, Brostrom O, Karlen P, et al. DNA aneuploidy in ulcerative colitis: reproducibility, topographic distribution, and relation to dysplasia. Gastroenterology 1992;102:1149–54.

197. Lofberg R, Lindquist K, Veress B, et al. Highly malignant carcinoma in chronic ulcerative colitis without preceding dysplasia or DNA aneuploidy. Report of a case. Dis Colon Rectum 1992;35:82–6.

198. Burmer GC, Levine DS, Kulander BG, et al. C-Ki-Ras mutations in chronic ulcerative colitis and sporadic colon carcinoma. Gastroenterology 1990;99: 416–20.

199. Harpaz N, Peck AL, Yin J, et al. p53 protein expression in ulcerative colitis-associated colorectal dysplasia and carcinoma. Hum Pathol 1994;25:1069–74.

200. Chang M, Tsuchiya K, Batchelor RH, et al. Deletion mapping of chromosome 8p in colorectal carcinoma and dysplasia arising in ulcerative colitis, prostatic carcinoma, and malignant fibrous histiocytomas. Am J Pathol 1994;144:1–6.

201. Greenwald BD, Harpaz N, Yin J, et al. Loss of heterozygosity affecting the p53, Rb, and mcc/apc tumor suppressor gene loci in dysplastic and cancerous ulcerative colitis. Cancer Res 1992;52:741–5.

202. Brentnall TA, Crispin DA, Rabinovitch PS, et al. Mutations in the p53 gene: an early marker of neoplastic progression in ulcerative colitis. Gastroenterology 1994;107:369–78.

203. Kern SE, Redston M, Seymour AB, et al. Molecular genetic profiles of colitis-associated neoplasms. Gastroenterology 1994;107:420–8.

204. Burmer GC, Rabinovitch PS, Loeb LA. Frequency and spectrum of c-Ki-ras mutations in human sporadic colon carcinoma, carcinomas arising in ulcerative colitis, and pancreatic adenocarcinoma. Environ Health Perspect 1991;93:27–31.

205. Viola M. Dysplasia and Cancer in Inflammatory Bowel Disease. Journal Found 1990; in press.

206. Schneider A, Stolte M. Differential diagnosis of adenomas and dysplastic lesions in patients with ulcerative colitis. J Gastroenterol 1993;31:653–6.

207. Levine DS, Rabinovitch PS, Haggitt RC, et al. Distribution of aneuploid cell populations in ulcerative colitis with dysplasia or cancer. Gastroenterology 1991;101:1198–210.

208. Bernstein CN, Shanahan F, Weinstein WM. Are we telling patients the truth about surveillance colonoscopy in ulcerative colitis? [see comments]. Lancet 1994;343:71–4.

209. Axon AT. Cancer surveillance in ulcerative colitis—a time for reappraisal. Gut 1994;35:587–9.

210. Lofberg, Brostrom O, Ost A, et al. Colonoscopic surveillance in longstanding total ulcerative colitis. A fifteen-year followup study. Gastroenterology 1990; in press.

211. Leidenius M, Kellokumpu I, Husa A, et al. Dysplasia and carcinoma in longstanding ulcerative colitis: an endoscopic and histological surveillance programme. Gut 1991;32:1521–5.

212. Jonsson B, Ahsgren L, Andersson LO, et al. Colorectal cancer surveillance in patients with ulcerative colitis. Br J Surg 1994;81:689–91.

213. Ransohoff DF, Riddell RH, Levin B. Ulcerative colitis and colonic cancer. Problems in assessing the diagnostic usefulness of mucosal dysplasia. Dis Colon Rect 1985;28:383–8.

214. Taylor BA, Pemberton JH, Carpenter HA, et al. Dysplasia in chronic ulcerative colitis: implications for colonoscopic surveillance. Dis Colon Rectum 1992;35:950–6.

215. Dood SM. Chronic ulcerative colitis complicated by atypical carcinoid tumor. J Clin Path 1986;39:913–6.

216. Owen DA, Hwang WS, Thorlakson RH, et al. Malignant carcinoid tumour complicating chronic ulcerative colitis. Am J Clin Pathol 1981;76:333–8.

217. Miller RR, Sumner HW. Argyrophilic cell hyperplasia and an atypical carcinoid tumor in chronic ulcerative colitis. Cancer 1982;50:2920–5.

218. Gillen CD, Andrews HA, Prior P, et al. Crohn's disease and colorectal cancer. Gut 1994;35:651–5.

219. Choi PM, Zelig MP. Similarity of colorectal cancer in Crohn's disease and ulcerative colitis: implications for carcinogenesis and prevention. Gut 1994;35:950–4.

220. Ekbom A, Helmick C, Zack M, et al. Increased risk of large-bowel cancer in Crohn's disease with colonic involvement. Lancet 1990;336:357–9.

221. Lashner BA. Risk factors for small bowel cancer in Crohn's disease. Dig Dis Sci 1992;37:1179–84.

222. Greenstein AJ, Sachar DB, Smith H, et al. Patterns of neoplasia in Crohn's disease and ulcerative colitis. Cancer 1980;46:403–7.

223. Hamilton SR. Colorectal carcinoma in patients with Crohn's disease. Gastroenterology 1985;89:398–407.

224. Greeinstein AJ, Meyers S, Szporn A, et al. Colorectal cancer in regional ileitis. Q J Med 1987;62:33–40.

225. Shorter RG. Risks of intestinal cancer in Crohn's disease. Dis Colon Rectum 1983;26:686–9.

226. Gyde SN, Prior P, McCartney JC, et al. Malignancy in Crohn's disease. Gut 1980;21:1024–9.

227. Korelitz BI. Carcinoma of the intestinal tract in Crohn's disease: results of a survey conducted by the national foundation for ileitis and colitis. Am J Gastroenterol 1983;78:44–6.

228. Petras RE, Mir-Madjlessi SH, Farmer RG. Crohn's disease and intestinal carcinoma. A report of 11 cases with emphasis on associated epithelial dysplasia. Gastroenterology 1987;93:1307–14.

229. Glotzer DJ. The risk of cancer in Crohn's disease. Gastroenterology 1985;89:438–41.

230. Traube J, Simpson S, Riddell RH, et al. Crohn's disease and adenocarcinoma of the bowel. Dig Dis Sci 1980;25:939–44.

231. Meltzer SJ, Ahnen DJ, Battifora H, et al. Protooncogene abnormalities in colon cancers and adenomatous polyps. Gastroenterology 1987;92:1174–80.

232. Michelassi F, Testa G, Pomidor WJ, et al. Crohn's disease and adenocarcinoma of the intestinal tract. Report of four cases. Dis Colon Rectum 1991;34:174–80.

233. Michelassi F, Testa G, Pomidor WJ, et al. Adenocarcinoma complicating Crohn's disease. Dis Colon Rectum 1993;36:654–61.

234. Nikias G, Eisner T, Katz S, et al. Crohn's disease and colorectal carcinoma: rectal cancer complicating longstanding active perianal disease. Am J Gastroenterol 1995;90:216–9.

235. Ribeiro MB, Greenstein AJ, Heimann TM, et al. Adenocarcinoma of the small intestine in Crohn's disease. Surg Gynecol Obstet 1991;173:343–9.

236. Simpson S, Traube J, Riddell RH. The histologic appearance of dysplasia (precarcinomatous change) in Crohn's disease of the small and large intestine. Gastroenterology 1981;81:492–501.

237. Craft CF, Mendelsohn G, Cooper HS, et al. Colonic "precancer" in Crohn's disease. Gastroenterology 1981;80:578–84.

238. Warren R, Barwick KW. Crohn's colitis with carcinoma and dysplasia: report of a case review of 100 small and large bowel resections for Crohn's disease to detect incidence of dysplasia. Am J Surg Pathol 1983;7:151–9.

239. Cuvelier C, Behaert E, De Potter C, et al. Crohn's disease with adenocarcinoma and dysplasia. Macroscopical, histological and immunohistochemical aspects of two cases. Am J Surg Pathol 1989;13:187–96.

240. Lofberg R, Brostrom O, Karlen P, et al. Carcinoma and DNA aneuploidy in Crohn's colitis—a histological and flow cytometric study. Gut 1991;32:900–4.

241. Porschen R, Robin U, Schumacher A, et al. DNA aneuploidy in Crohn's disease and ulcerative colitis: results of a comparative flow cytometric study. Gut 1992;33:663–7.

5 Endoscopic Evaluation

Aaron Brzezinski and Bret A. Lashner

The era of fiberoptic endoscopy began in 1958 when Hirschowitz reported the first gastroscopy using a semiflexible gastroscope, and in 1968 Arulliani reported the first complete examination of the colon. Since then the advances in gastrointestinal endoscopy have revolutionized evaluation and treatment of gastrointestinal diseases. Unlike radiology, endoscopy allows direct visualization of the mucosa and sampling of the tissue for histologic examination and assists in obtaining a definitive pathologic diagnosis.

The importance of establishing a precise diagnosis relates to the clinical issues of long-term prognosis and, more importantly, to surgical decisions related to colectomy. The decision of which type of surgery is most appropriate relies largely on whether the patient has ulcerative colitis, Crohn's disease, or indeterminate colitis. Endoscopy is the fundamental tool in establishing these distinctions and in excluding other diseases that can mimic inflammatory bowel disease.

Endoscopy in Ulcerative Colitis

Endoscopic examination is used in patients with ulcerative colitis to confirm the diagnosis, to determine the extent of the disease, to assess response to treatment, and for cancer surveillance. Determining the extent of disease and disease activity is a prerequisite for rational treatment of patients with ulcerative colitis (1). For those patients with disease limited to the rectum, topical treatment with suppositories is usually adequate. For those whose disease extends to the sigmoid colon, and even to the splenic flexure, high concentrations of 5-ASA or corticosteroids can be provided in the form of enemas and in those with universal colitis, oral treatment should be instituted (2). Regardless of extent, for those patients with more severe disease corticosteroids are the drugs of choice.

Histologic analysis is the most sensitive diagnostic method for determining the extent of ulcerative colitis, and endoscopy allows adequate sampling of the colonic mucosa. Furthermore, endoscopy is more sensitive than radiology in determining the extent of ulcerative colitis (3). Because extent of ulcerative colitis is the principal determinant of the natural history of the disease and the efficacy of treatment, colonoscopy with biopsies should be done in all patients with newly diagnosed ulcerative colitis unless there are specific contraindications. Patients that on initial presentation have universal ulcerative colitis are more likely to develop toxic dilation of the colon, be refractory to medical treatment, have extra-intestinal manifestations, develop colorectal cancer, and require surgery (4).

Diagnosis

Colonoscopy is the most sensitive method for elucidating the cause of mucosal inflammation and is preferred for that purpose by most gastroenterologists (5,6). Colonoscopy allows the colonic mucosa to be examined from the rectum to the cecum and into the terminal ileum in most patients. Colonoscopy is safe in most patients with ulcerative colitis and can be used as the initial method for diagnosis and staging of disease in patients with either acute or chronic disease (7). Op-

Fig. 5.1. Severe ulcerative colitis, ulcer with detached edges. (See color plate.)

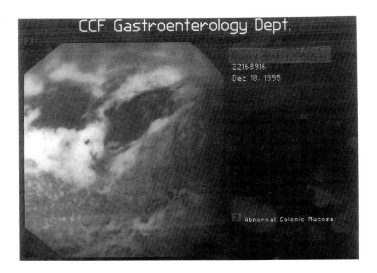

timal preparation of the colon is essential to adequately visualize the colonic mucosa. Colonoscopy can be safely done even in patients with severe ulcerative colitis, as long as there is no evidence of pneumoperitoneum (8) or toxic megacolon. In patients with an established diagnosis of ulcerative colitis, limited colonoscopy to the splenic flexure during an acute attack usually is adequate. Endoscopic evaluation will reveal that 92% of patients with severe colitis will have extensive deep ulcerations and mucosal detachments on the edge of these ulcerations, well-like ulcerations, and large mucosal abrasions distal to the splenic flexure, all of which are markers of severe disease (Fig. 5.1; see color plate). Patients with toxic megacolon or fulminant colitis need not be colonoscoped, unless endoscopic decompression is being attempted in the patient who has declined surgery. In such a

patient, a limited sigmoidoscopy, without colonic preparation, is sufficient to aid in the diagnosis and to sample the mucosa. Enemas with irritants should be avoided because they can cause transient mucosal erythema and can make differentiating between normal and abnormal mucosa difficult.

The healthy colonic mucosa is translucent, reflects some of the light from the endoscope, and allows visualization of the blood vessels. The vascular pattern is most marked in the rectum. Mucosal folds are present and are normally seen even after distending the colon with air (Fig. 5.2; see color plate). The mucosa of the terminal ileum has a velvety appearance and is not as translucent as that of the colon.

The earliest endoscopic manifestation of ulcerative colitis is an abnormal vascular pattern with prominent tortuous vessels and microaneurysms

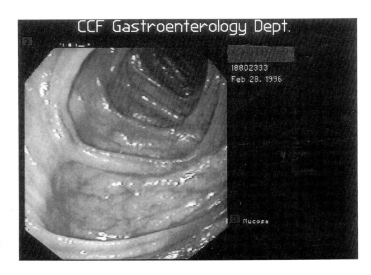

Fig. 5.2. Normal transverse colon. (See color plate.)

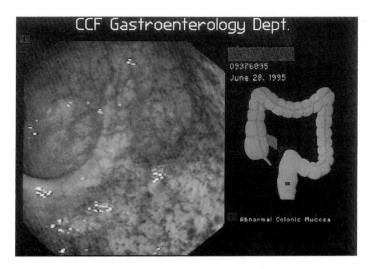

Fig. 5.3.   Mild ulcerative proctitis. (See color plate.)

(Fig. 5.3; see color plate). Trauma with the instrument tip produces submucosal petechiae. As the inflammation worsens, the mucosa becomes granular, opaque, and loses its sheen. The blood vessels cannot be seen and there is patchy erythema as a result of a local increase in blood supply. With disease progression, the vascular pattern is completely lost and the mucosa bleeds with even the slightest instrument trauma, a condition referred to as "mucosal friability" (Fig. 5.4; see color plate).

When ulcerative colitis is more severe, the inflamed mucosa is covered with a purulent exudate (Fig. 5.5; see color plate). In more severe cases, mucopus and blood are found in the lumen, and the mucosa is extremely friable. With disease progression, mucosal ulcerations can occur and can be confused with Crohn's disease of the colon. When an acute attack of ulcerative colitis subsides, the endoscopic appearance of the mucosa may return to normal, but some histologic abnormalities such as crypt atrophy and branched crypts persist (Table 5.1).

In chronic ulcerative colitis, the haustrae are commonly lost, so the colon has a tubular or "lead pipe" appearance and is shortened. The mucosa is opaque, granular, and friable, but purulent exudate or free bleeding is rare (Fig. 5.6; see color plate). Inflammatory polyps, commonly referred to as "pseudopolyps," occur as a result of exuberant mucosal regeneration or granulation tissue, which may epithelialize. Pseudopolyps are a nonspecific reaction that occurs in many colitides. Although classified as polyps, they are not neoplastic lesions. The presence of pseudopolyps signifies that an

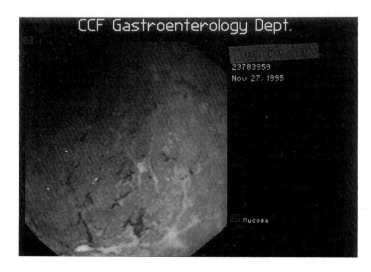

Fig. 5.4.   Moderate ulcerative colitis. (See color plate.)

Fig. 5.5. Severe ulcerative colitis, exudate. (See color plate.)

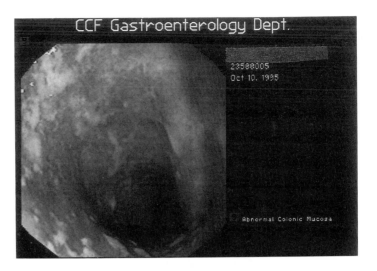

Table 5.1. Endoscopic grading of ulcerative colitis.[a]

Grade 0
Pale colonic mucosa with well-demarcated vessels
Fine submucosal nodularity with nodules identifiable beneath the normal colored mucosa (in healed or resolving colitis)
Tertiary arborization (neovascularization of the terminal arterioles)
Grade I
Edematous, erythematous, smooth, and glistering mucosa with masking of the normal vascular pattern
Grade II
Edematous, erythematous mucosa with a fine granular surface
Sporadic areas of spontaneous mucosal hemorrhage (petechiae)
Friability to gentle endoscopic pressure
Grade III
Edematous, erythematous, granular, and friable mucosa with spontaneous hemorrhage and mucopus in the lumen
Occasional mucosal ulceration

[a]From Miner PB, Peppercorn MA, Targan SR: Hosp Pract 28:1–24, 1993; with permission.

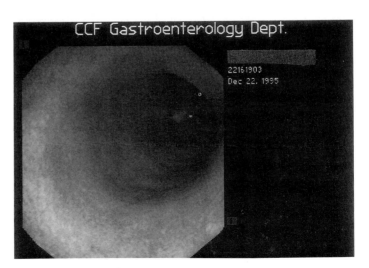

Fig. 5.6. Quiescent chronic ulcerative colitis. (See color plate.)

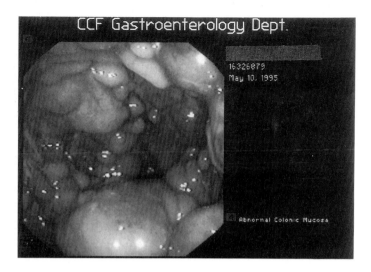

Fig. 5.7. Pseudopolyps in ulcerative colitis. (See color plate.)

area of mucosa has undergone a previous episode of severe inflammation with subsequent healing. Pseudopolyps can appear as multiple small polyps, large finger-like lesions, or, when contiguous, may fuse and become mucosal bridges or an irregular mass of tissue (Figs. 5.7, 5.8; see color plate).

Chronic ulcerative colitis can be complicated by strictures in 3% to 11% of patients. The incidence of adenocarcinoma among these patients has been reported to be as low as 0% and as high as 40% (9–11). Before the widespread use of endoscopy, strictures complicating ulcerative colitis were an indication for colectomy because the radiographic distinction between benign and malignant strictures is not reliable. Colonoscopy is essential in determining the nature of strictures in ulcerative colitis. Adenocarcinoma in strictures in ulcerative colitis

can occur in the absence of dysplasia in patients under surveillance programs (12). For diagnosis, multiple biopsies must be obtained. However, biopsies may be negative for dysplasia or cancer, either because the area was not adequately sampled or because the carcinomas have spread intramurally and are covered by intact mucosa. The three features that are strongly predictive of a carcinoma are: (1) strictures that occurs in patients with long-standing ulcerative colitis, (2) strictures located proximal to the splenic flexure, and (3) symptomatic strictures (13). In patients with one or more features predictive of carcinoma, and in patients with a tight stenosis that does not allow adequate sampling of the stricture or the mucosa proximal to it, colectomy should be seriously considered.

The severity of the attack in patients with ulcera-

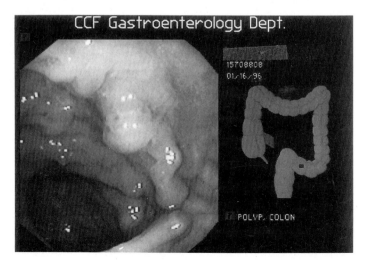

Fig. 5.8. Pseudopolyps in Crohn's disease. (See color plate.)

tive colitis determines medical treatment. Patients with mild or moderate attacks can be treated initially with 5-ASA compounds, whereas those with more severe attacks need treatment with corticosteroids. Multiple indices have been used to determine the severity of the attack. Truelove and Witts' criteria and the revised Oxford criteria are frequently used, but neither of these two includes endoscopic variables. Colonoscopy however, has a sensitivity of 95% for recognizing severe colitis, compared to 16% for Truelove and Witts' criteria and 73% for the modified Oxford criteria. The endoscopic findings seen in severe ulcerative colitis include deep and extensive ulcerations, mucosal detachment, well-like ulcerations, or total abrasion (14).

In ulcerative colitis, response to treatment is 4monitored clinically. The presence of edema and erythema at time of colonoscopy reportedly predicts symptomatic recurrence, and no histological features correlate with increased risk for recurrence (15). Currently, the role of endoscopy in assessing response to treatment is limited.

Surveillance for Colorectal Cancer

Colorectal cancer occurs in approximately 6% of patients with extensive ulcerative colitis and will be the cause of death in about 3%. The risk of developing colorectal cancer increases over time and is greater in patients with extensive disease, older age at the onset of symptoms, and in those with cholestatic liver disease and sclerosing cholangitis (16–18). There is no consensus that screening programs are cost-effective or that they decrease mortality from colorectal cancer in patients with ulcerative colitis. Failure to prevent cancer death may be related to poor patient adherence, sampling error, delaying colectomy in patients with low-grade dysplasia, or the fact that some cancers evolve rapidly and without detectable dysplasia preceeding the cancer. In spite of these limitations, the Inflammatory Bowel Disease/Dysplasia Morphology Study Group (IBD/DMSG) recommends surveillance colonoscopies in patients with extensive ulcerative colitis 7 to 10 years after the first symptoms of colitis and annual colonoscopy thereafter (19). Alternatively, based on hazard ratios to determine the most efficient screening schedule, the intervals between colonoscopies would be every 3 years during the first 12 years of disease, then every 2 years for the next 6 years, and then annually (20). A minimum of two biopsies, and preferably four, should be taken at 10 centimeter intervals. Biopsies should be read by an experienced pathologist. If

low-grade or high-grade dysplasia are detected and confirmed by a second pathologist, then proctocolectomy should be recommended (5).

The goal of surveillance in ulcerative colitis is to detect dysplasia or "precancerous" lesions because dysplasia is a strong predictor of cancer in patients with ulcerative colitis (21). Low-grade dysplasia progresses or is synchronous with cancer in 18% to 30% of patients, whereas high-grade dysplasia is found concurrent with cancer, or progresses to cancer, in 40% of patients (22,23). The positive predictive value for the coexistence or development of cancer given dysplasia is found at colonoscopy in patients with ulcerative colitis is 31%, whereas the negative predictive value for the development of such lesions in patients without dysplasia is 95% (24). Based on these results colectomy should be recommended to patients in whom dysplasia is detected, and patients in whom dysplasia is not detected can be reasonably reassured that cancer is unlikely, even though an estimated 0.7% to 4% of patients will develop cancer, despite no evidence of dysplasia on surveillance biopsies. The term "surveillance" in patients with ulcerative colitis refers to periodic endoscopy with biopsies to detect dysplasia and should not be applied when the colonoscopy is being performed because of a change in symptoms, bleeding, lack of response to treatment, or when it is done to evaluate a mass or stricture.

Patients with extensive Crohn's colitis have an 18-fold increase in colorectal cancer risk when compared with the general population. The risk is greater in those patients who developed colitis before 25 years of age. The absolute cumulative frequency of colorectal cancer is 8% after 22 years (25). In fact, when patients with ulcerative colitis and Crohn's colitis of similar anatomical extent are followed for a similar length of time, the increase in the risk of colorectal cancer is similar (26). In spite of the known increase in colorectal cancer in patients with Crohn's colitis, there are no surveillance guidelines for such patients. One of the reasons may be that the risk was recognized in latter years and also because patients with Crohn's colitis with symptoms refractory to medical treatment undergo colectomy early in the course of the disease.

Colonoscopy in Crohn's Disease

Crohn's disease differs from ulcerative colitis in the pattern and depth of inflammation. Crohn's disease can affect any segment of the gastrointestinal system in a discontinuous fashion. These areas of inflamed mucosa with intervening normal mucosa

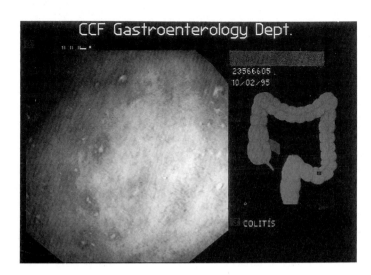

Fig. 5.9.   Aphtoid ulcers in the colon. (See color plate.)

create the characteristic pattern of "skip lesions." In the colon, the ulcers of Crohn's disease are characteristically surrounded by normal-appearing mucosa with a preserved vascular pattern. An early finding in Crohn's disease is "aphthoid ulceration," which consists of characteristically round, white, raised lesions 3 to 4 mm in size, surrounded by a rim of erythema (Figs. 5.9, 5.10; see color plate). In Crohn's disease the inflammation is transmural and produces deep, punched out, and discrete ulcers (Fig. 5.11; see color plate). Linear or serpiginous ulcerations that occur along the longitudinal axis of the colon are characteristic of Crohn's disease. "Cobblestoning" occurs when the deep ulcerations occur in a crisscross pattern, or when submucosal edema is surrounded by normal mucosa (Fig. 5.12; see color plate).

Intubation of the terminal ileum should always be attempted in patients with suspected Crohn's disease. It is successful in 80% to 95% of patients. Even if the mucosa in the terminal ileum appears to be normal, biopsies should be obtained since these can be abnormal and help establish the diagnosis of Crohn's disease (27).

Whereas endoscopy is important in the diagnosis of Crohn's disease, its role in monitoring response to treatment is uncertain. In patients with an acute attack of Crohn's disease, endoscopic grades do not correlate with the Crohn's Disease Activity Index (CDAI), and the endoscopic findings do not predict response to treatment (28) or the clinical course after steroid withdrawal (29). Furthermore, clinical and biological indices are virtually independent of endoscopic findings in pa-

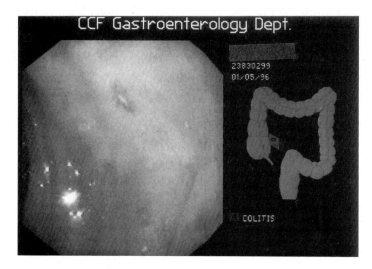

Fig. 5.10.   Aphtoid ulcers in the terminal ileum. (See color plate.)

Fig. 5.11. Crohn's disease ulcers. (See color plate.)

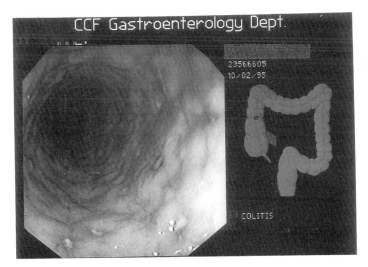

tients with quiescent or active colonic or ileocolic Crohn's disease (30). The discrepancy between endoscopic findings and clinical and biological markers of disease activity may be the result of transmural inflammation that is characteristic of Crohn's disease that cannot be assessed by endoscopy, where only the mucosa is visualized.

Intraoperative Endoscopy in Crohn's Disease

Surgery is a cornerstone in the management of most patients with Crohn's disease. Most surgeons agree that as much of the intestine as possible should be preserved and, in making such decision, the surgical strategy is governed primarily by pre-

operative information obtained from radiology and preoperative endoscopy, as well as by operative inspection of the intestine. External changes of the intestinal wall at time of operation do not reflect the extent of mucosal inflammation which is usually more extensive than the accompanying serositis or wrapping, whereas the bowel wall can be thickened without evidence of mucosal inflammation. Microscopic inflammation at the resection margin has no effect on postoperative recurrence rates (31).

Intraoperative endoscopy adds about 20 minutes to the operative time, and it has proven to be safe and not to increase postoperative complications. Currently, intraoperative endoscopy should be reserved for those patients in whom preoperative radiological findings are equivocal or in whom

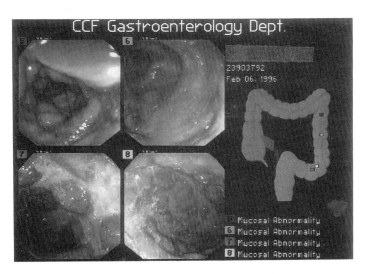

Fig. 5.12. Cobblestoning in Crohn's disease. (See color plate.)

the intraoperative findings do not account for the patients symptoms. In such patients, supplementary endoscopic information on the extent of mucosal involvement can influence surgical decisions in 47% to 60% of patients, usually saving the intestine from resection (32,33).

Differential Diagnosis

Crohn's Disease versus Ulcerative Colitis

The colonic mucosa has a limited repertoire of responses to injury, and it is often difficult to distinguish Crohn's disease from ulcerative colitis solely on the endoscopic appearance of mucosal lesions. Furthermore, in up to 15% of patients with colitis, there are no clinical, radiological, or endoscopic features to characterize the disease and such patients are labeled as having "indeterminate colitis." The differentiation between Crohn's disease and ulcerative colitis is especially important in those patients in whom a sphincter-saving proctocolectomy is being considered. On long-term follow-up, most patients with indeterminate colitis behave as having ulcerative colitis, rather than Crohn's disease (34).

Several endoscopic features however help to differentiate Crohn's disease from ulcerative colitis (Table 5.2). These features include:

1. Normal rectal mucosa. The finding of normal rectal mucosa and changes of inflammatory bowel disease proximal to the rectum in patients who have not been treated with suppositories or enemas strongly supports the diagnosis of Crohn's disease and almost certainly excludes ulcerative colitis (35).
2. Cobblestoning of the mucosa. Cobblestoning is seen in Crohn's disease and not in ulcerative colitis. Endoscopically, cobblestoning refers to areas of mucosal tissue that are heaped up as a result of a submucosal edema. The pattern is usually caused by deep ulcerations that occur in a crisscross, furrowed fashion, demarcating an area of inflamed mucosa. However, this lesion can occur independently of mucosal ulceration and should be distinguished from pseudopolyps and from raised dysplastic lesions associated with ulcerative colitis.
3. Aphthous ulcers. Aphthous ulcers originate in mucosa overlying lymphoid follicles. These ulcers are early lesions seen in patients with Crohn's disease and are 3 mm to 4 mm in diameter and often surrounded by a narrow red border of erythematous mucosa. Electron microscopy has confirmed these lesions to be submucosal lymphoid follicles penetrating the colonic mucosa with an inflammatory eruption through the superficial layer (36). Once thought to be pathognomonic of Crohn's disease, these ulcers may also be found in amebic colitis, tuberculosis, Yersinia enterocolitis, and in Behcets disease (37) but not in ulcerative colitis.
4. Skip lesions. In ulcerative colitis, ulcers never occur in an area of otherwise normal mucosa. Skip lesions are areas of normal mucosa in close proximity to areas of inflamed or ulcerated mucosa and are characteristic of Crohn's disease.
5. Terminal ileum involvement. In experienced hands, the terminal ileum can be intubated at the time of colonoscopy in up to 95% of patients (38). When intubated, the terminal ileum can provide important information, because it can be abnormal in up to two-thirds of patients with Crohn's disease. In patients with inflammatory bowel disease, ileal inflammation is usually diagnostic for Crohn's disease, the exception being patients with universal ulcerative colitis and backwash ileitis.

Table 5.2. Endoscopic features of ulcerative colitis and Crohn's disease.

Characteristics	Ulcerative colitis	Crohn's disease
Distribution	Symmetric	Asymmetric
Rectal involvement	Always	Variable
Skip lesions	No	Yes
Vascular pattern	Blunted	Frequently normal
Friability	Frequent	Infrequent
Erythema	Frequent	Less frequent
Aphthous ulcers	No	Yes
Linear ulcers	Rare	Frequent
Serpiginous ulcers	Rare	Frequent
Cobblestoning	No	Yes
Pseudo-polyps	Frequent	Frequent

Endoscopic findings can reliably distinguish Crohn's disease from ulcerative colitis in 90% of patients. It is more difficult to distinguish Crohn's disease from ulcerative colitis in patients with more severe disease (39). In those patients in which an initial diagnosis cannot be established, clinical follow-up with a repeat endoscopic evaluation can help determine whether the patient has Crohn's disease or ulcerative colitis. The histologic finding that is still considered specific for Crohn's disease and that is not found in ulcerative colitis is the presence of granulomas. Granulomas can be found in 15% to 30% of patients with Crohn's disease and are more commonly found at the edge of ulcers or in the upper gastrointestinal tract, even in the absence of endoscopic disease (40,41).

IBD versus Infectious Colitis

It is often difficult to distinguish clinically between early inflammatory bowel disease and infectious or acute self-limited colitis. The initial symptoms of fever and diarrhea in patients with inflammatory bowel disease can be acute in up to 40% of patients. In severe cases, it is extremely important to differentiate between inflammatory bowel disease and infectious colitis, because the treatment for inflammatory bowel disease is with corticosteroids, and these can have devastating results in patients with infectious colitis. The endoscopic findings of infectious colitis and of either Crohn's disease or ulcerative colitis can be indistinguishable. A careful clinical history, with emphasis on travel history and antibiotic use, stool studies, serologic studies, and the natural history of infectious colitis helps differentiate inflammatory bowel disease from infectious colitis.

Stool cultures take 48 to 72 hours and are positive in 40% to 72% of patients with infectious colitis (42). Endoscopic biopsies can help distinguish infectious colitis from inflammatory bowel disease. In infectious colitis, acute inflammatory cells predominate over chronic inflammatory cells, the neutrophils are found within the crypt epithelium rather than in the crypt lumen, and there is no crypt architectural distortion early in the course of infectious colitis. In infectious colitis caused by *Chlamydia, Campylobacter, Yersinia, Mycobacterium tuberculosis,* or *Schistosoma,* poorly circumscribed microgranulomas can be seen. Overall, 7% to 30% of patients with established infectious diarrhea can have biopsies suggestive of inflammatory bowel disease, and in 5% to 7% of patients with inflammatory bowel disease, the histologic features can resemble infection (Table 5.3) (43).

In intestinal tuberculosis caused by *Mycobacterium tuberculosis,* most of the lesions are seen in the cecum and the terminal ileum, although segmentary lesions through the colon have been reported (44). The endoscopic findings more commonly seen are ulcers of varying size, mucosal nodules, polypoid folds and strictures. A combination of histological features and culture helps in the diagnosis in up to 60% of patients.

Hemorrhagic colitis caused by *Escherichia coli O157:H7* is characterized by abdominal pain, bloody diarrhea, and low-grade fever and can cause hemolytic-uremic syndrome. Although it is usually reported as part of outbreaks related to improperly cooked hamburgers, outbreaks have also been reported from drinking water, person-to-person transmission, unpasteurized apple cider, milk, and lake water. The diagnosis is made by stool cultures and, when endoscopy is done, the findings are erythema, edema, and superficial or aphthous ulcerations in a patchy distribution. The endoscopic findings are more severe in the cecum and in the ascending colon (45). Pathologic analysis shows either an ischemic pattern, an infectious pattern, or both.

Patients with *Shigella dysenteriae* usually present

Table 5.3. Infections mimicking IBD.

Organism	Crohn's	U.C.	Specifics
Yersinia enterocolitica	Yes	Rare	Ulceration of TI, skip lesions or continuous
Yersinia pseudotuberculosis	Yes	No	Mesenteric adenitis, aphthoid ulcers
Shigella dysenteriae	Yes	Yes	Erythema, friability, exudate, skip ulcers, or continuous
Clostridium difficile	Yes	Rare	Pseudomembranes, skip lesions
Herpes simplex 1	Yes	Yes	Diffuse colitis, hemorrhage, erosions, and ulcers of different sizes
Cytomegalovirus	Yes	Rare	Terminal ileum, skip lesions
Mycobacterium tuberculosis	Yes	No	Patchy erythema, aphthous ulcers, skip lesions, mostly cecal
Schistosoma mansoni	Yes	Yes	Stools positive in <15%, always biopsy

with abdominal pain, diarrhea that can become bloody diarrhea, fever, and sometimes constitutional symptoms. Early in the course of the infection, the predominant endoscopic finding is mucosal edema. By the second week, the mucosa becomes friable and there are star-shaped mucosal ulcers. Later, there are punctate hemorrhagic spots with normal intervening mucosa and subsequent healing. The average duration of mucosal findings is 39 days. In more than 80% of patients, the entire colon is involved, and the more severe changes are in the sigmoid colon and descending colon (46).

Patients with *Yersinia enterocolitica* infection can present with a clinical picture resembling ileitis. Endoscopic examination reveals the terminal ileum to have round or oval elevations with or without ulcers and small ulcers in the cecum and the region of the ileocecal valve (47). Patients with *Yersinia enterocolitica* enterocolitis can also have edema, erythema, and aphthoid ulcers involving the left colon, making the differentiation from Crohn's disease difficult. The endoscopic changes usually resolve within 5 weeks.

In homosexual patients, infectious proctitis caused by *Neisseria gonorrhea*, *Chlamydia trachomatis*, herpes simplex, cytomegalovirus (CMV), or syphilis can mimic inflammatory bowel disease. In immunosuppressed patients, such as those with acquired immunodeficiency syndrome (AIDS) or those on immunosuppressive medication, CMV gastroenteritis can mimic inflammatory bowel disease (Fig. 5.13; see color plate). Endoscopically, the colonic mucosa may appear normal with the findings in the ileum of edema, erythema, extensive ulceration, and exudate. Patients with CMV proctitis present with severe anal pain and either single or multiple anal ulcers with raised edges. Pathologic analysis reveals CMV inclusions, and biopsies should be sent for viral cultures.

In patients with an established diagnosis of inflammatory bowel disease, infections can be responsible for exacerbations in up to 10% (48). When pseudomembranous colitis complicates the course of patients with inflammatory bowel disease, colonoscopy with biopsies is helpful in establishing the diagnosis, because in up to 10% of patients with pseudomembranous colitis (Fig. 5.14; see color plate), the flexible sigmoidoscopy and stool cultures can be negative.

IBD versus Ischemic Colitis

Ischemic injury to the colon usually occurs in the watershed area of the splenic flexure and less commonly in the sigmoid colon. In acute ischemia, the finding of a purplish mucosa with a sharp demarcation from normal mucosa helps to establish the diagnosis. However, the endoscopic picture is variable and includes erythema, friability, and gross ulceration, in which case acute ischemic colitis may be difficult to distinguish from acute self-limited colitis and inflammatory bowel disease. The rectum is not involved in patients with ischemic colitis, an important differential finding. In chronic ischemia, endoscopic findings include patchy ulcerations, stenosis, and pseudopolyps, making the distinction from Crohn's disease difficult. During the healing phase, strictures can occur. These strictures can also be found in rare patients that do not

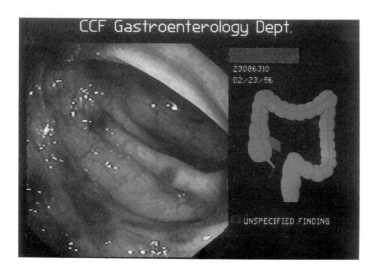

Fig. 5.13. CMV colitis. (See color plate.)

Fig. 5.14. Pseudomembranous colitis. (See color plate.)

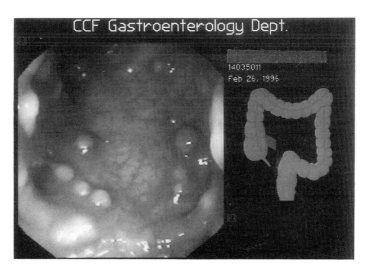

have symptoms during the acute phase of ischemic colitis. The strictures of ischemic colitis are usually long.

IBD versus Radiation Injury

Radiation colitis can usually be differentiated from inflammatory bowel disease by the medical history. The endoscopic findings associated with radiation colitis are friability, bleeding, and multiple telangiectasias (Fig. 5.15; see color plate).

IBD versus Solitary Rectal Ulcers

Solitary rectal ulcers typically presents as an irregular, flat ulceration covered with sloughs and surrounded by a rim of erythema. In 70% of patients, a single rectal ulcer is found, but in 30% of patients two ulcers can be detected. The ulcers are usually located on the anterior or on the anterolateral wall of the rectum, but they have also been described in the posterior or posterolateral wall. The ulcers are usually localized in the rectum and extend between 3 cm and 15 cm from the anal verge (49). Solitary rectal ulcers can occur secondary to the use of suppositories containing nonsteroidal anti-inflammatory drugs. Solitary rectal ulcers can also occur more proximal in the colon. The histological features of solitary rectal ulcers are characteristic and include fibromuscular obliteration of the lamina propria and thickening of the muscularis mucosa fibers.

Endoscopic Treatment Modalities in IBD

Therapeutic endoscopy has had a major impact in certain fields in gastroenterology. However, in the treatment of patients with either ulcerative colitis or Crohn's disease, the progress has been slow. Endoscopic colonic decompression has been used to treat toxic megacolon with variable success (50,51). However, because patients with toxic megacolon may have a paper-thin bowel wall, and the risk of perforation is so high, endoscopy should be reserved for patients who decline surgery.

Chronic bleeding is commonly seen in patients with either ulcerative colitis or Crohn's disease. However, massive bleeding is rare, and when it occurs, it is in Crohn's disease, when a deep ulcer erodes into a submucosal artery. If the bleeding is intermittent or slow enough to allow visualization of the bleeding site by endoscopy, then injection with epinephrine 1:10,000 or the use of thermal coagulation can be attempted. Massive bleeding in ulcerative colitis rarely occurs, it is usually diffuse in origin and is an indication for urgent colectomy (52).

Colonic strictures can occur in either ulcerative colitis or Crohn's disease. Small bowel strictures occur only in Crohn's disease. Strictures in long-standing ulcerative colitis are usually short and occur more commonly in the left and transverse colon. The presence of these strictures is of great

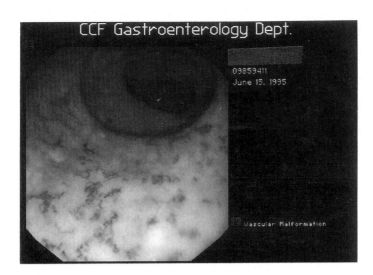

CCF Gastroenterology Dept.

09859411
June 15, 1995

Vascular Malformation

Fig. 5.15.   Telangiectasias in radiation proctitis. (See color plate.)

concern, because they may be malignant. Before considering endoscopic treatment with balloon dilatation, the entire colon should be carefully surveyed for dysplasia, including taking multiple biopsies of the stricture. If no dysplasia or malignancy is found, and the patient declines colectomy, then balloon dilatation of the stricture can be attempted.

In Crohn's disease, strictures can occur anywhere in the gastrointestinal tract. As in ulcerative colitis, the presence of a stricture should raise the possibility of malignancy because adenocarcinoma is detected in up to 7% of colonic strictures in patients with Crohn's disease (53). Therefore, before endoscopic treatment, adenocarcinoma should be excluded by taking multiple biopsies from the stricture. If the entire length of the stricture cannot be adequately sampled, then the stricture should be considered malignant, and surgical resection is the best treatment. Anal strictures are usually short, and a digital dilation or mechanical dilatation over a rigid dilator are usually successful. Rectal strictures can be treated with either rigid dilators or balloon dilators through a rigid endoscope or a flexible sigmoidoscope (54). Successful dilatation of colonic strictures has been variable. Balloons are the best choice among dilating devices (55). There are a few case reports of endoscopic balloon dilation of the pylorus or descending duodenum in patients with Crohn's disease strictures, but this modality as the initial treatment cannot be recommended because the experience is limited. The only type of stricture where balloon dilatation through the endoscope should be considered is the anastomotic stricture, where there is more experience and the results are acceptable (56). Other

techniques for stricture dilatation, such as electrocautery incision or laser therapy, have been used, but no conclusive data exist on its safety or usefulness, and the data available show a high rate of complications and early recurrence of the strictures.

Endoscopic Ultrasound

Endoscopic ultrasound, also known as endosonography, is widely used as a diagnostic technique in several medical specialties, such as urology, gynecology, cardiology, and gastroenterology. Transvaginal and transrectal endoprobes were first used in 1950. Since 1975, transrectal ultrasound has been widely used in the diagnosis and staging of prostatic carcinomas. In gastroenterology, the main role of endoscopic ultrasound has been in staging rectal carcinoma, esophageal carcinoma, and pancreatic neoplasms. Transrectal ultrasound can be performed with various types of instruments that differ in ultrasound frequency and scanning direction. Nonoptic instruments are most widely used for transrectal endosonography.

The main uses of endosonography in patients with inflammatory bowel disease is in assessing the anorectal area. Anorectal involvement in Crohn's disease is estimated to occur in 20% to 80% of patients. It is more commonly seen in patients with colonic involvement, but it occurs also in patients with disease limited to the small intestine. Furthermore, perirectal and perineal disease can be the presenting feature in 8% to 16% of Crohn's disease patients. Because perianal disease in patients with Crohn's disease can be painless, patients are commonly misdiagnosed as having hemorrhoids and are subject to surgery with disastrous results such as poor wound healing and damage to the anal sphincters with resultant fecal incontinence (57).

Endosonography is useful in diagnosing perianal and perirectal complications of Crohn's disease. It allows the detection and delineation of perianal, perirectal, and rectovaginal fistulae and abscesses with a sensitivity that has been reported to be as high as 100% (58–60). It also allows for anatomic evaluation of the anal sphincters (61). With transrectal endosonography, the size and location of abscesses or fistulae can be determined, and the anatomical relationship to the levator ani muscles and the anal sphincters can be described. When transrectal endosonography cannot be performed because of anal stenosis, severe rectal pain, or previous proctectomy, in women, transvaginal ultrasound may be used to determine and delineate the presence of fistulae or abscesses.

References

1. Camilleri M, Proano M. Advances in assessment of disease activity in inflammatory bowel disease. Mayo Clin Proc 1989;64:800–7.
2. Brzezinski A, Rankin GB, Seidner DL, et al. Use of old and new oral 5-aminosalicylic acid formulations in inflammatory bowel disease. Cleve Clin J Med 1995;62:317–23.
3. Holdstock G, DuBoulay CE, Smith CL. Survey of the use of colonoscopy in inflammatory bowel disease. Dig Dis Sci 1984;29:731–4.
4. Farmer RG, Easley KA, Rankin GB. Clinical patterns, natural history, and progression of ulcerative colitis: a long term follow up of 1,116 patients. Dig Dis Sci 1993;38:1137–46.
5. Fockens P, Tytgat GNJ. Role of endoscopy in follow-up of inflammatory bowel disease. Endoscopy 1992; 24:582–4.
6. Lichtenstein GR. Clinical advances in inflammatory bowel disease. Curr Opin Gastroenterol 1992;8:655–62.
7. Blomberg B. Endoscopic treatment modalities in inflammatory bowel disease. Endoscopy 1992;24:578–81.
8. Carbonnel F, Lavergne A, Lemann M, et al. Colonoscopy of acute colitis. A safe and reliable tool for assessment of severity. Dig Dis Sci 1994;39:1550–7.
9. Lashner BA, Turner BC, Bostwick DG, et al. Dysplasia and cancer complicating strictures in ulcerative colitis. Dig Dis Sci 1990;35:349–52.
10. Gumaste V, Sachar DB, Greenstein AJ. Benign and malignant colorectal strictures in ulcerative colitis. Gut 1992;33:938–41.
11. DeDombal FT, Watts J, Watkinson G, et al. Local complications of ulcerative colitis: stricture, pseudo-polyposis and carcinoma of the colon and rectum. Br Med J 1966;1:1442–7.
12. Reiser JR, Waye JD, Janowitz HD, et al. Adenocarcinoma in strictures of ulcerative colitis without antecedent dysplasia by colonoscopy. Am J Gastroenterol 1994;89:119–22.
13. Gumaste V, Sachar DB, Greenstein AJ. Benign and malignant colorectal strictures in ulcerative colitis Gut 1992;33:938–41.
14. Carbonnel F, Lavergne A, Lemann M, et al. Value of colonoscopy in assessment of severity of lesions in attacks of ulcerative colitis. Gastroenterology 1991;100:A201.
15. Courtney MG, Nunes DP, Bergin CF, et al. Colonoscopic appearance in remission predicts relapse of ulcerative colitis. Gastroenterology 1991;100:A25.
16. Lashner BA. Recommendations for colorectal cancer surveillance in ulcerative colitis: a review of research from a single university-based surveillance program. Am J Gastroenterol 1992;87:168–75.
17. D'Haens GR, Lashner BA, Hanauer SB. Pericholangitis and sclerosing cholangitis are risk factors for dysplasia and cancer in ulcerative colitis. Am J Gastroenterol 1993;88:1174–8.
18. Brentnall TA, Haggit RC, Rabinovitch PS, et al. Risk and natural history of colonic neoplasia in patients with primary sclerosing cholangitis and ulcerative colitis. Gastro 1996;110:331–8.
19. Riddell RH, Goldman H, Ransofhoff DF, et al. Dysplasia in inflammatory bowel disease: standardized classification with provisional clinical implications. Hum Pathol 1983;14:931–68.
20. Lashner BA, Hanauer SB, Silverstein MD. Optimal timing for colonoscopy to screen for cancer in ulcerative colitis. Ann Intern Med 1988;108:274–8.
21. Morson BC, Pang LSC. Rectal biopsy as an aid to cancer control in ulcerative colitis. Gut 1967;8:423–34.
22. Woolrich AJ, DaSilva MD, Korelitz BI. Surveillance in the routine management of ulcerative colitis: the predictive value of low-grade dysplasia. Gastroenterology 1992;103:431–8.
23. Lennard-Jones JE, Melville DM, Morson BC, et al. Precancer and cancer in extensive ulcerative colitis: findings among 401 patients over 22 years. Gut 1990;31:800–6.
24. Cohen RD, Argo C, Hanauer SB. The predictive value of colonoscopy in the evaluation for dysplasia and cancer in ulcerative colitis. Gastroenterology 1995;108(4):A799.
25. Gillen CD, Walmsley RS, Prior P, et al. Ulcerative colitis and Crohn's disease: a comparison of the colorectal cancer risk in extensive colitis. Gut 1994;35:1590–2.
26. Sachar DB. Cancer in Crohn's disease: dispelling the myths. Gut 1994;35:1507, 8.
27. Zwas FR, Bonheim NA, Berken CA, et al. Ileoscopy as an important tool for the diagnosis of Crohn's disease: a report of seven cases. Gastrointestinal Endoscopy 1994;40(1):89–91.

28. Modigliani R, Mary JY, Simon JF, et al. Clinical biological and endoscopic picture of attacks of Crohn's disease; evolution on prednisolone. Gastroenterology 1990;98:811–8.

29. Landi B, Nguyen Anh T, Cortot A, et al. Endoscopic monitoring of Crohn's disease treatment: a prospective, randomized clinical trial. Gastroenterology 1992;102:1647–53.

30. Cellier C, Sahmound T, Froguel E, et al. Correlations between clinical activity, endoscopic severity, and biological parameters in colonic or ileocolonic Crohn's disease. a prospective multi center study of 121 cases. Gut 1994;35(2):231–5.

31. Pennington L, Hamilton SR, Bayless TM, et al. Surgical management of Crohn's disease: influence of disease at margin of resection. Ann Surg 1980;192:311–8.

32. Smedh K, Olaison G, Nystrom PO, et al. Intraoperative enteroscopy in Crohn's disease. Br J Surg 1993;80:897–900.

33. Whelan RL, Buls JG, Goldberg SM, et al. Intraoperative endoscopy: University of Minnesota experience. Am Surg 1989;55:81–286.

34. Wells AD, McMillan I, Price AB, et al. Natural history of indeterminate colitis. Br J Surg 1991;78:178–81.

35. Spiliadis CA, Spiliadis CA, Lennard-Jones JE. Ulcerative colitis with relative sparing of the rectum: clinical features, histology and prognosis. Dis Colon Rectum 1987;30:334–6.

36. Rickert RR, Carter HW. The gross, light microscopic and scanning electron microscopic appearance of the early lesions in Crohn's disease. Scan Electron Microsc 1977;2:179–86.

37. Okada M, Maeda K, Yao T, et al. Minute lesions of the rectum and sigmoid colon in patients with Crohn's disease. Gastrointestinal Endoscopy 1991;37:319–24.

38. Zwas FR, Bonheim NA, Berken CA, et al. Diagnostic yield of routine ileoscopy. Am J Gastroenterol 1995;90:1441–3.

39. Pera A, Bellando P, Caldera D, et al. Colonoscopy in inflammatory bowel disease: diagnostic accuracy and proposal of an endoscopic score. Gastroenterology 1987;92:181–5.

40. Dancygier H, Frick B. Crohn's disease of the upper gastrointestinal tract. Endoscopy 1992;24:555–8.

41. Waye JD. Differentiation of inflammatory bowel conditions by endoscopy and biopsy. Endoscopy 1992;24:551–4.

42. Schumacher G, Sandstedt B, Kollberg B. A prospective study of first attacks of inflammatory bowel disease and infectious colitis. Clinical findings and early diagnosis. Scand J Gastroenterol 1994;29(3):265–74.

43. Morson BC, Dawson IMP, Day DW, et al. Gastrointestinal Pathology. Oxford: Blackwell Scientific Publications, 1990:477–549.

44. Shah S, Thomas V, Mathan M, et al. Colonoscopic study of 50 patients with colonic tuberculosis. Gut 1992;33:337–51.

45. Griffin PM, Olmstead LC, Petras RE. *Escherichia coli O157:H7*—associated colitis. A clinical and histological study of 11 cases. Gastroenterology 1990;99:142–9.

46. Khuroo MS, Mahajan R, Zargar SA, et al. The colon in Shigellosis: serial colonoscopic appearances in *Shigella Dysenteriae I*. Endoscopy 1990;22:35–8.

47. Matsumoto T, Iida M, Matsui T, et al. Endoscopic findings in *Yersinia-enterocolitica* enterocolitis. Gastrointest Endosc 1990;36:583–7.

48. Hermens DJ, Miner PB. Exacerbation of ulcerative colitis. Gastroenterology 1991;101:254–62.

49. Tandon RK, Atmakuri SP, Mehra NK. Is solitary rectal ulcer a manifestation of a systemic disease? J Clin Gastroenterol 1990;12:286–90.

50. Hoashi T, Tsuda S, Yao T, et al. A case of ulcerative colitis with toxic megacolon, successfully treated with colonoscopic decompression. Nippon Shokakibyo Gakkai Zasshi 1991;88:91–5.

51. Riedler L, Wohlgennant D, Stoss F, et al. Endoscopic decompression in "toxic megacolon." Surg Endosc 1989;3:51–3.

52. Robert JH, Sachar DB, Aufses AH Jr, et al. Management of severe hemorrhage in ulcerative colitis. Am J Surg 1990;159:550–5.

53. Yamazaki Y, Ribeiro MB, Sachar DB, et al. Malignant colorectal strictures in Crohn's disease. Am J Gastroenterol 1991;86:882–5.

54. Linares L, Moreira LF, Andrews H, et al. Natural history and treatment of anorectal strictures complicating Crohn's disease. Br J Surg 1988;75:653–5.

55. Blomberg B. Endoscopic treatment modalities in inflammatory bowel disease. Endoscopy 1992;24(6):578–81.

56. Blomberg B, Rolny P, Jarnerot G. Endoscopic treatment of anastomotic strictures in Crohn's disease. Endoscopy 1991;23:195–8.

57. Quinn PG, Binion DG, Connors PJ. The role of endoscopy in inflammatory bowel disease (review). Med Clin N Am 1994;78:1331–52.

58. Van Outryve MJ, Pelckmans PA, Michielsen PP, et al. Value of transrectal ultrasonography in Crohn's disease. Gastroenterology 1991;101:1171–7.

59. Wijers OB, Tio TL, Tytgat GNJ. Ultrasonography and endosonography in the diagnosis and management of inflammatory bowel disease. Endoscopy 1992;24:559–64.

60. Law PJ, Talbot RW, Bartram CI, et al. Anal endosonography in the evaluation of perianal sepsis and fistula in ano. Br J Surg 1989;76:752–5.

61. Law PJ, Bartram CI. Anal endosonography: technique and normal anatomy. Gastrointest Radiol 1989;14:349–53.

6 Radiographic Evaluation

Mark E. Baker and David M. Einstein

Radiologic studies are frequently used in patients with inflammatory bowel disease. Although endoscopy has replaced luminal contrast exams in many patients, especially in evaluation of the colon, imaging continues to play an important role in diagnosis and management of patients with these diseases. The purpose of this chapter is to discuss our approach to imaging in patients with inflammatory bowel disease rather than provide an exhaustive review of the potential radiologic tests used. We are radiologists who perform barium studies, ultrasound, computed tomography (CT), and magnetic resonance imaging (MRI) on patients with gastrointestinal diseases. Philosophically, we are organ system, disease-oriented radiologists rather than radiologists focused on technology. Therefore, we will discuss the appropriate use of imaging vis-à-vis clinical presentations, such as suspected inflammatory bowel disease, a patient with a fistula, or a toxic patient, rather than the use of a particular technology in patients with these diseases. Lastly, we have definite biases. Since this is a chapter focused on "how we do it," we will present those biases and make no apology in doing so. Unfortunately, the radiologic literature focuses on a technologic rather than a problem solving approach. As a result, there are very few, prospective studies to support our biases. We do best what works for us and what we do in large numbers. This chapter reflects what we do best.

Small Bowel Crohn's Disease

The small intestine is involved in up to 80% of patients with Crohn's disease; involvement is limited to the small bowel in 20%, whereas 60% of patients have combined colonic and small bowel pathology. Although colonoscopy has largely replaced the barium enema in the evaluation of colonic inflammatory bowel disease, the small bowel remains the province of the radiologist. The proximal portions of the small intestine are occasionally visualized with enteroscopy, but not routinely. The terminal ileum can often be intubated and examined at the time of colonoscopy. Endoscopy directly visualizes the mucosa and guides biopsies in this area. Small bowel radiography, however, visualizes the entire small intestine, and at the present time is the preferred method in patients with suspected or known Crohn's disease.

The distribution of small bowel Crohn's disease is relevant in determining the optimal method of radiographic examination. Although Crohn's disease is characterized by asymmetric involvement and intervening areas of normal bowel between lesions (skip lesions), the terminal ileum is involved in over 95% of cases. Disease may extend proximally for a variable length, but the jejunum is rarely involved to the degree seen in the ileum. Thus, any radiologic method used to examine the small bowel in Crohn's disease should be particularly capable of optimally demonstrating the distal ileum.

Crohn's disease is a chronic disorder, treated both medically and surgically, and is prone to recurrence following resection. Thus, depending on the clinical situation, a variety of questions may be addressed by the radiologist. These include:

1. Is disease present?
2. What is the anatomic distribution of the disease?

3. Are areas of stenosis present?
4. Is there evidence of small bowel obstruction?
5. Are fistulas present?
6. Is there recurrent disease at the anastomotic site?

Small Bowel Examination: Techniques

There are several radiologic techniques available to examine the small intestine. In patients with known or suspected Crohn's disease, the optimal method of examination depends on the radiologist's expertise, the clinical question, and the patient's condition. Close communication between the ordering physician and the radiologist leads to the best approach in each individual case. Information documenting the presence and extent of prior surgery and the type of anastomosis should be available to the radiologist whenever possible. The referring gastroenterologist or surgeon should be familiar with the strengths and limitations of the various techniques, as well as the preferences and capabilities of the radiologists with whom they work. In this way, the maximum amount of information can be obtained concerning each patient in the most expeditious and cost-effective manner.

Upper Gastrointestinal Exam with the Small Bowel Exam

Patients with Crohn's disease are commonly sent to the radiology department with a request for an upper GI and small bowel follow-through examination. Although Crohn's disease may involve the stomach and duodenum in up to 20% of cases, this almost always occurs in the setting of advanced ileocolic disease, and is rarely responsible for the patient's immediate problems. Unless specific information regarding the upper gastrointestinal tract is sought by the clinician, an examination tailored to the small intestine should be ordered. This is because the high-density barium used for a double contrast examination of the stomach is not optimal in evaluating the small bowel. The barium is far too dense, often resulting in markedly opaque loops of small bowel, obscuring the fine mucosal detail needed to diagnose early Crohn's disease. By omitting the upper GI portion of the examination, a more tailored study of the small intestine can be performed, resulting in a better exam at considerable savings in time and cost.

What Small Bowel Exam to Order

In many radiology departments, a small bowel series or follow-through examination consists solely of several timed overhead radiographs of the abdomen followed by a cursory fluoroscopic examination and spot-film of the terminal ileum. This practice should be condemned, as it is an incomplete method of examination of the small bowel, and accounts for many of the discouraging results reported in the literature for small bowel radiography.

Several authorities have proposed that enteroclysis, or small bowel enema, is the most accurate and thus the preferred method of examining the small bowel in patients with Crohn's disease and other small bowel diseases (1–5). We have not found this to be the case in most patients. Enteroclysis is a more involved method of examination, when compared to a routine small bowel study, requiring passage of a tube either via the nose or mouth into the duodenum. The exam is often very uncomfortable for the patient. The examination can be more time-consuming for the radiologist, especially if the radiologist is not familiar with the technique or if only a few are performed every month.

Enteroclysis tests the distensibility of the bowel more completely than a routine small bowel series and displays the bowel in double-contrast. This technique is reportedly more sensitive in detecting early disease, demonstrating fistulae, identifying skip lesions, and excluding the presence of disease (1,4). The degree of distention and quality of the double-contrast effect are often greater in the proximal small bowel than distally, however, limiting the usefulness of this technique in cases of early or limited Crohn's disease. In our practice, we reserve the use of enteroclysis to patients with known Crohn's disease in whom resection is planned, when more exact knowledge of the proximal extent of disease and the presence of skip lesions would alter the surgical approach.

Our preferred method of examining the small intestine is the dedicated small bowel series. This involves oral administration of a barium suspension optimized for the small bowel (we use Entrobar; Lafayette Pharmaceuticals, Lafayette, Indiana), followed by overhead radiographs every 15 to 20 minutes. Frequent fluoroscopic examination, with vigorous palpation and compression, oblique positioning, and spot-filming is also performed after each overhead film, not just when the barium column reaches the colon. These maneuvers elevate this technique above the routine small bowel series, yielding a more complete examination of the small intestine. Several reports have documented a sensitivity rate equal to that obtained with enteroclysis in the detection of Crohn's disease when carefully performed (6–8).

We have found an additional modification of this dedicated small bowel series to be of significant benefit in the evaluation of patients with suspected, known, or recurrent Crohn's disease: the peroral pneumocolon. This technique is a rapid, simple, and well-tolerated method of improving the visualization of the distal ileum. Once the barium column reaches the colon and routine spot-films of the terminal ileum have been obtained, a small Foley catheter is inserted into the patient's rectum and air is insufflated into the colon. By manipulating the patient's position, the air can be directed into the cecum, across the ileocecal valve, and into the ileum. This results in improved distention of the ileum and produces a double-contrast image analogous to that seen with double-contrast barium enemas. Early signs of Crohn's disease such as mucosal granularity and aphthous ulcers are thus more easily visualized (9).

In our experience, the peroral pneumocolon adds significant information in the following scenarios: improving visualization of a normal but initially poorly visualized or suspicious terminal ileum; demonstrating subtle, early signs of Crohn's disease in a terminal ileum previously thought to be normal; differentiating areas of spasm from fixed, stenotic lesions, and a more confident diagnosis of Crohn's disease when findings were initially thought to be equivocal (Fig. 6.1) (10–12). The peroral pneumocolon is particularly useful in patients with prior ileocolic resections, as the air passes freely into the neoterminal ileum owing to the absence of the ileocecal valve. Thus, the peroral pneumocolon is an integral part of our examination of the small bowel in patients with Crohn's disease.

Small Bowel Examination in Patients with a Colectomy and Ileostomy

In patients who have had an ileal resection and/or colectomy with an ileostomy, the small bowel is studied in a two-step fashion. First, retrograde injection of barium via gravity into the ileostomy through a Foley catheter optimally demonstrates the distal ileum, the most common site of recurrence. Injection of air via a 60-cc syringe or with an air bulb into the barium filled loops allows a detailed double-contrast examination to be performed, permitting the detection of subtle, early recurrent disease. Several feet of distal ileum can be adequately evaluated by this retrograde examination. Subsequently, oral administration of barium and a carefully monitored dedicated small

bowel series allows evaluation of the more proximal portions of the small intestine.

Small Bowel Crohn's Disease: Radiographic Findings

The radiologic appearances of Crohn's disease in the small intestine have been extensively documented elsewhere (1,2,9,13–15), but will be briefly reviewed here. Radiographic findings depend on the stage of disease, technique of examination utilized, and the presence of prior resection. The physician caring for a patient with Crohn's disease should recognize that the radiographic appearances often correlate poorly with the clinical condition of the patient and degree of disease activity.

Crohn's disease is characterized by transmural inflammation and ulceration, with a propensity for fistula formation, stricturing, and skip lesions separated by normal-appearing bowel. The radiographic findings can be divided into nonstenotic and stenotic phases.

Nonstenotic phase: The earliest radiographic manifestations of Crohn's disease are mucosal fold thickening (Fig. 6.2), aphthous ulcers, and diffuse mucosal granularity. The latter two require visualization of the en-face mucosal pattern, and are seen best with enteroclysis or peroral pneumocolon techniques. Aphthous ulcers, which appear as punctate collections of barium surrounded by a lucent rim of edema (Fig. 6.3), and diffuse mucosal granularity may be seen as the sole abnormality, or may be present proximal to areas of more severe ulceration or narrowing.

Deep ulceration is the hallmark of more advanced nonstenotic Crohn's disease, and appears initially as thin, fissure-like ulcers perpendicular to the bowel lumen or larger collar-button or rose-thorn ulcers. These ulcers often progress to an intersecting network of longitudinal and transverse ulcers. The inflamed but otherwise intact islands of mucosa between these ulcers form a pseudo-polypoid or cobblestone pattern (Fig. 6.4), another characteristic finding. Transmural inflammation at this stage leads to thickening of the bowel wall with separation of the individual loops of involved bowel from one another and from adjacent, normal loops. Segments of diseased bowel may become adherent to one another, to uninvolved loops of small or large bowel, or to adjacent structures such as the bladder or vagina. As the ulcerations progress and penetrate beyond the serosa, fistulae and sinus tracts may form. Abscess formation is a sequela of advanced Crohn's disease, but is best detected by CT rather than barium studies.

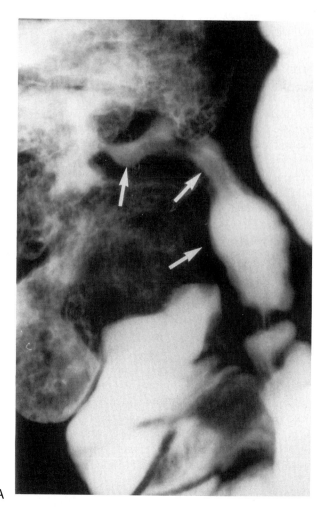

A

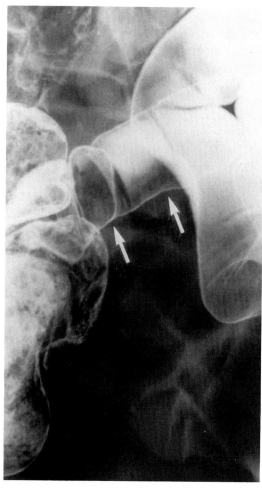

B

Fig. 6.1.   Thirty-five-year-old man with right lower quadrant pain and diarrhea, and a high level of clinical suspicion of Crohn's disease. (A) Spot film of the terminal ileum performed at the conclusion of a dedicated small bowel series suggests mild narrowing and irregularity (white arrows). (B) After performance of a peroral pneumocolon, the terminal ileum is well seen in double-contrast and is clearly normal (white arrows). (C) 29-year-old woman being evaluated for recurrent Crohn's disease. Spot film from a dedicated small bowel series demonstrates narrowing, irregularity, and nodularity of the neoterminal ileum. (D) Peroral pneumocolon more accurately demonstrates a short segment of mild narrowing with nodular mucosa. The degree of narrowing and length of involvement were overestimated on the initial film.

Stenotic phase: Some luminal narrowing is present in the majority of patients with small bowel Crohn's disease. Nonstenotic and stenotic phases may coexist in an individual patient at any given point in time. Progression from the nonstenotic to the stenotic phase may occur in one segment of bowel over the course of follow-up examinations. Initially, mild narrowing of the lumen is due to transmural inflammation and wall thickening. At this stage, the bowel may be devoid of any normal mucosal folds or markings, and appear as an irregular, featureless, rigid tube. Progression to fibrosis results in more marked, fixed areas of narrowing (Fig. 6.5). Strictures may be solitary or multiple, short or long, and when multiple are separated by varying lengths of normal-appearing or mildly inflamed bowel.

Long, markedly narrowed segments of bowel, termed the "string sign," are a hallmark of stenotic Crohn's disease. The stricture diameter is almost never completely secondary to a fixed process as spasm is invariably present in most. No prestenotic dilation indicates no significant obstruction despite the severe degree of narrowing. As a result, the string sign is rarely seen with enteroclysis, as the improved luminal distention inherent in the technique overcomes the spastic component. Similarly, air distention during peroral pneumocolon pro-

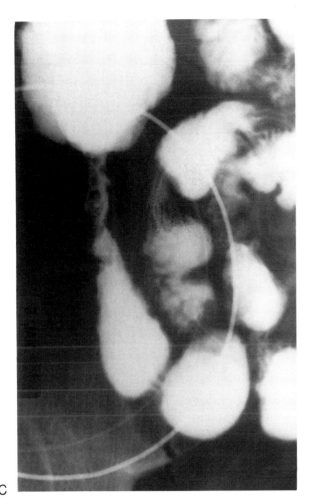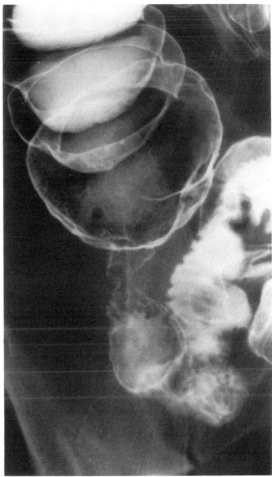

C   D

Fig. 6.1. *Continued*

vides a more accurate assessment of the degree of narrowing.

When the bowel is dilated proximal to a stricture, some degree of obstruction is present. The stenosis may result in intermittent episodes of partial small bowel obstruction, or progress to a high-grade obstruction requiring surgery. Importantly, a small bowel obstruction in a patient with Crohn's disease is not always due to the disease itself. If the patient has had prior surgery, the obstruction is often secondary to adhesions. Enteroclysis has been recommended as an accurate means of differentiating between these two etiologic possibilities, as optimal therapy will vary depending on the cause of the obstruction (2).

Fistulae and sinus tract development are characteristic of Crohn's disease. Fistulae can occur from the small bowel to the skin, colon, bladder, perineum, vagina, and even the urethra. Importantly, fistulae occur commonly with stenotic disease; the fistulae extend from the bowel just proximal to the stenotic segment. A common constellation of findings is stenotic disease in the terminal ileum with one or more fistulae from the small bowel to the right colon.

Segments of bowel involved by Crohn's disease are often separated from one another by intervening lengths of normal-appearing bowel (Fig. 6.6). These skip lesions are quite characteristic of Crohn's disease. Careful examination of the normal-appearing segments may show signs of early involvement such as diffuse mucosal granularity or aphthous ulcers. Accurate assessment of the full extent of involvement is desirable but not absolutely vital in the initial assessment or follow-up of patients with Crohn's disease, as these patients are usually managed medically. If surgery is contemplated, however, this determination becomes paramount, as it may be difficult for the surgeon to detect mild disease by inspection or palpation. Detecting skip lesions and the proximal extent of disease requires careful and systematic fluoroscopic observation, palpation, and compression during a dedicated small bowel series, or

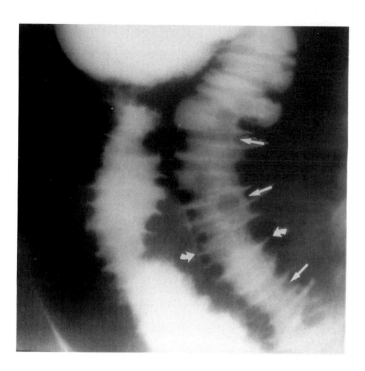

Fig. 6.2.   Crohn's disease. Spot film of the terminal ileum reveals regular mucosal fold thickening. The thickened folds are smooth, evenly spaced, and parallel one
another (white arrows). The edges of the barium filled
lumen are spiculated and mimic penetrating ulcers
(curved white arrow).

enteroclysis. Indeed, this is the main indication for performing enteroclysis in our Crohn's disease population.

Another hallmark of Crohn's disease is its propensity to recur following surgical resection, occurring in 50% to 80% of patients, usually within the first two years after surgery (13). Recurrence commonly occurs at the anastomosis, involving pri-

marily the neoterminal ileum. Many of the recurrences represent progression of very early, subtle disease which was not recognized radiologically, endoscopically, or by direct inspection. The peroral pneumocolon is a particularly helpful technique in detecting early signs of recurrence, as the air freely fills the neoterminal ileum resulting in an elegant double-contrast examination of the mucosa.

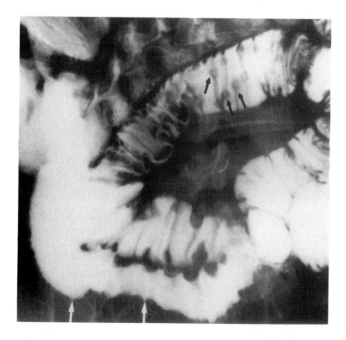

Fig. 6.3.   Crohn's disease. Several aphthous ulcers are seen
in a loop of distal ileum (black arrows). The more distal
ileum is more severely inflamed, with mild luminal narrowing and small ulcerations (white arrows).

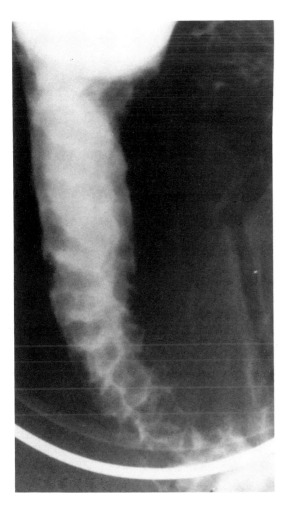

Fig. 6.4. Crohn's disease. Cobblestone pattern of the terminal ileum in Crohn's disease, caused by residual islands of mucosa protruding between an intersecting network of linear ulcers.

Differential Diagnosis of Radiographic Findings

Although several of the above radiographic findings are highly suggestive or characteristic of Crohn's disease, few are truly pathognomonic. The differential diagnosis of Crohn's disease based on the radiographic appearance alone is wide, and depends on the stage of disease. Diffuse mucosal granularity is a reflection of abnormal villi, and has been described in radiation enteritis, small bowel ischemia, and protein losing enteropathy in addition to Crohn's disease (16,17). Aphthous ulcers are also seen in Yersinia enteritis, Salmonella infection, tuberculosis, and Behcet's syndrome (9). Mucosal fold thickening in Crohn's disease may be regular or nodular, and thus mimic ischemia, hemorrhage, radiation enteritis, Whipple's disease, or

lymphoma. Ulceration, mucosal irregularity, and narrowing of the terminal ileum may be stimulated by lymphoma or tuberculosis, or adjacent pelvic inflammation such as appendiceal abscess or pelvic inflammatory disease (9). Solitary, short focal strictures in Crohn's disease may mimic those in primary or metastatic carcinoma or ischemia. Thus, the final diagnosis may often require integration of data from a number of sources, including clinical presentation, radiographic findings, laboratory tests, endoscopy, and biopsy.

Colonic IBD

Diagnosis: Endoscopy versus Barium Enema

The diagnostic approach to the patient with suspected or known colonic inflammatory bowel disease is more controversial than in small bowel Crohn's disease. Involvement of the colon is found in 80% of patients with Crohn's disease; isolated colonic Crohn's disease occurs in 20% of all patients. Ulcerative colitis by definition is primarily a disease of the large bowel. The terminal ileum is involved in 10% to 40% of cases of ulcerative colitis, but only in the setting of pancolitis. Single-contrast barium enema, double-contrast barium enema, sigmoidoscopy, and colonoscopy have all been used in the evaluation of Crohn's colitis and ulcerative colitis. Few direct comparisons between these methods have been performed, but at the present time the endoscopic methods have largely replaced radiologic evaluation.

When comparing the various diagnostic methods, it is important to consider the clinical question. In determining the *presence* or absence of disease, either Crohn's or ulcerative colitis, sigmoidoscopy and colonoscopy are clearly more sensitive than the barium enema. Direct mucosal visualization inherent in the endoscopic techniques allows earlier detection of subtle changes. Colonoscopy detects either Crohn's disease or ulcerative colitis in 17% to 36% of patients when a double-contrast barium enema is normal (18–21). In these series, the minor mucosal changes missed by the enema were felt to cause symptoms and usually were managed medically in a relatively aggressive manner (22). Thus, a normal, high-quality double-contrast barium enema does not exclude early, subtle colonic inflammatory bowel disease. It should also be noted that a small number of patients with a normal colonoscopic appearance of the colon will demonstrate histologic changes of

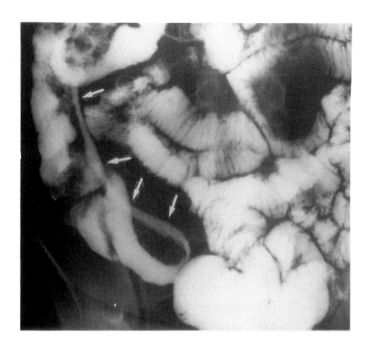

Fig. 6.5.   Crohn's disease. Long segment of narrowed, ulcerated terminal ileum in Crohn's disease (white arrows). Note the separation of loops indicative of bowel wall thickening and fibrofatty changes of the mesentery.

inflammatory bowel disease if random biopsies are taken at the time of colonoscopy.

Once colonic inflammatory bowel disease is diagnosed, some information concerning the *extent* of disease is usually desirable. Once again, colonoscopy has been found to be more accurate than double-contrast barium enema (19,23). Holdstock et al. studied a group of 149 patients with ulcerative colitis or Crohn's disease. Only 15% of patients had

evidence of pancolitis by barium enema, whereas 34% had pancolitis detected by colonoscopy and 62% by multiple biopsies (24). The addition of multiple biopsies improves the evaluation of disease extent over colonoscopy alone. Accurate knowledge of the extent of disease may not significantly alter patient management (24,25).

The final point of comparison between endoscopy and radiology involves correctly diagnosing

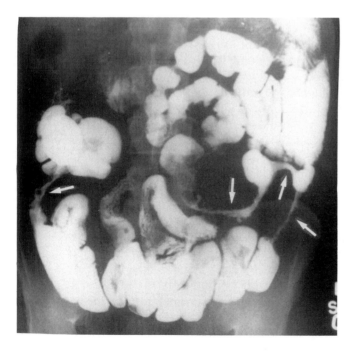

Fig. 6.6.   Crohn's disease. Multiple markedly narrowed segments of small bowel (white arrows) separated from one another by relatively normal regions.

the *type* of colitis. Here, radiology clearly performs better than in detecting the presence of disease or determining the extent. The double-contrast barium enema has been proven to allow accurate differentiation of ulcerative colitis from Crohn's colitis in virtually all cases of radiologically detectable disease (20,21,26,27). These studies reported few if any disagreements between endoscopy and double-contrast barium enema concerning the type of colitis present. This distinction is particularly accurate (95% to 98%) in early disease, as early ulcerative colitis and Crohn's colitis have distinctly different appearances, as will be detailed in a later section. Double-contrast barium enema has been shown to be vastly superior to the single-contrast examination in inflammatory bowel disease, particularly in detection and categorization of early disease.

The advantages of a barium enema over colonoscopy include lower cost and complication rate, higher rate of complete colonic visualization, improved detection of deep ulcers and fistulae, assessment of colonic distensibility and length, and the ability to visualize segments proximal to a tight stricture. Enema films create a permanent record for comparison to later studies, information vital when disease progression is suspected. The advantages of colonoscopy are direct visualization of the mucosa, detection of subtle disease as well as improved assessment of the extent of disease, both leading to superior sensitivity. The ability to perform biopsies is another major advantage, permitting the diagnosis of minimal colitis, dysplasia, and carcinoma. The latter is particularly crucial in patients with ulcerative colitis, as they have a substantial increased incidence of colon cancer, and thus require close, lifelong surveillance. Although double-contrast barium enema easily detects advanced carcinomas, dysplasia and early carcinoma are not reliably diagnosed. Biopsy may also provide information concerning the relative activity or chronicity of disease, information vital for management.

What, then, is the preferred method of studying the colon in patients with ulcerative colitis or Crohn's colitis? Although equivalent in differential diagnosis, colonoscopy is clearly superior in sensitivity. Many authorities thus recommend colonoscopy as the primary modality in colonic inflammatory bowel disease (18,24,28). The double-contrast barium enema, by virtue of its ability to demonstrate symmetric or asymmetric bowel involvement may be useful as a complementary study in the 5% to 10% of patients with endoscopically or histologically indeterminate colitis. Barium enema

would also be indicated for evaluation of the colon proximal to a tight stricture that prevents the passage of the colonoscope.

However, there are several gastroenterologists who continue to recommend the double-contrast barium enema, coupled with flexible sigmoidoscopy, as the preferred method of evaluating patients with colitis (25,29,30). In these authors' opinion, most patients with inflammatory bowel disease do not require colonoscopy. As ulcerative colitis virtually always involves the rectum, and Crohn's disease in over half of all patients, sigmoidoscopy and biopsy should detect disease in most patients. After sigmoidoscopy, a double-contrast barium enema would add information concerning the more proximal colon, and allow the diagnosis of Crohn's disease in those patients without rectal involvement. Colonoscopy would be the complementary examination, required in only a minority of patients for the following indications: cases of nondiagnostic sigmoidoscopy and barium enema and to biopsy any mass or stricture detected by barium enema, or for cancer surveillance in long-standing ulcerative colitis (30).

Double-contrast barium enema and colonoscopy are both useful and complementary examinations, and each has its proponents. The reality of the situation usually mandates that colonoscopy is the preferred examination, as the majority of clinicians who care for these patients perform colonoscopy. In the future, economic factors may play a role. Enemas are less costly as they do not require sedation, monitoring, and recovery and take less time. Nonetheless, it is much more convenient for clinicians and their patients to perform one examination at one time (colonoscopy), rather two exams at two different sites.

In our practice at the Cleveland Clinic Foundation, we perform more barium enemas on patients with Crohn's disease than ulcerative colitis. The vast majority of these are on patients with known, established disease; rarely is the diagnosis of ulcerative colitis or Crohn's colitis first made in the radiology department. Our clinicians feel strongly about the need for cancer surveillance in ulcerative colitis, and the superior sensitivity of colonoscopy for dysplasia and subtle changes of early carcinoma have justifiably made this the preferred examination in this patient group. Barium enema may be more suited for the follow-up of patients with Crohn's disease, due to its propensity for skip lesions, strictures, deep ulcerations, and fistulae. Double-contrast barium enema may also give useful information for differentiating the small minority of patients with an indeterminate colitis.

Contrast Enema Techniques

The double-contrast barium enema is superior to the single-contrast examination in the evaluation of inflammatory bowel disease. The single-contrast exam is capable of demonstrating advanced disease with deep ulcers, fistulae, areas of narrowing, and changes in haustration, but fine mucosal detail is not seen. The double-contrast exam permits evaluation of mucosal detail en face, and allows detection and characterization of the early phases of ulcerative and Crohn's colitis. Double-contrast barium enema can be safely performed in patients with inflammatory bowel disease in the majority of instances. An "instant enema," performed in the nonprepared bowel, often provides adequate information for diagnosis, as in active inflammatory bowel disease little fecal residue may remain in the colon (31). A bowel prep is preferable if the patient is able to tolerate it. A plain film of the abdomen is usually taken prior to performing the barium enema. This allows evaluation of the amount of residual stool, caliber of the colon, and the presence or absence of bowel wall thickening or nodularity. Barium enema is contraindicated if the plain film or clinical condition suggests a pancolitis, megacolon, or peritonitis/perforation. When a colonic perforation is suspected or possible with an enema, and a luminal exam is deemed necessary for patient management (an unusual occurrence), water soluble contrast media should be used.

Inflammatory Colitis: Radiographic Findings

As discussed previously, the double-contrast barium enema is a relatively sensitive examination in detecting the presence and extent of disease, and distinguishing ulcerative colitis from Crohn's disease in the vast majority of patients, even those with radiologically detectable mild or early disease. The radiographic findings in ulcerative and Crohn's colitis have been extensively detailed in the radiology, gastroenterology, and surgery literature (20,21,26–28,31,32–38). The salient features of each, emphasizing the differential features, will be discussed immediately. The radiographic manifestations of both ulcerative and Crohn's colitis depend on the stage at which the disease is studied. For purposes of simplicity, the findings will be divided into early and late stages for each disease.

Ulcerative colitis: Ulcerative colitis is primarily a disease of the mucosa. Involvement characteristically begins in the rectum and extends proximally for a variable distance, often involving the entire colon (pancolitis). The distal colon and rectum are involved in virtually all (95%) of cases. Diffuse, continuous, and symmetric involvement is a hallmark of ulcerative colitis, with essentially no areas of residual normal mucosa. Symmetry refers to circumferential disease involvement of the bowel. In ulcerative colitis, disease involvement is always symmetric at any particular point in the colon.

Early manifestations: The earliest radiographically detectable abnormality in cases of ulcerative colitis is a fine, diffusely granular appearance, reflecting mucosal edema and hyperemia (Fig. 6.7) (31). If the colon is "wet" or if the patient has been treated with steroid enemas these findings may be absent. Excessive fluid in the colon often prevents adequate coating of the surface even with high-density barium. Steroid enemas treat the superficial ulcers.

With further progression of disease, small, superficial ulcers are seen, imparting a coarse granularity or stippled appearance (Fig. 6.8). These ulcers often enlarge, progressing to deeper "collar-button" ulcers. These ulcers are always seen, however, on a background of abnormal, granular mucosa. Involvement of the colon continues to be symmetric and continuous, as opposed to the skip lesions seen in Crohn's colitis (Fig. 6.9). As the ulcers enlarge and interconnect, islands of residual inflamed mucosa become isolated, producing inflammatory pseudopolyps, similar to the cobblestone pattern of Crohn's disease. The caliber and length of the involved colon are usually maintained at this stage, although the haustral markings may become lost.

Late manifestations: More marked loss of the haustral markings occurs. Even though ulcerative colitis is essentially a mucosal disease, some degree of wall thickening is seen, predominantly due to hypertrophy of the muscularis mucosa and thickening of the lamina propria (37). The colon becomes mildly to moderately narrowed, again, in a diffuse, continuous fashion. An overall shortening of the colon is also often present, with loss of the hepatic and splenic flexures. The colon thus assumes the appearance of a fixed, rigid pipe (Fig. 6.10). In patients with a pancolitis, the terminal ileum may appear abnormal. This has been termed "backwash ileitis," suggesting that some toxic substance has been refluxed from the colon into the terminal ileum, causing it to become diseased. In reality, this more likely represents actual involvement of the terminal ileum by direct extension of the colonic inflammatory process. The ileocecal valve tends to be patulous and fixed in an open position, so the terminal ileum is readily visualized.

Fig. 6.7. Ulcerative colitis. (A) Fine, diffusely granular appearance of the mucosa in ulcerative colitis. Involvement is continuous and symmetric, involving the entire mucosal surface. (B) Contrast the appearance in A with this case of early Crohn's disease of the colon, which reveals aphthous ulcers scattered on a background of normal, featureless mucosa. Note the asymmetric involvement at a specific level when compared to the symmetric involvement in the case of ulcerative colitis (A).

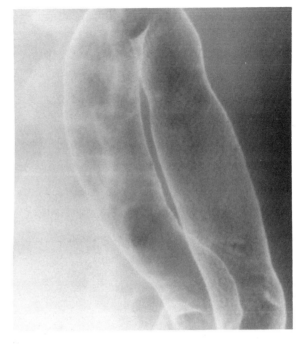

A

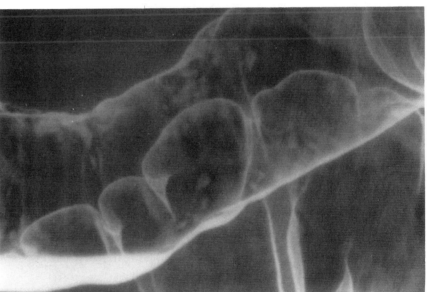

B

In Crohn's disease, the valve and terminal ileum are often spastic and/or stenotic.

Both benign and malignant strictures are seen in patients with ulcerative colitis. Benign strictures occur in 10% of patients, and like benign strictures in other diseases, demonstrate gradual, smoothly tapered margins. They are most common in the rectum and sigmoid, and may be multiple. Patients with ulcerative colitis have a significantly increased risk of developing colon cancer. Although often annular in appearance, these carcinomas in ulcerative colitis are often schirrous in nature and have a tubular, stricture-like appearance, requiring biopsy to differentiate them from a benign stricture. Thus, any stricture seen in the setting of long-standing ulcerative colitis must be viewed with suspicion.

Crohn's colitis: The radiographic hallmarks of Crohn's disease of the colon are similar to those seen in the small bowel. Pathologic changes and their radiographic counterparts are primarily those of extensive, deep ulceration and transmural involvement.

Early manifestations: The earliest radiographic finding in Crohn's colitis is the aphthous ulcer. These are seen as small, punctate collections of barium with a surrounding radiolucent halo of

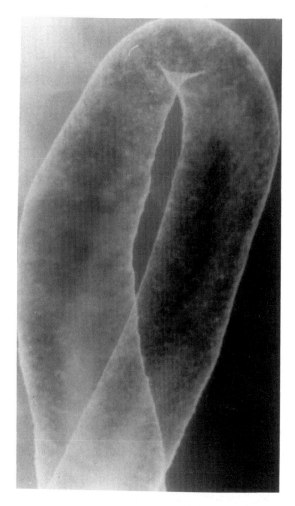

Fig. 6.8. Ulcerative colitis. Multiple diffuse small ulcers, visualized as round and linear collections of barium, distributed on a background of diffusely granular mucosa.

edema, scattered over a variable length of otherwise normal mucosa (Fig. 6.11). A prominent pattern of lymphoid hyperplasia may precede or accompany these aphthous ulcers. The ulcers may eventually enlarge to form deeper "rose-thorn" or "collar-button" ulcers (Fig. 6.12). The presence of aphthous or deeper ulcers on a background of normal mucosa is a key finding in the differentiation of Crohn's colitis from ulcerative colitis; the latter may have similar deep ulcers, but they are invariably seen on a background of abnormal, granular mucosa. Just as in Crohn's disease of the small bowel, an intersecting network or longitudinal and transverse ulcers may develop, isolating islands of residual mucosa, leading to the cobblestone pattern. This may mimic the pseudopolyps seen in ulcerative colitis, but other manifestations, including symmetric and continuous vs. asymmetric and discontinuous involvement, appearance of the

mucosal background, and distribution of disease usually allows differentiation. Long, paracolic fistulae and ulcers paralleling the lumen, termed the "double-tracking sign" are also occasionally seen, which mimic the findings of diverticulitis.

The distribution of disease in Crohn's colitis differs from that in ulcerative colitis, being asymmetric and discontinuous, with skip lesions frequently seen (Fig. 6.13). Crohn's disease more commonly involves the right side of the colon, often in continuity with terminal ileal involvement. In contrast to ulcerative colitis, Crohn's disease involves the rectum in only about 50% of cases. Perianal disease, with ulcers, abscesses, and fistulae, however, are common in Crohn's disease. These are rarely a component of ulcerative colitis.

Late changes: Fistulae to other segments of the colon, small bowel, bladder, vagina, psoas muscle, or other areas are a hallmark of Crohn's disease. Localized abscess may develop, which are best evaluated with CT, and often amenable to imaging-guided percutaneous drainage. Transmural inflammation and fibrosis lead to wall thickening and luminal narrowing. Focal strictures are seen in approximately 25% of cases of advanced Crohn's disease, and are often asymmetric and irregular. An increase incidence of carcinoma is present in patients with Crohn's colitis, but it is substantially less than that seen in ulcerative colitis.

Crohn's colitis vs. ulcerative colitis: Distinguishing radiologic features—several radiologic features, alone or in combination, allow an accurate degree of differentiation of the two major forms of inflammatory bowel disease (20,26,27,31,34,36,37):

1. Earliest manifestations—diffusely granular mucosa in ulcerative colitis; aphthous ulcers on a background of normal mucosa in Crohn's colitis.
2. Distribution—Rectal involvement with variable proximal extent in ulcerative colitis; right-sided predominance and frequent rectal sparing in Crohn's disease.
3. Continuous disease in ulcerative colitis; discontinuous disease with skip lesions in Crohn's disease.
4. Symmetry—at any given level of the colon, ulcerative colitis involves the intestinal segment in a symmetric fashion while Crohn's colitis will show asymmetric changes (Fig. 6.14). This is reflective of the continuous or discontinuous involvement characteristic of the two diseases.
5. Fistulae, sinus tracts, and perianal disease common in Crohn's disease; extremely rare in ulcerative colitis.

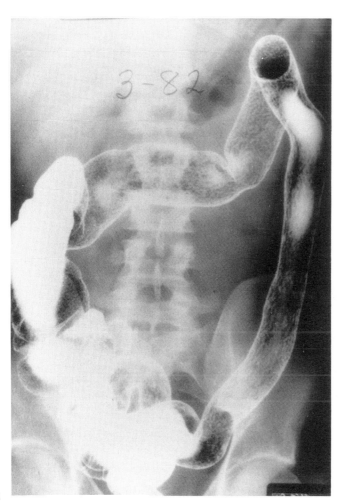

A

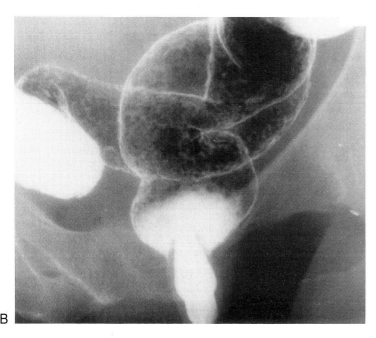

B

Fig. 6.9. Ulcerative colitis. Survey film of the entire colon (A) and spot film of the rectosigmoid region (B) from a double-contrast barium enema demonstrate a pancolitis, with diffuse, continuous, and symmetric involvement. Coarse mucosal granularity and multiple small ulcers are present.

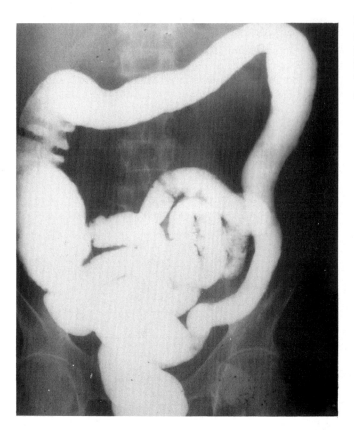

Fig. 6.10. Ulcerative colitis. Single-contrast barium enema demonstrates loss of haustral markings, mild narrowing, and shortening involving the majority of the colon. Relative sparing of the right side of the colon is present. This technique does not show the mucosal detail of the double-contrast examinations in the previous figures.

6. Deep penetrating (>3mm) ulcers—common in Crohn's disease; less common in ulcerative colitis.

7. Terminal ileal disease—common in Crohn's colitis, even with patchy colonic involvement; uncommon and seen only with pancolitis in ulcerative colitis. The findings in so-called back-wash ileitis in ulcerative colitis are distinctly different than those seen in Crohn's disease. The ileocecal valve is patulous and the abnormal terminal ileum is dilated with a fine granular mucosal pattern.

Several features, however, can be seen in either Crohn's disease or ulcerative colitis and are not particularly helpful in differentiating one from another. These include: strictures, pseudopolyps/cobblestoning, shape of deep ulcers, bowel wall thickening, pancolitis with or without megacolon. Just as differentiation may be impossible based on colonoscopic or even histologic examination, a small (5% to 10%) number of cases studied radiologically will also be called indeterminate (36). Crohn's disease is more frequently misclassified as ulcerative colitis, particularly in cases of pancolitis, than the opposite (31). When overlap in the radiologic features is found in an individual case, care-

ful evaluation of all the radiologic findings is required. Signs of early disease (granular mucosa in ulcerative colitis, aphthous ulcers in Crohn's colitis) are most distinctive, and should be carefully sought (Fig. 6.15) (37).

Differential diagnosis of colitis: The various radiologic manifestations of ulcerative colitis and Crohn's colitis are not pathognomonic, and can be seen in a number of other colitides (20). Aphthous ulcers may be seen in Behcet disease, ischemic colitis, and a variety of infectious colitides including those caused by entamoeba, *salmonella*, *shigella*, and cytomegalovirus. Deeper ulcers are present in ischemic colitis, amebic colitis, and strongyloides infection. Focal strictures have been found in colonic tuberculosis and ischemic colitis. Diffuse cobblestoning or pseudopolyps may mimic lymphoma, a polyposis syndrome, or pseudomembranous colitis. Doubletracking is commonly seen in both Crohn's disease and diverticulitis. Finally, toxic colitis or megacolon may be seen in ischemic, pseudomembranous, or amebic colitis.

Although characteristically a disease of adolescents and young adults, a second smaller peak incidence occurs over the age of 50 (31). In these patients, ischemic colitis is a particularly important differential consideration.

Fig. 6.11. Crohn's disease. Multiple small aphthous ulcers (black arrows) are asymmetrically located in a segment of the sigmoid colon, with an otherwise normal, featureless mucosa.

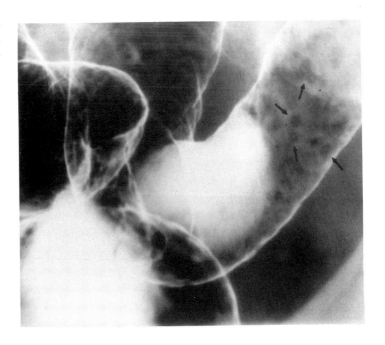

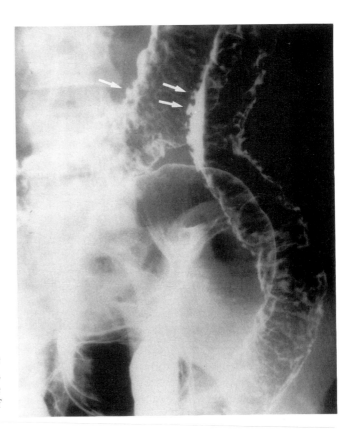

Fig. 6.12. Crohn's disease. Extensive involvement of the transverse colon, splenic flexure, and descending colon, with deep, collar-button ulcers (white arrows). Note the sparing of the rectosigmoid, distinguishing this case of Crohn's colitis from ulcerative colitis.

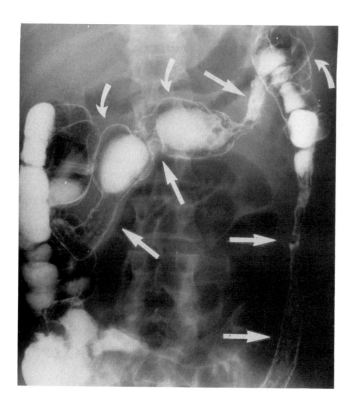

Fig. 6.13.   Crohn's disease. Discontinuous involvement of the colon, with several "skip lesions" of varying lengths (white arrows), separated by segments of normal-appearing bowel (curved white arrows).

Thus, a careful synthesis of clinical findings, laboratory tests, radiographic abnormalities, endoscopic appearance, and biopsy results may be required to arrive at the final diagnosis. Proper care of the patient with inflammatory bowel disease requires a multidisciplinary approach, with close cooperation of gastroenterologist, surgeon, and radiologist.

Radiologic Evaluation of a Toxic Patient: Pancolitis with or without Megacolon

The use of the term toxic megacolon is probably not appropriate from the radiographic point of view. First, toxicity can not be detected from a radiograph; toxicity can only be ascertained clinically. Further, patients can be toxic with a pancolitis and have a normal caliber colon. Lastly, the radiographic findings indicating a pancolitis can be present in a patient who does not meet the clinical criteria for toxicity. For plain film interpretation it is probably better to use the term(s) pancolitis with or without megacolon and reserve the additional modifier, toxic, when the clinical presentation is known. This complication of inflammatory bowel disease is uncommon and most often occurs in ulcerative colitis, but can occur in patients with Crohn's colitis as well as other colitides.

Toxicity is present when the following are found in a patient with inflammatory bowel disease: fever > 38.5°C, erythrocyte sedimentation rate of >30 mm/hour, leukocytosis (>10,500 wbc/me), tachycardia (heart rate > 100 beats/min) and anemia (39). When these signs are present, along with the radiographic changes of a pancolitis with or without dilation, then the diagnosis of a toxic pancolitis can be made.

The radiographic diagnosis of a "toxic megacolon" is most commonly made from characteristic findings on a plain radiograph of the abdomen (40). The "classic" appearance is a dilated colon demonstrating a nodular mucosa. On a routine supine view of the abdomen, the most common location is the transverse colon; a finding due entirely to patient position (the transverse colon is the most anteriorly located segment of the colon in the supine position). In many cases, most or all of the colon is equally affected. On decubitus views, either the ascending or descending colon may exhibit a similar appearance.

In the classic appearance, the internal diameter of the lumen may approach 8 to 10 cm, with any diameter over 5 cm considered abnormal. The nodules extending into the lumen may be relatively small (1 to 2 cm) or very prominent, large "thumbprints" (more often seen when the colon is not dilated). In some instances, the wall of the colon itself appears thick. However, pathologically, the

Fig. 6.14. Crohn's disease. Survey (A) and spot films of the transverse colon (B) from a double-contrast barium enema demonstrate asymmetric involvement in Crohn's colitis. Note the normal appearance of the superior border of the transverse colon, with ulcerations (black arrows) and rigidity of the inferior border. Areas of relatively uninvolved colon balloon out between the diseased segments, causing sacculations (white arrows). The ulcerations occur on a background of otherwise normal, featureless mucosa, as opposed to the diffuse mucosal granularity seen in ulcerative colitis.

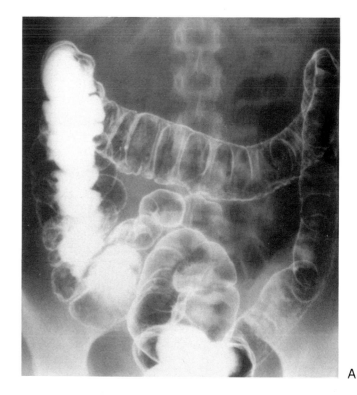

A

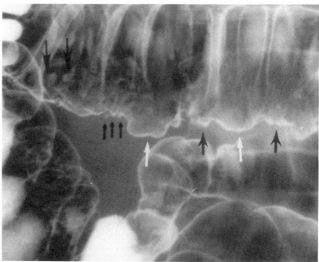

B

wall is thinned; the apparent thickening may be due to submucosal or mesenteric fat edema.

Dilation of the colon may not be present in a toxic patient with pancolitis (Fig. 6.16). A normal caliber colon may result from a perforation. However, in the absence of free air on upright or decubitus views, any colon with thickened haustra or mucosal nodularity should alert the radiologist to the possibility of a pancolitis.

A contrast enema in patients with toxic colitis especially with a megacolon is contraindicated. Barium should never be used if an exam will alter patient management. Water soluble enemas can be used to determine the presence of a perforation when free air is present. However, they (1) rarely show a leak as perforations are often small or seal rapidly, (2) are difficult to perform due to the large amount of air in the colon (an airlock is created when large volumes of air are present in the colon, often preventing the adequate opacification/distension of the colon), and (3) rarely change patient management.

The two most important radiographic findings other than those of a pancolitis are: (1) free intra-

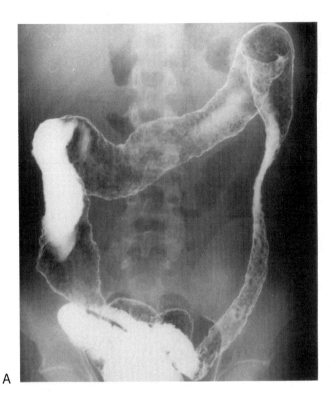

A

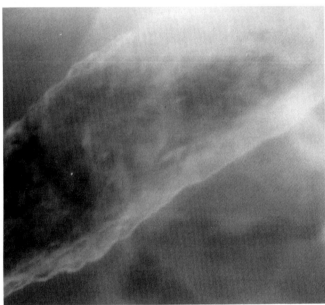

B

Fig. 6.15. (A) Double-contrast barium enema demonstrates a pancolitis, with diffuse ulceration, mild luminal narrowing and shortening, and continuous involvement. (B) Careful inspection of the pattern of involvement, however, reveals multiple aphthous ulcers asymmetrically located on a background of relatively normal mucosa, allowing a confident diagnosis of Crohn's colitis to be made.

peritoneal air, and (2) progressive dilation of the colon over time especially if the initial film shows no dilation. Surgery is most often indicated and performed in the following situations: (1) generalized peritonitis, (2) severe abdominal pain especially when localized, (3) septic shock, (4) colonic hemorrhage and (5) failure of medical treatment to resolve the clinical picture (39).

Abdominal CT can be very helpful in managing "toxic" patients with a severe pancolitis and may be the only appropriate radiographic study after plain films. The presence of an abscess detected by CT may explain the patient's symptoms. CT can also guide immediate, appropriate drainage of the abscess when detected. If an abdominal CT excludes an abscess, the clinician can safely assume that the signs and symptoms are wholly attributable to the colonic disease. Lastly, small amounts of free intraperitoneal air missed with plain radiography can be detected by CT.

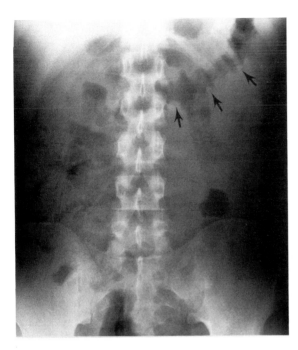

Fig. 6.16. Plain abdominal film shows a collapsed, nodular transverse colon (arrows) indicating a severe pancolitis without megacolon.

Fistula Studies: Fistulography versus Antegrade and Retrograde Luminal Exams

Patient's with Crohn's disease frequently present with bowel fistulas. Most of the time, the origin and extent of these fistulas is unknown, information which often alters management. Therefore, radiologists are often asked to evaluate these fistulas with radiographic techniques (41). Traditionally, radiologists take a passive role in the request for evaluation and the study requested is often not the best. We prefer to take an active role in the evaluation of these patients. Often a small bowel exam is requested, but the patient would be best examined with a transcutaneous study (a so-called fistulagram) or a cystogram.

The biggest challenge in fistulography is obtaining adequate pressure to fully evaluate the tract. The best approach is the one which produces the greatest pressure possible. For instance, if a entero or colo-vesical fistula is suspected, the best test is a cystogram rather than an antegrade small bowel study or a retrograde, water soluble contrast study. Our approach is as follows.

Entero-entero fistulas are almost always identified by an antegrade, barium study of the small bowel and as such are not a problem vis-à-vis appro-priate test request. If a left sided enterocolic fistula is suspected based on signs and symptoms, it is best to start with a water-soluble contrast enema (often referred to as a Gastrograffin enema). We do not use Gastrograffin as it is expensive and the same information can be obtained using a less-expensive water soluble contrast agent (Hypaque or any other inexpensive high-osmolar ionic contrast agent). Right sided enterocolic fistulae are best evaluated with an antegrade small bowel examination.

Entero- or colocutaneous fistulas are always best evaluated via a cutaneous approach if the tract can be adequately cannulated with an appropriately sized catheter. Therefore, the first attempt should be a fistulagram. To achieve adequate pressure, the radiologist must match the catheter size (ranging from a small 2 to 3 French pediatric feeding tube to a 30 French Foley catheter) with the size of the fistula tract; thus, achieving a seal. We prefer to pass the catheter as far into the tract as possible, often under fluoroscopic guidance, in order to achieve the best study. If this cannot be done, most of the contrast will leak out onto the skin. If there is a large, open wound, it will be necessary to probe the wound with a catheter looking for the site of leak. Unfortunately, an adequate seal is often impossible with large wounds and we must resort to a luminal study.

Despite the method of evaluation, oblique and lateral views must be obtained for adequate evaluation. Lastly, if an extensive fistulous tract is identified without bowel connection, it may be helpful to perform a postfistulagram CT exam without administration of oral contrast media. In a limited experience, we have found this to be very helpful in proving a bowel connection.

As previously stated, bowel fistulae to the urinary bladder should first be evaluated with a cystogram. This method achieves the greatest pressure, even greater than a water soluble enema especially if the ileocecal valve is incompetent or the patient cannot retain a large volume enema.

Vaginal fistulas can be particularly difficult to identify. The first study should probably be a water soluble enema especially if formed stool is identified in the vaginal vault. However, if this fails to identify the fistula, a vaginogram can be performed (42). The biggest challenge is achieving a seal at the vaginal introitus so that adequate pressure is generated. We use a large Foley catheter inserted into the outer vagina with the balloon inflated to at least 20 to 30 cc. The woman is then asked to cross her legs and gentle traction is applied to the catheter. This generally lodges the Foley balloon in the vagina. With the patient in a slight Trendelenberg

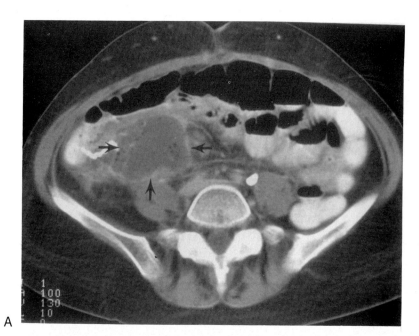

A

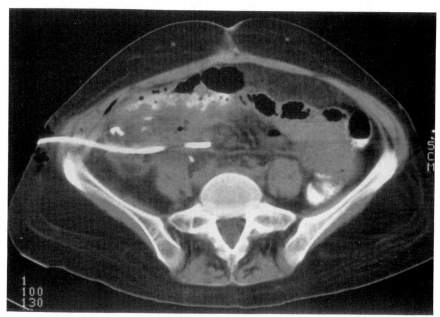

B

Fig. 6.17. (A) CT scan through false pelvis shows a well defined, water attenuation mass (arrows) in the mesentery indicating a probable abscess in this patient with Crohn's disease postileocolic resection. (B) Pyogenic material was obtained with CT-guided, needle aspiration and then the abscess drained with a percutaneous catheter. (C) A "tube-check" of the drain catheter one month later shows connection of abscess cavity (A) with the small bowel (arrowheads). (D) The percutaneous catheter was inadvertently pulled out three months after placement. A sinogram shows no connection to bowel.

position, water soluble contrast is injected into the Foley. We have found that injection, rather than gravity is best. In our experience, this technique often identifies the fistula and its source.

Lately, several centers have used magnetic resonance imaging to identify the course and extent of fistulous tracts, especially in presurgical planning. The unique advantage of MR lies in its multiplanar imaging capabilities (coronal, sagittal and oblique planes in addition to the traditional axial plane). These capabilities are especially helpful in the pelvis. In the pelvis, CT can only be performed in the axial plane. With current spiral scanners, coronal and sagittal reconstruction can be performed. But, unless specialized, narrow slice technique is used, the spatial resolution of the images is inferior to the images obtained with MR. These narrow slice routines are time consuming and add radiation dose; an issue which is more critical in evaluating young patients. In addition to its multiplanar capabilities, MR is more sensitive than CT in identifying muscular involvement by inflammatory processes. In several small series, MR was particularly helpful in depicting involvement of the supra and infralevator compartments as well as the pelvic side wall and musculature (43–45). With a focused

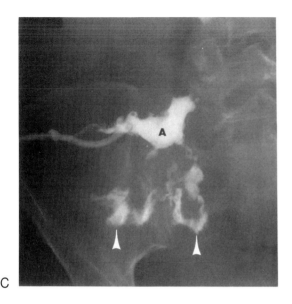

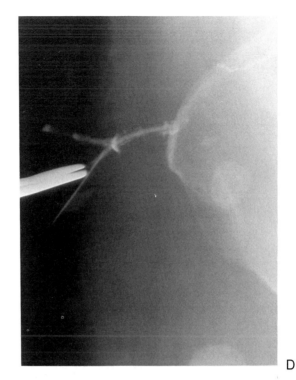

Fig. 6.17. *Continued*

imaging approach, using modern, fast scanners, the exam should not take more than 30 minutes. This time makes MR more cost-equivalent to CT than in the past. In selected cases, with the additional information provided, MR may be more cost-effective in patient management.

Abscess Detection and Treatment in Patients with Inflammatory Bowel Disease

Abdominal CT is a common radiologic study in patients with inflammatory bowel disease, especially Crohn's disease. Patients often present with fever, chills, abdominal pain and/or distension with an elevated white blood count and the clinical question is whether there is a complicating abscess. CT is the modality best suited for this dilemma because within 1 to 2 hours of the ingestion of oral contrast media, the question can be easily answered.

An abscess on CT is a near-water to water density "collection" that is not bowel (Fig. 6.17). We use the term collection rather than masses to avoid defining an abscess on the basis of a particular morphology. This is because our concept of an abscess has evolved over the years. Classically, an abscess is well-defined, rounded or oval and often has a definable wall. However, infected fluid collections can occupy an intra- or extraperitoneal space and not be well-defined (Fig. 6.18). Further, loculated, infected peritoneal fluid is relatively common and is classically not an abscess.

Because a localized loop of fluid filled bowel can mimic an abscess, oral contrast media ingestion before CT is extremely helpful. In fact, unless there is a bowel obstruction it is almost essential. In the presence of a bowel obstruction, the fluid filled, continuously dilated tubular bowel lumen can almost always be distinguished from an abscess. We administer a water soluble contrast enema if the colon is not opacified and when we cannot distinguish potentially unopacified colon from a possible abscess. However, it is not our routine to administer retrograde colonic contrast.

There are no characteristic findings that distinguish an infected from a noninfected fluid collection. Air in a collection is highly suggestive of infection but air can be present in a sterile, postoperative collection. The density of the fluid is not helpful in the differentiation. High density strongly suggests a hemorrhagic component. The only consistent means of determining the nature of a fluid collection is via aspiration.

Therefore, once a localized fluid collection is detected, if an infectious process is suspected an image guided, needle aspiration should be performed (Fig. 6.17). However, before aspiration is performed, the possibility of a drainage should be

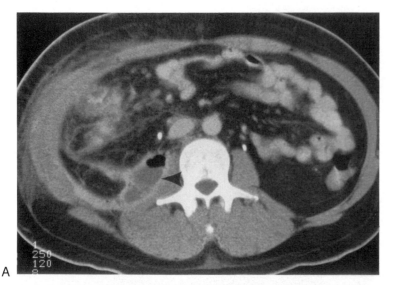

A

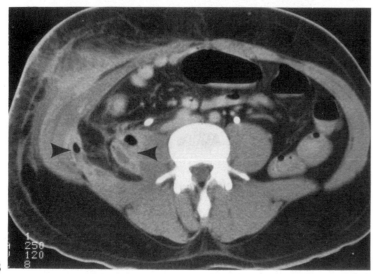

B

Fig. 6.18. (A) and (B) CT scans at two levels show extensive infected spaces in right retroperitoneum (arrowheads) in this patient with Crohn's disease of the small bowel. Two drain catheters were placed in this patient, one in the medial retroperitoneum and the other in the anterior abdominal wall (not shown). (C) "Tube check" of the medial drain catheter confirms the extent of the process in the retroperitoneum (arrows). A bowel communication was not confirmed. (D) CT scan performed after "tube check" (no oral or intravenous contrast media administered) shows contrast in small bowel (arrowheads) indicating a bowel connection to infected retroperitoneal process.

discussed. From our perspective, once pus is aspirated, we are obligated to percutaneously drain the collection with a catheter. Often, however, obvious purulent material is not obtained and the fluid is sent for gram stain and culture. Some advocate immediate gram stain of the material; if polymorphonuclear leukocytes or bacteria are identified then a catheter should be placed (46,47). In our practice, if the stakes are high enough with a patient, regardless of the appearance of the fluid, we place a catheter. If the fluid does not grow microorganisms over 36 to 48 hours, then the catheter can be removed. In patients who are stable, we often wait to place the catheter. In these cases, consultation between the radiologist and clinician is critical prior to procedure.

Some authors advocate the routine use of antibiotics before an aspiration and drainage is per-

formed (48–50). In our experience, most patients are already on antibiotics prior to the procedure. However, in our experience as well, those who are not almost never experience sepsis. We have seen sepsis only twice in draining well over 300 abscesses; one of these patients had a liver abscess and another had a large pancreatic abscess and experienced an episode of peritonitis right after the placement of the catheter.

Many radiologists use a trochar technique to place the catheter. However, it is very difficult to easily place a 12- or 14-French catheter using this approach. Our approach has been to use the standard Seldinger technique; entering the collection first with an 18-g needle, and then using a guide wire to place increasingly larger dilators and then the catheter. In experienced hands, this approach can be performed safely and quickly on the CT

Fig. 16.18.   *Continued*

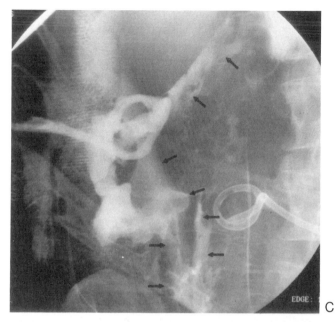

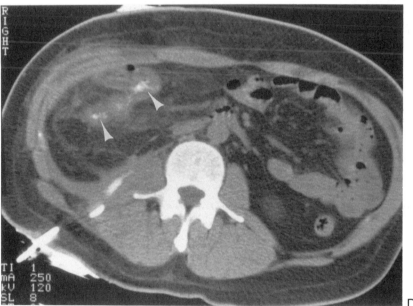

scanner without fluoroscopic guidance. In most cases, we can drain an abscess in less than 15 minutes.

Ultrasound and fluoroscopy can be used to guide percutaneous catheter placement. The method of choice for guidance should be left to the radiologist. There are many skilled radiologists who use sonography to guide needle and catheter placement with equivalent and even improved accuracy when compared to CT (51–53). When using fluoroscopy alone, the abscess must be relatively large and already identified with cross-sectional imaging. In most cases we utilize CT to guide catheter placement because the abscess is usually first

identified on CT. For convenience, the patient is left on the CT scanner table to drain the abscess after its identification. When vital structures must be avoided CT is the method of choice.

The dogma for abscess drainage is that the collection be well-defined, nonhemorrhagic, and accessible via an approach that does not traverse vital structures including overlying bowel. Outside the pelvis, a safe approach can almost always be found except with small, interloop collections. The pelvis is a particular challenge. The combination of the bony pelvis, bowel and other vital structures often prevents the easy insertion of a catheter. A variety of techniques have been developed to circumvent these problems including transvaginal and rectal techniques and the insertion of the catheter via the greater sciatic notch (54–60). Our experience is via the last approach, which if performed carefully is very effective and without significant complications.

Imaging guided, percutaneous drainage should be the treatment of choice for any abdominal abscess unless there is a compelling reason to perform immediate surgery (usually for another problem). Simply from a cost point of view, it is much cheaper to drain the abscess percutaneously rather than surgically. At the Cleveland Clinic, our direct professional and technical cost (not charge) for a CT guided drainage is approximately $410.00 (professional direct cost = $300; technical direct cost = $110) (includes nursing, sedation, and assumes a 40 minute procedure time). Total technical and professional, direct and indirect costs are $738. Our charges for a CT guided procedure are $1887.00. However with current reimbursement rates of 50% or less, we are only barely recovering our costs. Costs for an operative procedure are significantly greater than the percutaneous approach.

There are very few reasons why a radiologist should not attempt to drain a fluid collection. A catheter should not traverse a bowel loop. However, if an abscess needs draining and the patient is not a surgical candidate, bowel may be traversed safely (61). Coagulopathy should be corrected to at least tolerable levels; however, our "cut-off" for platelet count and PT/PTT levels is very dependent on the patient's condition and the necessity to drain the collection. Infected hematomas in general cannot be adequately drained via percutaneous catheters. However, there should be no reason why a trial of drainage should not be attempted as long as an appropriate end-point is understood by both the radiologist and the primary physician. The size of the catheter is largely irrelevant. Unless the collection contains very viscous material most collections can be completely collapsed with a 10- to 14-g catheter. It is common for a physician directly caring for the patient to request the placement of a larger catheter to promote further or more rapid drainage. More often than not, the failure of a catheter to function has less to do with the diameter of the catheter and more to do with the contents of the abscess (necrotic, particulate material, or stool) and the size of the catheter side holes. In general, the side-hole size does not increase dramatically from a 10- to 16-French catheter. Occasionally, large-bore (16 to 20 gauge) Mallecot catheters can be placed in stool filled abscesses. However, these cases are unusual and often

occur in patients who are not surgical candidates due to other comorbid conditions.

Catheter care post drainage is as important if not more important than the placement of the catheter. The most consistent reason for catheter "malfunction" is lack of care. Floor nurses (more commonly medical rather than surgical) often seem unable to care for catheters. Catheters must be flushed on a regular basis in order to maintain patency. In a busy ward, this often is forgotten. The radiologist must be vigilant and involved in the care of a catheter. Unfortunately, the culture of radiology does not promote this degree of physician involvement.

When a catheter stops draining, a management decision must be made based on the following criteria: the size of the abscess relative to the amount of drainage; the patient's condition; and, the suspected cause of the abscess. If the drainage seems appropriate to the estimated volume of the abscess before it was drained, and the patient is asymptomatic and a potential enteric connection to the abscess is not suspected, then the catheter can be removed without any imaging. However, if the drainage is not consistent with the size of the cavity, the patient remains symptomatic or if a bowel connection is a possibility, then a catheter-check must be performed (Figs. 6.17, 6.18). This involves injecting the catheter with iodinated contrast under fluoroscopic visualization. This simple test will show if the catheter is clogged (as is often the case), the relative size of the residual cavity and whether a bowel connection is present. It is common for a clinical service to request a repeat CT when the catheter drainage decreases or stops. In our experience this is unnecessary and expensive. CT will detect other collections or complications of a preexisting abscess such as a secondary liver abscess, but most of the time the information gleaned from the follow-up CT does not alter the patient's management. It is also common for a clinical service to reimage a collection in 7 to 10 days just to assess the progress of the drainage. In a patient who is improving clinically this is also unnecessary.

Patients with catheters do not need to be hospitalized long-term unless their clinical condition warrants this degree of care (62). With appropriate education, patients can manage their catheters at home. In addition to education, it is key that a consistent individual in radiology act as a focal point for contact. For the last six months we have had a biopsy/catheter nurse coordinating our interventions. One of her responsibilities is to educate patients before discharge and then follow-up on a periodic basis when the patients go home.

Virtually any collection can be drained; however, the success rate varies depending upon the patient's condition, the cause of the abscess and comorbid conditions. In a recent large series of image-guided, percutaneous pyogenic abscess drainage, the "success" rate approached 90%. However, one must define "success." In a review of 164 abdominal, nonsolid organ, pyogenic abscess drainage's (including postoperative, diverticular, appendiceal as well as Crohn's abscesses) the following was found: 59% cured (the patient returned to normal state of health; negative one-year follow-up); 16% temporized (resolution of abscess improved patient's condition prior to adjunctive surgery to remove the underlying cause; patient afebrile within 72 hours and signs and symptoms resolved); 16% palliated (symptomatic relief and defervescence); 9% failure (63). Therefore, in most cases, percutaneous drainage is instrumental in temporizing or resolving the patient's condition, with the abscess often completely cured.

Complications are uncommon to rare. In the above mentioned series, a total of 335 abscesses were drained with an overall complication rate of 9.8%. Sepsis was most common (4.2%). Malpositioned tubes (wrong position, tube requiring reposition or tube which "fell out") occurred 2.4% of the time (tubes almost never "fall out"; they are generally pulled out during patient motion). Bowel was transgressed or perforated in 1.2%. Hemorrhage occurred in less than 1%.

In patients with Crohn's disease, abscesses can be successfully drained with percutaneous catheters. Success rates vary depending upon the series but are generally between 70% to 90% (64–66). In the above mentioned series, there were 13 abscesses in 12 patients with Crohn's disease. Nine of 11 abscesses showed bowel communication. Of the nine with fistulous communication with the bowel, one was cured, seven were temporized and one failed. The temporized patients were treated for 2 to 5 weeks before undergoing bowel resection. The four abscesses without bowel communication were all cured. Therefore, percutaneous drainage can often be curative. However, in many the abscess often recurs due to underlying diseased bowel segment. Therefore, the drainage serves to "cure" the abscess and sterilize the surgical bed (much like the approach for diverticulitis surgery). In the four published series of 45 patients with Crohn's abscess, no enterocutaneous fistulae have resulted from the catheter placement despite the fact that the cavity commonly communicated with the bowel (90%–100%). It should be noted that if the abscess communicates with the bowel and abscess "cure" is

sought from a percutaneous drain, then it will be necessary to keep the catheter in place for weeks to months (Fig. 6.17).

Ileoanal Pouch Studies

In patients with chronic ulcerative colitis, the ileal pouch-anal anastomosis has become a common surgical treatment after a total proctocolectomy. At the Cleveland Clinic, the ileal-J pouch is the pouch of choice. Luminal studies of the pouch prior to closure of a temporary stome is routine (67,68). These "pouchograms" are performed approximately 8 to 12 weeks after pouch creation in order to determine the integrity of the pouch-anal anastomosis and of the oversewn "blind-end" of the pouch. We use a retrograde approach with water soluble contrast (Hypaque rather than Gastrograffin as it is 4 to 5 times cheaper). We use a small blue catheter without a balloon tip. Care should be taken in inserting the catheter as the anal anastomoses are often tight and insertion of the catheter painful.

Pouch leaks generally occur in two locations: at the anal anastomosis and at the "blind-end" of the pouch. Anal anastomotic leaks are often small, contained and extend lateral or posterolateral from the pouch-anal anastomotic site. They may only be seen after the enema tip has been removed as the tip may occlude the leak site during the exam. Larger leaks extend into the presacral space (Fig. 6.19).

Blind-end leaks occur at the oversewn end of the pouch. These leaks are detected during the filling or filled phase of the water soluble enema. A false-positive diagnosis of a leak can occur when contrast is trapped in outpouched mucosa of the blind-end. Blind-end leaks are often only seen when the lumen is adequately distended. Most patients with an ileal pouch have the proximal end of the pouch open to the ileostomy. Therefore, adequate distension may not be achieved via a retrograde approach because of the "pop-off" valve effect of the ileostomy. We have contemplated studying patients with an antegrade approach (via the ileostomy), but have little experience with this method. Other complications of ileal pouches include pouch-vaginal fistulas (Fig. 6.20).

The sole role of CT in the evaluation of patients with ileoanal pouches is in the search for an abscess. If a water density mass is identified in the pelvis, aspiration and drainage attempts should be performed. If an abscess is detected, a water soluble contrast enema is then required to detect a pouch leak as the source of the abscess. We have been

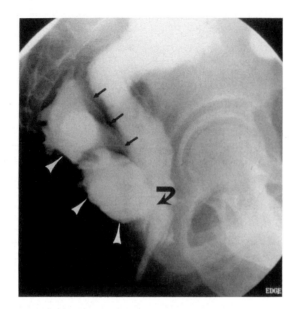

Fig. 6.19. Water soluble contrast enema of a J-pouch shows extravasation of contrast arising from the pouch-anal anastomosis (curved arrow) and extending into the presacral space (arrowheads). Note that the extravasated contrast is posterior to the pouch suture line (arrows).

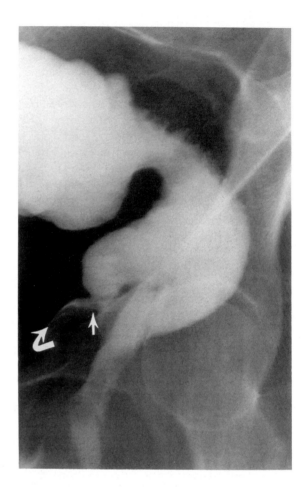

Fig. 6.20. Water soluble contrast enema of a J-pouch shows extravasation (arrow) of contrast anteriorly with fistulization into the vagina (curved arrow).

uniformly disappointed in the routine use of water soluble, pouch contrast before the CT is performed in order to identify extravasation. Fluoroscopy remains the best method to identify the presence and exact site of the leak.

A complication of a functioning pouch is "pouchitis." Luminal studies are rarely used to detect this complication as a safe endoscopy is more specific and can guide biopsy if necessary. Likewise, a complicating adenocarcinoma occurring in residual rectal mucosa is better detected with endoscopy and biopsy. Rarely, pouch-perianal fistulas occur and can be demonstrated with a water soluble contrast enema.

Summary

Crohn's disease and ulcerative colitis are complex clinical entities which require a multidisciplinary approach to patient management. The gastroenterologist, surgeon and radiologist must work together closely to optimally manage these patients. In terms of imaging, this is especially important as luminal and cross-sectional studies address different clinical questions even though they can provide complementary information. From a radiologist's point of view, we are most effective with imaging when presented with a clinical question and then are given the freedom to choose which imaging

study or studies best address that question or questions.

The following summary statements can be made concerning imaging:

1. An air-contrast barium enema is sensitive in the detection and classification of colitis but has been largely supplanted by colonoscopy which offers the advantages of direct visualization of the mucosa and biopsy of involved areas. In cases where the colitis is indeterminate by colonoscopy and biopsy, an air-contrast barium enema can provide a more specific diagnosis in some cases of Crohn's disease if the characteristic asymmetric and discontinuous changes are present.
2. For the small bowel, barium studies remain the primary imaging method of choice. A carefully performed, dedicated small bowel examination, liberally augmented with the peroral pneumocolon technique will identify the fol-

lowing: 1) the early changes of Crohn's disease; 2) the location and extent of disease; and 3) complications of fistula and sinus tract formation and bowel obstruction. More specialized radiologic examinations including enteroclysis, fistulography and vaginography may also have a role in evaluating selected patients with Crohn's disease.

3. While (CT) is blind to the bowel mucosa, it is ideally suited to evaluate extramucosal disease including bowel wall thickness, mesenteric fat changes and extraintestinal complications such as abscess formation. CT is the single best test for an acutely ill patient with Crohn's disease where the clinical question is abscess formation vs. an acute flare of mucosal disease. When an abscess is identified, a pro-active, aggressive abdominal radiologist plays a vital role in patient management by draining that abscess in a timely manner.

References

1. Herlinger H. The small bowel enema and the diagnosis of Crohn's disease. Radiol Clin North Am 1982;20:721–42.

2. Engelholm L, DeToeuf J, Herlinger H, et al. Crohn's disease of the small bowel. In: Herlinger H, Maglinte DDT, eds. Clinical Radiology of the Small Intestine. Philadelphia: W.B. Saunders Company; 1989:295–334.

3. Nolan DJ. Radiology of Crohn's disease of the small intestine: a review. J R Soc Med 1981;74:294–300.

4. Maglinte DDT, Chernish SM, Kelvin FM, et al. Crohn's disease of the small intestine: accuracy and relevance of enteroclysis. Radiology 1992;184:541–5.

5. Maglinte DDT, Lappas JC, Kelvin FM, et al. Small bowel radiography: how, when, and why? Radiology 1987;163:297–305.

6. Ott DJ, Chen YM, Gelfand DW, et al. Detailed peroral small bowel examination vs. enteroclysis. Part 2: radiographic accuracy. Radiology 1985;155:31–4.

7. Carlson HC. Perspective: the small bowel examination in the diagnosis of Crohn's disease. AJR 1986;147:63–5.

8. Trenkner SW, Hommeyer S. Practical imaging of the small bowel. The Radiologist 1995;2:127–37.

9. Glick SN. Crohn's disease of the small intestine. Radiol Clin North Am 1987;25:25–45.

10. Kelvin FM, Gedgaudas RK, Thompson WM, et al. The peroral pneumocolon: its role in evaluating the terminal ileum. AJR 1982;139:115–21.

11. Kressel HY, Evers K, Glick SN, et al. The peroral pneumocolon: technique and indications. Radiology 1982;143:414–6.

12. Wolf KJ, Goldberg HI, Wall SD, et al. Feasibility of the peroral pneumocolon in evaluating the ileocecal region. AJR 1985;145:1019–24.

13. Marshak RH. Granulomatous disease of the intestinal tract (Crohn's disease). Radiology 1975;114:3–22.

14. Marshak RH, Lindner AE. Regional Enteritis. In: Radiology of the Small Intestine. Philadelphia: W.B. Saunders Company; 2nd ed, 1976:179–245.

15. Herlinger H, Caroline DF. Crohn's Disease. In: Gore RM, Levine MS, Laufer I, eds. Textbook of Gastrointestinal Radiology. Philadelphia: W.B. Saunders; 1994:824–43.

16. Glick SN, Teplick SK. Crohn's disease of the small intestine: diffuse mucosal granularity. Radiology 1985;154:313–7.

17. Jones B, Hamilton SR, Rubesin SE, et al. Granular small bowel mucosa: a reflection of villous abnormality. Gastrointest Radiol 1987;12:219–25.

18. Durdey P, Weston PMT, Williams NS. Colonoscopy or barium enema as initial investigation of colonic disease. Lancet 1987;2:549–51.

19. Dijkstra J, Reeders JWAJ, Tytgat GNJ. Idiopathic inflammatory bowel disease: endoscopic-radiologic correlation. Radiology 1995;197:369–75.

20. Williams HJ, Stephens DH, Carlson HC. Double-contrast radiography:colonic inflammatory disease. AJR 1981;137:315–22.

21. Freeny PC. Crohn's disease and ulcerative colitis: evaluation with double-contrast barium examination and endoscopy. Postgrad Med 1986;80:139–56.

22. Elliott PR, Lennard-Jones JE, Bartram CI, et al. Colonoscopic diagnosis of minimal change colitis in patients with a normal sigmoidoscopy and normal air-contrast barium enema. Lancet 1982;1:650, 651.

23. Gabrielson N, Ganquist S, Sundelin P, et al. Extent of inflammatory lesions in ulcerative colitis assessed by radiology, colonoscopy, and endoscopic biopsies. Gastrointest Radiol 1979;4:395–400.

24. Holdstock G, DuBoulay CE, Smith CL. Survey of the use of colonoscopy in inflammatory bowel disease. Dig Dis Sci 1984;29:731–4.

25. Waye JD. Endoscopy in Idiopathic Inflammatory Bowel Disease. In: Kirsner JB, Shorter RG, eds. Inflammatory Bowel Disease, 3rd ed. Philadelphia: Lea & Febiger; 1988:353–76.

26. Laufer I, Hamilton J. The radiological differentiation between ulcerative and granulomatous colitis by double-contrast radiology. Am J Gastroenterol 1976;66:259–69.

27. Kelvin FM, Oddson TA, Rice RP, et al. Double contrast barium enema in Crohn's disease and ulcerative colitis. AJR 1978;131:207–13.

28. Gitnick G, ed. Inflammatory Bowel Disease: Diagnosis and Treatment. New York: Igaku-Shoin; 1991.

29. Salena BJ, Hunt RH. Diagnosis: an Endoscopist's Perspective. In: Targan SR, Shanahan F, eds. Inflammatory Bowel Disease—From Bench to Bedside. Baltimore: Williams & Wilkins; 1993:352–65.

30. Hogan WJ, Hensley GT, Geenen JE. Endoscopic evaluation of inflammatory bowel disease. Med Clin North Am 1980;64:1083–102.

31. Caroline CF, Evers K. Colitis: radiographic features and differentiation of idiopathic inflammatory bowel disease. Radiol Clin North Am 1987;25:47–66.

32. Fraser GM, Findlay JM. The double contrast enema in ulcerative and Crohn's colitis. Clin Radiol 1976;27:103–12.

33. Laufer I, Mellens JE, Hamilton J. Correlation of endoscopy and double-contrast radiography in the early stages of ulcerative and granulomatous colitis. Radiology 1976;118:1–5.

34. Laufer I. Air contrast studies of the colon in inflammatory bowel disease. Crit Rev Diag Imaging 1977;9:421–47.

35. Marshak RH, Lindner AE, Maklansky D. Granulomatous colitis. Mt Sinai J Med 1979;46:431–54.

36. Margulis AR, Goldberg HI, Lawson TL, et al. The overlapping spectrum of ulcerative and granulomatous colitis: a roentgenographic-pathologic study. AJR 1971;113:325–34.

37. Gore RM, Laufer I. Ulcerative and granulomatous colitis: Idiopathic Inflammatory Bowel Disease. In: Gore RM, Laufer I, Levine MS, eds. Textbook of Gastrointestinal Radiology. Philadelphia: W.B. Saunders; 1994:1098–1141.

38. Bartram CI, Laufer I. Inflammatory bowel disease. In: Laufer I, Levine MS, eds. Double Contrast Gastrointestinal Radiology 2nd ed. Philadelphia: W.B. Saunders; 1992:579–645.

39. Fazio VW. Toxic megacolon in ulcerative colitis and Crohn'ss' colitis. Clin Gastroenterol 1980;9:389–407.

40. Halpert RD. Toxic dilatation of the colon. Radiol Clin North Am 1987;25:147–55.

41. Alexander ES, Weinberg S, Clark RA, et al. Fistulas and sinus tracts: radiographic evaluation, management and outcome. Gastrointest Radiol 1982;7:135–40.

42. Cooper R. Vaginography: a presentation of new cases and subject review. Radiology 1982;143:421–5.

43. Koelbel G, Schmiedl U, Majer MC, et al. Diagnosis of fistulae and sunus tracts in patients with Crohn's disease: value of MR imaging. AJR 1989;152:999–1003.

44. Outwater E, Schiebler ML. Pelvic fistulas: findings on MR images. AJR 1993;160:327–30.

45. Myhr GE, Myrvold HE, Nilsen G, et al. Perianal fistulas: use of MR imaging for diagnosis. Radiology 1994;191:545–9.

46. van Sonnenberg E, D'Agostino HB, Casola G, et al. Percutaneous abscess drainage: current concepts. Radiology 1991;181:617–26.

47. van Sonnenberg E, D'Agostino HB, Sanchez RB, et al. Percutaneous abscess drainage: editorial comments. Radiology 1992;184:27–9.

48. Spies JB, Rosen RJ, Lebowitz AS. Antibiotic prophylaxis in vascular and interventional radiology: a rational approach. Radiology 1988;166:381–7.

49. van Waes PF, Simoons-Smit IM. Use of antibiotics in interventional radiologic procedures: an important lesson still to be learned. Radiology 1988;166:570, 571.

50. Hunter DW, Simmons RL, Hulbert JC. Antibiotics for radiologic interventional procedures. Radiology 1988;166:572,573.

51. Grønvall S, Gammelgaard J, Haubek A, et al. Drainage of abdominal abscesses guided by sonography. AJR 1982;138:527–9.

52. Jeffrey, RB Jr, Wing VW, Laing FC. Real-time sonographic monitoring of percutaneous abscess drainage. AJR 1985;144:469,470.

53. McGahan JP, Anderson MW, Walter JP. Portable real-time sonographic and needle guidance systems for aspiration and drainage. AJR 1986;147:1241–6.

54. Nosher JL, Needell GS, Amorosa JK, et al. Transrectal pelvic abscess drainage with sonographic guidance. AJR 1986;146:1047,1048.

55. Butch RJ, Mueller PR, Ferrucci JT, et al. Drainage of pelvic abscesses through the greater sciatic foramen. Radiology 1986;158:487–91.

56. Jacques PF, Mauro M. Drainage of pelvic abscesses through the greater sciatic foramen. Letters to the Editor. Radiology 1986;160:278,279.

57. Nosher JL, Winchman HK, Needell GS. Transvaginal pelvic abscess drainage with US guidance. Radiology 1987;165:872,873.

58. Gazelle GS, Haaga JR, Stellato TA, et al. Pelvic abscesses: CT-guided transrectal drainage. Radiology 1991;181:49–51.

59. van Sonnenberg E, D'Agostino HB, Casola G, et al. US-guided transvaginal drainage of pelvic abscesses and fluid collections. Radiology 1991;181:53–6.

60. Bennett JD, Kozak RI, Taylor BM, et al. Deep pelvic abscesses: transrectal drainage with radiologic guidance. Radiology 1992;185:825–8.

61. Pettit P, Bret PM, Lough JO, et al. Risks associated with intestinal perforation during experimental percutaneous drainage. Invest Radiol 1992;27:1012–9.

62. Rifkin MD, Heffelfinger D, Kurtz AB, et al. Outpatient therapy of intraabdominal abscesses following early discharge from the hospital. Radiology 1985;155:333,334.

63. Lambiase RE, Deyoe L, Cronan JJ, et al. Percu-

taneous drainage of 335 consecutive abscesses: results of primary drainage with 1-year follow-up. Radiology 1992;184:167–79.

64. Safrit HD, Mauro MA, Jaques PF. Percutaneous abscess drainage in Crohn's disease. AJR 1987;148: 859–62.

65. Casola G, vanSonnenberg E, Neff CC, et al. Abscesses in Crohn's disease: percutaneous drainage. Radiology 1987;163:19–22.

66. Lambiase RE, Cronan JJ, Dorfman GS, et al. Percutaneous drainage of abscesses in patients with Crohn's disease. AJR 1988;150:1043–5.

67. Kremers PW, Scholz FJ, Schoetz DJ, et al. Radiology of the ileoanal reservoir. AJR 1985;145:559–67.

68. Brown JJ, Balfe DM, Heiken JP, et al. Ileal J pouch: radiologic evaluation in patients with and without postoperative infections complications. Radiology 1990;174:115–20.

7 Medical Therapy

Stephen B. Hanauer and Robert B. Stein

Medical therapy of inflammatory bowel disease (IBD) continues to be a challenging endeavor for the clinician. The pathogenesis of ulcerative colitis (UC) and Crohn's disease (CD) remain unclear. Similar to other chronic inflammatory diseases a genetic predisposition is likely with susceptible individuals failing to down-regulate an over exuberant immuno-inflammatory response to, as yet, undefined environmental triggers (1,2).

Therapeutic regimens continue to be developed for treating active IBD and maintaining clinical remission. In this chapter we will review the spectrum of therapeutic options available to the clinician; from sulfasalazine and the newer aminosalicylate compounds to the immunomodulators including methotrexate, 6-mercaptopurine, azathioprine, and cyclosporine. In addition, we will review the expanding armamentarium of novel therapies under investigation for the management of IBD, and discuss medical management according to clinical presentations.

Aminosalicylates

Sulfasalazine and the 5-aminosalicyclic acid derivatives (5-ASA, mesalamine) are the most commonly prescribed medications for mild to moderately active UC and CD, and for patients with quiescent disease (3–7). Sulfasalazine was developed in the 1930s in an attempt to combine the anti-inflammatory properties of salicylates with the antibacterial properties of sulfa drugs (8). The compound links a sulfa moiety (sulfapyridine) to an anti-inflammatory salicylate (5-aminosalicylic acid) by an azo-bond. Once reaching the colon, sulfasalazine is cleaved by azo-reductases, liberating 5-ASA from the sulfapyridine carrier (9). The 5-ASA component accounts for virtually all of the therapeutic effects, whereas the sulfapyridine moiety exerts the majority of adverse effects (10).

The anti-inflammatory mechanisms of the aminosalicylates are complex and still not fully understood. There has been considerable investigation of the potential mechanisms of action including, the inhibitory effects on the cyclo-oxygenase and lipoxygenase pathways, scavenging of oxygen-free radicals, and inhibition of thromboxane synthetase and platelet activating factor synthase (1,9,11–13). In addition, mesalamine inhibits the production of interleukin-1 (IL-1) and reduces immunoglobulin production by plasma cells (9,13,14).

Although the mechanism of action is not completely understood, sulfasalazine has demonstrated clinical efficacy in the treatment of UC and CD (5,6,15–18). In the 1960s clinical trials confirmed the utility of sulfasalazine for the treatment of mild to moderately active UC (15,16,18). Subsequent studies have demonstrated a dose-response for the maintenance of remission. Clinical improvement or remission has been demonstrated at doses of 2 to 6 g/day in 56% to 93% of patients with mild to moderately active UC (18,19). Further, 71% to 88% of UC patients are maintained in remission at doses of 1 to 4 g/day, with increased effectiveness demonstrated at the 4 g/day dosage (5,6,11,18,19).

The efficacy of sulfasalazine in CD is more dependent on the site of gastrointestinal involvement due to the known metabolism of this drug, where colonic release of 5-ASA bypasses proximal sites of active small bowel disease. Two large placebo-controlled, multicenter trials demonstrated that sulfasalazine at doses of 3 to 5 g/day was beneficial in the treatment of mild to moderate ileo-icolitis or colitis, but had no benefit over placebo in treating isolated small bowel CD (17,20). Maintenance of remission at 12 months in CD ranges from 50% to 85%, although low dose sulfasalazine (2–2.5 gldar) is no better than placebo at prolonging clinical relapse (7,16,20,21).

The most common side effects of sulfasalazine are related to the sulfa component and are dose related including malaise, nausea, anorexia, dyspepsia, and headaches (22,23). Gradually increasing the dose, administering with meals, and enteric coated preparations may help to alleviate these symptoms. Other idiosyncratic reactions to the sulfa moiety have been documented including, fever, rash, hepatitis, bone marrow suppression, hypersensitivity pneumonia, hemolytic anemia, and reversible sperm abnormalities (22,23).

The development of sulfa-free aminosalicylates (mesalamine, olsalazine) has enhanced the efficacy of therapy with an improved side effect profile (24). Several formulations are available including topical preparations, alternative azo-bonded carriers, and pH-dependent or continuous release preparations.

Topical Preparations

Topical preparations of mesalamine have demonstrated clinical efficacy in mild to moderate UC. Placebo-controlled trials have shown a 60% to 89% response in patients with distal UC or proctitis using 700 mg to 4 g/day enemas and 400 mg to 2 g/day suppositories, respectively (15,19,25). In addition, maintenance of remission has been demonstrated in approximately 75% of patients treated with 1 to 4 g/nightly enemas, 4 g nightly enemas for one week/month, or 4 g enemas twice weekly (15,19,25). Topical mesalamine has not been formally evaluated for CD.

Oral Formulations

The oral formulations of mesalamine (5-ASA) have been shown to be more effective than placebo in the management of mild to moderately active UC and in patients with quiescent disease (15,26), although the dose-response has required higher doses than would be anticipated from other trials involving sulfasalazine. Olsalazine (Dipentum) is composed of two 5-ASA molecules linked by an azo-bond. Diarrhea occurs in 10% to 20% of patients taking this medication secondary to its secretory effect on the small intestinal mucosa (27). Other preparations include a resin coated formulation

(Asacol®) designed to release the active drug at a pH >7.0, and mesalamine encapsulated into ethyl-cellulose microspheres (Pentasa®), providing continuous release in the small and large intestine. Each of the aminosalicylate preparations have similar clinical efficacy to sulfasalazine where equimolar concentrations are given to treat active UC or quiescent disease (10,28).

Studies have demonstrated clinical improvement in approximately 40% to 75% of patients with mild to moderately active UC using 2 g/day of mesalamine, with improved results when doses of 3 to 4 g/day are utilized (15,26). The oral aminosalicylate preparations have also proved to be effective in maintenance of remission in UC, as trials have demonstrated remission rates ranging from 54% to 80% at 12 months while using 1.5 to 4 g/day of mesalamine compounds (15,18).

Data are also available demonstrating the efficacy of aminosalicylate formulations in active and inactive CD. In contrast to UC patients, the dosage requirements are higher in CD. In a large, multicenter trial Pentasa provided clinical improvement only at the 4 g/day dosage (29). Two large meta-analyses summarizing the clinical efficacy of mesalamine preparations in maintaining remission in CD demonstrated relapse-free rates at 12 months of 68% to 95% at 1.5 to 3 g/day dosage (16,30).

Corticosteroids

Corticosteroids are the most commonly employed agents to treat moderate to severe IBD. In contrast to the aminosalicylates, steroids have not been effective in maintaining remission in either UC or CD (3–6,19,31,32). The anti-inflammatory properties of glucocorticoids are many including, inhibition of arachadonic acid liberation from membranes, decreased cytokine release including interleukin-1 (IL-1) and interleuken-2 (IL-2), direct lymphocytotoxicity, and decreased adherence and chemotaxis of eosinophils, neutrophils, and monocytes (10,33–35).

The clinical efficacy of corticosteroids in IBD was first reported in uncontrolled trials in the 1950s. Truelove and Witts demonstrated a 75% response to cortisone compared to a 41% response from placebo in patients with active UC (36). Since then other investigators have described efficacy of steroids in mild to moderate UC with response rates ranging from 70% to 90% (18,19,21). There is a dose response between prednisone 20 mg to 60 mg daily, although in outpatients there is no advantage to dividing the dose, and the side-effects at 60 mg probably outweigh any marginal clinical advantage over 40 mg daily dosing (35–38). Although the comparative effects of ACTH, hydrocortisone, prednisolone, and prednisone for the treatment of UC have not been clearly elucidated, it appears that patients previously treated with steroids respond better to hydrocortisone, while steroid naive patients may responds better to ACTH (39,40).

Topical steroids are useful to treat patients with distal colitis or as an adjunct for treating more extensive disease (18,19,41,42). Despite available absorption, prolonged administration results in systemic toxicity including adrenal suppression (10,19). There is ongoing development of steroid preparations that are more rapidly metabolized and less well absorbed (31,43). These novel formulations should provide enhanced clinical efficacy while reducing the side effects (31).

Corticosteroids also are effective for the treatment of active CD. Initial uncontrolled trials report greater than a 75% response in moderate to severe CD (19). The National Cooperative Crohn's Disease Study demonstrated a 60% clinical remission rate in patients with active small bowel CD using prednisone at doses of 0.25 to 0.75 mg/kg/day, compared with a 30% placebo response (20). The European Cooperative Crohn's Disease Study further supported the use of steroids in the treatment of small bowel and large bowel CD (17). Parenteral steroids are used to treat severe CD (31). Greater than 75% of patients will respond to doses of 40 to 60 mg/day IV methylprednisolone within 7 to 10 days, given in multiple daily doses or as a continuous infusion (21,31,44).

Despite their proven effectiveness in moderate to severe CD and UC, corticosteroids have no utility as maintenance agents to prevent relapse in IBD (3,19,31). Therefore, steroids should be prescribed to gain control of moderate to severe IBD but not to maintain remission.

There are many known complications of corticosteroid therapy related to the dose and duration of treatment. The long-term complications include osteonecrosis, osteoporosis, posterior subcapsular cataracts, myopathy, systemic infection, and adrenal suppression (10,19,31). Not uncommonly patients develop a "pseudoarthritis" while attempting to withdrawal from steroid therapy. This condition must be distinguished from the extraintestinal manifestations of IBD and should not be treated with nonsteroidal anti-inflammatory drugs (NSAIDS), as they can induce exacerbation of IBD (45).

There have been several attempts to alter the composition of synthetic glucocorticoids to enhance mucosal delivery while reducing systemic

bioavailability (31,43). Budesonide, a rapidly metabolized corticosteroid, has demonstrated clinical improvement as an enema preparation to treat UC (46–48). Oral budesonide has also demonstrated clinical efficacy in active CD (49–51), but low-dose therapy has provided only marginal benefits in prolonging clinical remission (52). Further studies evaluating variable dosing of budesonide are needed to determine its longer-term efficacy in quiescent disease.

Immunomodulators

Azathioprine and 6-MP

It has been suggested that the host immune system plays a significant role in the pathogenesis of IBD (14). This has led to investigation of various immunomodulatory agents (immunosuppressives) in active and quiescent UC and CD. Azathioprine is an antimetabolite that is metabolized systematically to the purine analogue 6-mercaptopurine (6-MP) and other active metabolites that inhibit DNA synthesis (10,33). The mechanism of action of azathioprine and 6-MP remains unclear in IBD, but natural killer cell function and cytotoxic T-cell function are diminished in subjects receiving 6-MP (10,31). The clinical response is delayed, requiring 3 to 6 months for efficacy.

Both azathioprine and 6-MP are used as long-term therapy in UC patients who are steroid dependent (53–55). Clinical response, defined as a steroid sparing effect or endoscopic improvement, has been demonstrated in 65% of patients using from 2.0 to 2.5 mg/kg/day of azathioprine and 1.0 to 1.5 mg/kg/day of 6-MP (53,54). These agents are also effective for maintaining remission in patients with UC (19,31,55).

Immunomodulatory therapy has also proven to be efficacious in treating active and quiescent CD (56–58). A recent metaanalysis demonstrated a mean 56% response in patients with active CD using 1.5 mg/kg/day of 6-MP or 2 to 2.5 mg/kg/day of azathioprine (56). Maintenance of remission has also been shown in 57% to 84% of patients receiving azathioprine or 6-MP at 1 to 3 years (56). Others have demonstrated as high as a 95% relapse-free rate over an average of 3 years. These agents have also proven efficacy in the management in patients unable to be weaned off of corticosteroids, and in patients with perianal and fistulous CD (57,58).

Initial concerns over the possible long-term side effects of azathioprine and 6-MP have been assuaged in recent years. The most concerning toxicity is the potential for neoplastic disease, most notably lymphoma. A study in 1989 demonstrated only one case of lymphoma of 396 IBD patients being treated with these agents (59). The lack of carcinogenic effects has been further supported by case-control studies from the UK (60).

Potential complications from azathioprine and 6-MP can be minimized with appropriate monitoring. Nausea, which commonly occurs in the first month of therapy, often responds to dose reduction (10,28). Pancreatitis, which can occur in up to 15% of treated patients, appears to be a hypersensitivity reaction that resolves with cessation of therapy (10,31,61). Fever, arthralgias, rash, and hepatotoxicity are other possible allergic reactions (10,31,32). Bone marrow suppression is dose-related and can be delayed (62), thus necessitating weekly monitoring of complete blood counts initially, and quarterly monitoring for patients on long-term therapy.

Cyclosporine

The immunomodulatory benefits seen in organ transplant recipients being treated with cyclosporine has prompted examination of its benefit in IBD. Cyclosporine inhibits T-cell function by interfering with transcription of interleukin-2 (IL-2) and its receptor within helper T-lymphocytes (33). Initial uncontrolled trials in severe UC demonstrated a mean response of 80% within 7 to 14 days (63). Controlled trials demonstrate similar results at a dose of 4 mg/kg/day administered by continuous infusion (64,65).

Refractory CD has also been shown to respond to IV cyclosporine within 14 days (63). High dose cyclosporine has additionally shown benefit in patients with refractory fistulas (66,67). One recent study demonstrated an 83% response after a mean of 7.9 days of high dose parenteral therapy (66).

In contrast to its proven benefit in refractory UC and CD, oral cyclosporine has not demonstrated consistent efficacy in the management of mild to moderate or quiescent IBD (68,69). There are multiple potential side effects of cyclosporine including hypertension, hirsutism, gingival hyperplasia, paresthesias, opportunistic infections, tremors, nausea, and headache (10,32). The most common adverse effect is dose-related renal dysfunction (10,31). Seizures may also complicate therapy, most commonly in those patients with serum cholesterol levels below 120 mg/dl (31,65).

Methotrexate

Methotrexate (MTX) is a folate inhibitor that interferes with DNA synthesis and may mimic IL-1.

Trials have demonstrated that 38% to 71% of UC patients treated with 15 mg/wk of oral MTX or 25 mg/wk of subcutaneous MTX achieved partial or clinical remission (70,71). A recent multicenter, controlled trial of MTX in active CD demonstrated 39% of those receiving 25 mg/wk of subcutaneous MTX vs. 19% of those receiving placebo were in clinical remission after 16 weeks. A significant steroid sparing effect was also reported in the MTX group (72). The utility of MTX in maintaining quiescent CD remains to be assessed.

Ten percent of patients treated with MTX develop nausea, vomiting, diarrhea, or stomatitis (32,73). Folic acid supplementation may minimize these complications (74). More serious potential complications include hepatic fibrosis, hypersensitivity pneumonitis, and leukopenia (10,28). Treated patients require periodic evaluation of liver chemistry tests and complete blood counts. In addition, MTX is teratogenic and a known abortifacant and should be avoided in men and women planning conception (10).

Antibiotics

Although no specific microorganism has been identified as the causative agent in either UC or CD (75), antimicrobial agents are frequently utilized in IBD (75,76). Antituberculosis regimens using three or four drugs have demonstrated inconsistent response rates in patients with active CD (77,78), although some authors have demonstrated improved remission rates in CD patients receiving quadruple drug therapy over 9 months (79).

The most extensively studied antibiotic in the treatment of IBD is metronidazole. Although there has been no therapeutic benefit in active or quiescent UC (80), metronidazole has been used as empiric therapy in patients with severe UC (81), and has demonstrated efficacy in treating pouchitis complicating colectomy and ileoanal anastomosis (82).

The utility of metronidazole for CD is more clearly defined. Sutherland et al. compared metronidazole to placebo in patients with mild to moderate ileocolonic CD and demonstrated significant superiority of metronidazole at a dose of 20 mg/kg/day (83). Metronidazole is also beneficial in the treatment of perianal CD (84). Clinical remission following ileal resection can also be achieved with metronidazole as demonstrated by Rutgeerts et al. although this benefit seems to diminish after 24 to 36 months postoperatively (85).

There are many potential adverse effects of metronidazole including nausea, glossitis, metallic taste, disulfiram-like reaction when taken with alcohol, and reversible neutropenia (19). Peripheral neuropathy may occur in up to 50% of patients treated long-term and may be irreversible (19).

Alternative antibiotic regimens have been studied to treat patients with IBD with variable results (80,86,87). Ciprofloxacin has demonstrated some benefit in UC (87) as well as in treating perianal and fistulous CD (88). Additionally, ciproflaxacin or alternative antibiotics may be efficacious in treating those patients intolerant of metronidazole (31,32). Further clinical trials are needed to better assess the efficacy of these agents in treating IBD.

Nutritional Therapies

Fish oils contain omega-3 fatty acid (eicosapentanoic acid) which inhibits the formation of leukotriene B4, a known proinflammatory leukotriene (4,5,31). Several studies have reported benefit of relatively large doses of fish oils in the treatment of UC (89,90), but therapy has not been well tolerated by patients.

It has been shown that patients with IBD have decreased levels of colonic short chain fatty acids (SCFA), which serve as primary nutrients of colonic epithelium (31). One investigator treated UC patients with butyrate enemas and noted improvement in 11 of 12 patients (91). Other studies confirm the role of butyrate enemas in UC (92,93).

New Therapeutic Options

There are a multitude of investigational agents under study for the treatment of IBD (94). *4-aminosalicylic acid,* and other ASA preparations are among this group, and have demonstrated some benefit in UC (95). Topical *lidocaine* has been used to treat clinically active ulcerative proctitis, with an 83% response demonstrated in one small study (96). Results of a controlled trial of *clonidine* demonstrated a 60% response over 30 weeks in patients with UC (97).

The association between cigarette smoking and IBD is intriguing. Patients with UC appear to have an improved clinical course while smoking, which is in sharp contrast to CD patients, who may promote disease flares while smoking (32,98,99). A randomized trial of nicotine therapy in active UC demonstrated complete resolution of symptoms in 49% of treated patients compared with a 24% response of those treated with placebo (100). In contrast to its efficacy in active UC, nicotine has not

demonstrated significant benefit in patients with inactive disease (101).

Other miscellaneous approaches to IBD therapy include *chloroquine* and *hydroxychloroquine, omeprazole,* GM-CSF, *epidermal growth factor, tacrolimus,* and *immunoglobulin* (94). *Hyperbaric oxygen* therapy has been effective in the treatment of perianal CD (102), and *heparin* has demonstrated efficacy in an uncontrolled trial of patients with active UC poorly controlled on sulfasalazine and corticosteroids (103).

Novel immunomodulatory modalities are under intense examination in the treatment of IBD. *Lymphocytoplasmapheresis* reduces the number of circulating T-cells, and has demonstrated efficacy in inducing remission in refractory CD (104). A recent study of *antitumor necrosis factor alpha* (cA2) in refractory CD demonstrated a clinical response of 80% within 7 days of receiving a single infusion (105). Others have demonstrated encouraging results treating active CD patients with *anti*-CD4 *antibodies* (106), and the use of *cytokine antagonists* (e.g., IL-1 receptor antagonist) are currently under investigation in the treatment of active IBD (31,94).

Management of Clinical Syndromes

Ulcerative Colitis

Distal Colitis
Mild-moderate ulcerative proctitis or sigmoiditis may be treated with either oral or topical therapy (Table 7.1). Clinicians must be aware of the dose response to oral aminosalicylate and the superior efficacy of rectal applications, the latter being, at times, offset by the social compromise of continuing topical therapy (4,5). A combination of oral aminosalicylates with either rectal mesalamine or steroids improves the rate of response (4,5). Hydrocortisone foam or prednisolone suppositories also are useful for proctitis, whereas mesalamine enemas effectively treat disease distal to the splenic flexure (4,5,41). Although the short-term use of topical steroids is usually well tolerated, long-term use is complicated by significant absorption and systemic effects (10).

Maintenance therapy to prevent relapse of distal colitis is indicated for patients with resistant first attacks or repeated disease flares similar to patients with more extensive colitis (4,5). Continuation of oral or topical aminosalicylates will reduce the likelihood of relapse in quiescent disease in a dose-dependent manner (107). Disease flares which occur while on maintenance therapy should be retreated with higher dose oral or rectal steroid or

Table 7.1. Medical management of ulcerative colitis.

Active disease
  Mild-moderate disease
    Distal colitis
      Sulfasalazine or 5-ASA preparation (oral or rectal)*
      Topical corticosteroid‡
    Extensive colitis
      Sulfasalazine or oral 5-ASA preparation
  Moderate-severe disease
    Distal colitis
      Topical corticosteroid‡
      Prednisone
    Extensive colitis
      Prednisone
  Severe-fulminant disease
    Extensive colitis
      Parenteral corticosteroid
      Intravenous cyclosporine°
Inactive disease
  Distal colitis
    Sulfasalazine or 5-ASA preparation (oral or rectal)*
    Azathioprine or 6-MP§
  Extensive colitis
    Sulfasalazine or oral 5-ASA preparation
    Azathioprine or 6-MP§

*A topical 5-ASA preparation may be prescribed alone or in combination with an oral 5-ASA preparation or sulfasalazine.
‡A topical corticosteroid may be prescribed alone or in combination with an oral 5-ASA preparation or sulfasalazine.
°Cyclosporine therapy should only be initiated after a patient fails to respond to parenteral corticosteroid therapy of 7 to 10 days duration.
§Azathioprine or 6-MP is used to treat steroid-dependent patients and patients with refractory disease.

aminosalicylate applications, then maintained on a higher dose of mesalamine. Many patients who require topical mesalamine to achieve remission often need continuation of nightly or several times weekly topical therapy to prevent relapse (5).

Extensive Colitis
Ulcerative colitis extending proximal to the splenic flexure requires treatment with sulfasalazine or an oral aminosalicylate preparation for mild to moderate disease, or initiation of oral corticosteroids for moderate to severe disease (4,5). Treatment should be continued until symptomatic and endoscopic remission before reducing the dosage, as premature tapering often results in more persistent or refractory disease. Adjunctive therapy with topical mesalamine or steroids can improve symptoms of tenesmus or urgency even in the setting of more extensive disease.

Patients presenting with severe disease require hospitalization and an intensive regimen of parenteral corticosteroids (108). Stool cultures as well as repeated *Clostridium difficile* assays should be performed. Aggressive fluid and electrolyte management should be initiated and the patient's diet

should be restricted according to the symptoms and the desire to eat. Aminosalicylates are withheld until the patient has stabilized. Corticosteroids may then be tapered according to the rapidity of the initial response and oral aminosalicylate therapy is reinstituted or initiated (4,5).

Fulminant colitis or toxic megacolon are emergencies requiring experienced intensive medical and surgical teamwork (109). Colonoscopy should be avoided or performed only by experienced clinicians. Parenteral steroid therapy should be instituted along with fluid, electrolyte and blood replacement. Oral intake may be maintained unless there is nausea, vomiting, or severe abdominal pain or tenderness. However, most physicians are more comfortable with an initial period of bowel rest. Nasogastric suction is necessary for those patients with distended small bowel by radiographic examination. Significant colonic distention may be reduced by having the patient roll from side to side (5). Placing a rectal tube or having the patient assume the knee-chest position may assist in the evacuation of accumulated colonic gas (109). Broad spectrum antibiotics are usually administered despite lack of support from controlled trials. For those patients that fail to respond to intensive steroid therapy, recent investigation supports the use of intravenous cyclosporine to induce clinical remission in severe disease (110).

The inductive regimen is continued until bowel movements are formed without hematochezia. Feedings are slowly advanced and oral aminosalicylates are added. The steroid regimen is changed to an oral program of divided daily doses initially, and then a single daily dose as the remission is maintained (4,5). Although steroids should be tapered according to the individual patient's status, tapering initially by 5 mg/week, and then by 2.5 mg/week is an appropriate guideline. Patients who have received cyclosporine should continue on the oral preparation until steroids have been weaned. Although it is currently unclear how to manage long-term immunomodulation in these patients (5,63), most patients who require cyclosporine are transferred to long-term treatment with azathioprine or 6-MP (111) in conjunction with an aminosalicylate.

Refractory Colitis and the Timing of Surgery
Two long-term concepts in the treatment of chronic IBD are steroid-resistance and steroid-dependence (112). The former applies to patients who fail to respond to an acute course of steroids while the latter describes patients who have disease relapse when steroids are tapered. Steroid-resistant

patients will often respond to a longer course of intravenous corticosteroids at higher doses (108). Additionally, steroid-resistant patients with mild to moderate disease will often respond to azathioprine or 6-MP, while those with severe disease will often respond to intravenous cyclosporine (5,64,110). Steroid-dependent patients should be maintained on a higher dose of oral mesalamine (4 to 4.8 g/day) as well as chronic topical mesalamine therapy until steroids are tapered (4,5,19). Recurrent relapse should then be re-treated and those steroid-dependent patients can be treated with long-term immunomodulation with azathioprine or 6-MP (4,5). Occasionally, patients who repeatedly relapse at low-doses of prednisone (below 10 mg/day) may be treated with chronic, homeostatic, doses (113). This must be done with extreme caution, with close monitoring for potential chronic steroid toxicity, especially metabolic bone disease such as osteoporosis.

UC should always be approached as a curable disease (114). The indications for surgery in UC include steroid dependency or side effects precluding continued medical therapy, colonic perforation, intractable hemorrhage, unresponsive toxic megacolon, or evidence of mucosal dysplasia or cancer (114,115). In the past surgical "cure" required a proctocolectomy and ileostomy, necessitating a permanent stoma. Recent surgical alternatives have revolutionized the outlook and expectations of patients with the advent of sphincter-saving procedures, primarily colectomy and ileoanal anastomoses with pelvic ileal reservoirs (see chapter 10). Although improving the postoperative quality of life, these procedures are compromised by the potential for "pouchitis." This may become a chronic condition in some patients, necessitating intermittent or chronic immunomodulatory or antibiotic therapy (82).

Crohn's Disease

Crohn's disease of the *esophagus, stomach,* or *duodenum* is uncommon and usually occurs in the setting or more distal small bowel or colonic disease (114) (Table 7.2). The symptoms of gastroduodenal disease overlap with peptic ulcer disease and include: dyspepsia, nausea/vomiting or postprandial epigastric pain. Gastroduodenal erosions or aphthae are common and do not correlate with symptoms. Larger or deeper ulcerations can hemorrhage or evolve to gastric outlet obstruction. Milder symptoms usually respond to acid-reduction therapy, particularly omeprazole (115). More severe symptoms will respond to short-term

Table 7.2. Medical management of Crohn's disease.

Active disease
  Mild-moderate disease
    Sulfasalazine or oral 5-ASA preparation[*]
    Metronidazole or alternative antibiotic[§]
    Prednisone
    Azathioprine or 6-MP[¶]
  Severe disease
    Parenteral corticosteroid
    Intravenous cyclosporine[¥]
  Perianal or fistulizing disease
    Metronidazole or alternative antibiotic[§]
    Azathioprine or 6-MP
    Intravenous cyclosporine[¥]
Inactive disease
  Ileocolonic disease
    Oral 5-ASA preparation[Φ]
    Azathioprine or 6-MP

[*]Sulfasalazine can be used for Crohn's colitis.
[§]Use metronidazole as a first line antibiotic and alternative antibiotics (e.g., ciprofloxacin) in those patients intolerant of metronidazole.
[¶]Azathioprine or 6-MP are prescribed for steroid-dependent patients and for those patients with refractory disease.
[¥]Intravenous cyclosporine should be reserved for steroid unresponsive patients with refractory disease or those with severe perianal or fistulous disease.
[Φ]Oral mesalamine is effective in patients who have a response to oral 5-ASA therapy, and it prevents postoperative recurrence of disease.

steroid administration followed by long-term immunomodulation for frequent relapse (53). There is no data concerning mesalamine for gastroduodenal disease. Persistent or recurrent gastric outlet obstruction requires surgical gastrojejunostomy.

Jejunoiletis is an uncommon variant of Crohn's disease often accompanied by focal stricture formation and small bowel bacterial overgrowth (116). A metabolic sequelae is hypoalbuminemia primarily due to protein-losing enteropathy. There is little data regarding the value of mesalamine in this subtype which is poorly responsive to steroids. Diarrhea can be treated with alternating antibiotics to reduce bacterial overgrowth and most patients will respond to long-term therapy with an immunomodulator (6). Obstructing strictures should be treated with "stricturoplasty" rather than extensive resection.

Terminal ileitis may mimic appendicitis. Patients with more insidious onset with mild to moderate symptoms are treated with mesalamine (4 g/day) (29) or an antibiotic such as metronidazole (750 to 1500 mg/day) (83). After symptoms resolve there is increasing evidence in favor of "maintenance" therapy with mesalamine at doses above 2 g/day (3,30). Patients with more severe symptoms accompanied by fevers, weight loss or other systemic inflammatory features require a short course of steroids (6,20) followed either by mesalamine or 6-mercaptopurine/azathioprine maintenance (6,58). Elemental feeding provides equal short-term effects to steroids but relapse is also similar after resumption of normal feeding (117). Recurrent small bowel obstruction, evidence of ureteral compression (e.g., hydronephrosis), or symptomatic ileosigmoid fistulae require an ileal resection.

Mild-moderate *ileocolonic* Crohn's disease responds to sulfasalazine (4 to 6 g/day) (17,20), mesalamine (4 g/day) (26), or metronidazole (750 to 1500 mg/day) (83). Elemental feedings or short-term steroids are effective in alleviating more moderate attacks after which maintenance with sulfasalazine, mesalamine or an immunosuppressant should be added (3,4,6,58). Stricturing or fistulizing complications can be approached surgically if an isolated, limited segment (e.g., ileocecal) is identified. More extensive disease should be approached conservatively with long-term medical therapies including immune modifiers (6); with surgery limited to specific focal complications via short resections or stricturoplasty.

Crohn's colitis differs from ulcerative colitis at presentation by the presence of segmental (non-confluent), linear or aphthoid ulceration; or the presence of perianal skin tags, fistulae, or abscesses (118). The therapeutic options for Crohn's colitis include sulfasalazine, mesalamine and steroids; but also antibiotics, elemental feeding or parenteral nutrition (see "terminal ileitis" or "ileocolonic Crohn's disease"). Topical applications of mesalamine or corticosteroids are utilized for rectal disease similar to distal ulcerative colitis although they have not been evaluated in clinical trials. Maintenance therapy after an acute attack consists of either high dose aminosalicylates (sulfasalazine 4 to 6 g/day or mesalamine 3 to 4 g/day) or immune modifiers (6). Segmental surgical resections are associated with an inexorable relapse (119,120), whereas, colectomy and ileostomy, in the absence of small bowel involvement, has a good prognosis with only a 20% chance of ileal recurrence. The efficacy of medical maintenance after colon resections has not been adequately evaluated but the concepts and alternatives are identical to small bowel disease.

Perianal disease frequently is a symptomatic manifestation with frustrating psychosocial consequences. Chronic, suppressive medical therapy with metronidazole (84) (or alternative antibiotics) or azathioprine/6-mercaptopurine (56) can reduce the drainage from perianal or recto-vaginal fistulas once rectal disease or accompanying diarrhea have been treated (6). Short term intravenous cyclosporine also can treat active fistulization after which transfer to chronic immunotherapy is necessary to prevent relapse (66,67). Evidence of an abscess or purulence should be approached surgically. Fistulotomy is acceptable for superficial fistulas but deeper (suprasphincteric, transphincteric, or complex) fistulas should be drained and treated with setons. Persistent drainage requires chronic metronidazole or azathioprine/6-mercaptopurine. Relapse after cessation of metronidazole is common (84) whereas long-term treatment must be monitored for clinical (or subclinical) neuropathy. Hyperbaric oxygen therapy may be useful for resistant perianal disease (102).

Management of Postoperative Crohn's Disease

Surgery for Crohn's disease is rarely curative (119,120). Symptoms after ileal resections may be secondary to altered surgical anatomy/physiology or recurrent disease. There is increasing evidence that oral mesalamine therapy may delay or prevent endoscopic or clinical evidence of recurrence (3,30,121,122). Postoperative metronidazole (85) or 6-mercaptopurine (3,58) may provide additional or independent benefits. The differentiation of inflammatory from anatomic symptoms is based on evidence for clinical inflammation (fevers, bleeding, weight loss) or signs (fecal leukocytes or endoscopic, radiographic or scintigraphic findings). Ileocecal resections are frequently complicated by postoperative diarrhea secondary to bile salt malabsorption (after resections less than 50 to 100 cm) or steatorrhea (resection greater than 100 cm). Stool analysis for fecal fat is discriminating. The former is treated with cholestyramine (31), the latter with a low fat diet.

References

1. Podolsky DK. Inflammatory bowel disease (review article). N Engl J Med 1991;325:928–37, 1008–16.
2. MacDermott RP. Alterations in the mucosal immune system in ulcerative colitis and Crohn's disease. Med Clin North Am 1994;78:1207–31.
3. Sachar DB. Maintenance therapy in ulcerative colitis and Crohn's disease. J Clin Gastroenterol 1995;20:117–22.
4. Hanauer SB. Medical therapy of ulcerative colitis. Lancet 1993;342:412–7.
5. Hanauer SB. Medical therapy in ulcerative colitis. In: Kirsner JB, Shorter RG, eds. Inflammatory bowel disease. 4th ed. Baltimore: Williams & Wilkins, 1995:664–94.
6. Meyers S, Sachar DB. Medical therapy of Crohn's disease. In: Kirsner JB, Shorter RG, eds. Inflammatory bowel disease. 4th ed. Baltimore: Williams & Wilkins; 1995:695–714.

7. Stark ME, Tremaine WJ. Maintenance of symptomatic remission in patients with Crohn's disease. Mayo Clin Proc 1993;68:1183–90.

8. Svarts N. Sulfasalazine. II. Some notes on the discovery and development of salazopyrin. Am J Gastroenterol 1988;83:497–503.

9. Greenfield SM, Punchard NA, Teare JP, et al. Review article: the mode of action of the aminosalicylates in inflammatory bowel disease. Aliment Pharmacol Therapy 1993;7:369–83.

10. Hanauer SB, Meyers S, Sachar DB. The pharmacology of anti-inflammatory drugs in inflammatory bowel disease. In: Kirsner JB, Shorter RG, eds. Inflammatory bowel disease. 4th ed. Baltimore: Williams & Wilkins, 1995:643–63.

11. Klotz U, Maier K, Fischer C, et al. Therapeutic efficacy of sulfasalazine and its metabolites in patients with ulcerative colitis and Crohn's disease. N Engl J Med 1980;303:1499–502.

12. Eliakim R, Rachmilewitz D. Potential mediators on inflammatory bowel disease. Gastroenterol Intl 1992;5:48–56.

13. Grisham MB. Oxidants and free radicals in inflammatory bowel disease. Lancet 1994;344:859–61.

14. Lauritsen K, Laursen S, Bukhave K, et al. Inflammatory intermediaries in inflammatory bowel disease. Int J Colorectal Dis 1989;4:75–90.

15. Sutherland LR, May GR, Shaffer EA. Sulfasalazine revisited: a meta-analysis of 5-Aminosalicylic acid in the treatment of ulcerative colitis. Ann Int Med 1993;118:540–9.

16. Steinhart AH, Hemphill D, Greenberg GR. Sulfasalazine and mesalazine for the maintenance treatment of Crohn's disease: a meta analysis. Am J Gastroenterol 1994;84:2116–24.

17. Malchow H, Ewe K, Brandes JW, et al. European Cooperative Crohn's Disease Study (ECCDS): results of drug treatment. Gastroenterology 1984;86:249–66.

18. Margolin ML, Krumholz MP, Fochios SE, et al. Clinical trials in ulcerative colitis: II. Historical review. Am J Gastroenterol 1988;83:227–43.

19. Hanauer SB, Stathopoulos G. Risk-benefit assessment of drugs used in the treatment of inflammatory bowel disease. Drug Safety 1991;6:192–219.

20. Summers RW, Switz DM, Sessions JT Jr, et al. National Cooperative Crohn's Disease Study (NCCDS): results of drug treatment. Gastroenterology 1979;77:847–69.

21. Saloman P, Kornbluth A, Aisenberg J, et al. How effective are current drugs for Crohn's disease? A meta-analysis. J Clin Gastroenterol 1992;14:211–5.

22. Das KM, Eastwood MA, McManus JP, et al. Adverse reactions during salicylazosulfapyridine therapy and the relation with drug metabolism and acetylator phenotype. N Engl J Med 1973;289:491.

23. Taffet SL, Das KM. Sulfasalazine: adverse effects and desensitization. Dig Dis Sci 1983;28:833.

24. Thomson ABR. Review article: new developments in the use of 5-aminosalicylic acid in patients with inflammatory bowel disease. Aliment Pharmacol Ther 1991;5:449.

25. Marshall JK, Irvine EJ. Topical aminosalicylate (ASA) therapy for distal ulcerative colitis: a meta-analysis. Gastroenterology 1994;106:A1037.

26. Hanauer S, Schwartz J, Robinson M, et al. Mesalamine capsules for the treatment of active ulcerative colitis. Results of a controlled trial. Am J Gastroenterol 1993;88:1188–97.

27. Wadworth AN, Ritton A. Olsalazine. A review of its pharmicokinetic properties, and therapeutic potential in inflammatory bowel disease. Drugs 1991;41:647–64.

28. Hanauer SB, Baert F. Medical therapy of inflammatory bowel disease. Med Clin North Am 1994;78:1413–26.

29. Singleton JW, Hanauer SB, Gitnick GL, et al, and the Pentasa Crohn's disease study group. Mesalamine capsules for the treatment of active Crohn's disease. Results of a 16 week trial. Gastroenterology 1993;104:1293–301.

30. Messori A, Brignila C, Trallori G, et al. Effectiveness of 5-Aminosalicylic acid for maintaining remission in patients with Crohn's disease: a meta-analysis. Am J Gastroenterol 1994;89:692–98.

31. Hanauer SB. Drug therapy: inflammatory bowel disease. N Engl J Med 1996;334:841–8.

32. Cohen RD, Hanauer SB. Immunomodulatory agents and other medical therapies in inflammatory bowel disease. Curr Opin Gastroenterol 1995;11:321–30.

33. Hawthorne AB, Hawkey CJ. Immunosuppressive drugs in inflammatory bowel disease: a review of their mechanisms of efficacy and place in therapy. Drugs 1989;38:267–88.

34. Brattsand R. Overview of newer glucocorticosteroid preparations for inflammatory bowel disease. Can J Gastroenterol 1990;4:407–14.

35. Boumpas DT, Chrousos GP, Wilder RL, et al. Glucocorticoid therapy for immune-mediated diseases: basic and clinical correlates. Ann Int Med 1993;119:1198–208.

36. Truelove SC, Witts LJ. Cortisone in ulcerative colitis. Final report on a therapeutic trial. British Med J 1955;2:1041–8.

37. Meyers S, Sachar DB, Goldberg JD, et al. Corticotropin versus hydrocortisone in intravenous treatment of ulcerative colitis. Gastroenterology 1983;85:351–7.

38. Baron JH, Connell AM, Kanaghinis TG, et al. Outpatient treatment of ulcerative colitis: comparison between three doses of oral prednisone. Br Med J 1962;2:441–3.

39. Lennard-Jones JE. Toward optimal use of corticosteroids in ulcerative colitis and Crohn's disease. Gut 1983;24:177.

40. Meyers S, Janowitz HD. Systemic corticosteroid therapy of ulcerative colitis. Gastroenterology 1985;89:1189–99.

41. Sutherland LR. Topical treatment of ulcerative colitis. Med Clin North Amer 1990;74:119–31.

42. Mulder CJ, Tygat GN. Review article: topical corticosteroids in inflammatory bowel disease. Aliment Pharmacol Ther 1993;7:125–30.

43. Danielsson A, Lofberg R, Persson T, et al. A steroid enema, budesonide, lacking systemic effects for the treatment of distal ulcerative colitis or proctitis. Scand J Gastroenterol 1992;27:9–12.

44. Shepard HA, Barr GD, Jewel DP. Use of an iv steroid regimen in the treatment of acute Crohn's disease. J Clin Gastroenterol 1986;8(2):154–9.

45. Bjarnason I, Hayllar J, MacPherson A, et al. Side effects of nonsteroidal anti-inflammatory drugs on the small and large intestine in humans. Gastroenterology 1993;104:1832–47.

46. Bianchi Porro G, Prantera C, Campieri M, et al. Comparative trial of budesonide and methylprednisolone enemas in active distal ulcerative colitis. Eur J Gastroenterol Hepatol 1994;6:125–30.

47. Danish Budesonide Study Group. Budesonide enema in distal ulcerative colitis. A randomized dose-response trial with prednisolone enema as a positive control. Scand J Gastroenterol 1991;26:1225–30.

48. Danielsson A, Hellers G, Lyrenas E, et al. A controlled randomized trial of budesonide versus prednisolone retention enemas in active distal ulcerative colitis. Scand J Gastroenterol 1987;22:987.

49. Rutgeerts, P, Lofberg R, Malchow H, et al. A comparison of budesonide with prednisolone for active Crohn's disease. N Engl J Med 1994;331:842–5.

50. Greenberg GR, Feagan GB, et al, and the Canadian Inflammatory Bowel Disease Study Group. Oral budesonide for active Crohn's disease. N Engl J Med 1994;331:836–41.

51. Sachar DB. Budesonise for inflammatory bowel disease. Is it the magic bullet? N Engl J Med 1994;331:873–4.

52. Greenberg GR, Feagan BG, et al. Oral Budesonide as Maintenance Treatment for Crohn's Disease: a placebo-controlled, dose-ranging study. Gastroenterology 1996;110:299.

53. Adler DJ, Korelitz BI. The therapeutic efficacy of 6-Mercaptopurine in refractory ulcerative colitis. Am J Gastroenterol 1990;85:712–22.

54. Choi PM, Targan SR. Immunomodualatory treatment in inflammatory bowel disease. Dig Dis Sci 1994;39:1885–92.

55. Gearge J, Pou R, Bodain C, et al. 6-Mercaptopurine is effective in chronic ulcerative colitis but how long do you use it? Gastroenterology 1994;106:A686.

56. Pearson DC, May GR, Fick GH, et al. Azathioprine and 6-MP in Crohn's disease. A meta-analysis. Ann Int Med 1995;122:132–42.

57. Ewe K, Press AG, Singe C, et al. Azathioprine combined with prednisolone or monotherapy with prednisolone in active Crohn's disease. Gastroenterology 1993;105:367–72.

58. Present DH, Korelitz BI, Wisch N, et al. Treatment of Crohn's disease with 6-mercaptopurine: a long-term randomised, double-blind study. N Engl J Med 1981;302:981–7.

59. Present DH, Meltzer SJ, Krumholz MP, et al. 6-mercaptopurine in the management of inflammatory bowel disease: short and long term toxicity. Ann Intern Med 1989;111:641–9.

60. Connell WR, Kamm MA, Dickson M, et al. Long-term neoplasia risk after azathioprine treatment in inflammatory bowel disease. Lancet 1994;343:1249–52.

61. Haber DJ, Meltzer SJ, Present DH, et al. Nature and course of pancreatitis caused by 6-mercaptopurine in the treatment of inflammatory bowel disease. Gastroenterology 1986;91:982–6.

62. Connell WR, Kamm, MA, Ritchie JK, et al. Bone marrow toxicity caused by azathioprine in inflammatory bowel disease: 27 years of experience. Gut 1993;34:1081–5.

63. Sandborn WJ, Tremaine WJ. Cyclosporine treatment of inflammatory bowel disease. Mayo Clin Proc 1992;67:981–90.

64. Lichteger S, Present DH, Kornbluth A, et al. Cyclopsorin in severe ulcerative colitis refractory to steroid therapy. N Engl J Med 1994;330:1841–5.

65. Sandborn WJ. A critical review of cyclosporine therapy in inflammatory bowel disease. Inflammatory Bowel Dis 1995;1:48–63.

66. Hanauer SB, Smith MB. Rapid closure of Crohn's disease fistulas with continuous intravenous cyclosporin A. Am J Gastroenterol 1993;88:646–9.

67. Present DH, Lichtiger S. Efficacy of cyclosporine in treatment of fistula of Crohn's disease. Dig Dis Sci 1994;39:374–80.

68. Feagan BG, McDonald JWD, Rochon J, et al, for the Canadian Crohn's Relapse Prevention Trial Investigators. Low dose cyclosporin A for treatment of Crohn's disease. N Engl J Med 1994;330:1846–51.

69. Stange EF, Modigliani R, Pena AS, et al, and The European Study Group. European trial of cyclosporine in chronic active Crohn's disease: a 12-month study. Gastroenterology 1995;109:774–82.

70. Baron TH, Truss CD, Elson CO. Low-dose oral methotrexate in refractory inflammatory bowel disease. Dig Dis Sci 1993;38:1851–6.

71. Kozorek RA, Patterson DJ, Gelfand MD, et al. Methotrexate induces clinical and histological remission in patients with refractory inflammatory bowel disease. Ann Int Med 1989;110:353–6.

72. Feagan BG, Rochon J, Fedorak RN, et al. Methotrexate for the treatment of Crohn's disease. N Engl J Med 1995;332:292–7.

73. Weinblatt BE. Methotrexate for chronic disease in adults. N Engl J Med 1995;332:330–1.

74. Morgan SL, Baggott JE, Vaughn WH, et al. Supplementation with folic acid during methotrexate therapy for rheumatoid arthritis. Ann Int Med 1994;121:833–41.

75. Sartor RB. Microbial factors in the pathogenesis of Crohn's disease, ulcerative colitis, and experimental intestinal inflammation. In: Kirsner JB, Shorter RG, eds. Inflammatory bowel disease, 4th ed. Baltimore: Williams & Wilkins; 1995:96–124.

76. Ursung B, Alm T, Barany F, et al. A comparative study of metronidazole and sulfasalazine for active Crohn's disease: the cooperative Crohn's disease study in Sweden. Gastroenterology 1982;83:550–62.

77. Prantera C, Kohn A, Mangiarotti R, et al. Antimycobacterial therapy in Crohn's disease: results of a controlled, double-blind trial with a multiple antibiotic regimen. Am J Gastroenterol 1994;89:513–8.

78. Hampson SJ, Parker MC, Saverymuttu SH, et al. Results of quadruple antimycobacterial chemotherapy in 17 Crohn's disease patients completing six months of treatment. Gastroenterology 1988; 94:A170.

79. Swift GL, Srivastava ED, Stone R, et al. Controlled trial of anti-tuberculous chemotherapy for two years in Crohn's disease. Gut 1994;35:363–8.

80. Peppercorn MA. Are antibiotics useful in management of nontoxic severe ulcerative colitis? J Clin Gastroenterol 1993;17:14–7.

81. Chapman RW, Selby WS, Jewel DP. Controlled trial of metronidazole as an adjunct to corticosteroids in severe ulcerative colitis. Gut 1986;27:1210–2.

82. Sandborn WJ. Pouchitis following ileal pouch-anal anastamosis: definition, pathogenesis, and treatment. Gastroenterology 1994;107:1856–60.

83. Sutherland L, Singleton J, Sessions J, et al. Double blind, placebo controlled trial of metronidazole in Crohn's disease. Gut 1991;32:1071–5.

84. Brandt LJ, Bernstein LH, Boley SJ, et al. Metronidazole therapy for perineal Crohn's disease: a follow-up study. Gastroenterology 1982;83:383–7.

85. Rutgeerts P, Hick M, Peeters M, et al. Prevention of clinical recurrence after ileal resection for Crohn's disease with metronidazole: a placebo controlled study. Gastroenterology 1994;106:A764.

86. Peppercorn MA. Is there a role for antibiotics as primary therapy in Crohn's ileitis? J Clin Gastroenterol 1993;17:235–7.

87. Turunen U, Farkkila V, Hakala K, et al. A double-blind, placebo controlled six-month ciprofloxacin treatment improved prognosis in ulcerative colitis. Gastroenterology 1994;106:A786.

88. Turunen U, Farkkila V, Valtonen V, et al. Long-term outcome of ciprofloxacin treatment in severe perianal or fistulous Crohn's disease. Gastroenterology 1993;104:A793.

89. Stenson WF, Cort D, Rodgers J, et al. Dietary supplementation with fish oil in ulcerative colitis. Ann Intern Med 1992;116:609–14.

90. Hawthorne AB, Daneshmend TK, Hawkey CJ, et al. Treatment of ulcerative colitis with fish oil supplementation: a prospective 12 month randomised controlled trial. Gut 1992;33:922–8.

91. Breuer RI, Buto SK, Christ MI, et al. Rectal irrigation with short chain fatty acids for distal ulcerative colitis. Preliminary Report. Dig Dis Sci 1991;36: 185–7.

92. Steinhart AH, Brzezinski A, Baker JP. Treatment of refractory ulcerative proctosigmoiditis with butyrate enemas. Am J Gastroenterol 1994;89:179–84.

93. Scheppach W, Sommer H, Kirchner T, et al. Effect of butyrate enemas on the colonic mucosa in distal ulcerative colitis. Gastroenterology 1992;103:51–6.

94. Hanauer SB, Schulman M. Novel therapies for inflammatory bowel disease. Gastro Clin North Amer 1995;24:523–40.

95. O'Donnell LJ, Arvind AS, Hoang P, et al. Double-blind, controlled trial of 4-aminosalicylic acid and prednisolone enemas in distal ulcerative colitis. Gut 1992;33:947–9.

96. Bjorck D, Dahlstrom A, Johansson L, et al. Treatment of the mucosa with local anesthetic in ulcerative colitis. Agents Actions Special Conference Issue, C60, 1992.

97. Lechin F, van der Dijs B, Insausti CL, et al. Treatment of ulcerative colitis with clonidine. J Clin Pharmacol 1985;25:219–26.

98. Hanauer SB. Nicotine for colitis. The smoke has not yet cleared. N Engl J Med 1994;330:856–7.

99. Cottone M, Roselli M, Orlando A, et al. Smoking habits and recurrence in Crohn's disease. Gastroenterology 1994;106:643–8.

100. Pullan RD, Rhodes J, Ganesh S. Transdermal nicotine for active ulcerative colitis. N Engl J Med 1994;330:811–5.

101. Thomas GAO, Rhodes J, Mani V, et al. Transdermal nicotine as maintenance therapy for ulcerative colitis. N Engl J Med 1995;332(15):988–92.

102. Lavy A, Wwisz G, Adir Y, et al. Hyperbaric oxygen for perianal Crohn's disease. J Clin Gastroenterol 1994;19:202–5.

103. Gaffney PR, Doyle CT, Gaffney A, et al. Paradoxical response to heparin in 10 patients with ulcerative colitis. Am J Gastroenterol 1995;90:220–3.

104. Bicks RC, Groshart KW, Chandler RW. The treatment of severe chronically active Crohn's disease by T8 (suppressor cell) lymphaphersis. Gastroenterology 1985;88:A1325.

105. van Dulleman HM, van Deventer SJH, Hommes DW, et al. Treatment of Crohn's disease with anti-tumor necrosis factor chimeric monoclonal antibody (cA2). Gastroenterology 1995;109:129–35.

106. Stronkhorst A, Radema S, ten Berge I, et al. Phase I multiple-dose pilot study of chimeric monoclonal

M-T412 (anti-CD-4) antibodies is Crohn's disease. Gastroenterology 1993;104:A784.

107. Jarnerot G. New salicylates as maintenance treatment in ulcerative colitis. Gut 1994;35:1155–8.

108. Jarnerot G, Rolny P, Sandberg-Gertzen H. Intensive intravenous treatment of ulcerative colitis. Gastroenterology 1985;89:1005–13.

109. Present DH. Toxic megacolon. Med Clin North Am 1993;77:1129–48.

110. Actis GC, Ottobrelli A, Pera A, et al. Continuously infused cyclosporine at low dose is sufficient to avoid emergency colectomy in acute attacks of ulcerative colitis without the need for high-dose steroids. J Clin Gastroenterol 1993;17:10–3.

111. Hawthorne AB, Logan RFA, Hawkey CJ, et al. Randomised controlled trial of azathioprine withdrawal in ulcerative colitis. Br Med J 1992;305:20–2.

112. Munkholm P, Langholz E, Davidsen M, et al. Frequency of glucocorticoid resistance and dependency in Crohn's disease. Gut 1994;35:360–2.

113. Sternberg EM, Chrousos GP, Wilder RL, et al. The stress response and the regulation of inflammatory disease. Ann Int Med 1992;117:854–66.

114. Nugent FW, Roy MA. Duodenal Crohn's disease: an analysis of 89 cases. Am J Gastroenterol 1989;84:249–54.

115. Valori RM, Cockel R. Omeprazole for duodenal ulceration in Crohn's disease. Br Med J 1990;300:438–9.

116. Tan WC, Allan RN. Diffuse jejunoileitis of Crohn's disease. Gut 1993;34:1374–8.

117. Lewis JD, Fisher RL. Nutrition support in inflammatory bowel disease. Med Clin North Am 1994;78:1443–56.

118. Ogorek CP, Fisher RS. Differentiation between Crohn's disease and ulcerative colitis. Med Clin North Am 1994;78:1249–58.

119. Rutgeerts P, Ggeboes K, Vantrappen G, et al. Predictability of the postoperative course of Crohn's disease. Gastroenterology 1990;99:956–63.

120. Caprilli R, Castro M, Cirillo LC, et al. Postoperative recurrence in Crohn's disease: definition, prediction and monitoring. Gastroenterol Int 1993;6:145–8.

121. Brignola C, Cottone M, Pera A, et al. Mesalamine in the prevention of endoscopic recurrence after intestinal resection for Crohn's disease. Gastroenterology 1994;108:345–9.

122. McLeod RS, Wolff BG, Steinhart AH, et al. Prophylactic mesalamine treatment decreases postoperative recurrence of Crohn's disease. Gastroenterology 1995;109:404–13.

8 Indications for Surgical Treatment in Ulcerative Colitis and Crohn's Disease

Fabrizio Michelassi

Ulcerative colitis and Crohn's disease represent a disease spectrum with protean manifestations and complications. Although as many as half of all patients with inflammatory bowel disease require at least one surgical procedure to address complications derived from their disease, the decision in favor of a surgical approach and its timing is rarely an easy one. Important considerations entering in the final decision include the localization of the disease, the amount of diseased bowel, the length of grossly normal intestine, the feasibility of bowel-sparing procedures in Crohn's disease, the likelihood that a temporary or permanent stoma may be necessary and the changes in the quality of life that surgery may produce. Other factors such as personal or work-related commitments may also influence timing of the surgical treatment. Due to the need to balance objective findings with personal considerations, it is essential that the patient, the gastroenterologist and the surgeon, assisted by the radiologist and the pathologist, partake in the decision of the optimal treatment plan for the patient.

This chapter addresses indications for surgical treatment in ulcerative colitis and Crohn's disease. Rather than offering a lengthy description, this chapter is structured around Tables 8.1 and 8.2 each with appropriate explanatory paragraphs. Hopefully, this format will offer a quick and easy reference to the reader often confronted with the complexity of inflammatory bowel disease.

Ulcerative Colitis: Indications for Surgical Treatment

The most common indication for surgical treatment in chronic ulcerative colitis is failure of medical therapy, which comprises as many as three-fourths of patients in large series (1). Depending on the severity of the disease, up to 60% of patients with fulminant colitis fail to respond to intravenous steroid therapy (2,3), ACTH (4,5), or cyclosporine (6). A slow or incomplete response portends to colectomy in two-thirds of patients, often within one year. The majority of patients has recurrent attacks. Long-term maintenance of remission may be difficult and 30 percent of patients will require surgical intervention (1).

Fulminant colitis with acute abdomen occurs in approximately 10% of patients (1). The development of persistent abdominal pain and distention, diffuse abdominal tenderness and rebound, tachycardia, and fever indicate progression to an acute abdomen and the need for emergency surgical intervention. Fulminant colitis may be complicated by toxic megacolon or perforation. Although few patients with toxic megacolon may be successfully treated with corticosteroids, intravenous fluids and electrolytes, antibiotics and bowel rest, the majority requires surgical treatment. Increasing colonic dilatation with thumbprinting (edema of the colonic wall) or pneumatosis (air dissecting the bowel wall) indicates impending perforation. A free or walled-off perforation is a rare complication and usually represents the end result of an untreated toxic megacolon. If perforation occurs, the mortality rate with surgical treatment is as high as 50% (7).

Ulcerative colitis predisposes to the development of colorectal cancer. The risk of colorectal cancers developing in ulcerative colitis patients ranges from 0.3% to 1.0% (8). Although the progression of dysplastic epithelium to a colorectal

Table 8.1. Ulcerative colitis: indications for
surgical treatment.

- Failure of medical treatment
  ➤ Persistence of symptoms despite corticosteroid
     therapy
  ➤ Recurrence of symptoms when high-dose
     corticosteroids are tapered
  ➤ Worsening symptoms or new onset of complications
     while on maximal medical therapy
  ➤ Occurrence of steroid-induced complications
     (Cushingoid features, weight gain, systemic
     hypertension, diabetes, steroid myopathy, osteopenia,
     compression fractures, aseptic necrosis of femoral
     head, increased irritability, cataracts)
- Fulminant colitis with acute abdomen
  ➤ Without toxic megacolon
  ➤ With toxic megacolon
  ➤ With walled-off perforation
  ➤ With free perforation
- Malignant transformation
  ➤ Carcinoma
  ➤ Dysplasia
  ➤ DALM
- Hemorrhage

Table 8.2. Crohn's disease: indications for surgical
treatment.

- Failure of medical treatment
  ➤ Persistence of symptoms despite corticosteroid
     therapy for longer than six months
  ➤ Recurrence of symptoms when high-dose
     corticosteroids tapered
  ➤ Worsening symptoms or new onset of complications
     with maximal medical therapy
  ➤ Occurrence of steroid-induced complications
     (Cushingoid features, cataracts, glaucoma, systemic
     hypertension, aseptic necrosis of the head of the
     femur, myopathy, or vertebral body fractures
- Obstruction
  ➤ Intestinal obstruction (partial or complete)
- Septic complications
  ➤ Inflammatory mass or abscess (intraabdominal, pelvic,
     perineal)
  ➤ Fistula if
     — Drainage causes personal embarrassment (eg.
        enterocutaneous, enterovaginal fistula, fistula-in-
        ano)
     — Fistula communicates with the genito-urinary
        system (eg. entero- or colo-vesical fistula)
     — Fistula produces functional or anatomic bypass of
        a major segment of intestine with consequent
        malabsorption and/or profuse diarrhea (e.g.,
        duodenocolic or entero-rectosigmoid fistula)
     — Free perforation
- Hemorrhage
- Carcinoma
- Growth retardation
- Fulminant colitis with or without toxic megacolon

cancer has never been documented with certainty, the presence of dysplasia has been reported in a much higher percentage of specimens of ulcerative colitis complicated by cancer than ulcerative colitis without malignant transformation. In addition, accumulating evidence obtained with modern molecular biology techniques, supports the concept of an orderly progression from normal epithelium to dysplastic epithelium to an invasive cancer. In view of this modern evidence to established concepts of tumorigenesis, and considering the expected long duration at risk for many young patients, and the risk of failure by surveillance, unequivocal dysplasia should be considered an indication to surgical treatment. Cancer risk in the presence of a low-grade dysplasia has been calculated at 10% to 20%. When high-grade dysplasia is present, this risk is increased to 30% to 40%. If the dysplasia is associated to a mass (DALM), the risk of carcinoma is as high as 40% to 60% (9).

Massive hemorrhage is rarely an indication for emergency colectomy, rather a marker of the severity of the disease (10).

Crohn's Disease: Indications for Surgical Treatment

Due to the chronic and recurrent nature of Crohn's disease, most patients have been treated medically for some time before coming to the attention of a surgeon. Medical treatment is to be judged a failure and surgery considered (a) when high-dose corticosteroid therapy proves inadequate; (b) for those patients who may be asymptomatic while on high-dose corticosteroid therapy but develop recurrence of symptoms with tapering of the steroid dose; (c) when the disease progresses with worsening of symptoms or new onset of complications while on maximal medical therapy; and (d) in the presence of significant treatment-related complications.

Patients with worsening obstipation usually become candidates for a surgical procedure after failing medical treatment. As many as 22% of patients requiring surgical intervention for Crohn's disease fall into this category (11). Symptoms differ depending on the location of the disease in the gastrointestinal tract: delayed gastric emptying in gastroduodenal disease, postprandial cramps in ileo-jejunal disease, abdominal distention, pain and diarrhea in colonic disease and laborious defecation with anal strictures. Occasionally, acute obstruction is precipitated by a stricture or by a lengthy diseased segment and can be partial, high grade or complete. Although even a complete obstruction can usually resolve with bowel rest, nasoenteric suction and intravenous fluid resuscitation, the underlying high-grade obstructive lesion which has caused the partial or complete obstruction, should be treated surgically to avoid recurrence of the obstruction. Surgical treatment is undertaken, if possible, when the obstruction is resolved and consists of bowel resection or strictureplasty for intraabdominal disease. Mechanical anal dilatation may be all that is needed for isolated anal stenosis.

Inflammatory masses and abscesses occur in as many as 20% (11). The physical findings of an inflammatory mass should raise the suspicion that the patient may harbor an abscess. Inflammatory masses and abscesses usually indicate that the disease has reached a degree of severity to be unlikely to respond to medical treatment. Abscesses may be located in the abdominal cavity, in the retroperitoneum, in the pelvis or in the perineum. If in the abdominal cavity they may be under the abdominal wall (parietal), between loops (interloop) or intrahepatic.

Fistulas are common and present in as many as one third of patients undergoing surgery for Crohn's disease (11). Rarely are they the sole indication for surgical treatment. These instances are detailed in the table. Most commonly patients with fistulas present with symptoms related to the worsening of their Crohn's disease (anorexia, fatigue, weight loss) or to the development of complications (obstruction, inflammatory masses, abscess, sepsis).

Free perforation is rare, being reported as occurring in one to three percent of patients requiring surgical intervention for complications of Crohn's disease (10). Usually the result of a secondary rupture of an abscess into the abdominal cavity, it requires prompt surgical intervention with resection of the perforated segment of intestine.

Although occult gastrointestinal bleeding is common, massive hemorrhage is an extremely rare complication of Crohn's disease, occurring in approximately one percent of patients (12,14). If the bleeding does not stop after initial transfusion with four to six units of blood, a celiac and mesenteric angiogram should be obtained. Preoperative localization of the hemorrhage may help intraoperative decisions when faced with multiple separate segments of disease.

Current estimates show an observed prevalence of 0.3% for small bowel adenocarcinoma and 1.8% for colorectal carcinoma in patients with Crohn's disease (15). The risk of cancer increases with duration and extension of disease, treatment with immunosuppressants and in bypassed loops. The goal of surgical treatment includes curative resection of the cancer, if possible, or palliation when indicated, with removal of associated segments of inflammatory disease when necessary.

Growth retardation occurs in 15% to 30% of children affected by Crohn's disease (16). If it persists despite adequate medical and nutritional support, surgical treatment must be chosen before puberty, or meaningful longitudinal growth will not occur because of closure of epiphyses (17).

Fulminant colitis with or without toxic megacolon occurs in Crohn's disease at a lesser rate than ulcerative colitis. Symptoms, findings, and treatment are the same as in ulcerative colitis.

References

1. Michelassi F, Finco C. Indications for surgery in inflammatory bowel disease: the surgeon's perspective. Kirsner JB, Shorter RG, eds. Inflammatory Bowel Disease 4th ed. Baltimore: Williams & Wilkins; 1995: 771–83.

2. Kirsner JB, Palmer WL, Spencer JA, et al. Corticotropin (ACTH) and adrenal steroids in the management of ulcerative colitis: observations in 240 patients. Ann Int Med 1959;50:89.

3. Edwards FC, Truelove SC. The course and prognosis of ulcerative colitis. Gut 1963;4:299.

4. Korelitz B, Lindner AE. The influence of corticotrophin and adrenal steroids in the course of ulcerative colitis: a comparison with the presteroid era. Gastroenterology 1964;46:671.

5. Meyers S, Sachar DB, Goldberg JD, et al. Corticotropin versus hydrocortisone in the intravenous treatment of ulcerative colitis: prospective, randomized, double-blind clinical trial. Gastroenterology 1983;85:351.

6. Lichtiger S, Present DH, Kornbluth A, et al. Cyclosporin in severe ulcerative colitis refractory to steroid therapy. New Engl J Med 1994;330(26):1841–5.

7. Norland C, Kirsner JB. Toxic dilatation of colon (toxic megacolon): etiology, treatment and prognosis in 42 patients. Medicine 1969;48:229.

8. Ransohoff D. Colon cancer in ulcerative colitis. Gastroenterology 1988;94:1089.

9. Blackstone MO, Radial RH, Rogers BHG, et al. Dysplasia-associated lesion or mass (DALM) detected by colonoscopy in long-standing ulcerative colitis: an indication for colectomy. Gastroenterology 1981;80:366.

10. Edwards FC, Truelove SC. The course and prognosis of ulcerative colitis IV. Carcinoma of the colon. Gut 1964;5:15.

11. Michelassi F, Balestracci T, Chappell R, et al. Primary and recurrent Crohn's disease: experience with 1379 patients. Ann Surg 1991;214(3):230–40.

12. Farmer RG, Hawk WA, Turnbull RG Jr. Clinical patterns in Crohn's disease: statistical study of 615 cases. Gastroenterology 1975;68:627.

13. Crohn BB, Yarnis H. Regional ileitis. 2nd ed. New York: Grune & Stratton 1958.

14. Homan WP, Tang CK, Thorbjarnason B. Acute massive hemorrhagae from intestinal Crohn's disease. Arch Surg 1976;111:901.

15. Darke SG, Parks AG, Grogono JL, et al. Adenocarcinoma and Crohn's disease: a report of two cases and analysis of the literature. Br J Surg 1973;60:169–75.

16. McCafferty TD, Nasr K, Lawrence AM, et al. Severe growth retardation in children with inflammatory bowel disease. Pediatrics 1970;45:386.

17. Homer DR, Grand RJ, Colodny AH. Growth course and prognosis after surgery for Crohn's disease in children and adolescents. Pediatrics 1977;59:717.

Section II
Ulcerative Colitis

Part I
Operative Technique

9 Proctocolectomy with Ileostomy, Abdominal Colectomy with Ileostomy, and Abdominal Colectomy with Ileoproctostomy

Roger Hurst

Indications

Total proctocolectomy with permanent end-ileostomy is indicated for those patients who require surgical treatment of ulcerative colitis, yet are not candidates for restorative proctocolectomy with ileoanal anastomosis. For the most part this includes patients with preoperative anal incontinence, elderly patients, and those patients with rectal adenocarcinomas. In addition, a small number of patients will prefer to have total procto-colectomy with permanent end ileostomy over an ileoanal anastomosis. Concerns over functional results, risk of pouchitis, and need for multiple surgeries are commonly sighted reasons for patients to reject ileoanal anastomosis in favor of total proctocolectomy with permanent ileostomy (1).

Primary indications for proctocolectomy are failure of medical management and risk of carcinoma. Total proctocolectomy is mostly performed in an elective setting for stable patients. Patients suffering from acute complications of ulcerative colitis such as fulminant colitis, toxic megacolon, perforation, malnutrition, or hemorrhage are often too ill to undergo a total proctocolectomy and in general are best treated by abdominal colectomy with rectal-sparing (2). The proctectomy can then be performed several months later when the patient's overall condition has improved and after they have been weaned from systemic steroids. In very rare instances, patients with significant rectal bleeding or severe tenesmus may require proctectomy even in the urgent setting. Abdominal colectomy with rectal sparing is occasionally indicated as an elective procedure when the diagnosis of ulcerative vs. Crohn's pancolitis is in question. In this

unusual situation an abdominal colectomy with end ileostomy and Hartmann's pouch can be performed. If pathologic examination of the resected specimen reveals ulcerative colitis or indeterminate colitis, the patient can proceed to an ileoanal anastomosis procedure. If the pathology of the resected specimen is consistent with Crohn's proctocolitis, a completion proctectomy is required.

Abdominal colectomy with ileoproctostomy (ileo-rectal anastomosis), formerly a common procedure for the surgical management of ulcerative colitis, is rarely performed today (3). Restorative proctocolectomy with ileoanal anastomosis has virtually supplanted ileoproctostomy. Currently ileoproctostomy is reserved for the unusual situation in which a colectomy is indicated in the presence of a metastatic colon cancer or for cancer prophylaxis, yet the patient is unwilling to undergo an ileoanal anastomosis procedure. Abdominal colectomy with ileorectal anastomosis will eliminate the cancer risk in the colon, and allow for surveillance of the remaining mucosa at risk via proctoscopy. Even with repeated surveillance, however, rectal adenocarcinomas can develop in these patients. Hence this procedure represents a poor substitute for the preferred ileoanal anastomosis.

Preoperative Preparation

Prior to operation the surgeon should confer with the patient and family so that they understand the nature of the operation, the necessity for surgery, the treatment options including alternative therapies, operative hazards, possible complications, and potential benefits. Most importantly, the patient should have a thorough understanding of the

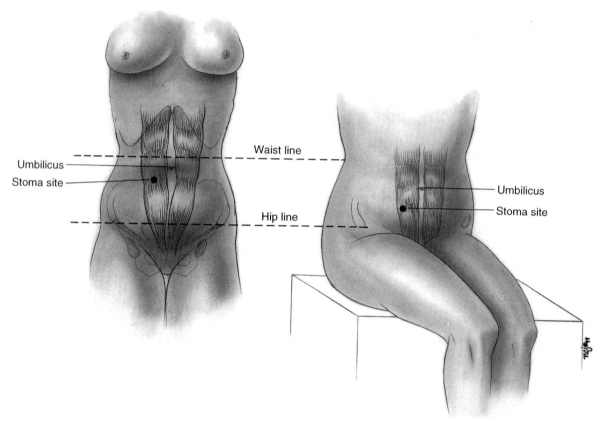

Umbilicus
Stoma site
Waist line
Hip line
Umbilicus
Stoma site

Fig. 9.1.   The stoma site is marked prior to surgery. The ileostomy should be located over the right rectus abdominus muscle on a flat area away from skin folds and bony prominences.

nature of an ileostomy and be aware of the possibility of impairment of sexual function. All appropriate candidates are given the opportunity for autologous blood donation. Additionally, male patients who may desire to father children in the future are advised to cryopreserve a sample of their sperm prior to operation.

Selection of the optimal placement of the ileostomy should be determined preoperatively. Proper stoma location in a critical step in the performance of total proctocolectomy as it will have a profound effect on the patient's adjustment to the ileostomy (4). Consultation with an enterostomal therapist should be made to assist in the placement of the proposed stoma. Ideally the ileostomy site should be located over the right rectus muscle on a flat area away from deep skin folds and bony prominences. The surface of the abdomen should be evaluated in both the sitting and standing positions as this will often demonstrate skin folds and creases not evident in the supine position (Fig. 9.1). Finally, the patient's belt line is determined and every effort is made to place the stoma below it. Once the optimal position of the stoma has been identified it is marked with an intradermal injection of meth-

ylene blue. This results in a temporary "tatoo" that remains visible for approximately two weeks.

Specific medical problems such as anemia, hyperglycemia and electrolyte abnormalities should be discovered and remedied prior to operation.

The bowel is mechanically cleansed with a combination of a clear liquid diet beginning 48 hours prior to operation and oral polyethylene glycol solution the evening before surgery. Patients recently treated with corticosteroids should be given intravenous stress dose hydrocortisone prior to induction of anesthesia and continued through the postoperative course (5). Intravenous prophylactic antibiotics should be administered one hour prior to surgery so that maximal tissue antibiotic levels are achieved at the time of the skin incision (6).

Pitfalls and Danger Points

Although total proctocolectomy with end-ileostomy does entail pitfalls and danger points, most are readily avoidable with proper technique. They include:

1. Injury to pelvic autonomic nerves with resultant sexual and urinary dysfunction.
2. Ureteral injuries.
3. Fecal contamination with resultant risk of intraabdominal sepsis and wound infections.
4. Improper plane of dissection along the sacrum resulting in injury to the presacral venous plexus and excessive blood loss.
5. Improper ileostomy placement and construction.
6. Splenic Injury

Operative Strategies

Ulcerative colitis is a disease that is limited to the mucosal lining of the colon and rectum, therefore complete removal of the colon and rectum is curative. Extraintestinal manifestations of ulcerative colitis such as cutaneous, joint, and vascular manifestations usually regress following total proctocolectomy. Total proctocolectomy however does not effect the clinical course of ulcerative colitis associated rheumatoid arthritis, ankylosing spondylitis, or sclerosing cholangitis which tend to progress even after extirpation of the colorectal mucosa (7,8).

Because ulcerative colitis is limited to the inner lining of the colon and rectum, wide surgical dissection with radical mesenteric resection is unnecessary and meddlesome. Unless the colon or rectum is known or suspected to harbor an invasive carcinoma the dissection should remain close to the bowel. This is particularly true for the pelvic dissection where close adherence to the wall of the rectum during the lateral and posterior dissection is necessary to avoid injury to the pelvic nerves.

Operative Technique

Position

The abdominal portion of the procedure is performed with the patient supine. Once the abdominal and pelvic dissections are complete, the patient is placed in the modified lithotomy position for the perineal dissection. It is therefore advantageous to position the patient with the buttocks at the break of the table prior to induction of anesthesia. While in the lithotomy position the legs are supported with Allen stirrups (Allen Manufacturing Company, Cleveland, OH). With ample padding, the patient's heel should rest flat in the well of the stirrups with a majority of the extremity's weight being placed on the sole of the foot. The thighs are flexed 45° and abducted to expose the perineum. To avoid pressure on the peroneal nerve the legs

should be internally rotated. The proper position is reached when the lower leg points in a direction overlying the contralateral shoulder (Fig. 9.2).

Incision

Total proctocolectomy is best performed through either a vertical mid-line incision or an infraumbilical transverse incision. Both of these incisions provide adequate access to the recesses of the abdomen and pelvis. The transverse incision has the advantages of excellent protection against fascial dehiscence and superior cosmetic healing, whereas the vertical mid-line incision is less time consuming and provides better exposure particularly in the obese patient. If a transverse incision is selected, it should be placed so as to avoid interference with the planed ileostomy site. If interference with the planned ileostomy site is not avoidable, a mid-line incision should be selected. Paramedian incisions should be avoided as they give less than ideal exposure, interfere with stomal placement, are time consuming, and provide for a very poor cosmetic appearance.

Exploration

Upon entering the abdomen it is important to fully examine the viscera looking for possible manifestations of Crohn's disease and synchronous pathology. The stomach, duodenum, and small bowel are closely examined. If small bowel Crohn's disease is detected then it can be concluded that the patient is suffering from Crohn's colitis rather than ulcerative colitis and the need for a total proctocolectomy should be reassessed.

Mobilization of the Right Colon

The right colon, cecum, and terminal ileum are fully mobilized by incising the lateral parietal peritoneum from around the cecum and superiorly to the hepatic flexure. This is best accomplished by lifting the peritoneum with a right angle clamp while the first assistant divides the peritoneum with the electrocautery using the coagulation current (Fig. 9.3). When encountered, small vessels are grasped with forceps and cauterized using a coaptive technique prior to their division. A thin layer of connective tissue referred to as the "fusion fascia" lies just underneath the peritoneum. This thin layer of tissue should be divided parallel to the incision in the peritoneal reflection. With this, the proper surgical plane is entered and the mesentery of the colon can be fully mobilized while the right ureter and gonadal vessels remain in their normal

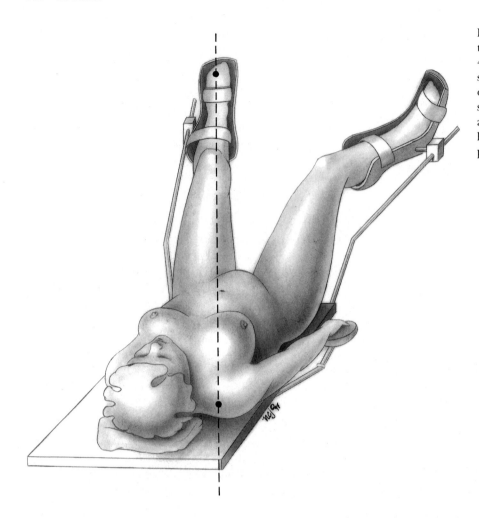

Fig. 9.2.   In the lithotomy position the thighs are abducted and flexed 45 degrees. The tip of the coccyx should be accessible from the end of the table. To avoid lateral pressure on the peroneal nerve, the legs are internally rotated and the lower legs are aligned in a direction that points to the contralateral shoulder.

retroperitoneal position. Incising the lateral peritoneum without dividing the fusion fascia results in a dissection plane that is too posterior causing the ureter to remain attached to the posterior surface of the mesentery.

With the mobilization of the right colon, the ureter and duodenum are identified and separated from the mesentery to prevent their injury at the time of division of the mesocolon. The hepatic flexure of the colon is mobilized by dividing the superior peritoneal attachments. This is accomplished by continuing the lateral peritoneal incision superiorly over the hepatic flexure. Care must be exercised not to injure the underlying duodenum. Division of the peritoneum is continued until the right lateral edge of the greater omentum is encountered.

Transverse Colon

The transverse colon is separated from its attachments to the greater curvature of the stomach. This can be accomplished with or without preservation

of the greater omentum. If the greater omentum is to be preserved it is dissected off the transverse colon and mesocolon by incising along the "avascular" space between the two structures. Preservation of the omentum is not generally associated with complications, although retention of an ischemic omentum may result in adhesion formation and resultant small bowel obstruction (8). For these reasons it is often best to resect the greater omentum with the transverse colon.

This is accomplished by first entering the lesser space through the gastrocolic ligament so that the omentum can be separated from the greater curvature of the stomach. The optimal site for entry into the lesser space is a point above the transverse colon and to the left of the middle colic vessels, along the left side or proximal end of the greater curvature of the stomach. The greater omentum is less likely to be fused with the transverse mesocolon at this location compared to a point to the right of the middle colic vessels. To preserve optimal gastric perfusion, the incision in the gastrocolic ligament is made caudal to the gastroepiploic vessels. The

Fig. 9.3. The right colon is mobilized by incising the peritoneal reflection and the underlying fusion fascia. This incision is carried from around the cecum to the suspensory ligament of the hepatic flexure (inset).

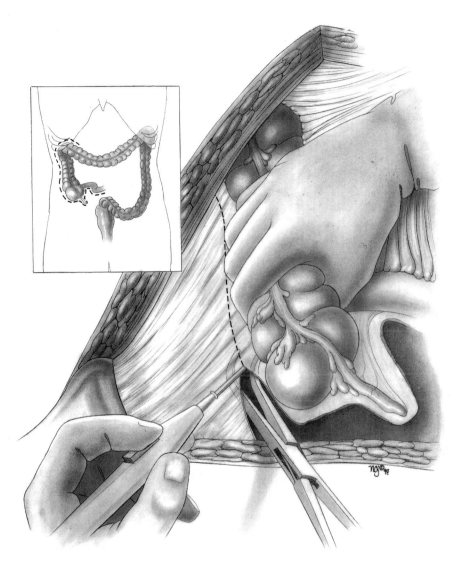

division of the omentum is carried proximally and distally along the transverse colon (Fig. 9.4). Proximally the omental dissection meets up with the peritoneal incision previously performed to mobilize the hepatic flexure. Distally the division of the greater omentum is carried towards the splenic flexure. However, full mobilization of the splenic flexure is only undertaken after the left colon has been mobilized.

With the mobilization of the transverse colon great care must be exercised to avoid splenic injury. Attachments of the greater omentum or colon to the capsule of the spleen often occur. Traction on the transverse colon or omentum places tension on these delicate attachments and can thus result in an avulsion injury to the splenic capsule. It is, therefore, important to inspect the area adjacent to the spleen and, if necessary, divide any omental adhesions prior to applying traction to the distal transverse colon and omentum.

Left Colon

Adhesions of the sigmoid colon to the left posterior lateral abdominal and pelvic walls are divided. As with the right colon the peritoneal reflection is then incised along the lateral reflection (line of Toldt) and the fusion fascia is likewise incised in a parallel fashion. The left ureter is identified to ensure its safety. Incision of the peritoneum and fusion fascia is carried superiorly towards the splenic flexure. With division of the peritoneal attachments of the left colon and completion of the division of the omentum from the greater curvature of the stomach, the splenic flexure is then approached as a triangle of intestine held at its apex by peritoneal attachments. The anterior suspensory ligament of the splenic flexure originates from the left margin of the gastrocolic ligament and extends to the diaphragm as the phrenocolic ligament. These attachments are coagu-

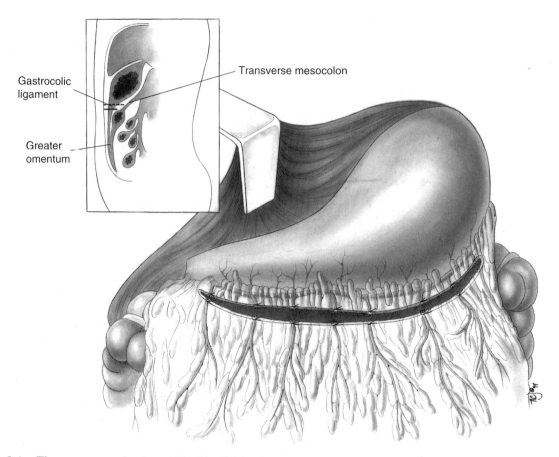

Fig. 9.4.   The transverse colon is mobilized by dividing the omentum from its attachments to the greater curvature of the stomach.

lated and divided. Full mobilization of the colon from terminal ileum to rectosigmoid junction is thus accomplished.

Division of the Mesentery

The terminal ileum is divided between bowel clamps or with a GIA stapling device and the mesentery of the colon is divided. The incision in the mesentery of the cecum, ascending transverse and descending colon is undertaken at a convenient distance from the bowel wall. Larger vessels are doubly ligated while avascular portions of the mesocolon can be incised with electrocautery (Fig. 9.5). To avoid injury, both ureters and the duodenum are visualized during the transection of the mesentery. To keep a safe distance from the hypogastric sympathetic neural plexus the division of the sigmoid mesentery is carried through the sigmoid arterial arcades, staying superficial to the inferior mesenteric artery.

Creation of Hartmann's Pouch or Ileoproctostomy

If rectal sparing with either Hartmann's pouch or ileorectal anastomosis is to be performed, the left colic and sigmoid branches of the inferior mesenteric artery are divided whereas the terminal branches of the inferior mesenteric vessels are preserved. This will assure a good blood supply to the remaining rectal stump and aid in the healing of Hartmann's pouch closure or the ileorectal anastomosis. Preservation of the main inferior mesenteric vessels and the superior rectal vessels also simplifies any subsequent proctectomy by keeping the pelvic sympathetic nerves free of surrounding scar tissue and by providing for a key anatomical landmark that will assist in the location of the appropriate presacral dissection plane for any future planned proctectomy.

With rectal sparing the rectosigmoid junction is divided at the level of the sacral promontory. If an

Fig. 9.5. Line of division of the mesentery of the colon.

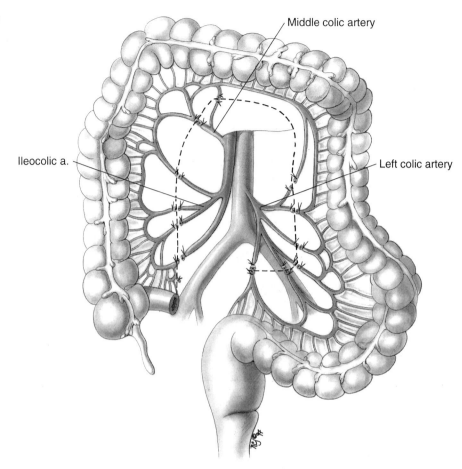

Middle colic artery

Ileocolic a.

Left colic artery

ileorectal anastomosis is to be performed, this can be accomplished in an end to end or side to end fashion utilizing any of the standard hand sutured or stapling techniques. To create a Hartmann's pouch the mesentery and pericolonic fat are cleaned from the bowel wall of the rectosigmoid junction. Approximately 2 cm of bowel is prepared in such a manner and the bowel is then closed with a TA stapling device utilizing 4.8-mm staples. The bowel is then divided proximal to the staple line. The staple line should be closely examined to ensure that the staples are in two rows of well formed "B"s and that they are not cutting into the muscularis propria of the bowel. To provide extra assurance against dehiscence, the staple line should be oversewn with interrupted 3-0 silk Lembert sutures (Fig. 9.6). These sutures should be carefully placed so that the anterior and posterior serosal surfaces are approximated without undue tension. In thickened and edematous bowel it is often necessary to invert a substantial amount of tissue to bring the closure together without excessive tension that may result in the sutures cutting through the tissue.

In a well constructed Hartmann's pouch, placement of pelvic drains are not necessary and can be harmful as their placement close to the suture line may promote a dehiscence. If the severity of disease or the presence of distal obstruction precludes a safe closure of a Hartmann's pouch then the creation of a mucus fistula should be considered. A mucus fistula requires a much larger segment of distal bowel and is associated with a greater risk of bleeding from the retained segment. Additionally a mucus fistula is unsightly and often generates a very foul odor.

If attempts to make a secure Hartmann's closure fail and the remaining rectal stump is too short to bring out as a mucus fistula, then the proximal rectum should be resected and the closure of the Hartmann's pouch should be performed just below the peritoneal reflection. In this situation closed suction drains should be placed in the deep pelvis and the peritoneum closed over the rectal stump. Such a short Hartmann's pouch, however, will make finding the rectal stump during a subsequent completion proctectomy and ileorectal anastomosis significantly more difficult.

164   R. Hurst

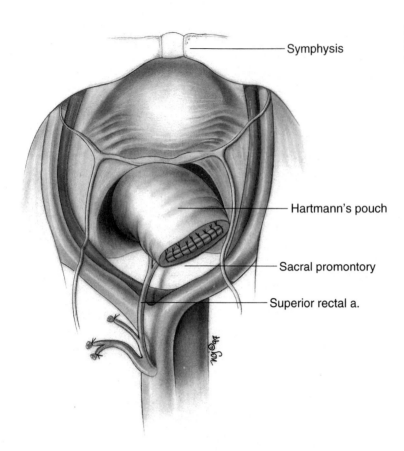

— Symphysis

— Hartmann's pouch

— Sacral promontory

— Superior rectal a.

Fig. 9.6.   Hartmann's pouch is created at the level of the sacral promontory with superior rectal vessels left intact.

Proctectomy

If a proctectomy is to be performed, the sigmoid colon is not stapled and the dissection is continued distally with the specimen still attached. The pelvic dissection of the rectum is greatly simplified if undertaken in an orderly and step wise fashion. The dissection begins with complete posterior mobilization of the rectum. This initial posterior mobilization allows for clear definition of the lateral rectal ligaments which are divided as the second step of the pelvic dissection. Division of the lateral ligaments in turn results in forward mobilization of the rectum and unravels the deep recess of the rectovaginal or rectovesicle pouch. This unraveling provides better exposure for the final anterior dissection.

After division of the sigmoid mesentery has reached a level below the sacral promontory the terminal branches of the inferior mesenteric artery, the superior rectal vessels, are ligated and divided. Since the sympathetic neural plexus lies directly behind the inferior mesenteric artery at the pelvic brim, the nerves are clearly identified at this point, dissected free of the vessels then the terminal branches of the inferior mesenteric artery and vein (superior rectal vessels) are divided with the undisturbed neural plexus in full view (Fig. 9.7). After

division of the superior rectal vessels at the level of the sacral promontory the parietal peritoneum is incised from the point of ligation of the superior rectal vessels inferior and laterally for a distance just sufficient to gain full access to the presacral space between the fascia propria of the rectum and the presacral fascia. The left and right ureters should again be clearly identified as they course inferolaterally across the true pelvis. The rectum is retracted anteriorly and the loose areolar tissue along the presacral space is divided under direct vision using electrocautery (Fig. 9.8). Care must be used to ensure that the dissection continues in the proper plane. The presacral venous plexus should remain covered by the presacral fascia, otherwise bleeding that can be difficult to control will occur. If the uncovered veins of the presacral venous plexus are seen, then the approach is too deep and the dissection should be carried closer to the rectum. Even when in the proper plane between the fascia propria of the rectum and the presacral fascia, small communicating vessels between the rectum and the presacral plexus can occur and for this reason, mobilization of the rectum blindly with blunt hand dissection is to be avoided (10). If bleeding from the presacral venous plexus occurs it can often be managed with suture ligation. Occasionally, how-

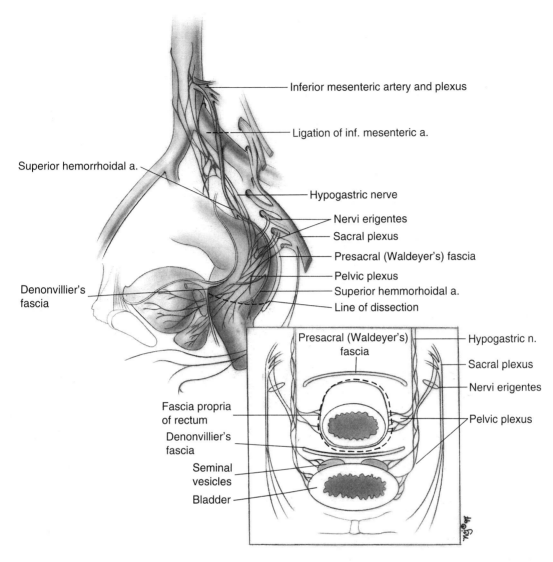

Inferior mesenteric artery and plexus

Ligation of inf. mesenteric a.

Superior hemorrhoidal a.

Hypogastric nerve

Nervi erigentes

Sacral plexus

Presacral (Waldeyer's) fascia

Pelvic plexus

Superior hemmorhoidal a.

Line of dissection

Denonvillier's fascia

Presacral (Waldeyer's) fascia

Hypogastric n.

Sacral plexus

Nervi erigentes

Pelvic plexus

Fascia propria of rectum

Denonvillier's fascia

Seminal vesicles

Bladder

Fig. 9.7.   Proctectomy dissection is maintained close to rectal wall to avoid injury to sympathetic and parasympathetic nerves.

ever, injured veins can retract into the bony substance of the sacrum and these vessels may require the use of titanium thumbtacks to control the bleeding (11).

Posterior mobilization of the rectum should extend beyond the level of the coccyx with Waldeyer's fascia being incised with electrocautery. The resultant complete posterior mobilization of the rectum defines the posterior surface of the lateral ligaments (Fig. 9.9).

The preaortic sympathetic nerves can be seen dividing into two major trunks in the upper sacral area. These branching sympathetic trunks continue laterally to the right and left walls of the pelvis, passing through the tissue of the lateral rectal ligaments. The sympathetic nerves are gently dissected off the posterolateral aspect of the fascia propria of the rectum and the lateral rectal liga-

ments are then approached posteriorly and divided as close as possible to the rectal wall. Division of the lateral ligaments close to the rectum also avoids injury to the more caudad sacral parasympathetic nerves. A majority of this pelvic dissection can be accomplished with electrocautery with larger vessels being ligated prior to division. To facilitate the division of the lateral rectal ligaments, anterior and superior traction is placed on the rectum with the aid of a sturdy right angle bowel clamp (Wertheim Cullen pedicle clamp). This upward retraction places tension on the lateral ligaments, further defining their attachment to the rectal wall (Fig. 9.10).

Following the posterior and lateral mobilization, superior traction of the rectum will result in the unfolding of the recesses of the rectovaginal or rectovesicle pouch. This unfolding greatly facili-

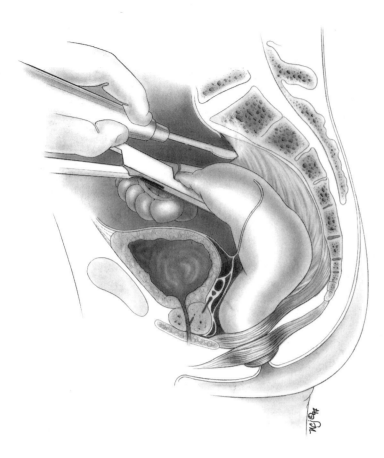

Fig. 9.8.   After division of the superior rectal vessels, the rectum is retracted forward and mobilized anteriorly by dissecting along the presacral space under direct vision.

tates the anterior dissection by providing better exposure and allowing for the efficient application of tension and counter tension at the point of dissection. The anterior peritoneum and underlying fatty tissue is incised to expose the longitudinal muscle fibers of the anterior wall of the rectum. At this level (posterior to Denonvilliers' fascia) the anterior dissection is undertaken in an inferior direction. The anterior dissection is greatly facilitated by sturdy traction on the rectum directed towards the sacral promontory. In the male the anterior dissection is continued to the level of the inferior border of the prostate and completion of the anterior dissection can be determined by palpating the Foley catheter as it passes through the membranous urethra. In the female patient the anterior dissection is continued until the thickening of the perineal body and anal sphincter mechanisms can be palpated. After the anterior dissection is complete additional lateral dissection may be necessary so that the rectum is circumferentially mobilized to the level of the levator ani muscles.

With completion of the pelvic dissection the distal rectum is stapled with a TA stapling device. The rectum is divided above the staple line leaving behind a short rectal stump (Fig. 9.11). A soft closed suction drain is placed deep into the pelvis over the remaining rectal stump and is brought out through a separate stab incision in the lower abdominal wall far from the planned ileostomy position.

Creation of the Ileostomy

In true idiopathic ulcerative colitis roentgenographic evidence for "backwash ileitis" with edema of the terminal ileum may occasionally occur. This nonspecific inflammation quickly resolves following removal of the inflamed colon and ileal resection is generally not necessary. Rarely, however, the terminal ileum may be sufficiently edematous that safe eversion of the lumen for creation of a Brooke ileostomy is not possible. Under such circumstances resection of a short segment of ileum may be necessary.

Over the marked ostomy site a circular incision is made two centimeters in diameter. The subcutaneous fat is divided transversely and the anterior rectus sheath is opened with a cruciate incision. The fibers of the rectus abdominus muscle are bluntly separated with the aid of hand-held retractors. The posterior rectus sheath and peritoneum are then incised. The cut end of the ileum

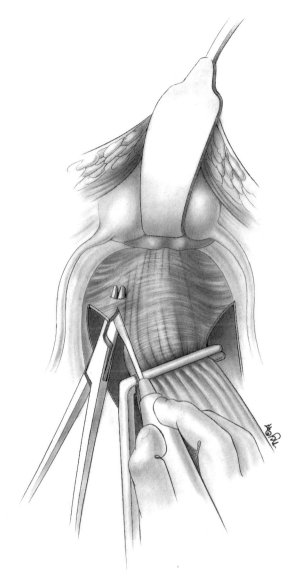

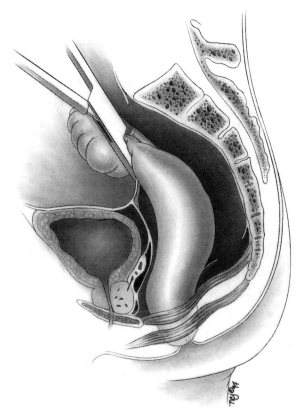

Fig. 9.10. Posterior dissection of the rectum is carried through Waldeyer's fascia (which can be seen transected over the levators) to lift the rectum from both the sacrum and the posterior aspect of the levator sling.

Fig. 9.9. The lateral ligaments are divided close to the rectal wall so as to avoid injury to the autonomic nerves.

is delivered through the ostomy incision so that approximately five centimeters of ileum extends above the surface of the skin (Fig. 9.12). To prevent stomal prolapse the mesentery of the ileum is sutured to the inner surface of the anterior abdominal wall. The right lateral gutter is then closed by suturing the peritoneum to the cut edge of the ileal mesentery, from the duodenum to the ostomy site.

After the delivery of the ileum through the abdominal wall, the abdominal cavity is then irrigated and the celiotomy incision is closed. The ileostomy is matured using interrupted 3–0 chromic sutures. An everting seromuscular suture is first placed at the antimesenteric edge of the ileum. Everting su-

tures are also placed at ninety degrees to the antimesenteric stitch. The suture at the mesenteric border needs to be placed carefully as to avoid injury to the mesenteric vessels (Fig. 9.13) and, at times, may be omitted. These sutures are placed with a full thickness bite of the open end of the ileum, a seromuscular bite of the ileum at the skin level, and a subcuticular bite of the skin. Once all everting sutures have been placed, they are then tied. The resultant stoma should protrude approximately two to three centimeters above the abdominal wall (Fig. 9.14). Simple sutures between the cut edge of the ileum and the dermis are then placed circumferentially to allow complete approximation of the mucocutaneous junction.

Perineal Dissection

If a complete proctocolectomy is to be carried out, the patient is placed in a lithotomy position and the rectal stump is gently irrigated with a povidine-

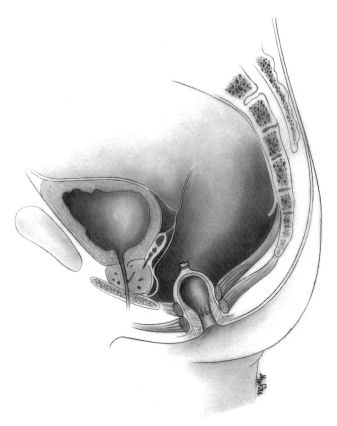

Fig. 9.11.   With completion of the abdominal and pelvic dissections, a short rectal stump remains.

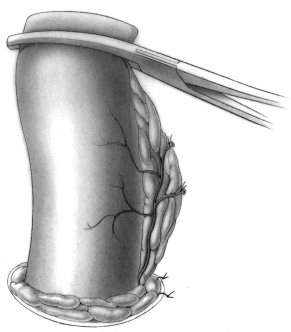

Fig. 9.12.   Five centimeters of ileum is delivered through the ileostomy incision.

iodine solution. A povidine-iodine soaked gauze is then placed into the rectal stump and the anus is sutured closed with a purse string suture placed at the level of the anal verge. The perineum is then shaved and sterilely prepped. In the female patient the vagina is also prepped.

Removal of the rectal stump is best carried out along the plane between the internal and external sphincters (Fig. 9.15). With a needlepoint electro-cautery, a circular incision is made over the palpable groove between the internal and external sphincters (Fig. 9.16). This intersphincteric plane is easiest to identify laterally. Thus, the dissection should commence on the left and right sides and then proceed to connect posteriorly and anteriorly. The dissection is carried upward and the pelvic cavity is entered first posteriorly and then working laterally to meet anteriorly. With this the rectal stump is completely excised. Through the perineal wound the closed suction drain can be identified and its proper position at the level of the levator-ani should be ensured. The perineal wound is closed by approximating the external sphincter mechanism in layers using absorbable suture. The skin edges are trimmed with a scalpel and the skin

closed with a nylon interrupted vertical mattress suture (Fig. 9.17).

Postoperative Care

The nasogastric tube can be removed in the operating room. In the absence of intraoperative contamination perioperative antibiotics are discontinued within twenty-four hours. Sequential compression stockings are continued until the patient is fully ambulatory. The Foley catheter is removed on the fourth postoperative day. The diet is advanced once output from the ileostomy has begun.

In the immediate postoperative period edema often accumulates in the ileostomy. Over time this edema subsides and significant shrinkage of the stoma occurs. It is therefore important that the patient be instructed on how to cut the opening of the stoma appliance to accommodate the changing size of the ileostomy.

Complications

Perineal Wound Infection

Perineal wound infection often manifests with fever, perineal pain, erythema, and purulent drainage. This complication is best avoided by proper bowel preparation, prophylactic antibiotics, and

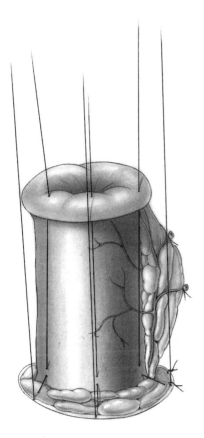

Fig. 9.13. Everting sutures are placed on the anti-mesenteric edge of the ileum at 90° on either side of this stitch and on the mesenteric border of the small bowel.

avoidance of fecal soilage. Intersphincteric perineal dissection as described above allows for effective closure of the perineal dead space and thus may also reduce the likelihood of this complication (12). When perineal wound infection occurs, the skin sutures are removed, purulent fluid is completely drained, necrotic tissue debrided, and the wound packed.

Urinary Retention

Postoperative urinary retention may result from the use of opiates, anticholinergic medication, pre-existing mechanical urinary obstruction, such as benign prostatic hypertrophy, or from intraoperative autonomic nerve injury. Overuse of opiates and the administration of anticholinergic medication should be avoided if the patient experiences difficulty voiding after urinary catheter removal. Patients with a history of symptoms consistent with urinary obstruction should be investigated prior to proctocolectomy.

Urinary retention due to autonomic nerve injury is uncommon and is best avoided by conducting the pelvic dissection as close to the rectum as possible. This is particularly true for the division of the lateral ligaments and the anterior rectal dissection. When urinary retention related to autonomic nerve injury it is best managed with intermittent catheterization. In most instances this is required for only a limited time as bladder function tends to recover. Long term intermittent self catheterization is rarely necessary.

Sexual Dysfunction

Impotence is an uncommon complication following total proctocolectomy and occurs in approximately 1% to 2% of male patients (13). Retrograde ejaculation, however, is more common and has been reported to occur in up to 5% of males. In women, mild dyspareunia is common, occurring in up to 30% of cases. When dyspareunia occurs after total proctocolectomy it is often transient and is usually not severe enough to limit sexual activity. Female fertility is perhaps diminished following total proctocolectomy, however, this procedure does not preclude full term pregnancy with normal vaginal delivery (14).

Misdiagnosis

Histologic examination of the removed colon and rectum may demonstrate features that are diagnostic for Crohn's disease. Even with histology consistent with ulcerative colitis, the diagnosis cannot be totally certain and manifestations of Crohn's disease in the small bowel may develop years after total proctocolectomy. All patients should be informed of this possibility.

Stomal Complications

Complications related to the ileostomy are common and include ischemia, peristomal hernia, prolapse, and stricture. Approximately 25% of patients undergoing total proctocolectomy with end Brooke ileostomy will require surgical revision of their stoma to deal with one or more of these complications (15).

Complications of the Hartmann's Pouch

Complications associated with a Hartmann's pouch include dehiscence with pelvic sepsis, bleeding from diseased mucosa, and severe tenesmus. Suture line dehiscence is best prevented by cautious closure of the stump. When dehiscence occurs drainage of pelvic sepsis is required. Per-

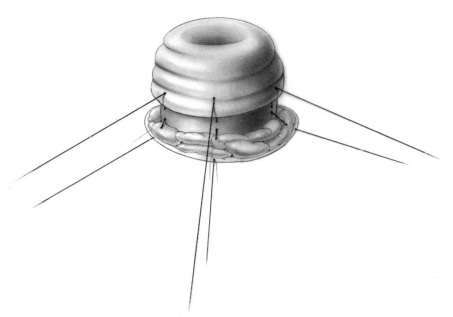

Fig. 9.14. The everting sutures are tied and simple sutures are placed between the cut edge of the ileum and the dermis.

cutaneous or transrectal drainage is occasionally possible, but operative drainage with reclosure of the pouch at the level of the peritoneal reflection is at times necessary.

Minor bloody drainage from the Hartmann's pouch is common, but severe bleeding requiring transfusions is rare. To control moderate bloody drainage, hydrocortisone enemas can be used. It may be necessary however to continue therapeutic

systemic steroids for two to three weeks so that the Hartmann's pouch can heal prior to instilling the hydrocortisone enemas.

Severe bleeding may require early proctectomy. Alternatively packing the rectal stump with gauze moistened with either saline or an alpha-agonist containing solution has been reported. Packing a rectal stump to tamponade bleeding, however, is likely to be very uncomfortable for the patient and

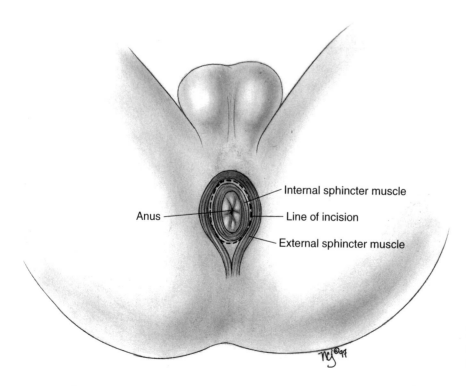

Fig. 9.15. The line of dissection is carried out between the internal and external anal sphincters.

Fig. 9.16. Line of incision for the perineal dissection.

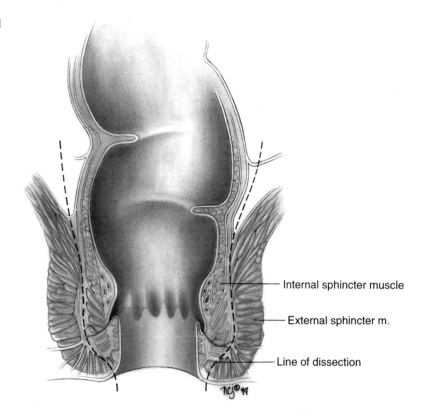

Internal sphincter muscle

External sphincter m.

Line of dissection

Fig. 9.17. Closure of the perineal wound.

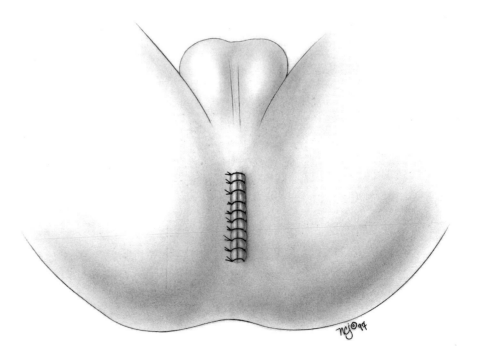

may result in perforation of the rectal stump closure.

In rare instances severe debilitating tenesmus may occur after abdominal colectomy with rectal sparing. If not controlled with pain medication and steroid therapy, severe tenesmus may necessitate early proctectomy.

Small Bowel Obstruction

Adhesive small bowel obstruction is not an uncommon complication following total proctocolectomy and appears to be more frequent than with other abdominal operations. Closure of the right lateral peritoneal space may help to reduce the likelihood of small bowel obstruction, but verification of this with clinical data is lacking (16).

Long-Term Results

The long-term results following total proctocolectomy for ulcerative colitis are good. With complete removal of the colon and rectum, patients can be weaned off corticosteroids and other anti-ulcerative colitis medications are discontinued. Patients, of course, have to live with the consequences of a permanent abdominal stoma. After a variable period of adjustment, however, almost all patients are able to resume their normal activities in both their personal and professional lives (17).

References

1. Hurst RD, Finco C, Rubin M, et al. Prospective analysis of perioperative morbidity in one hundred consecutive colectomies for ulcerative colitis. Surgery 1995;118:748–55.
2. Hawley PR. Emergency surgery for ulcerative colitis. World J Surg 1988;12:169–73.
3. Melville DM, Ritchie JK, Nicholls RJ, et al. Surgery for ulcerative colitis in the era of the pouch: the St Mark's Hospital experience. Gut 1994;35:1076–80.
4. Tomaselli N, Jenks J, Morin KH. Body image in patients with stomas: a critical review of the literature. J Enterostom Ther 1991;18:95–9.
5. Salem M, Tainsh RE, Bromberg J, et al. Perioperative glucocorticoid coverage. A reassessment 42 years after emergence of a problem. Ann Surg 1994;219:416–25.
6. Kaiser AB. Antibiotic prophylaxis in surgery. N Engl J Med 1996;315:1129–38.
7. Gravallese EM, Kantrowitz FG. Arthritic manifestations of inflammatory bowel disease. Am J Gastroenterol 1988;83:703–9.
8. Cangemi JR, et al. Effect of proctocolectomy for chronic ulcerative colitis on the natural history of primary sclerosing cholangitis. Gastroenterology 1989;96:790–5.
9. Parc RF, Balladur PM, Block GE, et al. Proctocolectomy. In: Block GE, Moossa AR, eds. Operative Colorectal Surgery. Philadelphia: W.B. Saunders, 1994:151–64.
10. Wang, QY, Shi WJ, Zhao YR, et al. New concepts in severe presacral hemorrhage during proctectomy. Arch Surg 1985;120:1013–20.
11. Navatvongs S, Fang DT. The use of thumbtacks to stop massive presacral hemorrhage. Dis Colon Rectum 1986;29:589, 90.
12. Berry AR, Campos RDE, Lee ECG. Perineal and pelvic morbidity following perimuscular excision of the rectum for inflammatory bowel disease. Br J Surg 1986;73:675.
13. Bauer JJ, Gelernt IM, Salky B, et al. Sexual dysfunction following proctocolectomy for benign disease of the colon and rectum. Ann Surg 1983;197:363–7.
14. Metcalf AM, Dozois RR, Kelly KA. Sexual function in women after proctocolectomy. Ann Surg 1986;204:624–7.
15. Ritchie JK. Ileostomy and excisional surgery for chronic inflammatory disease of the colon: a survey of one hospital region. Gut 1971;12:528–40.
16. Leong AP, Londono-Schimmer EE, Phillips RK. Lifetable analysis of stomal complications following ileostomy. Br J Surg 1994;81:727–9.
17. McLeod RS, Churchill DN, Audrey ML, Vanderburgh S, Cohen Z. Quality of life of patients with ulcerative colitis preoperatively and postoperatively. Gastroenterology 1991;101:1307–13.

10 Restorative Proctocolectomy with Ileoanal Anastomosis

Jeffrey W. Milsom

The restorative proctocolectomy (RP) for the treatment of ulcerative colitis evolved naturally as the goals of surgery for ulcerative colitis blossomed from preservation of life to preservation of function. The operation became the mainstay of therapy for most patients with ulcerative colitis during the 1980s, and represents one of the major technical achievements of modern gastrointestinal surgery, as it allows the majority of patients with ulcerative colitis requiring surgery to live without a permanent stoma. The operation also bequeathed major insights into pelvic floor and anal sphincter function, and into some of the subtleties of pelvic anatomy. In addition, the operation gave surgeons, gastroenterologists, their patients, and other medical experts deeper insights into small intestine adaptability, absorption, and motility. Many of the consequences of this operation, including pouchitis, dysplasia of remnant columnar epithelium, and the long-term outcome of the ileal pouch (decades postoperatively) will require further study before they are well understood, and these issues remain tantalizing research projects awaiting current and future investigators.

Although the quest for an "ideal" operation for ulcerative colitis remains as an important challenge to surgeons with an interest in inflammatory bowel disease, the role of the RP seems established: it is the operation of choice for both surgeons and patients if the diagnosis seems secure and there are no medical contraindications.

This chapter will attempt to situate the restorative proctocolectomy in its proper context in the management of ulcerative colitis. We will discuss the indications and contraindications for RP. Thereafter, some of the specific pitfalls and danger points of the RP operation will be highlighted. Controversial aspects of the operation will be discussed, such as the performance of the hand-sewn versus stapled anastomosis of the ileal pouch to the anal sphincters or the distal rectum. Finally, complications and long-term results will be assessed, and special circumstances considered (such as pregnancy after the RP procedure). This chapter, therefore, will attempt to place this procedure in its proper context under a wide variety of circumstances. The very important sections of Chapter 11 will thereafter give us deeper comprehension of various *designs* of the ileal pouch, and how they may be used to advantage in treating ulcerative colitis patients requiring surgery.

The evolution of the surgical management of ulcerative colitis did not stop with just the development of different pouch designs. Decreasing the length of the retained rectal muscular cuff (which originally was left at 8 to 10 cm as in the Soave procedure) to only 1 or 2 cms has lessened the incidence of pelvic (intramuscular) cuff abscesses (1). The efferent ileal limb of the S-pouch, if left longer than 1 to 2 cm, occasionally would not permit effective emptying of the pouch, requiring patients to pass drainage catheters transanally for effective bowel evacuation (2). Thus, we have learned that the efferent limb of the S-pouch should be kept to a size of less then 2 cm.

Concerns over preservation of sexual function have led surgeons to actively identify and preserve the pelvic nerves-both sympathetic and parasympathetic during proctectomy. Whereas surgeons in the 1970s believed that a nerve-preserving proctectomy necessitated performance of the posterior dissection close to the rectal wall (between the posterior rectal wall and the mesorectum) in order to preserve pelvic nerve function, we now know that effective pelvic nerve preservation is possible by directly identifying the hypogastric nerves posterior to the inferior mesenteric artery and sweeping them posterolaterally away from the mesorectum, thereafter dissecting in the avascular plane between the fascia propria of the rectum and the presacral fascia. Entry into this relatively bloodless plane greatly expedites the procedure without increasing the risk of retrograde ejaculation (due to hypogastric nerve injury). Therafter, by keeping the lateral margins of the resection close to the rectum as the "lateral stalks" are divided, the parasympathetic nerves are also preserved.

A recent technical refinement of major significance has been the preservation of the "anal transitional zone" or the distal 1 to 2 cm of the rectal columnar epithelium, to which the ileal pouch is anastomosed. First proposed by Johnston et al. of Leeds (3), as a means whereby fecal continence may be improved (with resultant decreased anal soiling), the procedure has become more popular because it permits a much more rapid ileoanal anastomosis to be effected, owing to the ability to use a transanally-placed circular stapler in lieu of performance of a hand-sewn anastomosis. The controversies over the use of a stapled versus hand-sewn ileoanal anastomosis will be discussed later in this chapter.

There is little question that further technical refinements will occur in the development of surgery for ulcerative colitis. The ability to treat patients in one stage, without the need for a temporary stoma, is currently popular in some centers and used sparingly or rarely in others. The role of the one stage operation in the management of most patients with ulcerative colitis patients is still being evaluated and will be discussed in detail later in this chapter.

There is little doubt that laparoscopy will also come to play a role in ulcerative colitis therapy, although the extensive nature of proctocolectomy with a restorative procedure has largely hindered current laparoscopic surgeons from treating ulcerative colitis patients. At our center, we are using laparoscopic techniques to perform total abdominal colectomy with ileostomy and temporary preservation of the rectum in selected cases of urgent surgery for nonperforated, nontoxic ulcerative colitis patients. The purpose of this study is to evaluate the feasibility and safety of performing laparoscopic colectomy in such patients. We are comfortable in performing laparoscopic total colectomy for other indications (familial polyposis, colonic inertia, and in selected cases of Crohn's colitis) and

have had good results in over 65 cases, totally mobilizing the colon and dividing the mesentery by laparoscopic techniques, then removing the specimen and inserting the center rod and anvil of a circular stapler into the terminal ileum by a right lower quadrant incision of 3 to 5 cm in length (or by forming an ileostomy in the usual location). Details of the operative strategy and clinical outcome on the first two dozen patients undergoing this extensive procedure for familial adenomatous polyposis have been published in 1997 (4).

Indications for the Surgical Management of Ulcerative Colitis

The decision to proceed with an operation as extensive as restorative proctocolectomy must not be taken lightly by either the patient or the surgeon. In addition to the extensive nature of the procedure, complication rates remain considerable (from 18% to 40%), although most are minor and very tolerable compared to disease activity of the ulcerative colitis. In addition, we believe the development of the RP with its prospect for a life without a stoma has permitted many patients to have a timely surgical referral, since the ultimate successful outcome for the vast majority of patients had made it easier for gastroenterologists and other primary care physicians to offer surgical therapy to their patients.

RP should be considered any time surgical therapy is necessary for ulcerative colitis. Contraindications to the procedure include poor anal sphincter function and locally advanced or metastatic rectal cancer complicating ulcerative colitis. In addition, a small number of patients will prefer a proctocolectomy with ileostomy because of concerns over functional results, risk of pouchitis and need for multiple surgeries and constant follow-up.

The RP should almost always be considered in the elective setting, thus its role in the treatment of toxic colitis or in the severely debilitated patient is controversial at least. There are several reports from centers performing large volumes of this type of surgery describing RP in acute fulminant colitis, including ours (5). These represent highly selected patients who were treated by experienced surgeons. What is safest for the patient is always the primary consideration, and a total abdominal colectomy with ileostomy and preservation of the rectal stump is nearly always the treatment of choice for the patient with an urgent or emergency indication for surgery. RP remains an option for these patients three to six months after full recovery from their colectomy.

Details of Elective Indications for Restorative Proctocolectomy

The most common indications for RP are listed in Table 10.1. Intractability is the commonest (6) this being defined as: 1) intolerable or medically threatening complications of the colitis such as diarrhea, anemia, dehydration, fatigue, tenesmus, or obstruction; or 2) inability to wean off high doses of corticosteroid therapy (generally > 10 mg of prednisone or its equivalent per day) without exascerbation of the colitis over a 9 to 12 month period.

When a colorectal carcinoma is diagnosed in ulcerative colitis patients, it is reasonable to consider performing an RP, provided the patient has curable disease and the cancer is located above the midrectum. Most experts agree that RP is not indicated if the operation proves to be palliative, i.e., life expectancy is less than one year.

Patients with reasonable sphincter function who manifest dysplasia, either high or low grade, on surveillance biopsies of the colon should be considered candidates for RP. We advocate that *low* grade dysplasia be an indication, as well as high grade dysplasia, based on the facts that: (1) repeat biopsies of the colon may be unreliable, (2) colorectal carcinoma is not preceded by dysplasia in up to 26% of cases (7,8), (3) interobserver variation between pathologists about presence or absence of dysplasia ranges between 4% and 8% (9), and (4) two different reports have attested to the fact that 15% to 18% of patients found to have low grade dysplasia on initial screening will develop a colorectal carcinoma within 2 to 10 years, regardless of the findings of subsequent surveillance colonoscopies (10,11).

The issue of prophylactic colectomy in ulcerative colitis patients at high risk for the subsequent development of colorectal carcinoma is also worthy of discussion. There is compelling evidence that patients with colitis extending proximal to the splenic flexure are at high risk for the development of a colorectal carcinoma after 8 to 10 years of

Table 10.1. Indications for elective restorative proctocolectomy in ulcerative colitis.

Intact and properly functioning anal continence mechanism and:
• Disease intractability
• Unacceptable complications or side effects of medical therapy
• Presence or serious risk of colorectal carcinoma (dysplasia)
• Age less than 65 (relative)

---

disease, and at least belong in a careful surveillance program (12). Patients at particularly high risk are those with onset of disease before age 15, with a 30% or greater chance of developing a carcinoma during their lifetime (13,14). These patients, even in the absence of dysplasia, should be considered for a prophylactic RP.

The course of action to pursue in patients with indeterminate colitis is a complex one. In at least 5% to 10% of patients who are operated on for ulcerative colitis, the final pathologic diagnosis will be indeterminate colitis. McIntyre et al. in 1995, reported on 1232 ulcerative colitis patients undergoing RP at the Mayo Clinic with a mean followup of 60 months. Seventy one patients were eventually diagnosed with indeterminate colitis, i.e., none of them had features of Crohn's disease at the time of their initial surgery. This study noted no increased incidence of pouchitis, no increase in functional problems compared to ulcerative colitis patients, but a long term failure rate of 19%, compared to a rate of 8% in ulcerative colitis patients (15). Thus 80% of patients with indeterminate colitis in this series had a successful outcome with RP in the long term. W.L. Koltun reported a high incidence of pouch failure especially related to perineal complications in a Lahey Clinic series of patients with indeterminate colitis (16).

A known diagnosis of Crohn's disease should prompt the surgeon to avoid RP. This issue will be fully discussed in Chapter 34.

Contraindications

It is fundamentally important to recognize that not every ulcerative colitis patient presenting with an indication for surgery will be a candidate for the RP (Table 10.2). Obviously, serious anal dysfunction or prior proctectomy with removal of all or part of the sphincters disqualifies the patient from undergoing a RP.

How does one assess adequacy of the anal sphincters? Clinical assessment, as in most disease evaluations, is the foundation of decision-making for anal sphincter function for the inflammatory bowel disease (IBD) surgeon as well. Thus a careful history focusing on any prior anal disease or surgery, and anal continence during exacerbations of the colitis is important. Most patients, even with severe pouchitis, maintain reasonable bowel control except during their worst periods of illness. Careful questions about control for gas, liquid, and solid stools should clue the surgeon in as to whether bowel control is a serious problem for the patient. A history of any serious anal infection, abscess, fissure, or problem requiring surgery should

Table 10.2. Contraindications to restorative procto-colectomy in ulcerative colitis.

Absolute
-Acute, fulminant colitis, especially with clinical toxicity, peritonitis, or perforation of the colon
-Known Crohn's disease at time of operation
-Severe anal sphincter dysfunction
-Carcinoma of the distal rectum

Relative contraindications
-Morbid obesity
-Severe malnutrition or debility
-Age > 65 years
-Psychologically impaired or patients at high risk for noncompliance

prompt a careful focus on the degree of bowel control and whether or not Crohn's disease is a diagnostic consideration. Women who have had multiple vaginal deliveries, difficult deliveries with episiotomies or known sphincteric injuries also require careful scrutiny.

Physical examination is also central to the sphincteric evaluation, beginning with an evaluation of the perianal skin searching for edematous, cyanotic-looking tags (Crohn's-like), scars, fissures, or fistulae. A digital exam by the experienced surgeon can assess resting tone and voluntary squeeze pressure, and also the pliability of the sphincters and whether or not any stricturing is present. The mere presence of anal disease does not disqualify a patient from consideration—up to 10% of patients with ulcerative colitis may have some history of an anal lesion (17). Completion of the physical examination using anoscopy and proctoscopy is of further value in assessing the patient for signs of Crohn's disease and for thoroughly evaluating the anal canal (the site of the ileo-anal anastomosis).

Anal manometry is also a useful test, readily performed as part of the initial clinical examination, which we use to provide objective parameters of anal and rectal function. Although absolute numbers cannot be assigned to qualify or disqualify a patient for a RP, low resting anal pressures with an inability to double the resting pressure on voluntary squeeze effort is a bad prognostic sign for the degree of postoperative continence. Additionally, signs of nerve damage indicated by pudendal nerve terminal motor latencies of greater than 2 to 2.5 milliseconds is also of concern. If there is a question of muscle disruption related to previous vaginal delivery, endoluminal ultrasonography may be considered to assess the sphincters. This may be extremely accurate in determining whether there has been any muscle disruption (18).

Cancer of the middle or lower rectum: In an instance of disseminated cancer with a rectal primary, there should be no consideration given for a RP. The patient should undergo the simplest possible procedure, usually a proctocolectomy with end ileostomy (a low Hartmann-type of procedure might be reasonable to simplify the rectal excision and postoperative healing). If the cancer is early by preoperative staging measures (Stage I or II), then it may be reasonable to consider an RP. We would perform a covering loop ileostomy because of the added factor of radiation to the pelvis involved in the healing process in a Stage II or III patient who had undergone preoperative adjuvant therapy.

If the patient is discovered to have a T3 or greater rectal cancer after surgery and has not received preoperative adjuvant therapy, then a difficult decision must be made about whether or not to add chemoradiotherapy to the treatment regimen of a pelvic pouch patient. It is likely that the ileum will tolerate the treatment poorly, since the ileum is extremely sensitive to the effects of radiation. Nonetheless, it is wise to consider all aspects of treatment in each individual very carefully, since what will give the patient the best possible chance for a cure must be considered as the primary consideration.

Finally, for cancers of the distal rectum, where distal clearance of the tumor is not possible without sacrifice of the sphincters, proctocolectomy with ileostomy should be considered the treatment of choice.

Obesity

Patients who are overweight, especially if they are male and/or have a narrow pelvis, present a particular challenge to the surgeon. Once patients are over a body-mass index (BMI) of 35 (calculated by dividing weight in kilograms by height^2[kg/m^2]), then a very cautious approach in recommending pouch surgery should be taken. It may be technically very difficult or even impossible to achieve an adequate mesenteric length to consider a RP in such patients, and the small bowel mesentery may not even fit into the pelvis. If the surgeon anticipates that the overweight patient may present a major technical challenge at surgery, then it is advisable to warn the patient that the RP procedure may not be possible at the initial operation. It may even be a major technical challenge to bring a loop ileostomy up to the skin of the abdominal wall in these patients.

Seeking professional guidance to help the patient to try and lose weight is reasonable, although our Department of Colorectal Surgery hasn't had much success in seeing patients achieve positive results, even under these circumstances. Patients requiring surgery for ulcerative colitis generally are not well enough to undergo postponement of their surgery for the six months or more that is needed for effective weight loss. After total abdominal colectomy, the mesentery of the terminal ileum may lengthen over time, so that a pelvic pouch may become feasible after a year or more. Thus, in an obese patient where RP is not initially feasible, it is wise to not sacrifice the anal sphincters, to leave a rectal stump in place, and preserve the possibility for a future RP if circumstances and the patient's overall health status permit this consideration. The regaining of health after the colectomy surgery may also serve as a tremendous motivating factor for the patient to lose weight.

Age Considerations

Although there is no absolute upper age limit for patients who are candidates for a RP, it has been shown that age at the time of operation does correlate with the eventual functional outcome (19–21). Oresland et al. showed there was a uniform decrement in overall function between the third to the seventh decades of life (assessed by a functional scoring system arbitrarily assigned to each patient) at both three and twelve months after operation in patients undergoing the RP operation (19).

The most common problems faced by patients who are over the age of fifty at the time of the operation are increase in the amount of soiling and an increase in the number of stools per day when compared to younger patients (22–25). Cohen et al. in a study examining the outcome and surgical complication rate in patients over the age of 40 compared to those under the same age found that the leak rate at the ileal pouch anastomosis was significantly higher in the older patients (24). Lewis et al. found that the resting and maximum squeeze pressures of the anal sphincters were not different between patients over or under the age of fifty, before and after the operation. Only very mild differences in the incidence of mucus leakage and the ability to discriminate flatus from feces were seen, and these were not significantly different between groups (23).

Although we do not have any absolute upper age limit for the performance of the RP, the many coincident medical illnesses that older patients may have should definitely influence the surgeon's judgement—with a definite increase in the number of complications that may occur after the RP (in the anastomotic region especially), older patients may be much less fit to withstand the opera-

tions that may be necessary to correct the complication. Furthermore, older patients may have less anxiety about the prospect of a permanent stoma and may be eager to have the simplest possible operation to cure their colitis. These facets of RP surgery need to be discussed fully with any patient over the age of fifty (26).

Psychological Impairment

Although there are quite a range of psychological difficulties that a patient may suffer coincident with or as a result of ulcerative colitis, patients who suffer with major mental illness or who may be severely psychologically unstable are unsuitable for the RP. This is because of the difficulty in both counseling them before the operation, as well as following them afterwards. A permanent ileostomy is safer and generally in the best interest of mentally disturbed or incompetent individuals. It should be considered that the impairment could be secondary to the incapacitating effects of the underlying IBD, thus it may be reasonable to perform a total abdominal colectomy and ileostomy with rectal preservation and await the return of a healthier state of the patient, off all steroid medications, before a final decision is made.

Operative Strategy: What Are the Major Issues Confronting the Ileal Pouch Surgeon?

Although the particular merits of each of the pouch designs will be discussed in Chapter 11, there are definitely a significant number of issues that the "ileal pouch" surgeon must understand in his/her quest to provide the best in care to each ulcerative colitis patient who is a candidate for the RP. This section will attempt to prepare the pouch surgeon to confront these issues.

Issue: Pouch Design J, S, W, H, and Other Alternatives

Despite the given popularity of one pouch design versus another that may exist at any given medical center, there are certainly reasonable arguments about what particular pouch may work best under certain given circumstances. No experienced pouch surgeon would claim to use only one pouch design under all circumstances, thus he/she must be familiar with the pros and cons of each design (Table 10.3).

Table 10.3. Differences among ileal pouch styles.

Pouch style	J	S	W	H
Advantages	Simple	Large volume	Largest capacity	Can use to convert straight ileoanal to pouch without disconnecting ileoanal anastomosis
	Reaches in nearly all patients	May give additional 1–2 cm reach to anal canal compared to "J"	?Better earlier postop functional results	
	Functional result as good as other designs after 6–12 months	Large volume pouch immediately after operation	Empties well	
Disadvantages	Smallest volume (first 6 months)	Takes longer to make at operation (must be hand-sewn)	May be quite bulky in narrow pelvis	Complex
	May not reach as well in unusual cases	Can have efferent limb (emptying) problems	Sutured, thus takes lots of time to construct	Used by few surgeons
				Can have efferent limb problems like the S-pouch

Despite the pros and cons of different pouches, in our department we have favored the J-pouch overall because of its inherent simplicity, rapidity of construction compared to other techniques, and because of its apparent functional similarity to other designs after a period of adaptation of several months, during which time the J-pouch probably dilates and enlarges to about the same functional size as the S- or W-style pouches. Of 812 patients with ulcerative colitis undergoing the RP between 1983 to 1993, 547 (68%) had a J-pouch and the remainder underwent an S-pouch (27). Nearly 90% of the patients undergoing RP in our department currently undergo the J-pouch, owing to the above advantages.

In addition to the pouches listed in the table, other less popular pouches or types of reservoirs or ileoanal anastomoses have been proposed (Table 10.4).

Many of the proposed designs have some merit, but would only be used under special circumstances. The straight ileoanal anastomosis has been associated with reasonably good results in children, but the facility with which an ileal J-pouch can be constructed, combined with its negligible morbidity, probably argue against the construction of a straight ileoanal anastomosis in even children.

Single- versus Multistage Ileoanal Pouches

With the increasing confidence in performing the RP operation over the past decade, there has been a natural interest in performing a single-stage pro-

cedure for certain patients who are not acutely ill (i.e., performing the RP with omittance of the temporary defunctioning ileostomy). Advantages of such an approach, if it is safe, are intuitively obvious: the patient will not have to have a stoma, only one hospitalization is required, and thus health care costs and overall disability may be lessened. This approach has been controversial because the RP is an extensive operation, with a high incidence of pelvic sepsis and anastomotic leakage even in experienced hands (28–31).

Some centers have reported that the one-stage procedure, with omission of the temporary loop ileostomy may not be associated with any major long-term sequella as compared to the two-stage procedure, with initial performance of the RP and a temporary loop ileostomy (to be closed several months later) (32–35). There is also a definite morbidity to the ileostomy itself, with a need for operative revision in up to 7% of patients (28,29). Anastomotic leakage may not be any less common with diversion, although the seriousness of it may be less when diversion is present. There are also the concerns about high stoma output that may appear after ileostomy creation, which may be much worse after the more more proximally sited stoma of the two-stage procedure.

Other centers, including ours, have taken a more cautious approach, with the view that pelvic sepsis can be a disastrous outcome for pelvic pouch patients, and the circumstances where any added risk can be perceived before or during the operation should lead the surgeon to plan for a diverting

Table 10.4. Alternative pouches, reservoirs, and so on.

Straight ileoanal anastomosis	Simple, but associated with unacceptably high incidence of fecal soiling and diarrhea in adults
B-pouch (64)	Has two or three interrupted anastomoses-attempts to decrease fecal stasis effects
Inverted U-pouch (65)	Converts a straight ileoanal to a pouch without disconnecting the ileoanal anastomosis
Ileocecal valve transposition (66)	Muscular component of the valve was preserved, then transposed upstream from a straight ileoanal anastomosis
Ileal myectomy (67,68)	Strips of muscularis and serosa are excised from a straight ileal segment, making a highly compliant "pouch"-like structure. Has not caught on
Balloon stretching of ileal segment (69)	Must be done over many weeks postop, and patient compliance (pain) a difficult issue to overcome

ileostomy at the time of the RP. In our analysis of RP in patients with and without diversion, even though in a nonrandomized series, we found that the pelvic sepsis rate was 14% in the one stage group, while 4% in the two stage group (31). Of major concern is a recent report from the General Infirmary at Leeds, reporting on 100 consecutive patients undergoing RP, 50 of whom underwent a one-stage procedure and 50 a traditional two-stage RP. Although the patients were not randomized, there were significantly more serious complications in the one-stage group, 11 of whom developed pelvic sepsis (7 required reoperation). Seven diverted patients developed pelvic sepsis, but none required reoperation (36). The authors stated that although this study was not a randomized one, there was likely bias toward a better outcome in the one-stage group, since these were patients chosen for a one-stage approach based on their overall low risk status by experienced IBD surgeons.

There are other concerns voiced about the one-stage approach by a variety of experts. The "first days syndrome," wherein the patients do recover without obvious serious postoperative complications, but are extremely fatigued and suffer from diarrhea and anal excoriations over the first several weeks to months after the RP, is a common scenario. Probably related to this is the usual need for these patients to stay in the hospital for a significantly longer period of time than two-stage patients (31–36).

Thus, although there still are no large prospective, randomized trials comparing the one and two-stage procedures, most experienced surgeons continue to recommend the one-stage approach only when the RP is done under elective circumstances, when the patient is in good overall health, on no or low dose steroids (less than 20 mg per day), and all aspects of the operation proceed smoothly. Williamson et al. also recommend that young women who are considering childbirth should have a diverting ileostomy in order to minimize the risks that pelvic sepsis poses to their fertility (36). In the final analysis, most surgeons and patients will endure the sequellea of the temporary ileostomy better than those of pelvic sepsis.

Ileoanal Anastomosis-Stapled versus Hand Sewn?

There is still considerable debate about how the last several centimeters of the distal rectal mucosa should be handled at the time of the RP procedure. This "anal transitional zone" was nearly always completely removed early in the development of RP procedures, much as in the Soave pull-through procedure for Hirschsprung's disease, with hand-sutured anastomosis of the ileal pouch to the dentate line. Many surgeons were dissatisfied with this aspect of the RP, since the anal canal needed to be dilated and traumatized to a considerable extent during the operation, and there remained a significant amount of postoperative incontinence and soiling, especially in the first few months after this operation.

In the late 1980s, a number of reports suggested that preservation of the "entire anal canal," including the columnar epithelium that lined the upper anal canal above the dentate line, would dramatically improve continence after the RP, and this operation also was very appealing because it permitted a circular-stapled anastomosis to be created, thus providing a simpler, more rapid anastomosis that likely also was less traumatic to the anal canal (37,38). The physiologic basis for the stapled anastomosis was that the anal transitional zone seemed to have a functional role in anal continence, with demonstrable sensitivity to pain, touch, and temperature. This is also where the "sampling reflex" for fecal continence has been shown to reside (39–41). Therefore it made sense that its preservation would be of value in patients undergoing the RP.

Table 10.5. Comparison of values of the hand-sewn versus double-stapled ileal pouch-anal anastomosis.

	Advantage	Disadvantage
Hand-sewn	All disease removed, ?no need for surveillance	?Decreased functional result
	Outcome is equivalent to that of stapled pouch (45,70,71)	?Increased risk of complications
Stapled	Simpler, faster	"Strip" colitis (rare)
	Improved functional outcome	Risk of cancer, need for surveillance
	Decreased complication rate (38,72–74)	

The values of the hand-sewn vs. stapled ileal-pouch anastomosis are compared in Table 10.5.

Advocates of the hand-sewn RP have noted that the measurable resting pressure of the anal canal falls postoperatively regardless of which procedure is performed. Nonetheless, in patients undergoing the stapled procedure, there is a significant rise in the resting anal canal pressure, return of the normal rectoanal inhibitory reflex, and fairly rapid improvement in the continence in the first 12 months after surgery (42). Similar improvements have not been seen after the hand-sewn RP by some authors (42). Some of the better comparative studies have shown no differences between the two techniques (44,45). Other arguments against there being proven differences in outcome between the two techniques have been that the published reports showing differences in favor of the stapled technique have not been randomized, and the historical hand-sewn controls used as a comparison group for the stapled patients were done early in the experience of the surgeons involved, and thus may not be valid as a comparison group.

Nonetheless, there have been surprisingly few strong arguments in favor of the hand-sewn technique. Despite the worry about dysplasia of the residual columnar epithelium in the stapled patients, there have been no reports to date on malignant degeneration of this zone after RP—in fact all of the known cases of cancer developing after RP have occurred after a hand-sewn procedure (46–50). At the Cleveland Clinic, Ziv et al. reported on the followup of 254 patients who underwent stapled RP with at least yearly biopsies. After an average of 2.3 years, there were eight patients in whom low grade dysplasia was found in the anal transitional zone (ATZ), but only two of these were found to have a

persistent finding of dysplasia on repeat biopsy. These two patients went on to have a complete mucosectomy with advancement of their pouch to the dentate line (i.e., with preservation of their pouches). Neither of these patients had any signs of malignancy in the excised portion of their ATZ, and both had either pre- or postoperative evidence of dysplasia or cancer in the excised colectomy specimen. In addition, there is little strength in the argument that the hand-sewn patients do not need surveillance after operation, since the long term sequella of this operation are still relatively unknown, and there is also the potential for the pouch itself to develop dysplasia (51). After mucosectomy as well, up to 20% of patients will have remnants of columnar epithelium when microscopic analysis of excised pouch specimens were examined (51).

Thus, although there are still many advocates of the hand-sewn procedure, it seems that the ease of construction of a stapled procedure, along with its likely better functional result (at least in the first several months after the operation) is preferred by most ileal pouch surgeons. It should be mentioned that there are still patients in whom the preservation of the distal columnar epithelium is *not* advised: those with dysplasia or malignancy elsewhere in the lining of the large intestine or those with familial polyposis.

Mesenteric Lengthening: What If the Pouch Does Not Reach?

Despite every aspect of the RP operation proceeding smoothly, there always remains the possibility that the pouch will not have a long enough mesentery to permit it to reach to the pelvic floor. There are clinical circumstances in which this possibility is more likely: in obese patients, in patients with a fatty and/or narrow pelvis, and in extremely tall patients.

There are several "rules of thumb" which surgeons have recommended in the course of the RP operation to gauge whether the terminal ileum has been sufficiently mobilized: the most common is to grasp the most dependent loop of the ileum and drape it down over the symphysis pubis-if it reaches to the inferior border of the symphysis, then it is likely to reach to the dentate line (52).

Steps to follow in order to maximize the mobility of the terminal ileum include: 1) completely mobilize the ileal mesentery posteriorly until the duodenum and the pancreas are freed from it; 2) be sure to find the most dependent loop of the ileum to use for the anastomosis; 3) divide the peritoneum over the superior mesenteric artery in small transverse incisions serially towards the dependent loop; 4) divide the superior mesenteric artery or the ileocolic artery at a point where there are many collaterals around it to the small bowel, i.e., not too distally, or to divide one or more distal arcades in the ileal mesentery (53). When all these manuevers fail to satisfy the surgeon that the ileum has been adequately mobilized, then an S-shaped not a J-shaped pouch configuration should be considered, since the S-pouch will likely permit 1 or 2 cm more extension into the pelvis with its efferent limb. If the J-pouch has already been made, then the distal end could still be divided to make an efferent spout of an additional 1 to 2 cm. Other considerations that could be entertained at the time of operation are: 1) to leave a slightly longer rectal cuff (3 to 5 cm rather than 1 to 2 cm) in cases without dysplasia or cancer; 2) make an ileostomy upstream of the pouch, place the pouch with the end closed off into the pelvis and consider reoperation in about one year; 3) make a Kock pouch (continent ileostomy) and consider converting this after a year or more (54).

Despite the fact that it may seem difficult to make the pouch reach in certain cases, it is an unusual circumstance when this is not predictable based on the patient's preoperative physical status. Using the above guidelines, nearly all situations can be managed successfully. It is wise to always forewarn the patient and their family of the rare possibility that the pouch may not reach and an alternative may need to be considered.

Indeterminate Colitis in the OR

It is worth considering what actions should be undertaken when there is some question about the diagnosis of ulcerative colitis in the operating theater, i.e., when the surgeon considers by intraoperative findings that either indeterminate or Crohn's colitis are a possibility. This may occur as a result of unusual thickening of the colon or its mesentery (perhaps with some fat wrapping) or by the discovery of some ileitis suspicious for Crohn's, or some worrisome anal pathology-fissuring, tags, or fistulae that was not appreciated preoperatively. Whenever there is this concern, initially total abdominal colectomy should be carried out to treat the disease process that brought the patient to the operating theater in the first place. If the patient has been recently on high dose steroids or debilitated from the disease, then the most conservative approach is to fashion an ileostomy and leave the rectum in place. This permits the patient to recover, and allows the pathologist to study the colon specimen thoroughly over several days to make the best histologic determination about what type of colitis may be present.

If the surgeon discovers what appears to be unequivocally Crohn's disease of the colon with relatively mild rectal disease present (and seeks confirmation of this with frozen section histology examination in the operating theaters), then a reasonable course of action would be to perform colectomy with ileorectal anastomosis.

It is wise to counsel patients and their families prior to operation about the possibility of indeterminate colitis (up to 5 to 10% of patients) and that when there are no features of Crohn's disease at or before the operation, the RP operation is very successful in the majority of patients even when indeterminate colitis is considered after final pathologic examination of the removed specimen. McIntyre et al. of the Mayo Clinic followed 71 patients undergoing RP for what was determined to be indeterminate colitis after the pouch operation. After a mean follow-up period of 56 months, the functional results were largely similar when compared to patients with ulcerative colitis. The major difference seen was in the long-term failure rate, which was 19% in the indeterminate group, and only 8% in the ulcerative colitis group (15). Even in patients ultimately found to have Crohn's disease, a study at the Cleveland Clinic found that in 15 of the 16 patients where no preoperative features of Crohn's were noted, the long term outcome (mean followup of 38 months) was good, and the pouch was able to be preserved (55).

Postoperative Care
Portal Hypertension/Primary Sclerosing Cholangitis

The RP operation has become a topic of considerable interest for patients with ulcerative colitis and primary sclerosing cholangitis (PSC) because of the fact that (1) PSC patients have a slowly progressive disease that may lead to portal hypertension, cirrhosis, and liver failure; (2) Over 70% of PSC patients have concomitant ulcerative colitis; and (3) after proctocolectomy and permanent end ileostomy, over 50% of these patients with concomitant portal hypertension will develop peristomal varices (56). Thus the RP has become a procedure which can avoid the need for an abdominal wall stoma with its potential for developing varices when portal hypertension is present in PSC.

The most extensive experience documented on this subject comes from the Mayo Clinic in a report from 1993, wherein Kartheuser et al. assessed outcome in 40 patients with ulcerative colitis and PSC who received a RP between 1980 and 1990 (56). They documented a high complication rate but no mortality and no liver failure after the procedure. There was a 10% rate of pelvic sepsis, and reoperation was necessary in four (10%) patients. There was an overall 55% complication rate within the first 3 years after the operation, with a transfusion requirement of 47%, nearly twice that of other patients undergoing the same procedure without PSC. Interestingly, pouchitis occurred in 57% of patients at 4 years followup, although there was no evidence of varices at the ileal pouch-anal anastomosis, and no bleeding from the anastomosis after a mean followup of 71 months. This report documents the high complication rate, but overall safety of the RP as a means of treating the sequella of ulcerative colitis in PSC patients, even though the course of the liver disease is not affected by the colectomy. In part due to the fact that no perianastomotic varices were seen in this series, it is reasonable to attempt the RP in most patients with ulcerative colitis requiring surgery. In certain patients with mild rectal disease and severe liver disease, it may be reasonable to consider the total colectomy and ileorectostomy as a simpler alternative.

Pregnancy

After RP, many female patients in their reproductive years (and their surgeons) are extremely concerned about the possibility of significant disturbances to the continence mechanism following vaginal delivery. This is a natural concern, but there is significant evidence that most women following RP can expect to undergo routine vaginal delivery. In a report from the Mayo Clinic in 1985, Metcalf et al. discussed six women who conceived after undergoing the RP procedure, four of whom were able to have vaginal delivery without perceptible alteration in subsequent continence (21). Their recommendation at that time was that route of delivery should be individualized in RP patients.

A more recent publication by Juhasz et al. documented the clinical course of 43 women who delivered children after the RP procedure, 24 vaginally and 19 by Cesarean section (57). Eighteen of the women undergoing vaginal delivery also had an episiotomy. Nearly all of the women had increased stool frequency, episodes of incontinence, and perineal pad usage during pregnancy, and this resolved in nearly all women after delivery. Length of labor, number of deliveries, and whether or not the delivery was vaginal seemed to have no effect on function. After a mean followup of almost two

and a half years, there was no apparent decrease in function seen in the women who had vaginal deliveries. Based on this information, it is reasonable to suggest that vaginal delivery in a woman after RP is safe. If there have been complicating factors related to the RP procedure, e.g., sphincteric dysfunction, a complex fistula that developed postoperatively, or if the surgeon believes that a particular patient has a high risk situation for the development of a perineal problem during childbirth (e.g., rigidity of the pelvic tissues on physical examination), then recommending a Cesarean section is probably reasonable.

Small Bowel Obstruction

One of the most common postoperative complications after removal of the colon and rectum, whether the RP procedure is done or not, is adhesive small bowel obstruction. The incidence ranges from 10% to 20%, although about half or more of patients get better with nonoperative therapy (28,58–60). One of the most common sites for the adhesions leading to obstruction is at the ileostomy closure site. Although a variety of recommendations have been made with regard to "preventative" measures, there is no proven method by which to decrease this incidence.

One clinical practice we use at our institution is that if the obstruction occurs in the interval between creation of the pouch and ileostomy closure, then we will check the pouch integrity with a water soluble contrast enema, and if this study shows good healing of the pouch, then to go on to close the ileostomy at the time of the operation for obstruction.

Metabolic Abnormalities

A reasonable concern after RP is whether there are significant metabolic abnormalities that may occur after the procedure. There have been several reports that a vitamin B_{12} deficiency can occur, that a microcytic anemia may develop, or that there may be a predisposition to impaired lactose or xylose absorption (22,61). Stelzner et al. suggested that there can be impaired carbohydrate, amino acid, or short-chain fatty acid absorption (62). Although there are documented reports of these abnormalities, there is no systematic evidence that these are to be expected consequences of the RP.

There is a definite increase in the incidence of nephrolithiasis in RP compared to the general population, but this incidence is less than that seen after total proctocolectomy and end ileostomy. In addition, there does not appear to be any increase in the incidence of gallstones as compared to the normal population (63).

Thus, although there may be some ileal impairment, this is largely clinically unimportant. Other than a concern for a greater than usual risk for dehydration, patients with the RP procedure should be encouraged that their bowel will largely function normally.

References

1. Cohen Z, McLeod RS, Stern H, et al. The pelvic pouch and ileoanal anastomosis procedure: surgical technique and initial results. Am J Surg 1985;150: 601–7.
2. Lindquist K, Liljeqvist L, Sellberg B. The topography of ileoanal reservoirs in relation to evacuation patterns and clinical functions. Acta Chir Scand 1984; 150:573–9.
3. Johnston D, Holdsworth PJ, Nasmyth DG, et al. Preservation of the entire anal canal in conservative proctocolectomy for ulcerative colitis: a pilot study comparing end-to-end ileo-anal anastomosis without mucosal resection with mucosal proctectomy and endo-anal anastomosis. Br J Surg 1987;74:940–4.
4. Milsom JW, Ludwig KA, Church JM, et al. Laparoscopic total abdominal colectomy with ileorectal anastomosis for familial adenomatous polyposis. Dis Colon Rectum 1997;40:675–8.
5. Ziv Y, Fazio VW, Church JM, et al. Safety of urgent restorative proctocolectomy with ileal pouch-anal anastomosis for fulminant colitis. Dis Colon Rectum 1995;38:345–9.
6. Farmer RG, Easley KA, Rankin GB. Clinical patterns, natural history, and progression of ulcerative colitis. A long-term follow-up of 1116 patients. Dig Dis Sci 1993;38:1137–46.
7. Ransohoff DF, Riddell RH, Levin B. Ulcerative colitis and colonic cancer. Problems in assessing the diagnostic usefulness of mucosal dysplasia. Dis Colon Rectum 1985;28:383–8.
8. Taylor BA, Pemberton JH, Carpenter HA, et al. Dysplasia in chronic ulcerative colitis: implications for colonoscopic surveillance. Dis Colon Rectum 1992;35:950–6.
9. Collins RH, Jr, Feldman M, Fordtran JS. Colon cancer, dysplasia, and surveillance in patients with ulcerative colitis. A critical review [Review] [49 refs]. New Engl J Med 1987;316:1654–8.
10. Lennard-Jones JE, Melville DM, Morson BC, et al. Precancer and cancer in extensive ulcerative colitis: findings among 401 patients over 22 years. Gut 1990;31:800–6.
11. Woolrick AJ, DaSilva MD, Korelitz BI. Surveillance in the routine management of ulcerative colitis: the predictive value of low-grade dysplasia. Gastroenterology 1993;103:431–8.
12. Nugent FW, Haggitt RC, Gilpin PA. Cancer surveillance in ulcerative colitis [see comments]. Gastroenterology 1991;100:1241–8.
13. Ekbom A, Helmick C, Zack M, et al. Ulcerative colitis and colorectal cancer. A population-based study. New Engl J Med 1990;323:1228–33.
14. Kewenter J, Ahlman H, Hulten L. Cancer risk in extensive ulcerative colitis. Ann Surg 1978;188:824–8.
15. McIntyre PB, Pemberton JH, Wolff BG, et al. Indeterminate colitis—long term outcome in patients after ileal pouch-anal anastomosis. Dis Colon Rectum 1995;38:51–4.
16. Koltun WA, Schoetz DJ, Jr, Roberts PL, et al. Indeterminate colitis predisposes to perineal complications after ileal pouch-anal anastomosis. Dis Colon Rectum 1991;34:857–60.
17. Mortensen NJ. Patient selection for restorative proctocolectomy. In: Nicholls J, Bartolo D, Mortensen N, eds. Restorative Proctocolectomy. Osney Med, Oxford: Blackwell Scientific Publications; 1993:7–11.
18. Hool G, Hull TL, Milsom JW. Use of endoanal ultrasonography. J Pelvic Disease 1997;3:251–9.
19. Oresland T, Fasth S, Nordgren S, et al. The clinical and functional outcome after restorative proctocolectomy. A prospective study in 100 patients. Int J Colorectal Dis 1989;4:50–6.
20. Metcalf A, Dozois RR, Beart RW, Jr, et al. Pregnancy following ileal pouch-anal anastomosis. Dis Colon Rectum 1985;28:859–61.
21. Liljeqvist L, Lindquist K, Ljungdahl I. Alterations in ileoanal pouch technique, 1980 to 1987: complications and functional outcome. Dis Colon Rectum 1988;31:929–39.
22. Pemberton JH, Kelly KA, Beart RW, Jr, et al. Ileal pouch-anal anastomosis for chronic ulcerative colitis. Long-term results. Ann Surg 1987;206:504–13.
23. Lewis WG, Sagar PM, Holdsworth PJ, et al. Restorative proctocolectomy with end-to-end pouch-anal anastomosis in patients over the age of fifty. Gut 1993;34:948–52.
24. Cohen Z, McLeod RS, Stephen W, et al. Continuing evolution of the pelvic pouch procedure. Ann Surg 1992;216:506–11.
25. Nicholls RJ, Pezim ME. Restorative proctocolectomy with ileal reservoir for ulcerative colitis and familial adenomatous polyposis: a comparison of three reservoir designs. Br J Surg 1985;72:470–4.
26. de Silva HJ, de Angelis CP, Soper N, et al. Clinical and functional outcome after restorative proctocolectomy Br J Surg 1991;78:1039–44.
27. Fazio VW, Ziv Y, Church JM, et al. Ileal pouch-anal anastomoses complications and function in 1005 patients. Ann Surg 1995;222:120–7.
28. Galandiuk S, Wolff B, Dozois RR, et al. Ileal pouch-anal anastomosis without ileostomy. Dis Colon Rectum 1991;34:870–3.
29. Feinberg SM, McLeod RS, Cohen Z. Complications of loop ileostomy. Am J Surg 1987;153:102–7.

30. Scott NA, Dozois RR, Beart RW, et al. Postoperative intra-abdominal and pelvic sepsis complicating ileal pouch-anal anastomosis. Int J Colorectal Dis 1988;3: 149–52.

31. Tjandra JJ, Fazio VW, Milsom JW, et al. Omission of temporary diversion in restorative proctocolectomy-is it safe? Dis Colon Rectum 1993;36:1007–13.

32. Grobler SP, Hosie KB, Keighley MRB. Randomized trial of loop ileostomy in restorative proctocolectomy. Br J Surg 1992;79:903–6.

33. Senagore A, Milsom JW, Walshaw RK, et al. Does a proximal colostomy affect colorectal anastomotic healing? Dis Colon Rectum 1992;35:182–8.

34. Mikkola K, Luukkonen P, Jarvinen HJ. Long-term results of restorative proctocolectomy for ulcerative colitis. Int J Colorect Dis 1995;10:10–4.

35. Sugarman HJ, Newsome HH, Decosta G, et al. Stapled ileoanal anastomosis for ulcerative colitis and familial polyposis without temporary diverting ileostomy. Ann Surg 1991;213:606–19.

36. Williamson MER, Lewis WG, Sagar PM, et al. One-stage restorative proctocolectomy without temporary ileostomy for ulcerative colitis—a note of caution. Dis Colon Rectum 1997;40:1019–22.

37. Johnston D, Holdsworth PJ, Nasmyth DG, et al. Preservation of the entire anal canal in conservative proctocolectomy for ulcerative colitis: a pilot study comparing end-to-end ileo-anal anastomosis without mucosal resection with mucosal proctectomy and endo-anal anastomosis. Br J Surg 1987;74:940–4.

38. Kmiot WA, Keighley MR. Totally stapled abdominal restorative proctocolectomy. Br J Surg 1989;79: 961–4.

39. Duthie HL, Gairns FW. Sensory nerve-endings and sensation in the anal region of man. Br J Surg 1960;47:585–95.

40. Miller R, Bartolo DC, Orrom WJ, et al. Improvement of anal sensation with preservation of the anal transition zone after ileoanal anastomosis for ulcerative colitis. Dis Colon Rectum 1990;33:414–8.

41. Holdsworth PJ, Johnston D, Chalmers AG, et al. Endoluminal ultrasound and computed tomography in the staging of rectal cancer. Br J Surg 1988;75:1019–22.

42. Sagar PM, Holdsworth D, Johnston D. Correlation between laboratory findings and clinical outcome after restorative proctocolectomy: serial studies in 20 patients after end to end pouch-anal anastomosis. Br J Surg 1991;78:67–70.

43. Becker JM, Raymond JL. Ileal pouch-anal anastomosis: a single surgeon's experience with 100 consecutive cases. Ann Surg 1986;204:375–81.

44. Choen S, Burnett S, Bartram CI, et al. Comparison between anal endosonography and digital examination in the evaluation of anal fistulae. Br J Surg 1991;78:445–7.

45. McIntyre PB, Pemberton JH, Beart RW, et al. Double-stapled vs. hand-sewn ileal pouch-anal anastomosis in patients with chronic ulcerative colitis. Dis Colon Rectum 1994;37:430–3.

46. King DW, Lubowski DZ, Cook TA. Anal canal mucosa in restorative proctocolectomy for ulcerative colitis. Br J Surg 1989;76:970–2.

47. Stern H, Walfisch S, Mullen B, et al. Cancer in an ileoanal reservoir: a new late complication? Gut 1990;31:473–5.

48. Puthu D, Rajan N, Rao R, et al. Carcinoma of the rectal pouch following restorative proctocolectomy report of a case. Dis Colon Rectum 1992;35:257–60.

49. Sequens R. Cancer in the anal canal (transitional zone) after restorative proctocelectomy with stapled ileal pouch-anal anastomosis. Int J Colorect Dis 1997;12:254–5.

50. Hoehner JC, Metcalf AM. Development of invasive adenocarcinoma following colectomy with ileoanal anastomosis for familial polyposis coli—report of a case. Dis Colon Rectum 1994;37:824–8.

51. Heppell J, Weiland LH, Perrault J, et al. Fate of the rectal mucosa after rectal mucosectomy and ileoanal anastomosis. Dis Colon Rectum 1983;26:768–71.

52. Smith L, Friend WG, Medwell SJ. The superior mesenteric artery. The critical factor in the pouch pull-through procedure. Dis Colon Rectum 1984;27: 741–4.

53. Thirlby RC. Optimizing results and techniques of mesenteric lengthening in ileal pouch-anal anastomosis. Am J Surg 1995;169:499–502.

54. Hulten L, Fasth S, Nordgren S, et al. Kock's pouch converted to a pelvic pouch. Report of a case. Dis Colon Rectum 1988;31:467–9.

55. Hyman NH, Fazio VW, Tuckson WB, et al. Consequences of ileal pouch-anal anastomosis for Crohn's colitis. Dis Colon Rectum 1991;34:653–7.

56. Kartheuser AH, Dozois RR, Wiesner RH, et al. Complications and risk factors after ileal pouch-anal anastomosis for ulcerative colitis associated with primary sclerosing cholangitis. Ann Surg 1993;217:314–20.

57. Juhasz ES, Fozard B, Dozois RR, et al. Ileal pouch-anal anastomosis function following childbirth. An extended evaluation. Dis Colon Rectum 1995;38: 159–65.

58. Senapati A, Nicholls RJ, Ritchie JK, et al. Temporary loop ileostomy for restorative proctocolectomy. Br J Surg 1993;80:628–30.

59. Marcello PW, Roberts PL, Schoetz DJ, et al. Obstruction after ileal pouch-anal anastomosis: a preventable complication? Dis Colon Rectum 1993;36: 1105–11.

60. Mathey P, Ambrosetti P, Morel P, et al. The Swiss experience of the ileoanal anastomosis with reservoir: complications and functional results. Ann Chir 1993;47:1020–25.

61. Nicholls RJ, Belliveau P, Neill M, et al. Restorative proctocolectomy with ileal reservoir: a pathophysiological assessment. Gut 1981;22:462–8.

62. Stelzner M, Fonkalsrud EW, Buddington RK, et al. Adaptive changes in ileal mucosal nutrient transport following colectomy and endorectal ileal pull through with ileal reservoir. Arch Surg 1990;125:586–90.

63. Keighley MRB, Grobler S, Bain I. An audit of restorative proctocolectomy. Gut 1993;34:680–4.

64. Slors JF, Taat CW, Brummelkamp WH. Ileal pouch-anal anastomosis without rectal muscular cuff. Int J Colorectal Dis 1989;4:178–81.

65. Nelson RL, Prasad ML, Pearl RK, et al. Inverted U-pouch construction for restoration of function in patients with failed straight ileoanal pull-throughs. Dis Colon Rectum 1991;34:1040–2.

66. Johnston D, Holdsworth PJ, Smith AH. Preservation of the ileocecal junction and entire anal canal in surgery for ulcerative colitis—a two-sphincter operation. Dis Colon Rectum 1989;32:555–61.

67. Accarpio G, Scodamaglia R, Mignone D, et al. Total colectomy with ileoanal anastomosis and myotomy in the treatment of patients with colonic diseases. Coloproctology 1983;5:263–5.

68. Sagar PM, Holdsworth PJ, Salter GV, et al. Single lumen ileum with myectomy: an alternative to the pelvic reservoir in restorative proctocolectomy? Br J Surg 1990;77:1030–5.

69. Telander RL, Perrault J. Colectomy with rectal mucosectomy and ileoanal anastomosis in young patients: its use for ulcerative colitis and familial polyposis. Arch Surg 1981;116:623–9.

70. Luukkonen P, Jarvinen HJ. Stapled vs hand-sutured ileoanal anastomosis in restorative proctocolectomy—a prospective, randomized study. Arch Surg 1993;128:437–40.

71. McIntyre PB, Pemberton JH, Wolff BG, et al. Comparing functional results one year and ten years after ileal pouch-anal anastomosis for chronic ulcerative colitis. Dis Colon Rectum 1994;37:303–7.

72. Tuckson W, Lavery I, Fazio V, et al. Manometric and functional comparison of ileal pouch-anal anastomosis with and without anal manipulation. Am J Surg 1991;161:90–5; discussion 95–6.

73. Gozzetti G, Poggioli G, Marchetti F, et al. Functional outcome in hand-sewn vs. stapled ileal pouch-anal anastomosis. Am J Surg 1994;168:325–9.

74. Gemlo BT, Belmonte C, Wiltz O, et al. Functional assessment of ileal pouch-anal anastomotic techniques. Am J Surg 1995;169:137–42.

11 Ileal Reservoirs

Fabrizio Michelassi, Danny Takanishi,
Robin S. McLeod, Bruce A. Harms,
James R. Starling, and Eric W. Fonkalsrud

Historical Aspects of Surgery for Ulcerative Colitis

Before the start of the twentieth century, ulcerative colitis was largely a mysterious disease. Endoscopy (rigid proctoscopy) was infrequently performed, and surgical therapy consisted of attempts to irrigate the colon with anti-inflammatory liquids through an appendicostomy or later cecostomy (1). Part of this therapy was based on the lack of knowledge about safe anesthesia, antisepsis, and antibiotic therapy.

With improvements in surgery and anesthesiology, bypass operations (loop ileostomy, colostomy, or combinations thereof) became more commonplace. Nonetheless, there were no reliable stoma appliances in the first half of the twentieth century, and the construction of a safe ileostomy that could be managed effectively awaited the innovations of Alfred Strauss of Chicago in the 1940's (2), Sir Brian Brooks of the United Kingdom (3), and Rupert Turnbull (4) of The Cleveland Clinic in the 1950s.

Proof that the removal of the entire colon and rectum (proctocolectomy) was effective and safe in the management of ulcerative colitis was not apparent until Strauss and Strauss presented their results on this approach in 1944 (2). At the same time, these surgeons described a rubber appliance that could be bonded and sealed to the skin with rubber adhesions, and supported with an elastic belt. Ulcerative colitis patients could thereafter expect to lead a reasonably active lifestyle. The formation of an enterostomal therapy school in the late 1950s at The Cleveland Clinic helped stoma patients achieve even better quality of life by training dedicated nurses in the art of stoma care, stoma ap-

pliance development, and in patient and family education. The development of nurses specially trained in this field ranks as one of the most important achievements in improving the quality of life in ulcerative colitis patients.

By the 1960s, intraabdominal surgery had become safe and routine throughout most of the developed countries of the world. The focus of surgeons quite naturally shifted to further improvements in *function* and lifestyle of their ulcerative colitis patients. Following the proctectomy phase of the operation, with excision of the anus and pelvic floor, management of the perineal wound before the 1970s largely consisted of packing open the pelvis from the perineal aspect, thereafter leaving it to close by secondary intention. This healing process could take many months to years. Part of the reason for this slow healing process was that proctectomy, even for benign disease, entailed wide excision of the skin and soft tissues of the perineum including the sphincters and pelvic floor. Around this time, Lytle and Parks reasoned that preservation of the pelvic floor and anal sphincters was very possible during proctectomy for benign disease, and they described the "intersphincteric" proctectomy as an effective means of retaining pelvic soft tissue and levator muscles, thus permitting primary perineal closure and high rates of healing in their patients (5).

The next major step in ulcerative colitis surgery consisted of an adaptation of a urostomy procedure to an intestinal one by Nils Kock of Göteburg, Sweden. He initially described the formation of an intraabdominal reservoir procedure for a urinary ileal conduit, folding a U-shaped ileal segment back on itself, then sewing it together and placing it just below the abdominal fascia, upstream of the ileal spout to the skin. This did not succeed in improving "continence" for ileostomates until he thereafter, in the 1970s added a nipple valve to the reservoir. When the procedure worked, it permitted patients to function without an ileostomy appliance, instead intubating and draining the ileal reservoir every 3 to 6 hours at their convenience. Unfortunately, the procedure proved to be extremely complex, and was associated with "nipple valve" slippage leading to incontinence in nearly 50% of patients in the 1970s. With further modifications of the procedure, certain centers proved capable of reducing nipple valve slippage to 10% or better (6–8). Even so, the high technical requirements necessary have restricted performance of the Kock pouch procedure to institutions with a special interest in it.

The concept of the ileoanal anastomosis was introduced at least a century ago. Hochenegg and Vignali (9) attempted such a procedure at the turn of the nineteenth century for rectal carcinoma. Nissen and later Ravitch and Sabiston performed total proctocolectomy with ileoanal anastomosis in dogs. They soon thereafter reported on several patients, although poor functional results dampened enthusiasm for further development of the procedures (10). In the 1950s several surgeons experimented with the concept of an ileal "reservoir" being attached to the anal sphincters or low rectum in order to improve function: Valiente and Bacon constructed a triple loop (pantaloon) pouch of ileum in dogs, anastomosing it to the anal canal (11). Karlan et al. later described a double-barreled isoperistaltic pouch in a dog model, and showed that this was effective in maintaining continence (12).

Borrowing on the concept of the Soave procedure (coloanal anastomosis) used in the treatment of Hirschsprung's disease, which entailed rectal mucosectomy with pull-through of the normal proximal colon and anastomosis to the dentate line, the *straight* ileoanal anastomosis was successfully applied to four young patients with familial polyposis (13) with reasonably good results.

A major milestone in the development of the restorative proctoclectomy then came in 1977, when the pediatric surgeon Lester Martin of the University of Cincinnati reported on satisfactory short and long-term results in 17 young patients with ulcerative colitis who underwent straight ileoanal anastomotic procedures (14). This series was the first documentation that the ileoanal procedure could be a viable alternative to ileostomy in the management of patients, at least pediatric patients, with ulcerative colitis.

High rates of fecal incontinence, soiling, and perianal skin irritation prevented the straight ileoanal anastomotic procedure from being acceptable to most adult patients with ulcerative colitis. Thus, the reservoir concept was first applied to a small group of patients in the mid 1970s by Sir Alan Parks and John Nicholls of St Mark's Hospital in London (15). They described formation of an S-shaped reservoir anastomosed to the dentate line after distal rectal mucosal stripping, with a protective temporary loop ileostomy. Good to excellent fecal continence was seen in nearly all of their patients, and this procedure has remained popular up to the present time, with only several technical modifications since it was first described.

Although the concept of the pouch has been maintained, its configuration has been changed by a number of other surgical innovators, including Utsunomiya of Japan (16), Fonkalsrud of Los Angeles (17), and again Nicholls (18). They respectively designed J-, H-, and W-shaped pouches (Fig. 11.1), all for a variety of advantages or indications that will be described in this chapter. The advantages between them seem slight, especially over the long-term, and most surgeons seem to favor use of the J-shaped reservoir owing to its simplicity and ease of construction.

This chapter will focus on the surgical strategy in forming the ileoanal reservoir and anastomosis and attempts to place the different pouch designs in their proper context for the surgeon performing ileal pouch surgery, because all of the designs may have a role in restorative surgery for ulcerative colitis.

Operative Strategy

An important step in the performance of the pelvic ileal reservoir pouch procedure is assessing whether the end of the small bowel will reach the anus so that an ileoanal anastomosis can be performed adequately and safely and secondly, which pouch configuration will accomplish this best. Thus, prior to constructing the pouch, the small bowel mesentery is stretched beyond the pubic symphysis along the axis of the superior mesenteric vessels. If there is inadequate length, further mobilization of the small bowel mesentery may be required. Ease of reach is one of the factors to be considered in the selection of pouch design along with patient body habitus, size of pelvis and adequacy of terminal ileum length.

In the average patient, if a J-loop trial descent demonstrates adequate reach to the anal canal, there is no contraindication against proceeding with a J-pouch construction. This pouch is technically the easiest and the fastest to construct, it avoids problems with evacuation and functions well overall. This pouch is also the least bulky and may be best suited for a narrow pelvis or an obese patient. In addition, as passage of an EEA circular stapler into the distal outlet of an S- or an H-pouch may be technically difficult, a J-pouch configuration is preferred when a stapled ileoanal anastomosis is selected. In these cases, since length is not as great of a concern in the performance of a double stapled anastomosis, the S- or H-pouch do not offer any specific advantage over the J-pouch configuration.

If the J-loop trial descent suggests that the reach is inadequate after appropriate and complete mesenteric mobilization, an S- or H-pouch may be the preferred option where in association with a full mucosectomy. The S- or H-pouch, with the distal outlet, usually allows easier reach than the J- or W-pouch. The disadvantage of these pouches is that they take longer to construct than the J-pouch. A second concern is that patients may have difficulty emptying the pouch. However, this is a relatively rare complication as long as a short outlet is created.

The W-pouch has several definite advantages over other reservoir designs in patients presenting with partial loss of the distal ileum from a previous resection. In such patients, creation of a standard J-pouch would result in significant reduction of pouch capacity, as the first limb would be short. Similarly, an S-pouch design may not be feasible because of loss of the distal ileum, which is utilized to create the S-pouch outlet. A modified W-pouch construction can be performed with a shortened first limb and standard second, third, and fourth limb in this subgroup of patients.

Another distinct subset of patients who may benefit from a W-pouch are patients who have failed straight or J-pouch ileoanal reconstruction with poor functional results as reflected by high stool frequency. Harms et al. reported on a series of six patients presenting with failed straight ileoanal and J-pouch reconstruction (19). These patients typically demonstrate low volume, poorly compliant reservoirs with high stool frequency and nighttime incontinence problems, but adequate anal manometry pressure profiles. If normal sphincter pressure profiles are present, a successful conversion to W-pouch can be accomplished. Converting a low-volume reservoir system to a higher-capacity pouch significantly decreases overall stool frequency.

The lateral H-pouch has been used extensively in the past for children and for many adults with good long-term results, providing that the ileal spout was short and the pouch was less than 12 cm in length

(20). The lateral pouch was designed to place the two adjacent segments of ileum in an isoperistaltic position to enhance peristaltic contractions and the efficiency of pouch emptying. Subsequent myoelectric evaluation of various types of pouch construction in experimental animals has shown no benefit in isoperistaltic compared to antiperistaltic loops (21). As a simplified technique, the end of the terminal ileum is doubled back on itself as with a J-pouch, the ileum is then divided at the apex of the loop and the lower end of the distal segment is advanced inferiorly one centimeter. As the spout of the lateral pouch provides an additional one to two centimeters length compared to the J-pouch, the H-pouch should be considered an alternative for those patients with a short ileal mesentery in whom it is difficult to obtain sufficient length with a J-pouch to reach the anus without tension.

The J-Pouch*

Operative Technique

The J-pouch, created by folding the terminal ileum onto itself, can be constructed by hand suturing (22) or stapling techniques (23–25). The vascular supply to the terminal part of the ileum is checked for integrity prior to pouch construction. The apex of the pouch is then appropriately selected by positioning the ileum over the pubis to identify the longest section of mesentery and a stay suture is inserted on the antimesenteric side to identify this point (Fig. 11.2). The pouch should be at least 15 cm in length. Sutures are then placed between the distal and proximal limb of the J-pouch at the ileomesenteric junction (Fig. 11.3). These sutures not only serve the purpose of approximating the two limbs, but they also facilitate subsequent pouch formation and assist in avoiding the inadvertent inclusion of the ileal mesentery between the forks of the stapler. A noncrushing clamp is then applied on the small intestine proximal to the pouch to avoid spillage of intestinal contents during pouch preparation. A longitudinal enterotomy is performed on the proximal limb opposite to the end of the distal limb for a length that equals one-half the circumference of the intestine. The intestinal clamp, occluding the terminal ileum, is then released and the lubricated forks of an 80 mm linear stapler are inserted (Fig. 11.3A) and locked (Fig. 11.3B). Alternatively, if a stapler had been used to transect and close the terminal ileum at its junction with the ileocecal valve, a small enterotomy is performed to allow one of the forks of the linear stapler.

---

*Fabrizio Michelassi and Danny Takanishi

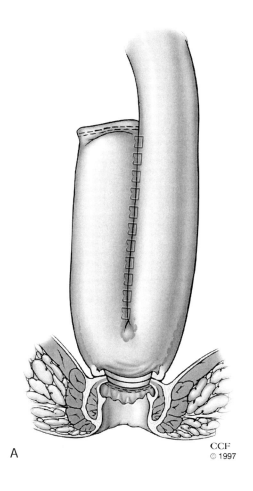

A

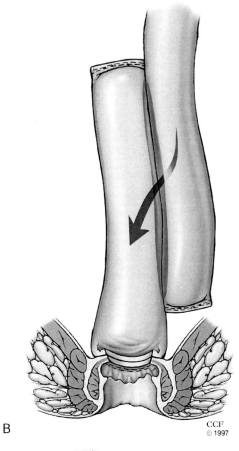

B

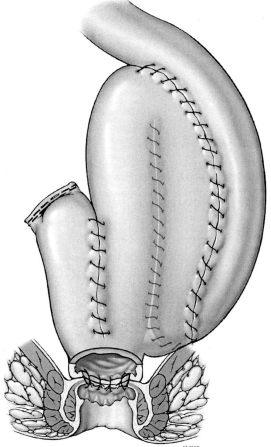

C

Fig. 11.1. (A) Design of the J-pouch using stapling instruments and preservation of the anal transitional zone. (B) Design of the H-pouch, the lateral ileoanal reservoir first described by Fonkalsrud. (C) The W-shaped pouch has the largest capacity of any reservoir and may permit the deepest reach into the pelvis of any pouch design.

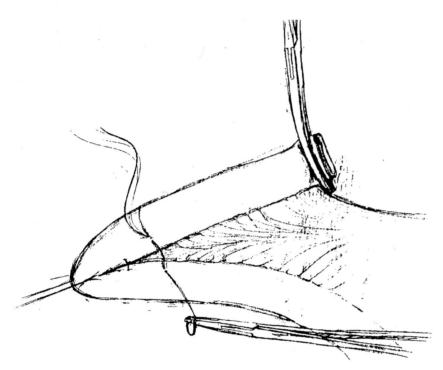

Fig. 11.2.   The apex of the pouch is selected and a stay suture is inserted on the antimesenteric side. Stitches are then applied between the distal and proximal limb of the J-pouch at the ileal mesenteric junction.

The mesentery of the terminal ileum is checked to make sure that it has not been included in the stapler (Fig. 11.4), after which the instrument is fired. The stapler is opened and removed, and by applying Babcock clamps on the suture lines, the pouch is everted (Fig. 11.5) until the remaining intact septum is reached and a new 80 mm stapler is inserted (Fig. 11.6). Usually, three 80 mm linear staplers are needed to construct a 15-cm pouch. The pouch is further everted after each subsequent firing by the Babcock clamps. The eversion of the pouch is helped by pulling the edge of the original enterotomy over the tip of the pouch. It is common to require a 50-mm linear stapler to suture and divide the most distal portion of the septum (Fig. 11.7). Once the pouch is totally everted, the two staple lines are inspected for bleeding (Fig. 11.8), which can be easily controlled by the use of electrocoagulation or suture ligation. The pouch is then reduced by gentle traction on the apical stitch and countertraction on the edge of the original enterotomy (Fig. 11.9). If a stapled ileoanal anastomosis is to be performed, the anvil of the EEA is introduced through the enterotomy and the stem is pushed through the apex of the pouch. Stay sutures are then applied at the end of the linear suture lines to aid in the closure of the remaining enterotomy (Fig. 11.10). Although such closure can be performed with a linear stapler, the asymmetry of the defect appears to be better compensated by a hand-sewn closure.

As soon as the enterotomy is sutured, the proximal intestinal clamp is removed. If a stapled ileoa-nal anastomosis is to be performed, the stem of the anvil is ready to be inserted in the docking device of the EEA, after it has pierced the wall of the stapled anorectal stump. If a hand-sewn anastomosis is to be performed, silk traction sutures are placed at the apex of the pouch and they are grasped with a long ring forceps inserted through the anus. The abdominal operator then guides the pouch into the pelvis, ensuring that the pouch is convexity lines up with the sacral concavity and that the efferent loop to the pouch lies on top of the superior mesenteric vessels rather than between the vessels and the sacral promontory. In addition, care must be paid so that other structures (i.e., ovaries, vagina, uterus, bladder, proximal small bowel) are not drawn into the pelvis. The perineal operator aids in the final positioning of the pouch initially by pulling gently on the silk traction sutures and later on by pulling on the pouch, after having grasped its apex gently with ring forceps. During the descent of the pouch into the pelvis, the perineal operator pays attention to maintaining the spacial orientation of the silk traction sutures, as confirmatory evidence that the pouch is not twisted.

Once the pouch has reached its final position, a hand-sewn anastomosis is performed between the dentate line and the pouch using twelve interrupted 4–0 vicryl stitches. The apex of the pouch is then opened in a circular fashion. A closed-suction drain may be used in the pelvis to drain serum and blood and it is usually removed within 48 hours.

The avoidance of any apical enterotomy allows

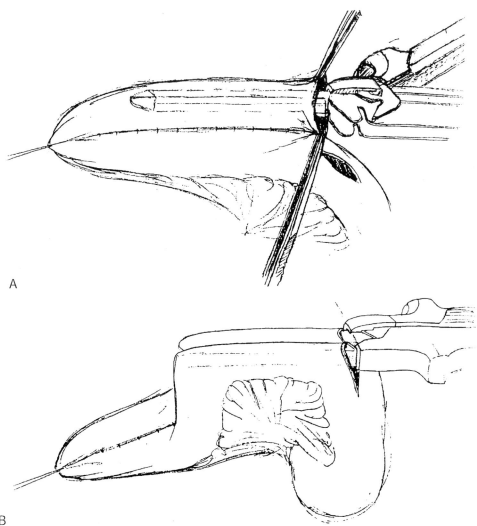

A

B

Fig. 11.3.   A longitudinal enterotomy is performed on the proximal limb opposite to the end of the distal limb for a length that approximately equals one half the circumference of the intestine. (A) the lubricated forks of an 80 mm linear stapler are inserted and (B) locked.

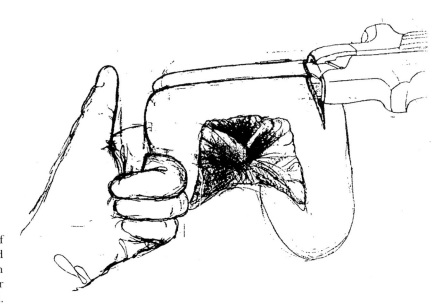

Fig. 11.4.   The mesentery of the terminal ileum is checked to make sure it has not been included in the stapler, after which the instrument is fired.

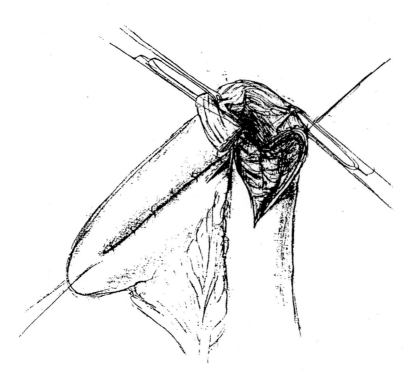

Fig. 11.5. After removal of the stapler, the pouch is everted by applying Babcock clamps until the remaining intact septum is reached.

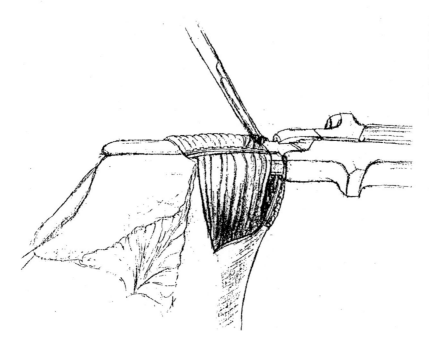

Fig. 11.6. A new 80 mm stapler is inserted. This maneuver is repeated three or four times, as necessary. The pouch is everted more after each subsequent firing by way of application of the Babcock clamps.

the pull-through of the pouch into the pelvis while still intact, minimizing the potential for pelvic contamination and the development of a pelvic or cuff abscess. Additionally, avoiding the apical enterotomy until the pouch is in its definitive position allows for creation of an enterotomy in the most optimal location and of proper size for construc-

tion of the ileoanal anastomosis, if a hand-sewn anastomosis is chosen. The eversion of the pouch allows for multiple applications of the linear stapler without the need for creating midpouch enterotomies that have been associated with postoperative dehiscences. Furthermore, there is no need for telescoping the intestine over the forks of the in-

Fig. 11.7.   It is common to require a 50 mm linear stapler to suture and divide the most distal portion of the septum, which has been encircled by passage of a right angle clamp.

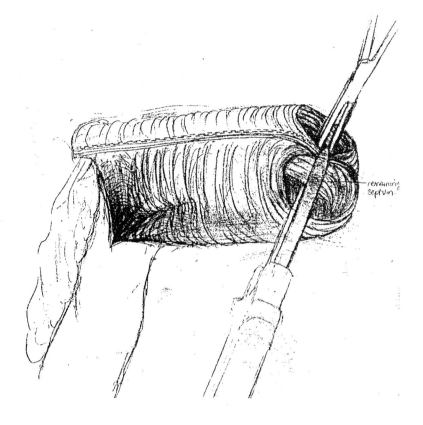

Fig. 11.8.   Once the pouch is totally everted, the two suture lines are inspected for hemostasis.

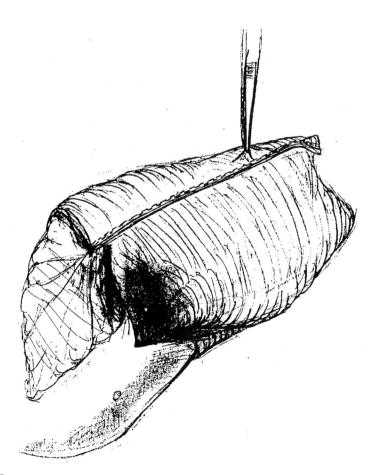

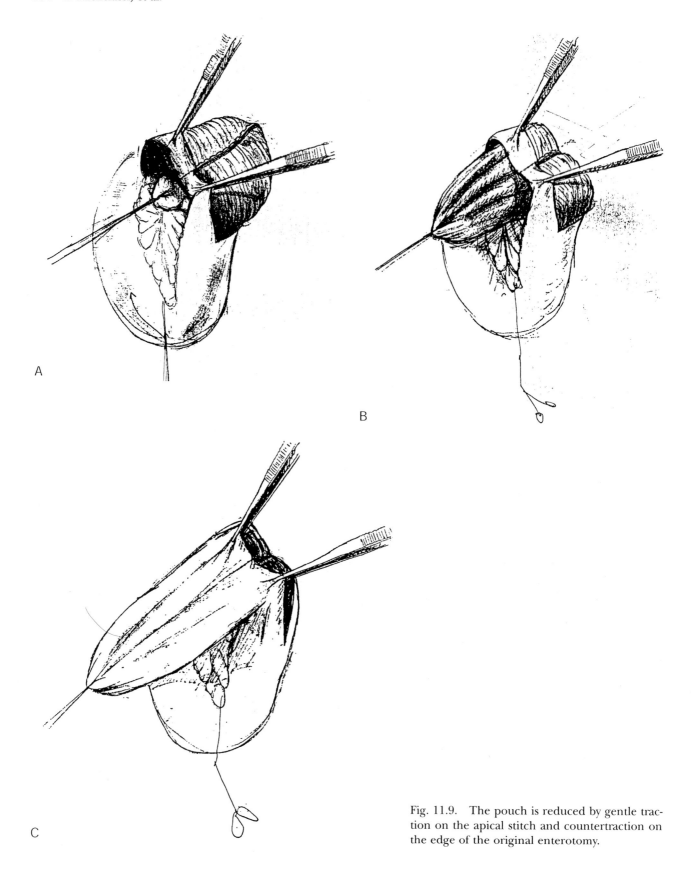

A

B

C

Fig. 11.9.   The pouch is reduced by gentle traction on the apical stitch and countertraction on the edge of the original enterotomy.

Fig. 11.10. Stay sutures are applied at the end of the linear suture lines to aid in the closure of the remaining enterotomy. Although such a closure could be performed with a linear stapler, the asymmetry of the defect can be better compensated by a hand-sewn closure.

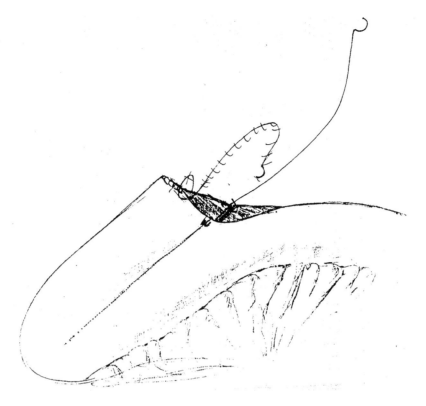

strument that can prove on occasion to be technically difficult.

The University of Chicago Experience with the J-Pouch

As of December, 1997, close to 300 restorative proctocolectomy with J-pouch ileoanal procedures have been performed at the University of Chicago. There has been no hospital mortality. The mean length of the pouch is 16.3 ± 2.4 cm. With a follow-up ranging from two months to 17 years, all but five patients retain their pouch. Pouch loss was due to chronic pouchitis in two, development of Crohn's complication in the pouch in two and poor pouch function in one.

All patients evacuate spontaneously. Frequency of bowel movements at 3, 12, and 24 months is 6.3 ± 2.1, 5.1 ± 1.9, and 5.9 ± 1.6 per day, respectively, without urgency. The majority of patients have fewer than six bowel movements per day, with three-fourths of them being pasty or formed. These results are obtained despite the fact that at least 40% of all our patients follow no specific dietary restrictions and 86% do not take any drugs to alter stool frequency.

Although only one fourth of our patients are able to distinguish flatus from stool, the majority is able to defer a bowel movement for longer than two hours. Only 11% are incontinent of stool in the first three years after surgery with continence improving substantially by two years. Acute pouchitis has occurred at least once in half of our patients by four years.

The S-Pouch*

Operative Technique

The ileum should be divided immediately proximal to the ileocecal valve to preserve the entire small bowel. Since the end of the ileum will be the lead point (unlike in a J-pouch where the apex approximately 15 cm proximal to the divided small bowel is the lead point), it is especially important to conserve all of the small bowel. In patients who have had a previous colectomy and ileostomy and have a pelvic pouch performed at a subsequent operation, care must be taken in taking down the ileostomy to avoid enterotomies. The ileostomy should be desuscepted to preserve all of the small bowel.

The mesentery of the small bowel is fully mobilized to the third part of the duodenum and the head of the pancreas in order to achieve maximum length. The overlying peritoneum is usually not serially divided to minimize the risk of disrupting a

---

*Robin S. McLeod

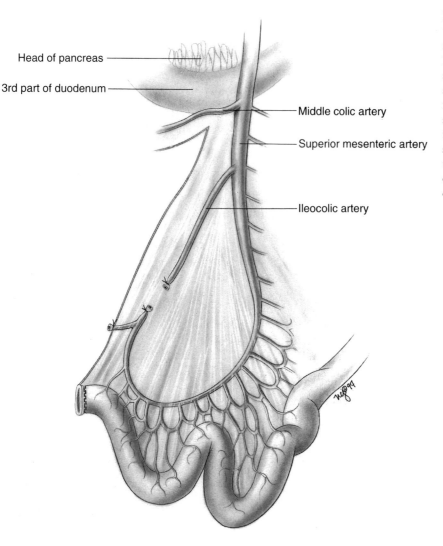

Head of pancreas

3rd part of duodenum

Middle colic artery

Superior mesenteric artery

Ileocolic artery

Fig. 11.11. The superior mesenteric, ileocolic and marginal vessels along the small bowel form an avascular triangle of mesentery. To construct the S-pouch, the ileocolic vessels are transected and the avascular mesenteric triangle is incised. This straightens the end of the terminal ileum so that the small bowel usually stretches several centimeters beyond the pubic symphysis. In doing this, one must be cautions that there is not excessive tension to avoid vessel tear.

major vessel when the pouch is pulled by the perineal operator. There is an avascular triangle bordered by the superior mesenteric vessels, the marginal vessels of the distal 15 to 20 cm of small bowel and the ileocolic vessels. The ileocolic vessels are divided at a point proximal to its division into the ileal and colonic branches. By dividing the mesentery close to the marginal vessels and along the superior mesenteric vessels, the distal end of the terminal ileum can be straightened (Fig. 11.11). It is this maneuver which contributes the extra several centimeters of length for a tension free anastomosis. Generally, if the end of the terminal ileum can stretch several centimeters beyond the pubic symphysis, the apex of the pouch outlet will reach the anus without difficulty.

The pouch is created using three loops of small bowel each approximately 10 cm in length. An outlet of approximately 1 to 2 cm is left (Fig. 11.12). The distal centimeter of the outlet is cleared of

mesentery to facilitate performance of the ileoanal anastomosis. To make the pouch, the second limb is positioned cephalad to the first limb and the third limb cephalad to the second. The position of the loop of bowel is maintained using Babcock clamps. The first and second loop of bowel are sutured together using a running 3–0 absorbable suture, placing the suture line approximately 1 cm from the mesenteric margin of each limb. Similarly, the second and third loop are sutured together. This second suture line on the second limb of bowel should be placed approximately 1 cm from the first suture line (Fig. 11.11). Then an enterotomy is made using electrocautery and in doing so the posterior wall of the pouch is created (Fig. 11.13). A second running layer of absorbable suture is inserted beginning on the posterior wall and continuing anteriorly to complete the anastomosis. Finally a second row of sutures is inserted on the anterior wall of the pouch (Fig. 11.14).

Fig. 11.12. A three limb pouch is created with each limb measuring approximately 10 cm in length. A 1 to 2 cm efferent outlet is left. A continuous suture is inserted between the first and second limb and the second and third limb to create the posterior wall of the pouch. Once this is completed, an enterotomy is made.

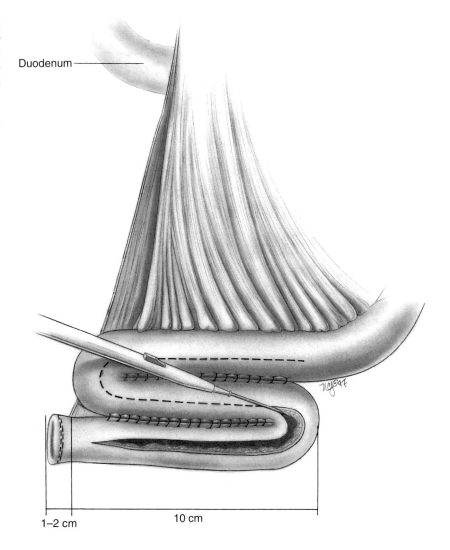

Duodenum

1–2 cm   10 cm

Once completed, a long Babcock clamp is inserted through the anus and the apex of the pouch outlet is grasped. The pouch is rotated so the mesentery lies to the right and anteriorly and the pouch itself lies in the hollow of the sacrum (Fig. 11.15). Once the pouch has been positioned adequately, the perineal operator excises a few millimeters of the outlet which contains the staple line. Then a hand-sewn ileoanal anastomosis at the dentate line is performed. A Jackson Pratt drain is inserted through a separate stab wound through the lower abdominal wall and laid 1 to 2 cm away from the ileoanal anastomosis. This drain, placed to avoid postoperative blood accumulation in the pelvis, is removed within 48 to 72 hours.

The University of Toronto Experience with the S-Pouch

Since 1982, over 900 pelvic pouch procedures have been performed at the Mount Sinai Hospital at the University of Toronto. Just over 25% have been constructed as S-pouches. Between 1984 and 1989, the S-pouch was our preferred design and was performed almost exclusively. In 1989, we began doing the ileoanal anastomosis using a double stapled technique and with this, performed a stapled J-pouch.

We believe the main advantage of the S-pouch is that we can obtain extra length which is often crucial when a mucosectomy and hand-sewn anastomosis are performed. As discussed previously, the distal few centimeters of terminal ileum can be straightened by dividing the ileocolic vessels and the avascular triangle of tissue that is bordered by the marginal, superior mesenteric and ileocolic vessels. Thus, although a J-pouch with a stapled ileoanal anastomosis is now performed in most patients, our preference is still to perform a S-pouch where a mucosectomy is essential such as patients with familial adenomatous polyposis or ulcerative colitis complicated by dysplasia.

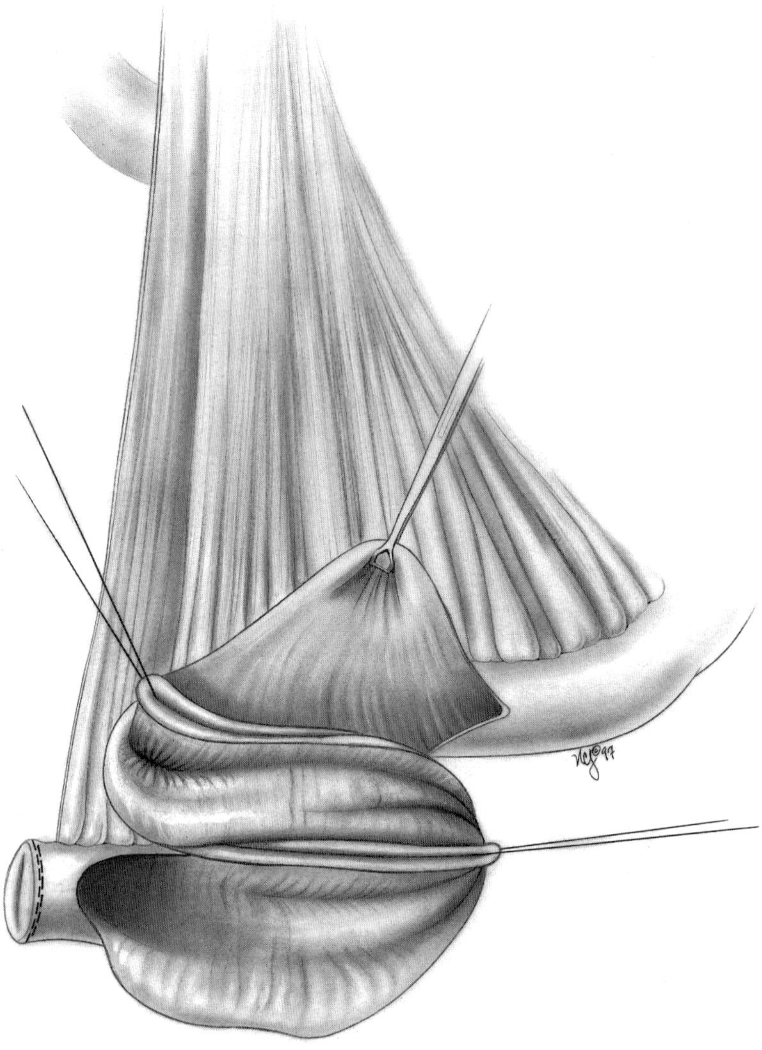

Fig. 11.13. The posterior wall of the pouch has been completed and the pouch has been opened. A second layer of running absorbable suture will be inserted.

Of the 251 S-pouches created between 1982 and 1989, the indication for surgery was ulcerative colitis in 209 (83%), familial adenomatous polyposis in 23 (9%), indeterminant colitis in 3 (1%) and Crohn's disease in 15 (6%). There were 144 males and 107 females with a mean age of 41.1 years. The latter cases were presumed preoperatively to have ulcerative colitis and we would not advocate performing a pelvic pouch in patients with known Crohn's disease. The ileoanal anastomosis was hand-sewn in 246 (98%) and stapled in 5 (2%). A defunctioning ileostomy was performed in all but 4 (1.6%) patients. Thirty-six (14.3%) patients with a S-pouch developed ileoanal anastomotic (IAA) dehiscence compared to an overall IAA leak rate of 10.2%. Our data suggest that there is a higher leak rate with a hand-sewn IAA and therefore the difference in leak rate is probably attributable to this rather than the difference in pouch construction per se. In addition, most S-pouches were constructed in our early experience so the higher leak rate may in part be due to our lack of experience with the procedure.

The functional results overall have been excellent. In a survey of 404 patients, of whom 129 had a S-pouch, the mean number of bowel movements was 5 to 6/24 hours. Overall 13 patients (3.5%) reported that they intubated their pouches on a regular basis but this complication was not reported exclusively in those with S-pouches. Sixty-five percent of patients were fully continent during the day and 50% fully continent during the night. Only 1 and 2% respectively of the remaining complained of major incontinence with the majority having

Fig. 11.14. The anterior wall of the pouch is being completed.

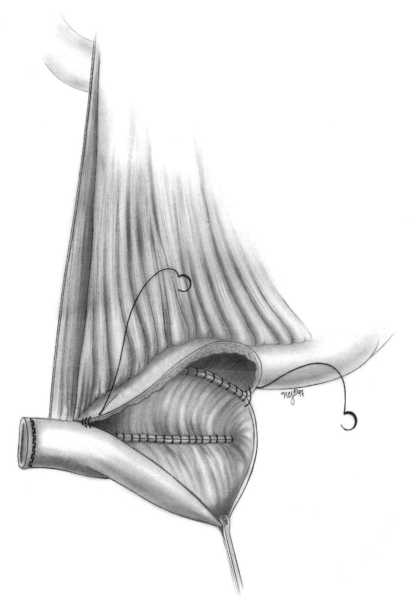

minor problems with seepage of mucus or small amounts of feces. When a multivariate analysis of the data was performed, there was no significant difference in the stool frequency or continence rate between patients who had S- or J-pouches.

In conclusion, it is our view that surgeons who perform the pelvic pouch procedure should be familiar with the construction of the various pouch designs. Depending on the circumstances, it may be technically easier to perform one pouch or the other. In the long-term, however, functional results do not seem to differ. The major disadvantage of the S-pouch is that it must be sutured and is thus more time consuming to perform. It is for this reason that our preference now is the stapled J-pouch and reserve the S-pouch for situations where a

mucosectomy and hand-sewn ileoanal anastomosis are indicated.

The W-Pouch*

Operative Technique

The modified W-pouch technique essentially consists of two, staggered, side-by-side J-loops (Fig. 11.16). The construction of the modified W-pouch is straightforward if several principles are followed. First, the W-pouch is constructed essentially as a J-pouch with extra side limbs to increase reservoir capacity. Second, the apex of the adjacent, second

---

*Bruce A. Harms and James R. Starling

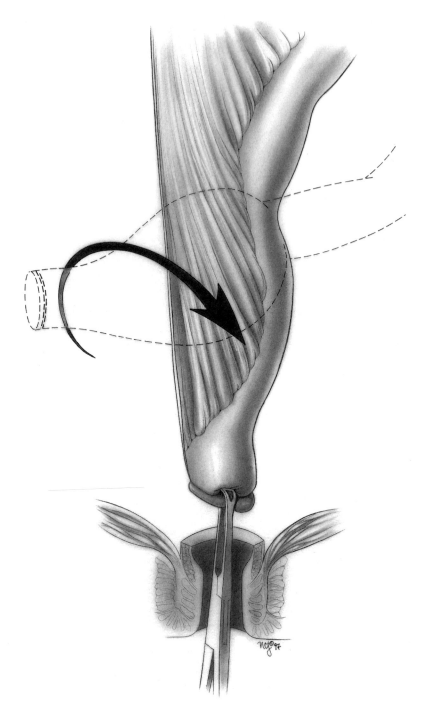

Fig. 11.15. After the mucosectomy has been completed, the outlet of the pouch is grasped by a Babcock clamp which is inserted through the anus. As the pouch is brought down into the pelvis, it is rotated so the pouch lies posteriorly in the hollow of the sacrum, the mesentery to the right and anteriorly and the afferent limb enters the pouch on the left side.

J-loop is positioned three centimeters proximal to the pouch outlet on the first loop to create a nipple effect on the end of the pouch and thereby expedite engagement into the anal canal. In such patients, it has been our experience that a modified W reservoir with smaller first and second limb and larger third and fourth limb will result in successful pouch construction with functional results nearly identical to those patients in whom standard equal length limbs are employed.

As with all types of pouch constructions, the ileum is divided flush with the cecum to maximize limb length. The ileocolic artery is identified and divided at its proximal takeoff with preservation of the distal branch of the superior mesenteric artery arcade to the ileum. The W-pouch outlet is identified and marked approximately 10 to 12 cm from the ileal division. Routine measurements are made on medium tension with a trial descent of the first J-loop, performed by a two surgeon approach. If the initial trial descent confirms that the reach is adequate and the pouch can be constructed with-

Fig. 11.16. Initial layout of W-pouch with staggered first and second J-loop.

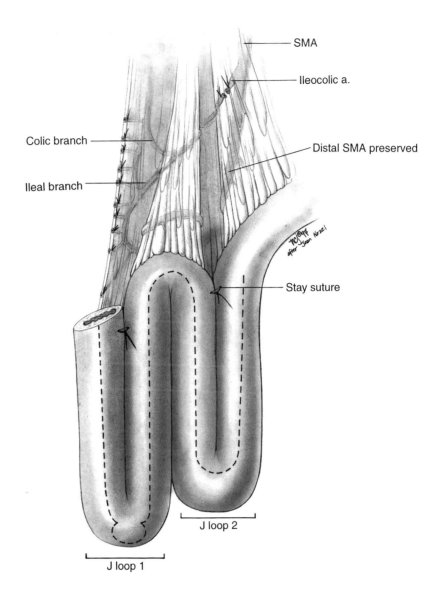

out mesenteric foreshortening, the W-pouch will reach the anal canal for the pouch-anal anastomosis. If the reach is not adequate with the test descent of the first J-loop, an alternative is to shorten the first limb of the initial J-loop. This places the outlet more distally, thereby improving reach into the anal canal.

The outline of the W-pouch is laid out with limb lengths averaging 11 cm (Fig. 11.16). The total length of the ileal pouch upon completion in the adult patient is approximately 15 cm. A needle-point electrocautery instrument is used to cut an ellipse out of the terminal J-loop to form the pouch outlet. The distal portion of the pouch outlet is then opened up along the antimesenteric portion of the first and second limbs (Fig. 11.17). It is help-

ful to tag the ends of the anastomotic lines with silk sutures to facilitate corner identification. The first of three posterior anastomotic lines is accomplished with running 3–0 polydioxanone suture. An alternative to running 3–0 polydioxanone suture for closure of the posterior anastomosis is a staple technique, with two firings of a Proximate Linear Stapler 90 (Ethicon Endo Surgery Inc., Cincinnati, OH). The success of this technique is equal to that of the standard running suture technique; operative time saved is insignificant. The second anastomotic line is completed in similar fashion, after opening the antimesenteric portion of the terminal ileum (Fig. 11.18). When opening up the ileum at the tip of the second J-loop, it is helpful to drift toward the mesentery. This improves the sec-

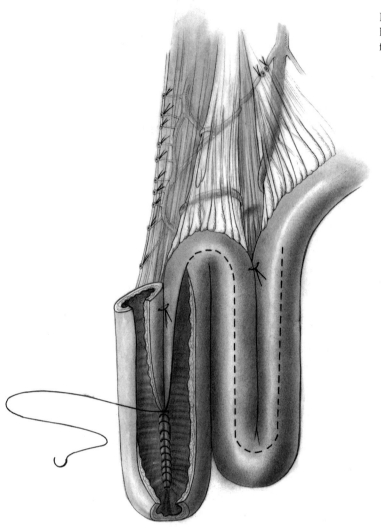

Fig. 11.17. Opening of the first two limbs and pouch outlet; construction of first posterior suture line.

ond J-loop reach and avoids any potential foreshortening problems upon final engagement into the anal canal. The second posterior anastomotic line is completed in the same fashion as the first with running 3–0 polydioxanone suture or staples. The pouch outlet is measured to not exceed 3 cm on tension. This avoids the dysfunctional evacuation problems that were encountered with the initial S-pouch design. The final posterior anastomotic line is accomplished by opening up the fourth and final limb (Fig. 11.19).

Completion of the pouch is performed with running 3–0 polydioxanone suture for the anterior anastomotic line (Fig. 11.20). The only variance from the running technique is a series of everted, interrupted 3–0 polydioxanone sutures placed along the distal 2 to 3 cm of the outlet. The aim of this modification is to prevent a partial disruption of the anterior suture line when sutures are used to create the pouch anal anastomosis. In early experi-

ence with the W-pouch, continuous running polydioxanone sutures were used to complete the entire anastomosis. In several patients, however, this resulted in a partial distal anterior anastomotic disruption over several centimeters that was attributed to unraveling of the distal anterior anastomosis. This can be prevented by the distal closure of the anterior anastomotic line with a series of interrupted sutures.

The pouch is routinely inflated with saline to ensure water tight suture lines. The W-pouch will hold 150 to 200 mL of saline. For a hand-sewn ileo-anal anastomosis, we routinely place 2–0 vicryl sutures in each quadrant of the pouch outlet to help engagement and to maintain spatial orientation. The W-pouch is then engaged into the anal canal utilizing a two surgeon approach with one surgeon working from the abdominal aspect and another surgeon working from the perineum (Fig. 11.21). A hand-sewn anastomosis is performed with twelve

Fig. 11.18. Opening of the second and third limb and construction of second posterior suture line. Note the opening at the apex of each loop is close to the mesentery to maximize adjacent loop reach.

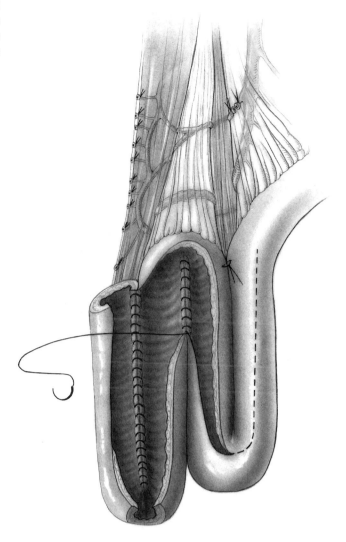

simple interrupted 2–0 vicryl sutures. An alternative is a stapled technique with an EEA stapler, which we have used with equal success.

The University of Wisconsin Experience with the W-Pouch

The most important aspects of W-pouch construction relate to functional results as reflected in stool frequency and continence results. As reported by Oresland et al., lower stool frequency is probably not just a reflection of pouch design, but of the length of terminal ileum utilized for pouch construction. Early experience by Nicholls and Pezim with the W-pouch documented a low stool frequency. This has been supported in our series and others' with experience in W-pouch construction (19,26). Clearly, pouch capacity does have an important impact on stool frequency and functional results which has been confirmed when low volume

J-reservoirs have failed and were converted to W-pouches. The significant decrease in stool frequency can be attributed only to an increase in pouch capacity. The difference between reservoir designs is probably small over the long term. In our experience, no significant difference has been demonstrated over the long term between S- and W-pouch functional results or stool frequency in contrast to Sagar et al., who demonstrated a functional advantage in the W vs. S design. Similarly, when physiologic parameters such as volume and pressure profiles were assessed, no major differences were evident between these pouch designs (Fig. 11.22) (27). Reports from surgeons with significant W-pouch construction experience show a consistent low stool frequency with an average range from 3.3 to 5.0 stools per day.

Continence results are equally as important as stool frequency (28,29). Reports have varied from no significant difference in continence between

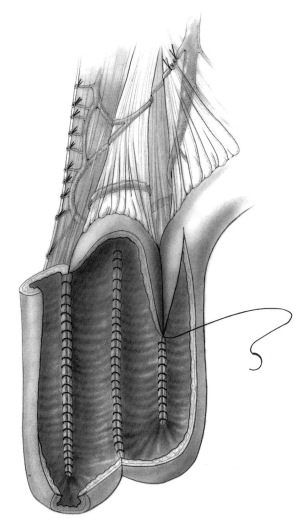

Fig. 11.19.   Opening of third and fourth limb for third posterior suture line.

W-pouch patients and other pouch designs to a significant improvement in both day and night-time continence (30). The relationship between intrapouch pressure at a given volume and the associated anal canal pressure probably play a major role in determining continence. This pouch-anal pressure gradient provides a safety zone at mid-to-low volumes that optimizes continence (Fig. 11.23) (29). Oresland et al., documented the importance of this relationship and implicated pouch capacity as a major factor in optimizing continence. The relationship between pouch and anal pressures provides evidence to suggest that to achieve optimal continence, ileal pouches should not be constructed with limited capacity regardless of pouch design. The overall excellent continence results reflected in W-pouch reports is not surprising given the larger pressure difference between the anal canal and intrareservoir space.

The spectrum of perioperative complications following W-pouch restorative proctocolectomy does not vary significantly between reports comparing W and other reservoir designs (27,31). Beginning with the initial report by Nicholls and Pezim no increase in operative morbidity has been attributed to selection of the W-pouch as an option for reconstruction. Table 11.1 summarizes the reported complications among W-pouch series. Major complications include small bowel obstruction (range 0 to 12.5) and anastomotic problems (dehiscence vs. stricture); their frequency is equivalent to that of other types of pouch designs (30). The W-pouch failure rate which ranges from 0 to 2.9% in reported series, is also equivalent to those of other designs (30).

The H-Pouch*

Operative Technique

The ileal mesentery is mobilized into the upper abdomen with the dissection carried immediately adjacent to the superior mesenteric vessels in order to provide sufficient length for the distal ileum to reach the anus. Extensive dissection along the mesenteric vessels may be necessary to minimize tension on the ileoanal anastomosis. The ileum is transected approximately 14 cm from the distal end, carefully preserving the vascular supply to the distal segment. The proximal ileum is advanced to a position adjacent to the distal segment and a small transverse incision is made through the antimesenteric side of the distal ileum, approximately 1 cm from the end (Fig. 11.24). A lateral isoperistaltic anastomosis is performed between the antimesenteric sides of each segment of ileum using the general intestinal anastomosis (GIA) stapling device. The upper end of the pouch is closed with staples or a running inverted absorbable suture (Fig. 11.25). The lower open end of the pouch is closed with a running inverting suture of 3–0 Maxon (Ethicon, Somerville, NJ). A second layer of running, and/or interrupted absorbable suture is placed circumferentially around the entire reservoir anastomosis. A spout of less than 1 cm extends from the inferior end of the pouch to the open end of the distal ileum (Fig. 11.26).

As a safe, satisfactory and slightly simplified alternative technique, the end of the distal 14 cm of ileum is doubled back on itself as with a J-pouch. The ileum is then divided at the apex of the loop

---

*Eric W. Fonkalsrud

Fig. 11.20. Completion of anterior suture line. Note the interrupted and running suture completion of the most distal 2 to 3 cm of the outlet (inset).

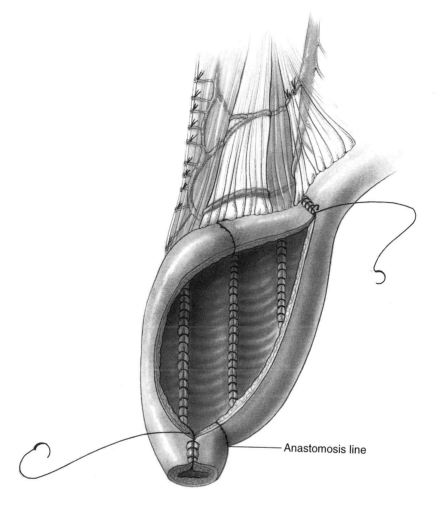

Anastomosis line

and the lower end of the distal segment is advanced inferiorly 1 cm. The pouch construction is then completed as noted above. This type of pouch construction with one antiperistaltic segment has functioned equally well as the lateral isoperistaltic pouch construction.

Silk traction sutures are placed through the ileal spout and the pouch is then drawn through the pelvis and rectal muscle canal such that the end of the spout extends to the anus (Fig. 11.26). The ileal mesentery is placed in a posterior position, and care is taken to avoid twisting or kinking the pullthrough segment. The ileal spout is sutured to the anoderm and underlying muscularis circumferentially with interrupted absorbable sutures (2–0 Vicryl). Approximately 24 sutures are used to complete the anastomosis. It is helpful to place quadrant sutures through the anal mucosa before bringing the pouch to the anus to facilitate proper placement of the remaining sutures. The pelvis is

drained transabdominally with a Jackson-Pratt catheter for four days.

The UCLA Experience with the H-Pouch

During the past 18 years, 561 patients (493 with ulcerative colitis, 59 with colonic polyposis, six with Hirschsprung's disease, and three with neuronal intestinal dysplasia) have undergone colectomy and mucosal proctectomy with endorectal ileal pullthrough operations at the UCLA Medical Center. An initial J-pouch was used for 313 patients, a lateral pouch for 221, an S-pouch for 16, and a straight ileal pullthrough for 20 patients. Nine patients with a straight pullthrough were converted to a J-pouch at a later time and seven additional patients were reconstructed to a lateral pouch.

Between 1977 and 1985, 111 patients underwent construction of a lateral isoperistaltic ileal reservoir with an ileal spout of 2 to 4 cm in length,

206   F. Michelassi, et al.

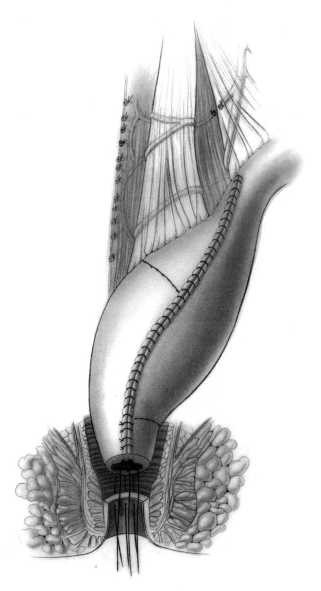

Fig. 11.21. Completed W-pouch construction and engagement into anal canal.

and the pouch measuring from 16 to 26 cm in length. The rectal muscle cuff in these patients varied from 5 to 9 cm in length. After January 1986, 117 patients underwent construction of a lateral reservoir of 13 cm length or less, with an ileal spout not exceeding 1.5 cm, and a rectal muscle cuff of 4 to 5 cm. After 1988, only 12 isoperistaltic lateral ileal reservoirs were constructed and since 1991 a J-pouch has been used routinely.

In reviewing the results with 228 lateral ileal reservoirs, there were no deaths related to the operation in the perioperative period or in long term follow-up. Major complications relating to the pouch included partial outflow obstruction from the pouch due to spout elongation with reservoir enlargement causing stasis in 43%, outflow obstruction due to spout elongation alone in 19% and pouch inflammation (pouchitis) in 18%.

Although stool frequency averaged 6.8 per 24 hours one year after the operation in the initial 111 patients, many developed a gradual increase in stool frequency and a sensation of incomplete emptying accompanied by an increase in gas, diarrhea, and nocturnal incontinence during the ensuing years. Several of these patients experienced episodes of pouchitis most of which resolved with administration of oral metronidazole, rectal irrigations with tap water, and occasional Rowasa enemas. Administration of antiperistaltic medications, such as loperamide (Imodium), diphenoxylate hydrochloride with atropine (Lomotil), or codeine, provided transient relief of stool frequency, but led to habituation with higher tolerance thresholds and were ineffective in relieving pouchitis. It became apparent that pouch stasis, whether due to a large poorly contractile pouch, outflow obstruction from a true stricture, or functional obstruction from an elongated ileal spout, was the cause of an increase in bacterial growth, decreased water absorption, and development of chronic mucosal inflammation and diarrhea, with increased stool frequency, urgency, and soiling.

During our early clinical experience, four of the 111 lateral isoperistaltic reservoirs were removed from 13 to 68 months postoperative and a permanent ileostomy was constructed because of persistent symptoms. Since it became apparent that additional patients would require return to an ileostomy, abdominoperineal reconstruction with shortening and tapering of the pouch and removal of the spout with debridement of obstructive pelvic scar tissue was performed on 82 of these 111 patients. A diverting ileostomy was used on only six of these patients. Mobilization of the pouch from the pelvis was performed with remarkable technical ease in the majority of patients, facilitated by the use of Bovie forceps. Transrectal mobilization of the ileal spout was commonly performed more easily than the original rectal mucosectomy. The ileal mesentery extending to the pouch was almost invariably lengthened by a few centimeters compared to the initial operation, making the reconstructed ileoanal anastomosis feasible without tension in almost all cases. Enlarged lymph nodes in the distal ileal mesentery and pelvic scar tissue often associated with an elongated muscle cuff commonly caused compression of the ileal spout and lower end of the pouch and were removed whenever feasible.

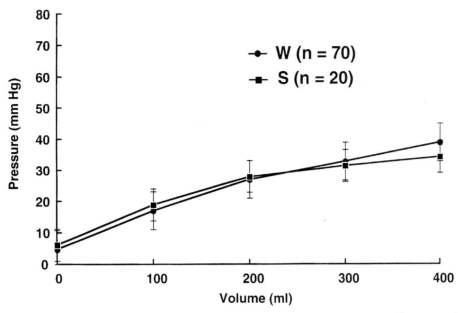

Fig. 11.22. Physiologic profile of S- and W-pouch volume and corresponding intrareservoir pressure. No significant difference demonstrated between S- and W-designs.

Reconstruction consisted of resection of the distal pouch and the entire spout to make the final pouch approximately 10 to 14 cm in length (Fig. 11.27). The antimesenteric side of the pouch was tapered in order to make the lower open end of the pouch of appropriate size for the ileoanal anastomosis. The repair was performed with two layers of interrupted absorbable 2–0 vicryl suture, and the ileoanal anastomosis was constructed with a single layer of interrupted vicryl sutures. Six of the 82

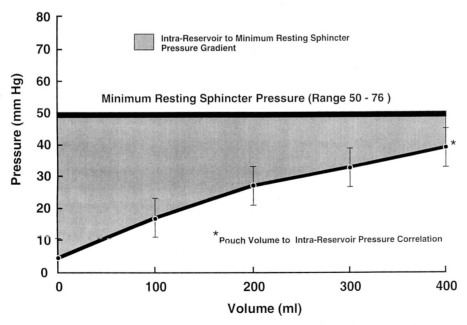

Fig. 11.23. W reservoir pouch anal pressure gradient between minimum resting sphincter pressure and intrareservoir pressure in 40 patients. With increasing volume up to 400 mL, intrareservoir pressure remains below minimum resting sphincter pressure.

Table 11.1.   Complication frequency in published W-pouch series.

	# Pt	Obstruction (%)	Anastomotic Dehiscence (%)	Anastomotic Stricture (%)	Failure (%)	Pelvic Infection (%)	Other (%)
Nicholls	64	12	6	6	1	0	6.7 (Bleeding)
Harms	109	7.9	3.4	8.9	0	0	3.4 (DVT/PE*, Bleeding) 5.6 (Prolonged Ileus)
Hatakeyama	16	12.5	6.3	18.8	0	6.3	6.7 (Pouch Fistula)
Keighley	15	0	0	20	0	1	6.7 (Pouch Fistula)
Hewett	35	11.4	0	0	2.9	2.9	2.9 (Pouch Fistula)

*Deep Venous Thrombosis/Pulmonary Embolus

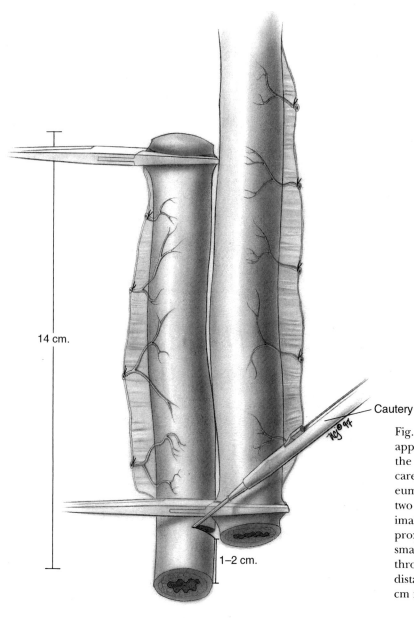

Cautery

Fig. 11.24.   The distal ileum is divided approximately 14 cm from its end and the mesentery to the distal segment is carefully preserved. The proximal ileum is advanced downward so that the two segments are side by side. The proximal and distal ileum are rotated to approximate the antimesenteric sides. A small transverse incision is made through the antimesenteric side of the distal ileal segment approximately 1–2 cm from the end.

14 cm.

1–2 cm.

Fig. 11.25. The GIA stapling device is inserted to construct the reservoir. The upper open end of the pouch is closed with the stapling device or with sutures.

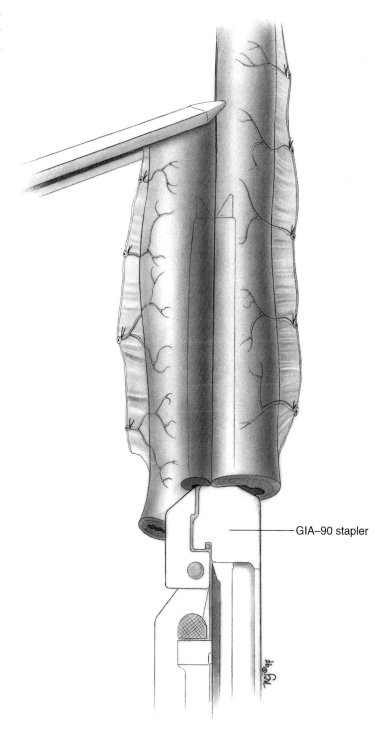

GIA–90 stapler

patients underwent diverting ileostomy because of poor general health at the time of operation or because of complexity of the reconstruction. Pelvic drainage and the postoperative care were carried out in the same manner as performed for the initial pullthrough operations, although in the majority of patients no steroids were used. Within four to six weeks, rectal dilatation with a size 19 Hegar dilator

was initiated and carried out twice weekly for several weeks or months if necessary.

For 16 of the initial 111 patients with an ileal spout exceeding 2.5 cm, and a pouch less than 15 cm in length, transanal resection of the spout with reanastomosis of the lower end of the pouch to the anus was performed. Transanal drainage of the pouch with a No. 30 Foley catheter for four to six

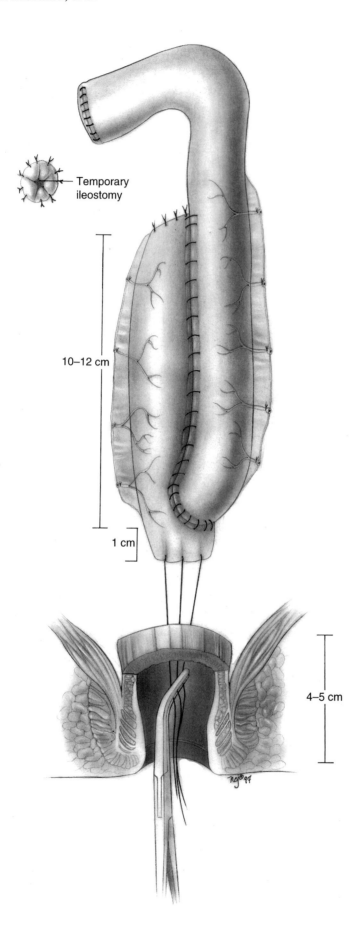

Temporary
ileostomy

10–12 cm

1 cm

4–5 cm

Fig. 11.26.   The lower end of the pouch is reconstructed with sutures. The staple and suture lines are supported with seromuscular absorbable sutures. The ileal spout is drawn through the rectal muscle cuff to the anus with traction sutures. The end of the ileal spout is sutured to the anus with interrupted absorbable sutures.

Fig. 11.27. Elongated and broad lateral ileal pouch with long spout, causing outflow obstruction and stasis. The pouch is mobilized from the pelvis and the lower end is resected to leave a residual pouch of 12–14 cm length. The distal end of the pouch is tapered using the GIA stapler or with absorbable sutures (A) such that the distal end is appropriate size for the ileoanal anastomosis (B).

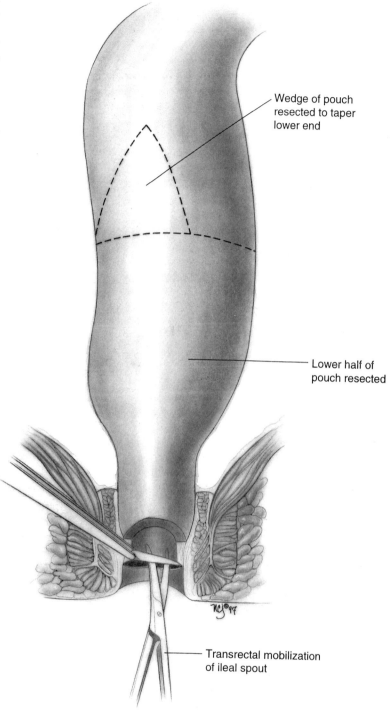

Wedge of pouch resected to taper lower end

Lower half of pouch resected

Transrectal mobilization of ileal spout

A

days was used for each of these patients. None of these patients with transanal pouch reconstruction required a temporary diverting ileostomy or pouch removal.

Learning from this initial experience, we modified the technique of pouch construction to minimize pouch stasis and enhance the efficiency of emptying. Since long and/or broad pouches do not empty as efficiently as short pouches with two loops, we reduced the length of the pouch to 8 to 12 cm, depending on the age of the patient (32), and we shortened the spout to 1 cm. This change in surgical technique resulted in fewer patients requiring later reconstruction: of 117 patients, 15 required an abdominoperineal reconstruction with anastomosis of the lower end of the tapered pouch

Fig. 11.27.   *Continued.*

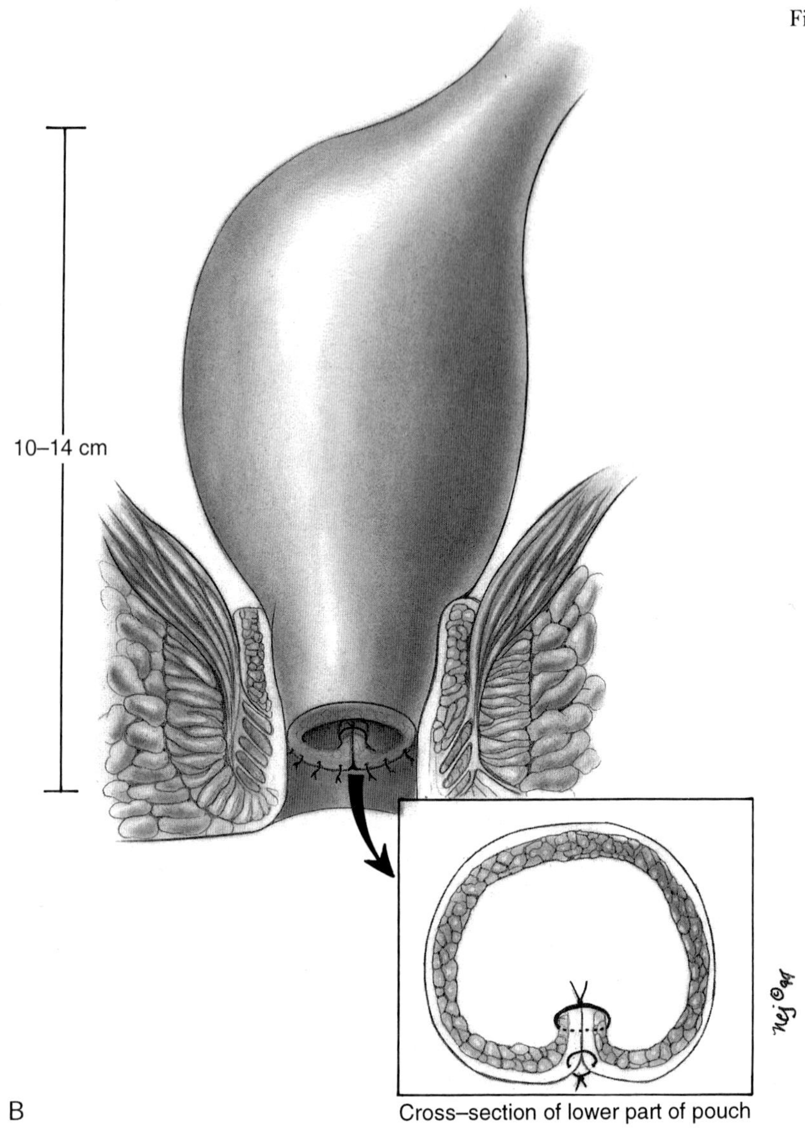

10–14 cm

B

Cross–section of lower part of pouch

to the anus and 28 underwent transanal resection of the spout with reanastomosis to the anus. Thus 141 of the 228 patients with a lateral ileal reservoir (62%) have undergone late reconstruction of the pouch because of persistent symptoms. One of these patients died within three days of the abdominoperineal reconstruction following a massive pulmonary embolism. In addition to the initial four patients who underwent pouch removal, eight additional patients have been returned to a permanent ileostomy because of chronic pouch malfunction. The pouch failure rate of 5.2% among these 228 patients with a mean follow-up of over 12 years is consistent with the results reported from other large centers using other pouch configurations. In contrast, only six of the 313 patients with a J-pouch have undergone pouch removal (1.9%) with a mean follow-up of 3.9 years. Seven of the

18 patients undergoing pouch removal were found to have histologic features of Crohn's disease in the resected specimen.

Review of 205 of the 228 patients with a lateral ileoanal pouch pullthrough procedure (137 reconstructed) with a mean follow-up of 12.8 years, showed that the long-term functional results are very similar to those observed in our hospital with the J-pouch. The average number of movements per 24 hours at three months is 5.9 and at six months is 4.8. Less than 6% have more than two staining or soiling episodes per week at four months. Ninety-three percent are functioning well from 3 to 17 years postoperation. Eighty-four can delay defecation for up to 1½ hours after the initial urge. Eighty-two percent can urinate without having a simultaneous defecatory movement; 64 percent can pass flatus without having a movement.

Ninety percent routinely take less than two minutes to empty. When examined after voluntary defecation, the residual stool volume in the pouch as determined by sigmoidoscopy, rarely exceeds 15 mL. Twenty-four females have delivered babies following lateral ileoanal pouch pullthrough, 13 by vaginal route. The majority of patients have unlimited physical activity.

References

1. Brown JY. Value of complete physiological rest of large bowel in treatment of certain ulcerations and obstetrical lesions of this organ. Surg Gynecol Obstet 1913;16:610–6.

2. Strauss AA, Strauss SF. Surgical treatment of ulcerative colitis. Surg Clin North Am 1944;24:211–24.

3. Brooke BN, Camb MC. The management of an ileostomy including its complications. Lancet 1952; 102–3.

4. Turnbull RB. Management of an ileostomy. Am J Surg 1953;86:617–24.

5. Lyttle JA, Parks AG. Intersphincteric excision of the rectum. Br J Surg 1977;64:413–6.

6. Dozois RR, Kelly KA, Beart RW, et al. Improved results with continent ileostomy. Ann Surg 1980;192: 319–24.

7. Gerber A, Apt MK, Craig PH. The kock continent ileostomy. Surg Gynecol Obstet 1983;156:345–50.

8. Fazio VW, Church JM. Complications and function of the continent ileostomy at the Cleveland Clinic. World Journal of Surgery 1988;12:148–54.

9. Hochenegg J. Meine operationerfolge bei rectum carcinoma. Wein Klin Wocheschr 1900;13:394–404.

10. Ravitch MM, Sabiston DC. Anal ileostomy with preservation of the sphincter—a proposed operation in patients requiring total colectomy for benign lesions. Surg Gynecol Obstet 1946;1095–9.

11. Valiente MA, Bacon HE. Construction of pouch using 'pantaloon' technique for pull-through following total colectomy. Am J Surg 1955;90:6621–43.

12. Karlan M, McPherson RC, Watman RN. An experimental evaluation of fecal continence-sphincter and reservoir in the dog. Surg Gynecol Obstet 1959;108: 469–75.

13. Safaie-Shirafi, Soper RT. Endorectal pull through procedure in the surgical treatment of familial polyposis coli. J Pediatr Surg 1973;8:711–6.

14. Martin LW, LeCoultre C, Shubert WK. Total colectomy and mucosal proctectomy with preservation of continence in ulcerative colitis. Ann Surg 1977;186: 477–80.

15. Parks AG, Nicholls RJ, Belliveau P. Proctocolectomy with ileal reservoir and anal anastomosis. Br J Surg 1980;67:533–8.

16. Utsunomiya J, Iwama T, Imajo M, et al. Total colectomy, mucosal proctectomy, and ileoanal anastomosis. Dis Colon Rectum 1980;23:459–66.

17. Fonkalsrud EW, Ament ME. Endorectal mucosal resection without proctocolectomy as an adjunct for abdominoperineal resection for non-malignant condition: clinical experience with five patients. Ann Surg 1978;67:533–8.

18. Nicholls RJ, Lubowski DZ. Restorative proctocolectomy: the four loop (W) reservoir. Br J Surg 1997;4: 564–6.

19. Harms BA, Andersen AB, Starling JR. The "W" ileal reservoir: long-term assessment following proctocolectomy for ulcerative colitis and familial polyposis. Surgery 1992;112:638–48.

20. Fonkalsrud EW. Surgical management of ulcerative colitis in childhood. Semin Pediat Surg 1994;3: 33–8.

21. Takamatsu H, Albert A, Mulvihill S, et al. Electrical activity and motility in the isoperistaltic side-to-side ileal reservoir. Surg Gynecol Obstet 1985;161:425–530.

22. Becker JM, Raymond JL. Ileal pouch-anal anastomosis. Ann Surg 1986;204:375–83.

23. Ballantyne GH, Pemberton JH, Beart RW, et al. Ileal J pouch-anal anastomosis: current technique. Dis Colon Rectum 1985;28:197–202.

24. Rolfsmeyer E, Rothenberger DA, Goldbert SM. Ileoanal pullthrough. In: Colon Rectal and Anal Surgery: current techniques and Controversies. In: Kodner IH, Fry RD, and Roe JP ed. St. Louis: CV Mosby; 1958.

25. Soper NJ, Becker JM. A stapled technique for construction of ileal J pouches. Surg Gynecol Obstet 1988;166:557–9.

26. Hatakeyama K, Yamai K, Muto T. Evaluation of W pouch-anal anastomosis for restorative proctocolectomy. Int J Colorectal Dis 1989;4:150–5.

27. Harms BA, Pahl AC, Starling JR. Comparison of clinical and compliance characteristics between S and W ileal reservoirs. Am J Surg 1990;159:34–40.

28. Michelassi F, Stella M, Block GE. Prospective assessment of functional results after ileal J pouch-anal restorative proctocolectomy. Arch Surg 1993;128: 889–95.

29. Pescatori M. The results of pouch surgery after ileoanal anastomosis for inflammatory bowel disease: the manometric assessment of pouch continence and its reservoir function. World J Surg 1992;16: 872–9.

30. Nicholls RJ. Restorative proctocolectomy with various types of reservoir. Word J Surg 1987;11:751–62.

31. Grotz RL, Pemberton JH. The ileal pouch operation for ulcerative colitis. Surg Clin North Am 1993; 73(5):909–32.

32. Stelzner M, Fonkalsrud EW, Lichenstein G. Significance of the reservoir length in the endorectal ileal pullthrough with ileal reservoir. Arch Surg 1988;123: 1265–8.

12 Proctocolectomy with the Kock Pouch

Zane Cohen and Robin S. McLeod

The Kock Pouch was developed by Professor Nils Kock in Göteborg, Sweden, in 1969. Professor Kock had been working with a continent urinary pouch in cats for approximately 7 years prior to first doing a continent ileostomy in humans. Initially, and during the early 1970s, multiple authors had reported on the outcome of patients undergoing a Kock pouch procedure. The indications at that time were specifically for patients not wishing to have a conventional ileostomy, as this was one alternative to total proctocolectomy and ileostomy. It provided the patient with a mechanism for continence, and overcame a significant number of psychosocial problems related to a conventional ileostomy. However, the procedure itself was, and still is, a complex one, with numerous complications. In fact, initially, the revision rate due to leakage from the continent ileostomy was reported in the 50% range. Initially, the outlet valve from the Kock Pouch was brought out obliquely through the rectus muscles in order to provide a mechanism of continence: in the early 1970s the "nipple" valve was introduced for the same purpose. However, there were problems with stabilization and sliding of the valve which required reoperations.

The Kock Pouch has undergone many modifications over the past 25 years. Some of these modifications include using a fascial sling around the outlet, various types of mesh around the outlet, different-shaped pouches, and different lengths of the nipple valve itself.

Despite these many modifications, patients must be informed prior to undertaking the Kock Pouch procedure that numerous complications are still possible, and revisionary surgery is still in the range of 15% to 20%. On the other hand, the procedure does provide an appliance-free existence, which is often a significant improvement to patients whose only other option might be a conventional Brooke ileostomy and external appliance.

The following will provide some detail of the Kock Pouch procedure.

Indications and Contraindications

Indications for the continent ileostomy are similar to those for patients undergoing a restorative proctocolectomy with pouch-anal anastomosis. The most frequent indications are patients who are seeking an alternative to a conventional ileostomy owing to skin problems or psychosocial and sexual difficulties or to a failed ileoanal pouch procedure. A firm histological diagnosis of ulcerative colitis is mandatory as the procedure is contraindicated in those patients with Crohn's disease. Anal sphincter dysfunction, or the presence of a low rectal cancer in conjunction with ulcerative colitis are contraindications to the pelvic pouch and may make the patient a candidate for the Kock pouch. The relative contraindications for the construction of a Kock pouch include previous resection of a significant amount of small bowel, age of the patient over 60 years, obesity, and significant psychiatric illness.

Preoperative Preparation

The most important aspect of preoperative preparation is to impart to the patient a knowledge of the surgical procedure. The patient must be explained the benefits and potential complications involved in constructing the Kock pouch and method of intubation and irrigation. The patient must also be informed as to how to react to problems that might arise. The patient must be extremely well motivated to undergo a Kock pouch procedure as there is still a relatively high reoperation rate associated with this procedure. Therefore the suggestion is to provide the patient with as much literature to read as possible, to allow the patient to view a video of the procedure if desired, and most importantly, to speak to other patients who have had both good and poor results from the Kock pouch procedure. This would give the patient an overall perspective of the Kock pouch operation. Patients are informed of preoperative bowel preparation, routine use of antibiotics, and routine use of Heparin anticoagulation. A consent is obtained from the patient based on their knowledge of the procedure and with the information that in a very small number of patients the Kock pouch procedure may not be technically feasible once the abdomen is opened.

Pitfalls and Danger Points

When taking down the ileostomy, the maximum amount of small intestine must be preserved. Devascularization of the outlet can occur by indiscriminately severing too many of the terminal ileal branches. As well, the vascular supply of the nipple valve can be avoided by not placing the stapling device across the mesentery of the intussuscepted segment. The free edge of the mesentery should be mobilized so that construction and placement of the Kock pouch does not produce any undue vascular compromise. Any type of mesh encirclement of the outlet should be avoided as in our experience this has caused erosion and fistula formation in an excessive number of cases. When the Kock pouch is being created in a patient with familial polyposis then the mesentery of the nipple valve should be checked to ensure that there is no desmoplastic reaction present. If it is present, it will make construction of an adequate length nipple valve almost impossible. Upon opening the small bowel limbs used to construct the pouch, the distal-most limb should be opened first to ensure that the mucosa is normal and that one is not dealing with an occult inflammatory process.

Operative Strategy

In most cases a previously made abdominal incision would once again be utilized. The final stoma site can be either at the site of the conventional end ileostomy site or a new site can be chosen, usually on the right side just above the pubic hairline. When a Kock pouch is constructed in conjunction with total proctocolectomy, a midline incision is preferred. One should inspect the entire small bowel before undertaking the procedure, once again to ensure that no occult inflammatory disease exists.

Operative Technique

Take Down of Ileostomy

On entering the abdomen adhesions are taken down, and the entire small bowel is freed and inspected. The ileostomy is taken down by making a circumferential incision around the mucocutaneous site. The everted segment is desuscepted and as much of the small bowel as is possible is preserved. A Kocher clamp or a linear cutting stapler is used across the distal most part of the small intestine to minimize spillage during the operative procedure.

Measurement of the Small Bowel for Creation of the Kock Pouch

Approximately 50 cm of the small bowel will be utilized for the procedure (Fig. 12.1). The distal

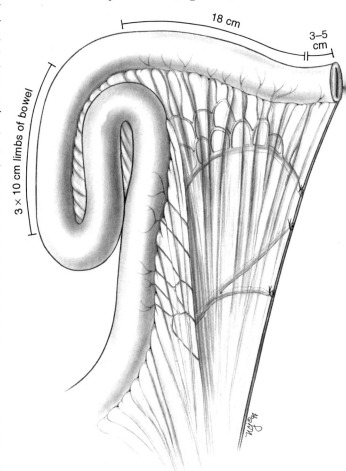

Fig. 12.1. Approximately 50 cm of the small intestine must be used for the Kock pouch procedure.

Fig. 12.2. Careful clearance of the mesentery from the 18 cm segment of small intestine to be intussuscepted greatly increases the possibility of safely forming the valve.

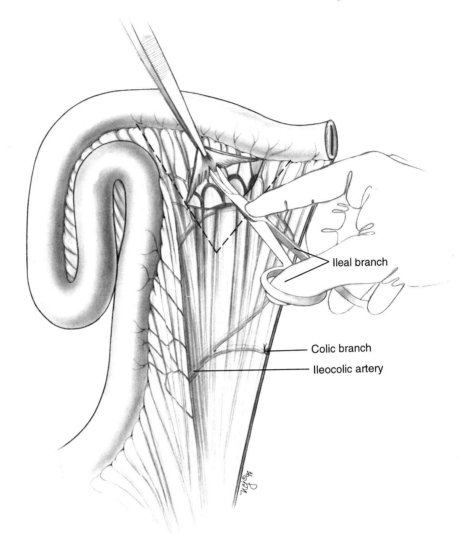

Ileal branch

Colic branch
Ileocolic artery

most 3 to 5 cm will be used for the outlet. This will be somewhat dependent on the thickness of the patient's abdominal wall. The next 18 cm proximal to this will be utilized for construction of the nipple valve and approximately 30 cm will be utilized for the Kock pouch.

Clearance of the "Nipple Valve" Mesentery

The 18 cm segment of the small intestine is isolated to be used for the nipple valve. Using transillumination, the vascular supply to the nipple valve segment can be easily seen and the peritoneum and mesentery over the vascular supply to this segment is excised on both sides of the vessels (Fig. 12.2). This is an important step in the procedure. Skeletonizing the vessels will minimize the thickness of tissue that must be intussuscepted in order to construct the nipple valve.

Creation of the Kock Pouch

There are several different pouch configurations utilized. The originally described Kock pouch (U-shaped pouch) or an S-pouch can be utilized. We have had experience with both pouch configurations and we do not favor any particular type of pouch configuration. More recently we have been using an S-shaped or triplicated pouch. It is important to fold each of the 10-cm limbs with one more cephalad to the other. This will prevent twisting and possible devascularization of the segment of the small intestine on completion of the pouch. The S-shaped pouch is best constructed using two layers of absorbable suture material. The sutures can be placed fairly close to the antimesenteric border of the middle limb but very close to the mesenteric border of the two outer limbs (Fig. 12.3). An incision is then made in the small bowel starting from the most distal portion and progressing proximally. A second posterior layer of absorbable suture material is utilized and su-

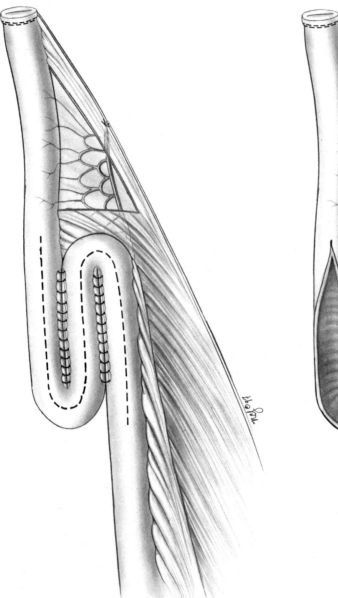

Fig. 12.3.   A triple loop pouch design is commonly used for the Kock pouch. The enterstomy on the middle limb is exactly antimesenteric, while those on the adjacent (outer) loops are tailored to be closer to the mesenteric border near the seromuscular suture line.

Fig. 12.4.   A two-layered closure running of the Kock pouch with absorbable suture is used in forming the pouch.

turing progresses towards the distal portion of the bowel where the intussusception of the nipple valve will occur (Fig. 12.4).

At this point in the operation we utilize either buscopan or glucagon as a muscle relaxant prior to intussuscepting the small intestine and creating the nipple valve. We have recently more successfully used a longer "nipple valve" that we feel decreases the postoperative complication of nipple valve slippage. Therefore approximately a 9-cm nipple valve is created and secured in position with three passes of the GIA 90 stapler without the knife (Fig. 12.5).

The first two passes of the stapler are placed on either side of the mesentery thus causing a bulging effect of the mesentery. The third pass of the stapler is placed on the more anterior aspect of the nipple valve. The anterior aspect of the pouch is then completed again using two layers of absorbable suture material. A row of interrupted sutures is then placed between the outlet and the pouch circumferentially but avoiding the mesentery that has been intussuscepted (Fig. 12.6). These sutures will take the pressure off of the staple line and help to maintain the nipple valve in position. The pouch is now

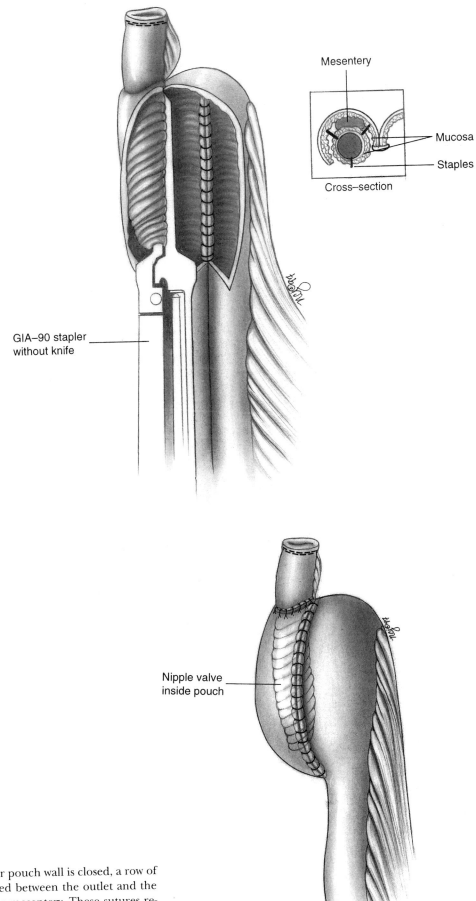

Fig. 12.5. The nipple valve is anchored to the pouch using three firings of a 90 mm gastrointestinal stapler without the knife. *Inset:* Note that placement of the staples are 120 degrees apart, carefully avoiding the mesentery.

Mesentery

Mucosa

Staples

Cross–section

GIA–90 stapler without knife

Nipple valve inside pouch

Fig. 12.6. Once the anterior pouch wall is closed, a row of interrupted sutures are placed between the outlet and the pouch, carefully avoiding the mesentery. These sutures reduce tension on the nipple valve and help hold the valve in position.

completed and can be tested for continence and integrity by inserting a foley catheter or a medina catheter through the outlet and instilling saline or air. A noncrushing intestinal clamp is placed on the afferent limb just above its entrance into the pouch prior to this maneuver. The pouch having been completed, is now ready to be secured to the abdominal wall after fashioning the stomal aperture.

Creation of the Stoma Aperture

If a previous ileostomy has been taken down and the aperture is not too large, then the same site can be utilized for the Kock pouch stoma. If another site is to be chosen, then a site lower in the right lower quadrant can be utilized. There is no necessity to preselect the stoma site in the patient as no appliance will be worn postoperatively. If a new stoma site is chosen, the old site is closed from within as well as from outside the abdominal cavity. A small dime sized circular incision is made in the skin and deepened through the subcutaneous

tissue. A cruciate incision is made in the fascia and the rectus muscle is split longitudinally. It is important to bring the stoma through the rectus muscle at a slightly oblique angle for more support to the stoma sight itself. The peritoneum is then punctured below the rectus muscle. The stoma aperture is widened to approximately two fingerbreadths. A Babcock clamp is then used from the outside and enters through the stoma site. The outlet is grasped and brought loosely through the stoma site. Sutures are then placed on both the lateral and medial aspects of the undersurface of the stoma site and sutured to corresponding points on the pouch itself (Fig. 12.7). These are then tied, in order to secure the pouch to the abdominal wall. The outlet is then placed on slight tension and transected at an appropriate point so that the matured stoma will be flush with the skin. The stoma is matured with either interrupted or continuous absorbable suture material. The pouch is placed dependently in the abdomen on the right side and extending down towards the pelvis.

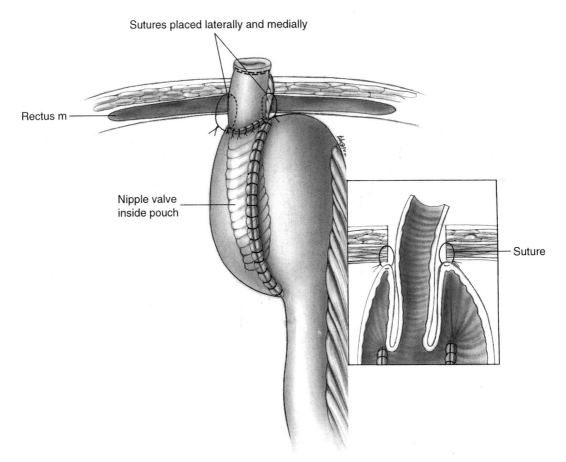

Fig. 12.7.   Completing the Kock pouch procedure involves placement of 4–6 nonabsorbable sutures circumferentially between the pouch outlet and the posterior sheath of the abdominal wall.

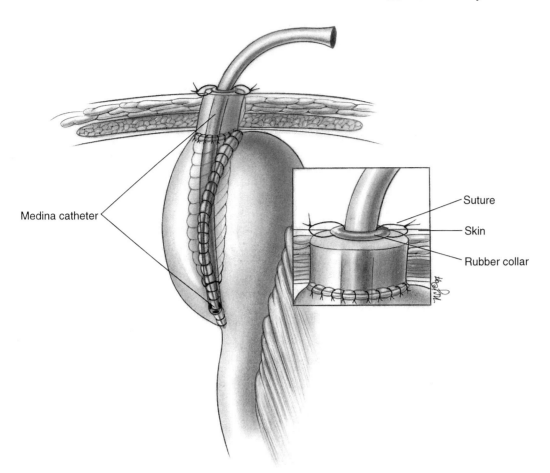

Medina catheter

Suture

Skin

Rubber collar

Fig. 12.8. A curved Medina catheter (a specially designed soft elastic catheter) is inserted into the most dependent portion of the pouch and secured to the abdominal skin using sutures attached to an outer rubber ring adjusted to lie at skin level.

Positioning of the Medina Catheter

A curved Medina catheter is used if possible. A rubber outer ring is placed over the Medina catheter, approximately halfway up the catheter. The catheter is then lubricated and placed within the pouch. One can easily feel when the tube enters the bottom part of the valve and into the pouch. It is very important to note at this point, that there is very little room between the bottom of the valve and the bottom part of the pouch. However, it is essential that the opening in the bottom of the Medina catheter lies beyond the bottom of the valve so that the stool contents can drain from the pouch. The tube is then secured in position by suturing the rubber collar on the Medina catheter to the skin in order to fix the position of the catheter within the pouch (Fig. 12.8). The Medina catheter is then connected to a straight drainage bag. No attempt is made to close the mesenteric defect in the right paracolic gutter. The wound is then closed in the usual manner. An intraabdominal drain is not usually required.

Postoperative Care

The postoperative care of the Kock pouch patient relates mainly to the care of the Medina catheter. In general terms, most of the patients do not require a nasogastric tube. The foley catheter that had been inserted preoperatively is usually removed within 24 to 48 hours. Antibiotics are given for three doses only.

One must be extremely diligent in caring for the Medina catheter. The catheter should be gently irrigated with small amounts of saline to ensure its patency, three times daily, starting the day after the operation. The nurse doing this irrigation must take any dressings from around the stoma away from stoma site so that he/she can assure that there is no irrigation fluid coming up beside the Medina catheter and spilling onto the skin. If this is the case then it can be assumed that the Medina catheter's bottom most opening is either blocked or that the Medina catheter itself is not in the pouch and has slipped back into the valve segment. The Medina catheter is left in situ for 24 days. The patient will usually be discharged from the hospital between the seventh and tenth postoperative days. The patient is instructed to leave the Medina catheter to straight drainage for the first 14 days postoperatively. Thereafter, the catheter is clamped for increasing periods of time to allow for expansion of the Kock pouch. The patient then returns on an outpatient basis on the twenty-fourth postoperative day and the Medina catheter is then removed, the patient is taught the methods of intubation and irrigation and a band aid or simple gauze dressing is placed over the stoma. The patient is once again instructed regarding the potential complications of the pouch and to return immediately if she/he cannot intubate the pouch. Instruction is given with regards to a diet. Initially a post ileostomy low fiber diet is utilized but gradually patients will be able to eat almost all foods. The patients are instructed to empty the pouch on a regular basis at least every four hours for the first two to three

weeks and then at least three to four times daily thereafter. Irrigation is not mandatory unless there is difficulty with the thickness of the stool.

Complications

Slippage of the Nipple Valve

Slippage or desusception of the nipple valve has been the most common complication of the continent ileostomy procedure. It usually occurs within the first three months following surgery but may occur years later. Slippage of the valve usually presents with difficulty or even inability to intubate the pouch. In addition, the pouch usually becomes at least partially incontinent. When patients state that they have difficulty with intubation or that they have a feeling that the tube butts against an end point, and they then have to twist and turn the tube in order to enter the pouch, it usually signifies partial or complete slippage of the nipple valve (Fig. 12.9).

Intact nipple valve

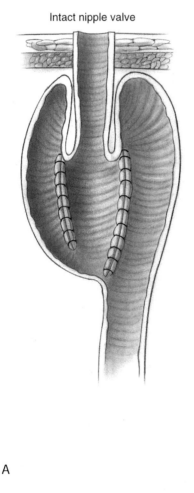

Slippage of nipple valve

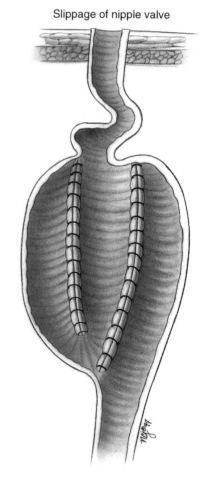

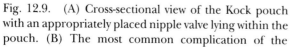

A   B

Fig. 12.9.   (A) Cross-sectional view of the Kock pouch with an appropriately placed nipple valve lying within the pouch. (B) The most common complication of the Kock pouch is the nipple valve slippage, which actually represents "desusception" of the nipple valve, leading to incontinence of the pouch and difficulty intubating it.

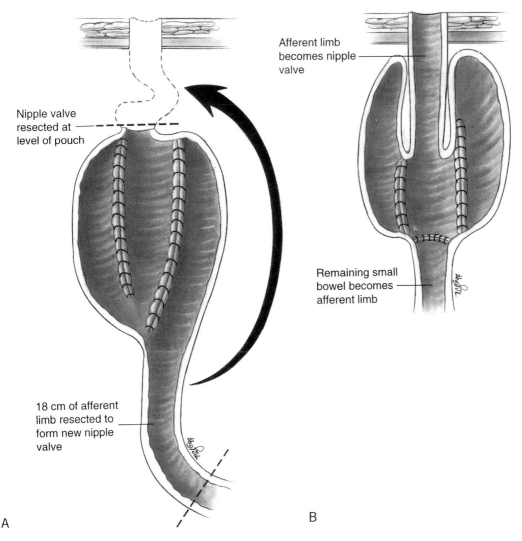

Fig. 12.10. Surgical correction of nipple valve slippage commonly involves resecting the pouch outlet and valve, then rotating the pouch and reforming the afferent limb into the new valve and outlet.

The diagnosis can be confirmed by digital examination of the outlet, or by intubation by the surgeon. Hypaque dripped into the outlet and valve will usually confirm the "hockey stick" deformity that is characteristic of slippage. Placement of a Medina catheter tube to achieve continuous drainage will relieve the problem temporarily, but a definitive solution usually requires surgical intervention. The pouch must be taken down from the abdominal wall, opened, and the nipple valve secured once again, usually with staples. If there is enough length of the nipple valve the same nipple valve can be used as part of reconstruction. The pouch is much larger at this stage than when it was initially constructed. Therefore, the top portion of the pouch can be used as an encirclement around the outlet similar to a Nissen fundoplication to further help secure the valve in place. If, on the other

hand, the valve is too short to reuse, then the nipple valve must be resected and a new one constructed from the afferent limb. The pouch must then be turned 180° around and the afferent limb is anastomosed to the pouch to complete the operation (Fig. 12.10).

Fistulae
These can occur internally or externally and are encountered in 8% to 10% of patients. There is a greater incidence of fistulae when mesh is used in conjunction with the Kock pouch procedure. A fistula through the base of the valve or from the reservoir to the abdominal wound or ileostomy opening may be encountered. A fistula through the base of the valve usually causes incontinence but unlike slippage of the valve the patient has no difficulty with intubation. A fistula may be encoun-

tered at any time after the operation but usually occurs within the first few months. Fistulae from the reservoir to the abdominal wound or to the stoma site can be caused by a leak from the sutures used to secure the reservoir to the abdominal wall or from mesh which may erode at the base of the outlet and result in fistulization. Fazio and Church reported their experience on 168 patients. They encountered 17 fistulae, 12 of which required surgical revision of the continent ileostomy. In six of their 17 fistulae no associated predisposing factor could be established, whereas Crohn's disease and the mesh were considered the cause in four and three patients respectively. Treatment of valve fistulae usually consists of reoperation, excision of the valve, and construction of a new valve using a technique similar to the one described above. Fistulae are more often encountered in those patients with Crohn's disease that inadvertently have Kock pouch after an initial diagnosis of ulcerative colitis. On occasion a complex fistula may require pouch excision.

Intestinal Obstruction

This commonly reported complication is usually secondary to adhesions and is not specific to the procedure. However, early in the postoperative period stool may obstruct the indwelling catheter. In addition, there may be volvulous of small bowel around the continent ileostomy causing obstruction, perforation, and peritonitis. The overall incidence of intestinal obstruction is 6% to 15%, which is comparable to the rate encountered after total proctocolectomy and conventional ileostomy.

Pouchitis

This disorder is a syndrome characterized by crampy abdominal pain, increased watery ileostomy output, discharge, bloating, and general malaise. In severe circumstances the condition might also be associated with weight loss, fever, arthralgias, anemia, increased sedimentation rate, and low serum iron and albumin. The clinical presentation can vary from a minor flu like illness to severe ileitis with general toxicity. The diagnosis should be considered on the basis of the history taken from the patient and confirmed by endoscopy biopsy and histology. The endoscopic appearance usually reveals various degrees of reddened mucosa with contact bleeding and numerous small ulcerations. The etiology of this condition is unknown but its prompt response to broad spectrum antibiotics such as metronidazole suggests it could be bacterial. Reports on the incidence of pouchitis vary considerably from 8% to 40 % depending on the

definition. The risk of developing an episode of pouchitis seems to be highest during the first two years after surgery and patients who do not experience an episode during the first four to five years following surgery are likely to represent a low risk group. Treatment is usually with antibiotics such as Flagyl. This treatment will usually eradicate the problem after a two week course. However, on occasion, pouchitis can be resistant to Flagyl and we have found that a combination of Flagyl and Ciprofloxacin is often effective. In more resistant cases we tend to keep the patient on antibiotics for at least three months. In very severe cases, when all medical therapy has been tried, pouch excision may be necessary.

Valve Necrosis

This complication is attributed to ischemia resulting from excision of the peritoneum and the mesentery from the segment of intestine to be used for the valve or from placement of staples across the mesentery supplying the nipple valve. Necrosis of the valve will produce a failure of the operation in that the patient will be incontinent. The only recourse to this is further surgery and creation of a new valve from the afferent limb as described above.

Volvulous of the Small Bowel

Volvulous of the small bowel around the pouch has been described. This may result in vascular compromise to the small bowel or to the pouch itself. As with any acute vascular compromise, the patient must be urgently operated upon.

Crohn's Disease

Crohn's disease may occur in the reservoir necessitating its ultimate excision. Our own series as well as others, suggests that the complication rate amongst patients with Crohn's disease is significantly higher than patients undergoing the procedure for chronic ulcerative colitis. The subsequent complications because of Crohn's disease may necessitate excision of the pouch. However, a number of patients with Crohn's disease will be able to be maintained on anti-Crohn's disease medication and/or antibiotics while maintaining good pouch function. On at least four occasions we have seen what appears to be typical Crohn's disease in the afferent limb leading into the pouch with relative sparing of the pouch itself. In these cases it is possible to resect the affected portion of the afferent limb and create a new afferent opening into the pouch. The mainstay of treatment of this complication is to avoid reoccurrence by carefully selecting the patients for the continent ileostomy procedure and not performing it in patients with histologically established Crohn's disease or those clinically suspected of having Crohn's disease despite a histological diagnosis of ulcerative colitis. In cases where Crohn's disease has been diagnosed after construction of the pouch and complications encountered of sufficient magnitude, pouch excision may have to be considered.

Outflow Tract Problems

Stenosis and stricture of the outflow tract usually occur at the skin level. These complications can also occur at the junction of the afferent limb and the pouch. When stenosis occurs at the skin level, a local revision can be carried out. When it occurs at the afferent limb and the pouch, a strictureplasty of the valve can be performed. Prolapse and eversion of the valve with incontinence are further complications encountered. Complete prolapse of the valve results in incontinence. It occurs in the presence of a large discrepancy between the diameter of the outflow tract at the base of the valve where the pouch meets the abdominal wall, and the diameter of the ileostomy itself. Stretching of the abdominal wall such as in excessive weight gain or pregnancy may result in prolapse of the valve because of the larger than normal stomal aperture. To deal with this troublesome but infrequent problem, surgical intervention is often necessary. In these situations, the pouch is opened, the valve is secured in its normal position, and if warranted, the stomal aperture is made smaller.

Bibliography

1. Arges MV, Dozois RR, Beahrs OH. Volvulus of the Kock pouch with obstruction and perforation: a case report. Aust N Z J of Surg 1981;51:311–3.
2. Cranley B. The Kock reservoir ileostomy: a review of its development, problems and role in modern surgical practice. Br J Surg 1983;70:94–9.
3. Dozois RR, Kelly KA, Ilstrup D, et al. Factors affecting revision rate after continent ileostomy. Arch Surg 1981;116:610–3.
4. Fazio VW, Church JM. Complications and function of the continent ileostomy at the Cleveland Clinic. World J Surg 1988;12:148–54.
5. Gottlieb LM, Handelsman JC. Treatment of outflow tract problems associated with continent ileostomy (Kock pouch). Report of six cases. Dis Colon Rectum 1991;34:936–40.
6. Handelsman JC, Gottlieb LM, Hamilton SR. Crohn's disesae as a contraindication to Kock pouch (continent ileostomy). Dis Colon Rectum 1993;36:840–3.
7. Kock NG. Ileostomy without external appliances: a survey of 25 patients provided with intra-abdominal intestinal reservois. Ann Surg 1971;173:545–50.
8. McLeod RS, Churchill DN, Lock AM, et al. Quality of life of patients with ulcerative colitis preoperatively and postoperatively. Gastroenterology 1991;101:1307–13.
9. Palmu A, Sivula A. Kock's continent ileostomy: results of 51 operations and experiences with correction of nipple valve insufficiency. Br J Surg 1978;65:645–8.
10. Schrock TR. Complications of continent ileostomy. Am J Surg 1979;138:162–9.

Section II
Ulcerative Colitis

Part II
Surgical Treatment of Specific Complications

Color Plate I

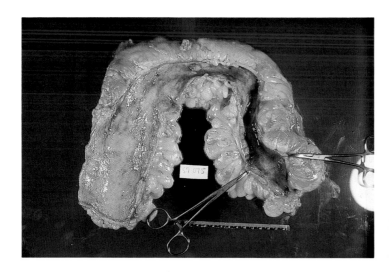

Fig. 4.4. Ulcerative colitis with quiescent disease proximally but with blood oozing from the mucosa distally.

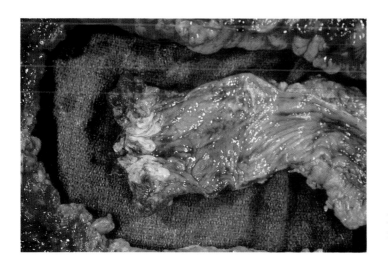

Fig. 4.7. Active ulcerative colitis but with relative rectal sparing at resection ascribed to cecal steroid enemas.

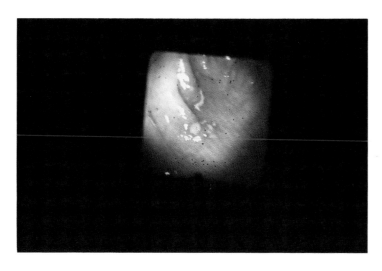

Fig. 4.8. (A) Crohn's disease with aphthoid ulcers forming snail tracks.

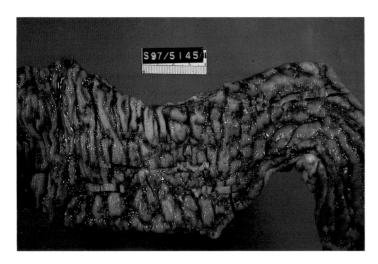

Fig. 4.8. (B) Resected colon showing cobblestoning and aphthoid ulcers some of which have linked up to form transverse and longitudinal ulcers.

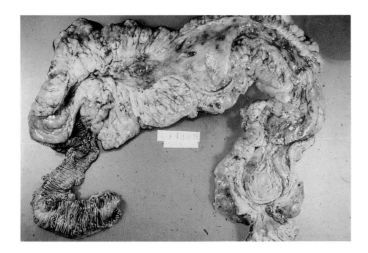

Fig. 4.10. Multiple large bowel strictures in Crohn's disease.

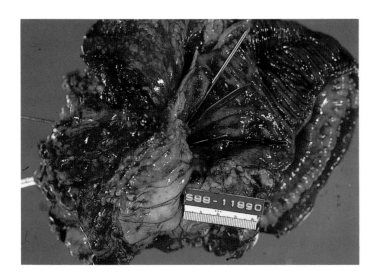

Fig. 4.12. Crohn's disease with multiple fistulas.

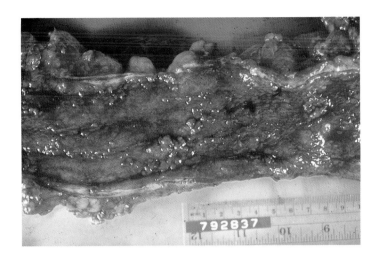

Fig. 4.14. Crohn's disease masquerading as ulcerative colitis. Despite the diffuse colitis there were transmural granulomas histologically.

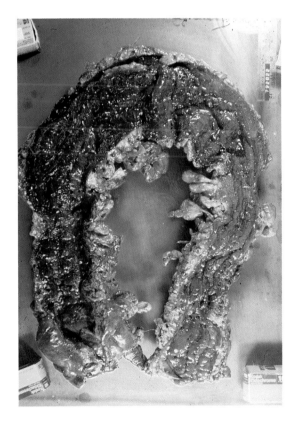

Fig. 4.16. Fulminant ulcerative colitis with disease that is most severe on the left side and with dilatation in the transverse colon.

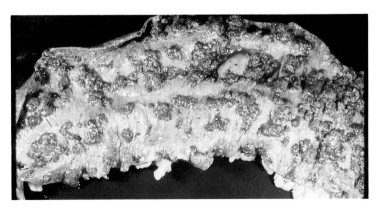

Fig. 4.18. Fulminant colitis (A) Residual mucosal islands and ulceration down to the visible circular muscle.

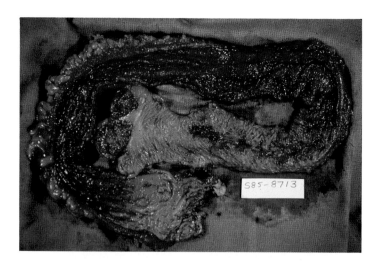

Fig. 4.19. Indeterminate colitis (colitis of unknown etiology), here resulting from rectal sparing (lower right), a transition to apparently diffuse disease but with longitudinal ulcers more proximally, and at the proximal limit of disease multifocal ulcers.

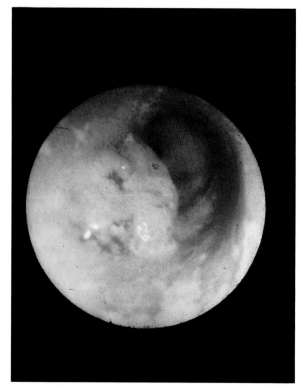

Fig. 4.23. Endoscopic nodular irregularity that was dysplastic on biopsy but proved to be an invasive carcinoma when resected—a so-called dysplasia-associated mass.

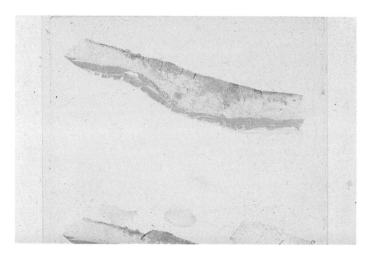

Fig. 4.24. Flat colitis carcinoma that is infiltrating into and expanding the submucosa, and which was an incidental finding in a resection for dysplasia.

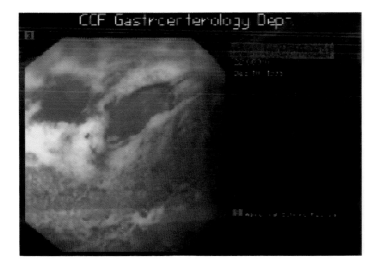

Fig. 5.1. Severe ulcerative colitis, ulcer with detached edges.

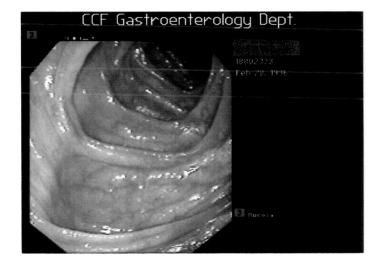

Fig. 5.2. Normal transverse colon.

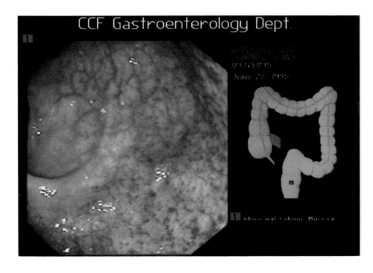

Fig. 5.3. Mild ulcerative proctitis.

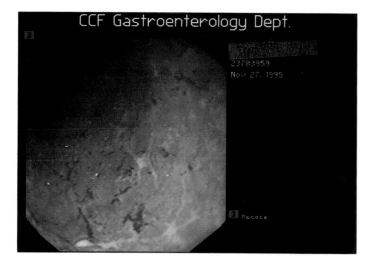

Fig. 5.4. Moderate ulcerative colitis.

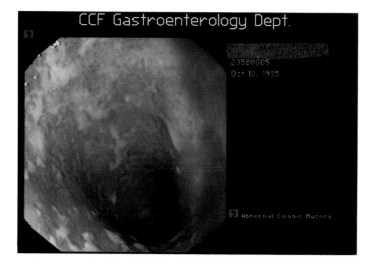

Fig. 5.5. Severe ulcerative colitis, exudate.

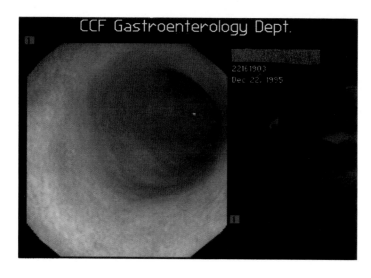

Fig. 5.6. Quiescent chronic ulcerative colitis.

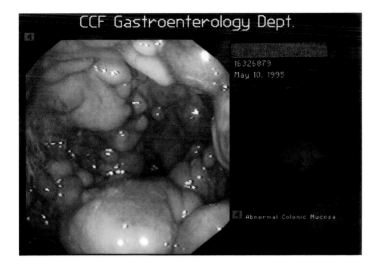

Fig. 5.7. Pseudopolyps in ulcerative colitis.

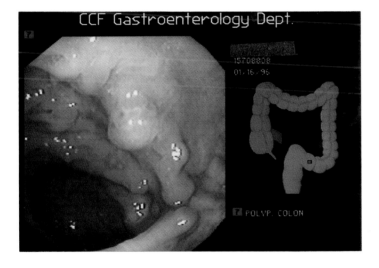

Fig. 5.8. Pseudopolyps in Crohn's disease.

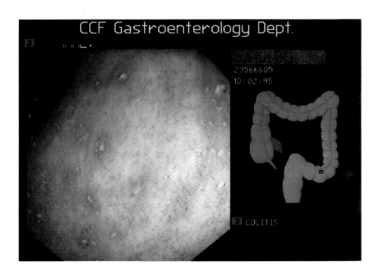

Fig. 5.9. Aphtoid ulcers in the colon.

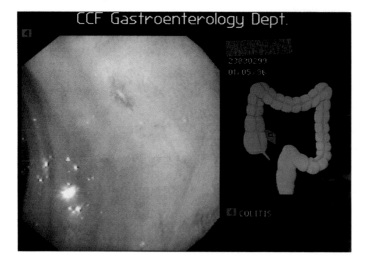

Fig. 5.10. Aphtoid ulcers in the terminal ileum.

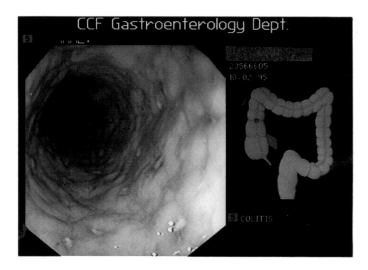

Fig. 5.11. Crohn's disease ulcers.

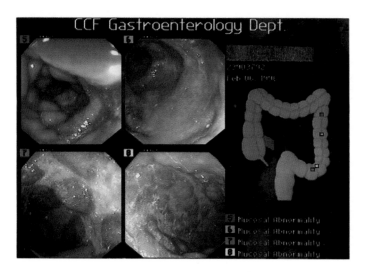

Fig. 5.12. Cobblestoning in Crohn's disease.

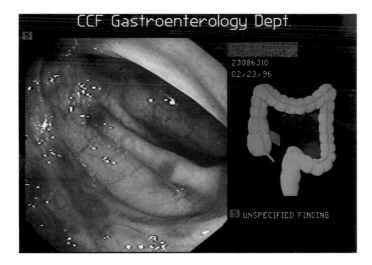

Fig. 5.13.   CMV colitis.

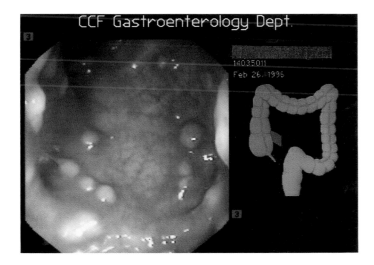

Fig. 5.14.   Pseudomembranous colitis.

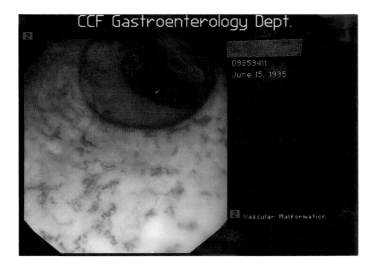

Fig. 5.15. Telangiectasias in radiation proctitis.

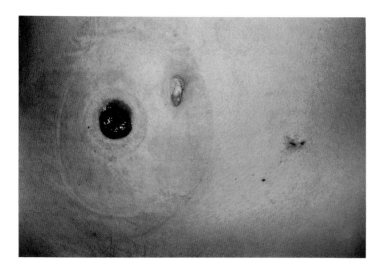

Fig. 23.1. A diverting loop ileostomy may be performed laparoscopically using only two puncture sites, one for the stoma and one in the left lower quadrant.

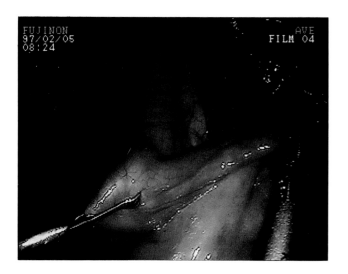

Fig. 23.2. The entire length of the small bowel may be examined laparoscopically by carefully grasping it in a "hand over hand" fashion using laparoscopic graspers.

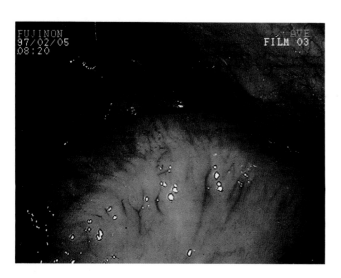

Fig. 23.3. An isolated segment of jejunal Crohn's disease is detected laparoscopically.

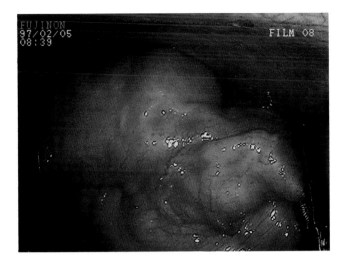

Fig. 23.4. An ileal stricture with proximal dilation is seen laparoscopically.

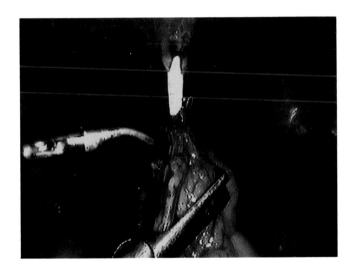

Fig. 23.5. Crohn's disease patients requiring prior percutaneous drainage of a mesenteric abscess may still be approached laparoscopically, carefully dissecting down adhesions with laparoscopic instruments.

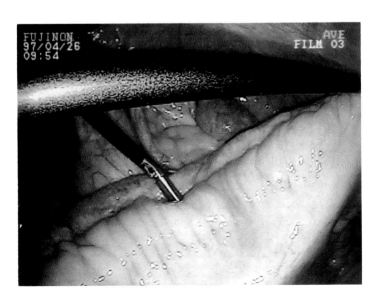

Fig. 23.8. Friability of affected segments of small bowel Crohn's disease mean special care must be taken when grasping with laparoscopic instruments.

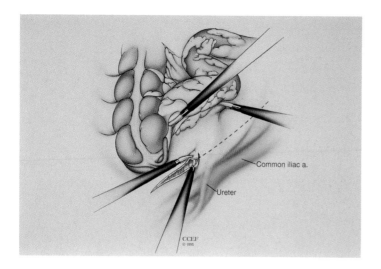

Fig. 23.9. The mesentery of the cecum and ascending colon is dissected retroperitoneally, so a tunnel is created beneath the mesentery in this avascular plane. Using this maneuver, the duodenum, ureter, gonadal vessels, and Gerota's fascia can be readily swept away from the dorsal aspect of the right colonic mesentery.

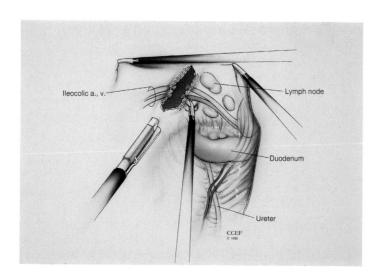

Fig. 23.10. The ileocolic pedicle is isolated from the retroperitoneum. The duodenum and ureter are especially protected and swept clear of the ileocolic vessels.

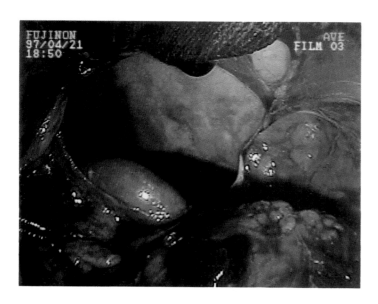

Fig. 23.11. A laparoscopic paddle retractor (at top) holds the intestine anteriorly so dissection of posterior and lateral attrachments may be expedited.

13 Management of Hemorrhage

Rolland Parc, Vianney Roger, and
Christophe Penna

Rectal bleeding is a frequent symptom of ulcerative colitis (1). Although diffuse oozing of blood from the actively diseased bowel does occur in the majority of patients with ulcerative colitis (2), severe or massive hemorrhage is encountered infrequently, but may lead to emergency surgery.

Mild or Moderate Hemorrhage

In the initial phase of the disease, patients complain of passing fresh blood, or bloody mucus, either separately from the stool, or on the surface of the movement. This symptom will often be considered as bleeding hemorrhoids, but patients, particularly those with proctitis, often pass a blood-stained mucus, causing frequent bowel evacuations (pseudodiarrhea), and may even be incontinent of it. When the disease progresses beyond the rectum, blood will be mixed with stool or bloody diarrhea, and frequency of rectal bleeding will decrease from 70% in proctitis to 35% in left-sided colitis or pancolitis as the frequency of diarrhea and abdominal pain will increase (3). When the disease is severe, patients pass a liquid stool containing blood, pus, and feces.

Edwards and Truelove (4) reported that in 20% of the patients with ulcerative colitis, hemoglobin level was under 60% of the normal level (9 g/dL), and in almost all patients, hemoglobin level was between 60% and 80% of the normal level.

Persistent or recurrent blood loss from the bowel may produce anemia of variable severity. The cause of the anemia can be the chronic mild loss of blood that escape attention and will lead to an iron deficiency anemia, but it can also be a severe degree of anemia arising in a short time during the course of an acute attack of colitis, even in the absence of any frank episode of severe bleeding from the bowel.

Other factors that may contribute to the development of anemia in ulcerative colitis include: colonic or rectal carcinoma; hemorrhoids; portal hypertension and coagulopathy resulting from associated liver disease such as sclerosing cholangitis or chronic hepatitis; autoimmune disorder such as thrombocytopenic purpura or hemolytic anemia.

Management of Mild or Moderate Hemorrhage

The management of hemorrhage at this step of the disease is essentially medical. It is the treatment of the active colitis with corticosteroids and then sulfalazine or one of the newer salicylate drugs to maintain remission. For patients with distal colitis, topical therapy with hydrocortisone or 5-aminosalicylic acid (5-ASA) enemas may be effective in decreasing rectal mucosa inflammation and rectal bleeding.

Specific management of hemorrhage include the correction of the anemia. It can be succesfully obtained with iron which sometimes needs to be given parenterally because oral iron is liable to be irritating to the bowel in patients with ulcerative colitis. Only when anemia is severe, blood transfusions are necessary. The risks of blood transfusion should be balanced against the risk of surgery.

Surgical treatment has to be proposed when medical treatment is unable to provide a long-lasting control of the symptoms, and before severe anemia in order to avoid blood transfusion. In this case, a restorative proctocolectomy with J-pouch ileoanal anastomosis is the procedure of choice because it eradicates the disease and it confers good functional results (2–13).

Total colectomy with ileorectal anastomosis provides good functional results when the rectum is relatively spared from the disease, or well controlled by topical steroid administration. This is a rare circumstance. The remaining rectal mucosa carries the risk of neoplastic degeneration estimated to be 10% and 15% respectively at 25 and 30 years (5–7). Thus a close surveillance of the rectal segment is necessary for the patient's life time. In our experience, among 197 patients with ileorectal anastomosis, 25% developed flares up of the disease with rectal bleeding and a secondary rectal excision or rectal exclusion has been necessary in 21% of patients after a 8.6 years median follow-up (7). In the Cleveland clinic experience between 1960 and 1982, the rate of rectal excision in patients having a ileorectal anastomosis after a subtotal colectomy for acute colitis was 30% after a mean follow-up of 8 years (8). Ileorectal anastomosis is indicated when there are doubts as to whether the patient is suffering from ulcerative colitis or Crohn's disease or in older patients. Its place in the treatment of ulcerative colitis today is minimal.

Management of Severe Hemorrhage

In our experience, severe acute hemorragic colitis has been encountered in 2.4% of all ulcerative colitis and 10% of severe acute colitis (14). In a French retrospective multicentric surgical study, including 698 patients operated on for ulcerative colitis, 4.2% of the patients had a severe acute hemorrhagic colitis and 13.6% of the severe acute colitis were hemorrhagic (15). The frequency of severe hemorrhage reported in the literature depends on the definition of severe hemorrhage given by the authors. Some of them, such as Edwards and Truelove (4) considered massive hemorrhage any hemorrhage necessitating transfusion before the acute situation is eventually controlled. They encountered 21 such cases among 624 colitis (3.4%) (4). Others, such as Goligher (16), have reserved the expression "massive hemorrhage" for cases in which the bleeding continues despite transfusion and is an indication for operation. Three such cases among 465 operated ulcerative colitis (0.6%) were encountered in this series (16). In the Mount Sinai experience 25 patients with severe hemorrhage in ulcerative colitis were reported (1.4% of all ulcerative colitis), and among them, 11 patients with massive hemorrhage requiring emergency

colectomy were identified (17). Thus, among patients with severe acute colitis, about 10% have a severe acute hemorrhagic colitis (8,14,15,17,18).

Severe or massive hemorrhage occurs early in the course of the disease with a mean of 2.6 years (17). Most patients with severe hemorrhage have an extensive colitis and almost all patients with massive hemorrhage have a pancolitis (17,18). Inversely, the frequency of severe hemorrhage is the highest among patients with pancolitis (3). Severe bleeding defined as hemorrhage associated with hemoglobin level below 11 g/dL or the need of 4 blood cell units, is a factor associated with extension of the disease (3). These observations tend to suggest that the severity of hemorrhage in ulcerative colitis is related to the extent as well as the severity of the desease.

This is an important differentiation from Crohn's disease. In ulcerative colitis, the bleeding may be diffuse, from large areas of ulcerated mucosa, though in Crohn's disease, the bleeding is often from a localized source and is caused by erosion of a blood vessel within multiple deep ulcerations that extend into the submucosa or deeper layers of the intestinal wall.

Management of Massive Hemorrhage

A dramatic reduction in postoperative mortality associated with surgery in complicated acute ulcerative colitis (toxic megacolon, fulminant colitis, and massive hemorrhage) has been obtained by an earlier referral of patients for operation (14,16). In severe acute hemorrhagic colitis, the intensive medical care with close surveillance, the timing for surgery, the choice of an appropriate surgical procedure are all of importance to a satisfactory outcome.

The preoperative management in hemorrhagic severe acute colitis is based on adequate fluid resuscitation, blood transfusions, correction of electrolyte and coagulation abnormalities, monitoring of hemodynamic parameters, urine output, and peripheral perfusion (14,19).

Hemorrhage responsible for anemia below 6 g/dL and/or requiring 4 to 6 units of packed red cells are indications for urgent surgery. Massive hemorrhage with shock resistant to resuscitation is an indication for immediate operation. Sometimes, toxic megacolon is associated with massive hemorrhage. Such association in patients with ulcerative colitis requires surgery within 6 hours after intensive resuscitation.

Bowel preparation is contraindicated. The patient is informed of the procedure and its consequences. He or she must also know that a restorative procedure will need to be performed at a later date. The site of the stoma is marked preoperatively.

The goal of surgery in emergency is not to eradicate all the diseased mucosa, but to extricate the patient from a life-threatening situation. Although, subtotal colectomy with ileostomy and mucous sigmoid fistula is now considered as the procedure of choice in emergency, massive hemorrhage arises the question as to whether resection of the rectum will be necessary to control the hemorrhage. Several procedures have been proposed to treat life-threatening fulminant ulcerative colitis.

Total Proctocolectomy with Ileostomy

Many years ago, proctocolectomy was advised as the operation of choice for patients requiring elective colectomy for ulcerative colitis. This procedure was also recommended in the emergency situation by many authors (20,21). Surgeons who advocated emergency subtotal colectomy in severe attacks of ulcerative colitis in hemorrhagic forms of severe colitis recommended a total proctocolectomy in order to avoid persisting hemorrhage from the rectum (22,23). The advantage lyes in treating the disease completely using a one stage procedure and in eradicating the possibility of further hemorrhage. However, the reported mortality has been high, varying from 8% (20), 9% (18), to 14% (23). In addition, this procedure eliminates the chance for a subsequent sphincter-saving operation (ileorectal or ileal-pouch-anal anastomosis). Thus, we do not advocate this operation as the initial procedure in the treatment of hemorrhage from ulcerative colitis.

Total Colectomy, Ileostomy, and Hartmann's Procedure

This procedure offers the possibility of a subsequent sphincter saving operation and it is the procedure of choice used by many surgeons. However, the previous colectomy may cause a higher incidence of small bowel obstruction and poorer functional results of the subsequent ileal-pouch-anal anastomosis (24). Despite a shorter rectal remnant, this procedure is associated with a high rate of persistent hemorrhage, compared with subtotal colectomy, ileostomy, and sigmoidostomy (25). A persistent hemorrhage in the remnant rectum is

difficult to control. In addition, a subsequent proctectomy with ileal-pouch-anal anastomosis is more difficult if the rectum is transected in the pelvis and the pouch is left short. For this reason it is advisable to transect the rectum in front of the sacral promontory. Hartmann's procedure may be indicated in cases of patients with recurrent intractable hemorrhage early after subtotal colectomy when the general status of the patient would make an ileal-pouch-anal anastomosis dangerous. In such cases, the level of rectal section should be low in order to avoid recurence of hemorrhage, but should also preserve the sphincter, in order to allow a subsequent ileal-pouch-anal procedure.

Subtotal Colectomy with Ileorectal Anastomosis

This procedure has been advocated in acute colitis in order to preserve the rectum. The long-term rate of secondary proctectomy is higher when ileorectal anastomosis has been performed in patients with a severe acute colitis than in elective patients (8). When severe hemorrhage is the indication for an emergency operation, an ileorectal anastomosis should not be considered because continued bleeding is inevitable and is associated with a high rate of anastomotic dehiscence (26).

Subtotal Colectomy, Ileostomy, and Sigmoid Mucous Fistula

This procedure has been adopted as the procedure of choice by many teams (8,19,25,27). It is a quick and easy procedure, removing the majority of the diseased mucosa and eradicates the toxic syndrome. The anal sphincter is preserved, giving the choice of a subsequent sphincter-saving procedure. It allows histologic examination of the colon, and adapted surgery: ileorectostomy for Crohn's colitis and ileal-pouch-anal anastomosis for ulcerative colitis. The mortality and morbidity rates are reduced by avoiding emergency rectal excision (28). In our experience, this procedure did not increase the morbidity of subsequent ileal-pouch-anal anastomosis and was associated with a more rapid functional recovery (19). The risk of persistent massive rectal bleeding, requiring emergency proctectomy is estimated between 4% (27) and 12% (17). In the Mount Sinai experience, 17 patients were operated on for severe bleeding and had a subtotal colectomy. Continued massive rectal bleeding requiring immediate proctectomy was not seen in any patient after subtotal colectomy (17).

In our experience, the surgical management of acute hemorrhagic colitis is the emergency subtotal colectomy, ileostomy and sigmoid mucos fistula. Persistent significant bleeding in the remaining colon and rectum is rare and can be treated with saline enemas with epinephrine (1 mg in 100 mL of saline) or by tamponading the rectal stamp with an epinephrine-soaked gauze. In most cases, hemorrhage will be controlled with this procedure, and an ileal-pouch-anal anastomosis will be considered 2 to 4 months later. In extremely rare cases, an intractable hemorrhage may have to be treated with an emergency completion abdominal proctectomy with transection of the rectum at the level of the levator muscles and preservation of the anal sphincter for further use in a J-pouch ileoanal anastomosis.

Conclusion

Rectal bleeding is the main symptom of ulcerative colitis. Its management is based on the treatment of ulcerative colitis: first medical and then surgical in persistent forms. Massive hemorrhage is a rare life-threatening complication that may lead to emergency surgery. In our experience, massive hemorrhage occurs in about 10% of patients with severe acute colitis. The preferred acute surgical management is a subtotal colectomy, ileostomy and sigmoidostomy or a total colectomy, ileostomy and Hartmann pouch.

References

1. Both H, Torp-Pedersen K, Kreiner S, et al. Clinical appearance at diagnosis of ulcerative colitis and Crohn's disease in a regional patient group. Scand J Gastroenterol 1983;18:987–91.

2. Farmer RG, Hamilton SR, Morson BC, et al. Ulcerative colitis. In: Haubrich WS, Kalser MH, Roth JLA, Schaffner F, eds. Gastroenterology. Berk EJ, ed. W B Saunders 1985:2137–221, vol 5.

3. Farmer RG, Easley KA, Rankin GB. Clinical patterns, natural history, and progression of ulcerative colitis. A long term follow-up of 1116 patients. Dig Dis Sci 1993;38(6):1137–48.

4. Edwards FC, Truelove SC. The course and prognosis of ulcerative colitis. Gut 1964;5:1–22.

5. Aylet AO. Cancer and ulcerative colitis. Br Med J 1971;1:203.

6. Baker WN, Glass RE, Ritchie JE, et al. Cancer of the rectum following colectomy and ileo-rectal anastomosis for ulcerative colitis. Br J Surg 1978;65:862–8.

7. Parc R, Legrand M, Frileux P, et al. Comparative clinical results of ileal-pouch-anal anastomosis in ulcerative colitis. Hepato-gastroenterol 1989;36:235–9.

8. Oakley JR, Lavery IC, Fazio VW, et al. The fate of the rectal stump after subtotal colectomy for ulcerative colitis. Dis Colon Rectum 1985;28:394–6.

9. McIntyre PB, Pemberton JH, Wolff BG, et al. Comparing funtional results one year and ten years after ileal-pouch-anal anastomosis for chronic ulcerative colitis. Dis Colon Rectum 1994;37:303–7.

10. Daudé F, Penna C, Tiret E, et al. Résultats de l'anastomose iléo-anale avec mucosectomie et réservoir en J dans la rectocolite hémorragique. Gastroenterol Clin Biol 1994;18:462–8.

11. Fazio VW, Ziv Y, Church JM, et al. Ileal-pouch-anal anastomoses complications and function in 1005 patients. Ann Surg 1995;222:120–7.

12. Penna C, Dozois R, Tremaine W, et al. Pouchitis after ileal-pouch-anal anstomosis for ulcerative colitis occurs with increased frequency in patients with associated primary sclerosing cholangitis. Gut 1996;38:234–9.

13. Truelove SC, Witts LJ. Cortisone in ulcerative colitis: final report on a therapeutic trial. Br Med J 1955;2:1041–8.

14. Lévy E, Cosnes J, Bognel JC, et al. Le syndrome de colite aigüe grave et ses éléments de pronostic (100 cas). Gastroentérol Clin Biol 1979;15:123–7.

15. Bérard P, Parc R, Frileux P, et al. Le traitement de la recto-colite ulcéro-hémorragique. Paris: Masson, 1984:93. (Chirurgie AFd, ed. Monographies de l'Association Française de Chirurgie; vol 1).

16. Goligher JC, Duthie HL, Nixon HH. Surgery of the anus, rectum and colon. 3rd ed. London: Baillere Tindall, 1980.

17. Robert JH, Sachar DB, Aufses AH, et al. Management of severe hemorrhage in ulcerative colitis. Am J Surg 1990;159:550–5.

18. Binder SC, Miller HH, Deterling RA. Emergency and urgent operations for ulcerative colitis. The procedure of choice. Arch Surg 1975;110:284–9.

19. Penna C, Daudé F, Parc R, et al. Previous subtotal colectomy with ileostomy and sigmoidostomy improves morbidity and early functional results after ileoanal anastomosis for ulcerative colitis. Dis Colon Rectum 1993;36:4, 343–8

20. Goligher JC, Hoffman DC, DeDombal FT. Surgical treatment of severe attacks of ulcerative colitis with special reference to the advantages of early operation. Br Med J 1970;4:703–6.

21. Binder SC, Patterson JF, Glotzer DJ. Toxic megacolon in ulcerative colitis. Gastroenterology 1974;66:909–15.

22. Albrechtsen D, Bergan A, Nygaard K, et al. Urgent colectomy for ulcerative colitis: early colectomy in 132 patients. World J Surg 1981;5:607–15.

23. Block GE, Moossa AR, Simonowitz D, et al. Emergency colectomy for inflammatory bowel disease. Surgery 1977;82:531–6.

24. Zenilman ME, Soper NJ, Dunnegan D, et al. Previous abdominal colectomy affects functional results after

ileal-pouch-anal anastomosis. World J Surg 1990;14:
594–9.

25. Carter FM, McLeod RS, Cohen Z. Subtotal colectomy for ulcerative colitis: complications related to the rectal remnant. Dis Colon Rectum 1991;34(11): 1005–9.

26. Mann CV. Total colectomy and ileo-rectal anastomosis for ulcerative colitis. World J Surg 1988;12: 155–9.

27. Korelitz BI, Dyck WP, Klion F. Fate of the rectum and distal colon after subtotal colectomy for ulcerative colitis. Gut 1969;10:198–201.

28. Hawley PR. Emergency surgery for ulcerative colitis. World J Surg 1988;12:169–73.

14 Toxic Colitis and Perforation

Joe J. Tjandra

Ulcerative colitis may range in severity from chronic and low-grade clinical condition to an acute and fulminating surgical emergency. It may involve the rectum only (proctitis), where the disease usually starts, or extend proximally to involve contiguously part or whole of the colon. This chapter is specifically concerned with patients in whom an emergent or urgent colectomy is needed because of toxic colitis and/or perforation. The colon itself may or may not be dilated in the toxic state, and thus the term megacolon may be misleading.

Acute Fulminant Colitis

The terms "acute," "toxic," and "fulminant" are used almost synonymously to describe very ill patients with ulcerative colitis. Acute colitis is characterized by the abrupt onset of bloody diarrhea, urgency, abdominal colic, and anorexia. Patients often are ill with severe anemia and dehydration. Overall, this condition occurs in approximately 10% of patients with ulcerative colitis. Severe attacks may occur as the first manifestation of the disease or during the course of a chronic illness.

A patient is considered to be toxic if, in addition to severe colitis, at least two of the following are present:

1. Tachycardia > 100/min.
2. Temperature > 38.6°C.
3. Leukocytosis > 10.5×10^3/L.
4. Hypoalbuminemia < 3.0 g/100 mL.

These patients often present with frequency and urgency in passing stool, dehydration, fever, tachycardia, anemia, hyponatremic, and hypokalemic al-

kalosis (1). Aggressive medical therapy should be initiated immediately. If their clinical status does not improve significantly within 24 to 48 hours, or if deterioration develops, surgery should be undertaken. With such an aggressive and effective coordinated approach, the mortality of fulminant colitis has fallen to less than 3% (2).

Toxic Megacolon

Toxic megacolon usually occurs in patients with extensive colitis but may also develop in those with only left-sided colitis. It represents the most serious and life-threatening complication that can occur in patients with acute fulminant colitis. It is part of the spectrum of an acute severe attack of colitis rather than a separate entity. Toxic dilatation or "megacolon" is generally defined as a diameter of the transverse colon exceeding 5.5 cm on a supine plain radiograph of the abdomen. However, dilatation may also affect the cecum, descending, and sigmoid colon. These patients usually are severely ill with abdominal distension and tenderness, increased stool frequency, fever, tachycardia, severe dehydration, and leukocytosis. However, signs of septicemia may be masked by the use of steroids resulting in a delayed diagnosis. The definition of acute fulminant colitis is not a rigid one, as patients may develop toxicity without megacolon or megacolon without severe toxic signs. These patients may not fulfill all the listed criteria for an acute severe attack but require the same aggressive management.

Toxic colitis used to occur in about 6% of hospitalized patients with ulcerative colitis (3) but its incidence is falling with more effective and coordinated medical and surgical management. Contributing factors include hypokalemia, anticholinergics and barium sulfate from barium enema. Toxic colitis or "megacolon" may also be the initial manifestion of ulcerative colitis. Other less common causes of toxic colitis include Crohn's disease, infection, ischemia, and pseudomembranous colitis. Toxic colitis is more common in ulcerative colitis than in Crohn's disease (4), and it tends to occur after a longer duration of illness and at an older age than with Crohn's colitis (5).

Toxic colitis or "megacolon" has a high risk of colonic perforation and consequently high mortality. The overall mortality is 30% with perforation compared with 4% without perforation (6). Urgent surgery is generally indicated after a period of medical stabilization and optimization. Whereas 30% of patients with toxic megacolon may respond to conservative therapy, thereby avoiding emergency surgery (7), most would ultimately have a colectomy because of repeated episodes of toxic dilatation (8) or incapacitating chronic symptoms (9).

Perforation

This occurs in 2% of patients with ulcerative colitis and is usually associated with toxic colitis or "megacolon" (10). The risk of perforation is highest at the time of the first attack and correlates with the extent and severity of the disease. Toxic megacolon with mucosal islands indicates impending perforation. Diagnosis may be delayed as the signs of peritonism may be masked by high dose steroids. There is generally increasing abdominal or shoulder pain but the only indication may be increased toxicity with fever and tachycardia. The clinician should maintain a high index of suspicion for perforation in monitoring the progress of any patient with toxic colitis.

Initial Investigations

Patients with an attack of severe colitis should be admitted to the hospital. Initial investigations include a complete blood count, a serum biochemical profile, blood cultures and coagulation studies. A plain radiograph of the abdomen and a chest x-ray in the upright position is obtained to detect colonic dilatation and any free intraperitoneal gas from colonic perforation.

If an infectious etiology is likely, an urgent stool culture is collected and tested for *Campylobacter, Salmonella, Shigella*, pathogenic *Escherischia Coli*, amoeba, and *Clostridium difficile*. A limited proctoscopic or flexible sigmoidoscopic examination with superficial biopsy is performed, especially in patients without a prior diagnosis of inflammatory bowel disease, so as to rule out pseudomembranous colitis and ischemic colitis. Colonoscopy and barium enema are contraindicated in acute fulminant colitis. Specific therapy for inflammatory bowel disease should be commenced prior to results of stool cultures and rectal biopsy, unless there are doubts about the diagnosis.

Medical Management

Adequate medical management and preparation for surgery is mandatory. Except in extreme urgency, psychological counselling with explanation of the surgical options should be provided since stoma is usually necessary. Narcotics are used with caution as they may obscure signs of peritonitis and may exacerbate toxic dilatation. Antidiarrheal agents are contraindicated as they may further exacerbate toxic megacolon.

Resuscitation

Intravenous fluids and electrolytes are initiated to correct dehydration, hyponatremia, and hypokalemia. Normal saline with potassium supplements are the most commonly used solutions. Blood transfusion is sometimes given to patients with profound anemia especially if surgery is contemplated. A central venous catheter is sometimes inserted for hyperalimentation and for monitoring hydration. A nasogastric tube is not used routinely unless the ileus is profound.

Steroids

Intravenous steroids are the mainstay of specific medical treatment for toxic megacolon. Hydrocortisone 100 mg is given every 6 hours intravenously. In patients achieving a good response, the steroid dose is gradually reduced after 4 to 5 days and changed to oral prednisone. Immunosuppressive agents have little place in the treatment of toxic megacolon, although there are reports describing the use of cyclosporine under carefully controlled circumstances leading to an acute remission in the majority of patients (11).

Antibiotics

With toxic megacolon, the bowel is friable and is associated with microperforation. Antibiotics effective against aerobic and anaerobic organisms are used although there is no convincing report that they alter the course of the disease process.

An effective parenteral regime includes a second or third generation cephalosporin and metronidazole.

Monitoring

Regular clinical evaluation is performed together with monitoring of pulse, blood pressure, temperature, stool frequency and consistency, hydration, abdominal girth, plain radiographs of the abdomen, and routine blood tests including complete blood count and serum biochemical profile. On our unit, we attempt to perform a clinical examination at least every 4 to 6 hours.

Indications for Surgery

Emergency surgery is indicated if there is free perforation or generalized peritonitis (11). Development of a true toxic megacolon (with transverse colon diameter greater than 5 cm on plain abdominal radiograph) is usually, but not always, an indication for early surgery. Surgery is indicated if there is no clear improvement after initiation of adequate medical management or if there is deterioration at any time after admission, such as increasing colonic dilatation and abdominal tenderness or worsening signs of toxicity. Plain radiograph of the abdomen is performed twice daily initially. An increasing colonic dilatation is a sinister event and calls for an urgent surgery. A paradoxical reduction in stool frequency may result from increasing ileus secondary to worsening toxicity rather than an overall improvement.

If, after 5 to 7 days, the improvement has been minor and there are still signs of toxicity such as tachycardia, fever, leukocytosis, and frequent bloody diarrhea, surgery is still indicated as there is little likelihood of sustaining a long-term remission. Some patients respond to medical management but continue to have low-grade active disease requiring high dose oral medications. Most of these patients ultimately require elective surgery.

Perioperative Preparation

The patient and family are counselled jointly by the gastroenterologist and the colorectal surgeon. The need for a stoma is discussed and the stoma site marked preoperatively. The stoma is usually temporary rather than permanent unless Crohn's disease is suspected because of associated anorectal suppuration. The patient is counselled that ileal pouch-anal anastomosis surgery may be feasible 3 to 6 months after the initial operation, provided that recovery has been satisfactory and the diagnosis of Crohn's disease has been satisfactorily ruled out.

Nutritional requirements are important, especially if a period of bowel rest appears likely. Patients requiring urgent surgery are often malnourished and may benefit from hyperalimentation perioperatively. Fluid and electrolytes should be fully replenished. Parenteral antibiotics are given perioperatively. Mechanical bowel preparations are contraindicated in urgent surgery.

Intermittent pneumatic compression stockings are routinely used. Steroids are continued after surgery and tapered gradually over several months if a patient has taken steroids within 12 months before surgery.

Choice of Operations

The optimal operation for both toxic megacolon and perforation is *subtotal colectomy with end ileostomy* (11). It is a simple procedure that removes most of the diseased large bowel and avoids an anastomosis in a critically ill patient. In acute colitis, differentiation between ulcerative colitis and Crohn's disease in the newly diagnosed cases may be confusing, even following histopathologic examination of the colectomy specimen (12). A staged procedure with colectomy and ileostomy preserves the anorectum and allows subsequent restorative ileoanal pouch surgery electively when the patient is healthy and on minimal anticolitic medications (13). Occasionally, persistent bleeding from the retained rectal stump may occur following colectomy, requiring topical and rarely parenteral steroids for control.

The principal alternative is *total proctocolectomy and permanent ileostomy*. This was once a popular treatment for acute colitis (14). It now has little place in the acute setting because of the increased morbidity and mortality associated with urgent or emergency proctectomy (2). The pelvic dissection is associated with major blood loss because of active proctitis. There is also an increased risk of pelvic sepsis, small bowel obstruction and damage to pelvic autonomic nerves. It is important nowadays to preserve the anal sphincter mechanism for possible later ileoanal pouch surgery. Total proctocolectomy and a permanent ileostomy may have a limited role in toxic colitis with profuse bleeding from the rectum. Even then, an ultralow Hartmann's closure of the rectum at the level of the levator floor with preservation of the anal sphincters is preferred. An "ultralow" Hartmann's procedure is preferable to a formal proctocolectomy because it avoids a perineal wound and may still permit a delayed ileoanal pouch surgery in the future. However even this more conservative option is not without its problems in severe inflammatory bowel disease (15), as, the tissues may be so friable that a stapled or sutured closure is not possible.

Subtotal Colectomy and Ileostomy—The Procedure

Preparation

The patient is anesthetized and a gentle examination under anesthesia with a rigid sigmoidoscope is performed to assess the degree of rectal inflammation. Evidence of perianal disease should be noted. The patient is placed supine and the abdomen is cleansed with antiseptic skin preparation and draped in the standard fashion. A nasogastric tube is helpful to decompress the stomach.

Laparotomy

A vertical midline incision is made based on the umbilicus, so as not to compromise potential sites of future stomas. It is not necessary to extend the incision distally as far as the pubic tubercle, as rectal dissection is not performed. Any free fluid is taken for culture and the presence of a feculent odor suggests a free colonic perforation. The colon is handled with extreme care and presence of any potential perforation is noted. This usually manifests itself as dense serosal attachment of the colon to omentum, parietes or other viscera. Careless mobilization of the colon in this situation may lead to colonic disruption and massive and uncontrolled fecal spillage. Sometimes, sealed perforations are present on the retroperitoneal aspect of the colon, becoming obvious only after full mobilization.

With extreme gaseous distension, gentle decompression of the colon through the rectal tube is helpful. Rarely, a decompressive colotomy in the transverse colon may be necessary. Careful placement of large mops to quarantine the surrounding strictures is essential prior to decompressive colotomy. A soft and curved noncrushing clamp may be more effective than a pursestring in the control of a decompressive colotomy in a friable bowel to avoid fecal spillage.

The entire small bowel from the duodenojejunal flexure to the terminal ileum is carefully examined for evidence of unsuspecting Crohn's disease. If a segment of omentum or peritoneum is adherent to a friable colon, the omentum or a segment of the pericolic peritoneum are resected together with the colon to minimize risk of iatrogenic perforation.

Colectomy

The colon is usually very distended and may be easily perforated even with careful handling. The most likely points of perforation are the splenic and hepatic flexures. Extreme care is essential and a densely adherent omentum should not be disturbed as it may contain a sealed perforation.

The colectomy is started by mobilizing the right colon and the peritoneum below the terminal ileum. A large pack is placed over the small bowel that is displaced towards the left. The terminal ileum is mobilized only enough to allow the small bowel to reach the anterior abdominal wall as an end ileostomy. The peritoneal reflection on the lateral side of the right colon is divided and by gentle finger dissection, the right colon and the mesentery are mobilized medially from their retroperitoneal position. Care is taken to avoid trauma to the duodenum.

The transverse colon is next mobilized. If the omentum is adherent to the transverse colon, it is resected with the colon by dividing the epiploic vessels from the gastroepiploic vessels. If not adherent, the greater omentum may be preserved by dissecting it from the transverse colon. This is started to the left of the middle colic vessels as it is easier to enter the lesser sac in that site. Dissection is then carried towards the hepatic flexure. Dissection in the lesser sac should be relatively avascular. The extreme right side of the omentum is resected which allows easier mobilization of the hepatic flexure.

The sigmoid and descending colon are next mobilized, prior to mobilizing the splenic flexure. The small bowel is transferred to the right side, wrapped in a large laparotomy pad. The sigmoid colon is held in the surgeon's hand. The lateral congenital adhesions and peritoneal reflection are carefully divided in the avascular plane, taking care to preserve the gonadal vessels and the left ureter.

Several large laparotomy pads are placed in the left paracolic gutter and over the small bowel to quarantine the splenic flexure region prior to its mobilization. This is a common site for iatrogenic perforation, particularly if the colon is grossly distended and the splenic flexure is excessively high. A second assistant next lifts up the left costal margin to fully expose the splenic flexure region. The incision may be extended cephaled if necessary. Mobilization of the left side of the transverse colon

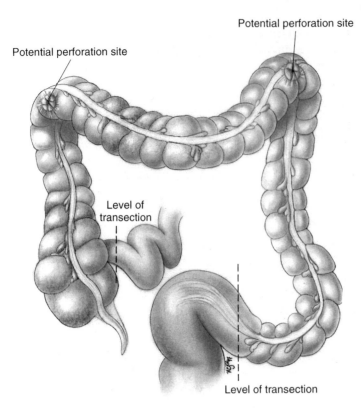

Potential perforation site

Potential perforation site

Level of
transection

Level of transection

Fig. 14.1.　Abdominal colectomy and preservation of rectal stump.

with division of the extreme left of the greater omentum is performed. The ileocolic ligament is divided and the splenic flexure gently teased away from the spleen. If a sealed perforation is present, the relevant segment of omentum or peritoneum is excised in continuity.

The mesenteric vessels are then ligated and divided close to the colon, taking care to preserve the main ileocolic and superior mesenteric vessels for future ileoanal pouch construction. The right and left branch of the middle colic vessels are divided separately. The upper and lower left colic vessels are also divided. The sigmoid arcades are divided close to the colon and the main inferior mesenteric vessels are preserved so as not to traumatize the preaortic sympathetic nerves (11). Little or no dissection is performed in the pelvis to minimize risk of sepsis and to facilitate a future ileoanal pouch. Once the mesenteric vessels are divided, the bowel ends are divided between clamps or staples (Fig. 14.1). The proximal line of division is just before the ileocecal valve and the terminal ileum is maximally preserved as construction of an ileal pouch may be done in the future. Distally the colon is transected just proximal to the rectosigmoid junction, leaving enough length of the sigmoid colon to allow it to reach the anterior abdominal wall.

Distal Rectosigmoid Stump

Management of the distal rectosigmoid stump is controversial. It may be closed and implanted subcutaneously at the lower end of the abdominal incision (16) or through a separate paramedian site (17). Alternatively it is exteriorized as a mucous fistula at the distal end of the abdominal wound (18) or through a separate site away from the main wound so as to minimize risk of wound infection (2,19) or left as a Hartmann's pouch (20).

We favor staple-transection of the distal sigmoid colon using a linear stapler, at a level that the retained rectosigmoid stump will reach the lower end of the midline incision without tension (Fig. 14.2). Advantages of leaving a long rectosigmoid stump include easier identification of the stump, fewer pelvic adhesions and thus easier pelvic mobilization, less operative blood loss and shorter operating time (21). By contrast, there is no apparent advantage between a long (25 cm) or ultralong (35 cm) rectosigmoid stump (22). The rectosigmoid stump is extraperitonealized by suturing the seromuscular layer of the bowel circumferentially to the peritoneum. The stump may also be exteriorized above the rectus sheath and implanted subcutaneously. The skin overlying this site is left open. In the event that the rectosigmoid stump

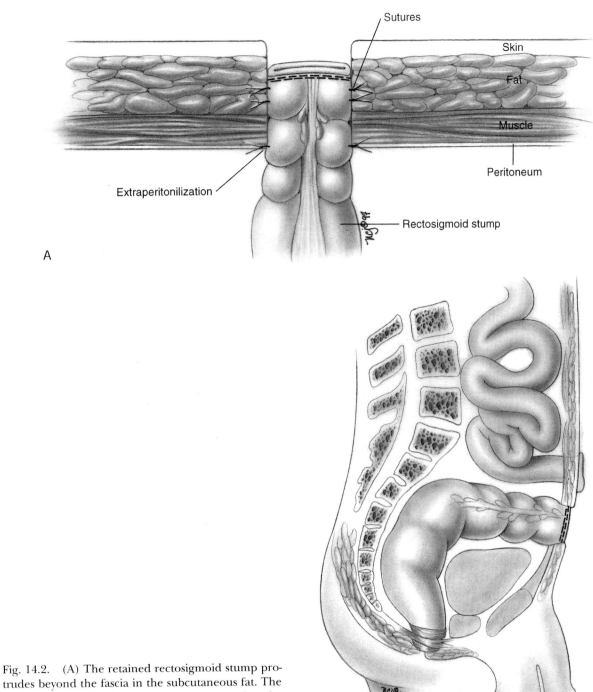

Fig. 14.2. (A) The retained rectosigmoid stump protrudes beyond the fascia in the subcutaneous fat. The peritoneum is closed around the stump so that the bowel end is extraperitonealized. (B) Lateral view showing the end ileostomy and the implanted rectosigmoid stump.

dehisces, drainage will occur through the skin wound rather than causing an intraperitoneal abscess. By implanting the rectosigmoid stump at the lower end of the midline incision rather than through a separate fascial opening in the left iliac fossa (17), we have not noted any increased wound infection rate. This technique of subcutaneous im-

plantation avoids a discharging and malodorous mucous fistula and the buried rectal stump is easily identifiable at a future laparotomy for ileoanal pouch.

If the rectosigmoid stump is severely diseased and friable, a formal mucous fistula is constructed through the lower end of the midline wound. If the bowel is too friable to hold sutures, a 5 to 7 cm stump is left protruding beyond the skin level and wrapped snugly with a gauze roll to provide anchorage to the abdominal wall. After a period of 7 to 10 days, the rectosigmoid stump becomes sufficiently adherent to the abdominal wall and is amputated at the skin level to allow maturation of the mucous fistula. Occasionally, delayed subcutaneous closure of the mucous fistula can be performed after resolution of fulminating inflammation (23).

It is preferable not to leave a closed and short rectal stump within the pelvis because of the risk of serious pelvic sepsis if the stump dehisces (17). Identification and mobilization of the short rectal stump during subsequent ileoanal pouch surgery can be difficult as the tissue planes are distorted and the risk of pelvic nerve injury and presacral hemorrhage is increased (17,24,25). A recent study (17) also shows that subsequent proctectomy is more difficult following an intraperitoneal closure of the rectum.

End Ileostomy

The ileostomy site is marked preoperatively (26). A circumferential incision is made around the pre-marked stoma site, about 2 to 2.5 cm in diameter. The skin disc is excised but the subcutaneous fat is preserved. This reduces the size of the subcutaneous dead space. A vertical incision is made with electrocautery through the subcutaneous fat, Scarpa's fascia and the anterior rectus sheath. The rectus muscle is split vertically, carefully avoiding the inferior epigastric vessels. Finally the posterior rectus sheath and peritoneum are incised vertically with electrocautery. The maneuver is facilitated by an upward pressure from within the peritoneal cavity under the ileostomy aperture using a sponge over the surgeon's hand. An optimal stoma aperture will accommodate snugly two fingers of a surgeon wearing size 7 or 8 gloves.

A Babcock clamp is passed through the aperture to grasp the distal end of the ileum, so that the ileal mesentery lies in a cephaled direction to facilitate closure of the lateral space. A length of approximately 6 cm of ileum is exteriorized through the stoma site and matured using 3–0 chromic catgut sutures between full-thickness bowel edge and the subcuticular skin (Fig. 14.3). The sutures should not go through the epidermis as islands of ileal mucosa may be implanted to the skin causing mucus leaks. Stabilizing sutures between the seromuscular layer of the ileum and the subcutaneous fat are rarely used.

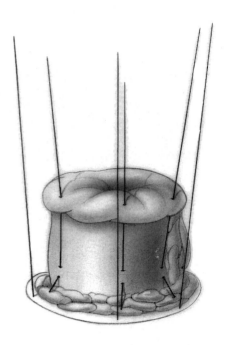

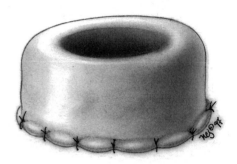

Fig. 14.3.   Construction of an end ileostomy. Radial sutures are placed and tied, producing eversion of the stoma.

Closure

If adequate hemostasis is achieved, suction drains are rarely used. If the rectal stump is very friable, a soft intraluminal rectal catheter is left in situ for 5 days. The abdominal wall fascia is then closed using standard techniques.

Postoperative Management

Intravenous fluids are continued until the ileus is resolved. Considerable depletion of fluid and electrolyte may occur from the stoma and should be carefully monitored. In the very malnourished, total parenteral nutrition for 4 to 5 days may be considered. Prophylactic antibiotics are continued postoperatively for 1 to 5 days depending on the extent of intraabdominal sepsis. A reducing regime of intravenous hydrocortisone is prescribed. As soon as fluids are absorbed by mouth, this is changed to oral prednisone. Depending on the period of steroid dependence, the steroid dose is gradually tapered postoperatively. Analgesia is provided with intravenous infusion of narcotics for 4 to 5 days. The urethral catheter remains in place until the patient is ambulant, usually for 4 days. Antithrombotic prophylaxis is recommended and early mobilization is generally encouraged.

As soon as possible, usually about the third postoperative day, stoma education is commenced. Prior to discharge, dietary advice relevant to an ileostomy is given as well.

Special Postoperative Complications

Subtotal colectomy with rectal preservation is a safe procedure even in malnourished patients with severe colitis receiving high doses of steroids (27).

Infection

Malnourished and immunosuppressed patients are particularly at risk. Common risk factors include serum albumin levels of less than 20 g/L, steroid therapy, and fecal contamination (28). Signs of sepsis may be subtle without fever or leukocytosis. Symptoms may be vague with anorexia, hypoalbuminemia and prolonged ileus. Wound infection especially in the lower end of the incision may signify a dehisced rectosigmoid stump. The skin sutures should be removed to facilitate drainage.

Rectal Bleeding

Minor bleeding from a friable rectum is common whereas massive bleeding is rare. Most of these may be controlled with topical and/or parenteral steroids and, if necessary, epinephrine enema. Rarely, an urgent proctectomy is needed (29).

Bowel Obstruction

About a third of patients have at least minor episodes of adhesive subacute small bowel obstruction after a colectomy (30). The reoperation rate is much lower, reported as 13% (31).

Diverting Loop Ileostomy and Decompressive "Blowhole" Colostomy

This technique was described by Turnbull and colleagues from the Cleveland Clinic for long-standing toxic megacolon complicated by walled-off perforations. It is used rarely, and has largely become a procedure of historical interest. This avoids manipulation of the colon with potential risk of major fecal spillage and tides the patient over this critical period. Definitive surgery, usually proctocolectomy, is then performed 4 to 6 months later when the patient is in a better physical state. With more coordinated modern medical and surgical management, emergency colectomy can now be performed safely in most patients and is the preferred surgical option.

This lesser procedure of ileostomy-colostomy should still be considered when the patient is critically ill with multiple sealed-off colonic perforations, massive colonic dilatation and a high splenic flexure.

A short lower midline incision is initially made. The terminal ileum just proximal to the cecum is identified by noting the fold of Treves. A full display and manipulation of the cecum is not necessary. A tape is placed around a loop of distal ileum within 5 to 7 cm of the ileocecal valve. The afferent and efferent limbs of the loop are clearly identified with marking sutures on either side of the tape. The ileal loop is then delivered through the stoma site using gentle traction on the tape. Twisting of the bowel is to be avoided. The afferent or functional end lies caudal and the efferent or nonfunctional end lies cephaled. A supporting plastic rod is passed through the mesenteric window and replaces the tape.

Through the lower midline incision, the site of the dilated transverse colon is noted and a separate 5 cm midline incision is made directly over the dilated transverse colon in the upper abdomen. The incision is deepened through the peritoneal cavity. The lower midline incision is now closed and covered with a sterile dressing (Fig. 14.4). The loop ileostomy is then constructed. An incision is made through the antimesenteric surface of the efferent or distal limb of the loop about 5 mm above the skin level (Fig. 14.5). About four fifths of the circumference of the bowel is incised. Sutures are applied between full-thickness of the cut edge of the bowel and the subcuticular layer of the skin, so that the afferent or proximal limb is everted over the rod. In this way, the afferent limb becomes the dominant functional end.

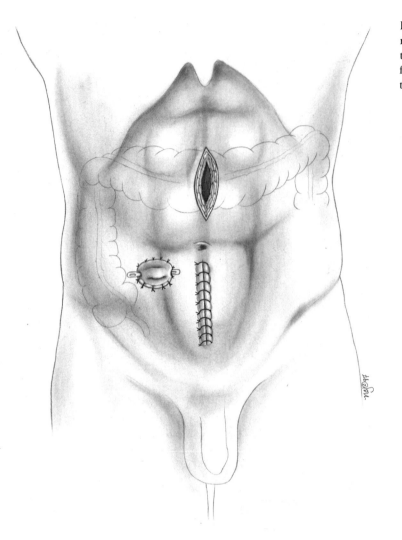

Fig. 14.4. After closure of the lower midline incision and construction of the loop ileostomy, they are draped off from the upper midline incision over the distended transverse colon.

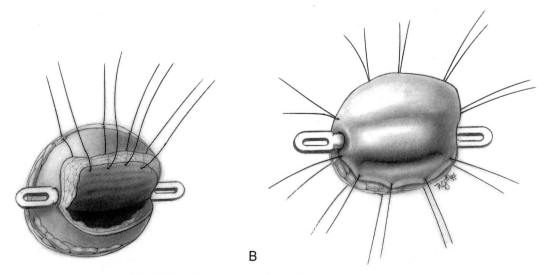

A B

Fig. 14.5. Construction of loop ileostomy.

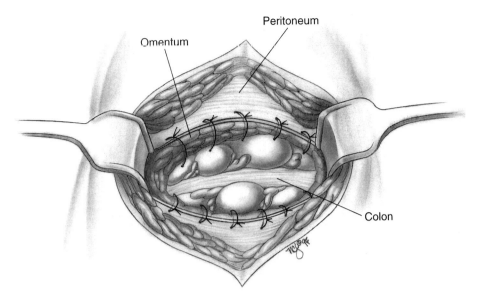

Fig. 14.6. Quarantining sutures are placed between the serosa of transverse colon and the peritoneum.

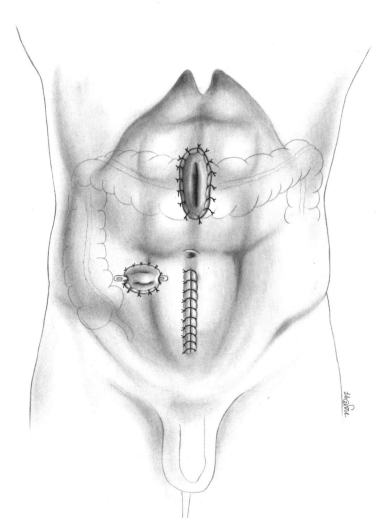

Fig. 14.7. Loop ileostomy and skin-level blowhole transverse colostomy.

The skin level blow-hole colostomy is then constructed. Through the upper midline incision, an edematous omentum overlying the transverse colon is incised with cautery and careful suture ligation. The serosa of the transverse colon is exposed. The peritoneum and the omentum and seromuscular layer of the colon are then carefully approximated using 3–0 vicryl sutures so as to quarantine the area from the general peritoneal cavity (Fig. 14.6). The colon is handled with care so as to avoid major disruption. A small transverse colotomy is made within the quarantined area and the gas and mucopurulent material are sucked away. The cut edges of the colon are then sutured to the skin edges with 3–0 vicryl sutures (Fig. 14.7). If there is excessive tension, the sutures are placed on the abdominal wall fat instead. Appliances are then placed over the stomas.

Patients usually improve rapidly after surgery and the mortality is low. Persistence of profuse watery or bloody diarrhea through the blow-hole colostomy indicates intractable colitis and is an indication for early colectomy.

Emergency Restorative Proctocolectomy and Diverting Ileostomy

This is associated with a significant operative morbidity and septic complications as many patients are on high-dose steroids (32). In general, such extensive surgery is best avoided in the critically ill patients (24,25).

Conclusion

Subtotal colectomy and end ileostomy with rectal preservation is the preferred surgical approach in emergency surgery for toxic megacolon and/or perforation.

References

1. Buckell NA, Lennard-Jones JE. How district hospitals see ulcerative colitis. Lancet 1979;1226–9.
2. Hawley PR. Emergency surgery for ulcerative colitis. World J Surg 1988;12:169–73.
3. Greenstein AJ, Sachar DB, Gibas A, et al. Outcome of toxic dilatation in ulcerative colitis and Crohn's colitis. J Clin Gastroenterol 1985;7:137–44.
4. Farmer ARG, Hawk WA, Turnbull RB. Clinical patterns in Crohn's disease: a statistical study of 615 cases. Gastroenterology 1975;68:627–35.
5. Fazio VW, Verschueren RCJ. Ileostomy-colostomy for toxic megacolon. In: Nyhus LM, Baker RJ, Fischer JE, ed. Mastery of Surgery. Boston: Little Brown, 1997;1227–34.
6. Heppell J, Farkouh E, Dube S, et al. Toxic megacolon: an analysis of 70 cases. Dis Colon Rectum 1986;29:789–92.
7. Norland CC, Kirsner JB. Toxic dilatation of the colon: etiology, treatment and prognosis in 42 patients. Medicine 1969;48:229–50.
8. Marshak RH, Korelitz BL, Klein SH, et al. Toxic dilatation of the colon in the course of ulcerative colitis. Gastroenterology 1960;38:165–80.
9. Grant CS, Dozois RR. Toxic megacolon: ultimate fate of patients after successful medical treatment. Am J Surg 1984;147:106–10.
10. Keighley MRB. Acute fulminating colitis and emergency colectomy. In: Keighley MRB, Williams NS, ed. Surgery of the Anus, Rectum and Colon. London: WB Saunders, 1993;1379–97.
11. Tjandra JJ. Emergency colectomy for fulminating colitis. In: Allan RN, Keighley MRB, Alexander-Williams J, Fazio VW, Hanauer S, Rhodes JM, eds. Inflammatory Bowel Disease. London: Churchill Livingstone, 3rd ed. 1997;727–32.
12. Price AB. Overlap in the spectrum of non-specific inflammatory bowel disease: colitis indeterminate. J Clin Pathol 1978;31:567.
13. Fazio VW, Tjandra JJ, Lavery IC. Techniques in pouch construction. In: Nicholls J, Bartolo D, Mortensen N, ed. Techniques to Restorative Proctocolectomy. Oxford: Blackwell Sci Pub 1993;18–33.
14. Binder SC, Miller HH, Deterling RA Jr. Emergency and urgent operations for ulcerative colitis. Arch Surg 1975;110:284–9.
15. Talbot RW, Ritchie JK, Northover JM. Conservative proctocolectomy: a dubious option in ulcerative colitis. Br J Surg 1989;76:738–9.
16. Motson RW, Manche AR. Modified Hartmann procedure for acute ulcerative colitis. Surg Gynecol Obstet 1985;160:463–4.
17. Carter FM, McLeod RS, Cohen Z. Subtotal colectomy for ulcerative colitis: complications related to the rectal remnant. Dis Colon Rectum 1991;34:1005–10.
18. Flatmark A, Fretheim B, Gjoine E. Early colectomy in severe ulcerative colitis. Scand J Gastroenterol 1975;82:531–6.
19. Lee EG, Truelove SC. Proctocolectomy for ulcerative colitis. World J Surg 1980;4:195–201.
20. Kyle SM, Steyn RS, Keenan RA. Management of the rectum following colectomy for acute colitis. Aust NZ J Surg 1992;62:196–9.
21. Ng RL, Davies AH, Grace RH, et al. Subcutaneous rectal stump closure after emergency subtotal colectomy. Br J Surg 1992;79:701–3.
22. Ozuner G, Strong S, Fazio VW. Effect of rectosigmoid stump length on restorative proctocolectomy after subtotal colectomy. Dis Colon Rectum 1995;38:1039–42.

23. Fazio VW, Turnbull RB. Ulcerative colitis and Crohn's disease of the colon: a review of surgical options. Med Clin North Am 1980;64:1135–59.

24. Tjandra JJ, Fazio VW. Indication for and results of ileal pouch. Curr Practice in Surg 1993;4:22–8.

25. Tjandra JJ, Fazio VW. Complications of the ileoanal pouch. In: Mazier WP, Levien DH, Luchtefeld MA, Senagore AJ, eds. Surgery of the Colon, Rectum and Anus. Philadelphia: WB Saunders 1995;893–903.

26. Fazio VW, Tjandra JJ. Prevention and management of ileostomy complications. J ET Nurs 1992;19:48–53.

27. Penna C, Daude F, Parc R, et al. Previous subtotal colectomy with ileostomy and sigmoidostomy improves the morbidity and early functional results after ileal pouch-anal anastomosis in ulcerative colitis. Dis Colon Rectum 1993;36:343–8.

28. Oakley JR, Lavery IC, Fazio VW, et al. The fate of the rectal stump after subtotal colectomy for ulcerative colitis. Dis Colon Rectum 1985;28:394–6.

29. Ganchrow MI, Facelle TL. Control of hemorrhage from a mucous fistula with foley catheter tamponade. Dis Colon Rectum 1992;35:1001–2.

30. Morowitz DA, Kirsner JB. Ileostomy in ulcerative colitis: a questionnaire study in 1803 patients. Am J Surg 1981;141:370–5.

31. Ritchie JK. Ulcerative colitis treated by ileostomy and excisional surgery. Br J Surg 1972;59:345–51.

32. Heyvaert G, Penninckx F, Filez L, et al. Restorative proctocolectomy in elective and emergency cases of ulcerative colitis. Int J Colorect Dis 1994;9:73–6.

15 Dysplasia and Cancer

Gilberto Poggioli, Luca Stocchi, and Antonino Cavallari

The risk of cancer in ulcerative colitis (UC) is well known and this topic has been thoroughly discussed in Chapter 4 (Riddell). In the past this risk was considered to increase exponentially with the duration of disease. In fact, it was considered to be 25% at 20 years and 34% to 43% over 25 years (1,2). These data were gathered from patients admitted to referral centers. Further prospective studies on patient populations in circumscribed areas have led to a lower figure (3–6). Moreover, the routine use of endoscopy and the widespread knowledge of histopathological premalignant patterns such as dysplasia (7,8) have deeply modified the attitude of physicians. In fact, many centers are carrying out programs of endoscopic and histologic surveillance in long-standing colitis attempting to better detect malignant modifications in their early stages. The dicussion has arisen in the past and still continues today about the usefulness of such programs and their cost-effectiveness (9–12).

The management of dysplasia and cancer associated with UC has been strongly influenced by the considerable progress in the surgical treatment of the disease that has taken place in the last decades.

Surgeons are aware that standard treatment of UC implies total proctocolectomy. During the 1950s and the 1960s the ileorectal anastomosis represented a reasonable compromise between the need of total removal of the target organ and the desire for a normal route of evacuation (13,14). The description of ileal-pouch-anal anastomosis (IPAA) has markedly modified such an attitude. At the beginning and during the first years of its use (15) (from the end of the 1970s to the first half of the 1980s) the problem of technical difficulties and consequent surgical failures proved to be the "dark side" of the procedure (16). Increased experience and widespread use has led to a dramatic decrease in postsurgical complications (17). Accordingly, the functional results have improved so much that some have argued that there is little difference in function and morbidity rate between ileoanal and ileorectal anastomosis (18). By now IPAA has become the procedure of choice in ulcerative colitis—even in selected cases complicated by dysplasia or cancer associated with UC.

Dysplasia and Ulcerative Colitis

Dysplasia is a definite precancerous lesion but its precise role in the therapeutic management of UC is not completely defined. In fact, many authors believe there is a direct progression from low grade dysplasia to high grade dysplasia to carcinoma (7). In contrast, others such as Jonsson (19) who started from the observation that two patients with high grade dysplasia that refused the operation were in good health and without dysplasia after 13 and 4 years respectively, suggest that the natural history of dysplasia is not completely understood.

There are two main problems which determine the operative strategy in the presence of dysplasia in UC:

1. Is the presence of dysplasia an absolute indication for surgery?
2. Should the dysplasia modify the surgical strategy and technique?

Dysplasia and Indications for Surgery

The presence of long-standing ulcerative colitis, especially if it extends proximal to the splenic flexure

(20,21), is a high-risk condition for the development of cancer. Major referral centers for inflammatory bowel diseases have established surveillance programs trying to detect early cancers or premalignant conditions such as dysplasia. These programs are mostly based on repeated colonoscopies on a yearly basis. Such recommendation has been endorsed since 1986 by the American College of Physicians (22) that stated that patients affected by long-standing extensive ulcerative colitis should have a colonoscopy every year. Nonetheless, it is difficult to definitively answer how best to conduct surveillance in long-standing ulcerative colitis because the results are controversial. The St. Mark's Hospital experience (23) revealed a significantly longer cumulative survival rate at 5 years of the 16 patients who developed cancer in UC during the surveillance program vs. the 104 patients with colitis-associated carcinoma who had not been included in the surveillance program, (87.1% vs. 55%, $p = 0.024$). In a prospective cohort study on 65 patients followed by the gastroenterologists of our hospital (24), 15 patients (23.1%) refused the surveillance program and two of them developed invasive cancer four and six years after the last follow-up colonoscopy, while out of the 46 patients who continued the surveillance, 4 developed early stage cancer. In contrast, a recent analysis (11) of 12 reports of endoscopic surveillance programs for long-standing colitis showed that only 12 cases out of 93 cancers (13%) were discovered at an early stage as a result of the endoscopic program. The success rate doubled (26%) when clinical evaluation and radiological tests were added to colonoscopy.

According to most authors (25), including ourselves, the number of early cancers detected cannot be listed as the only success index for a surveillance program. In fact, we must also consider patients where the dysplasia was discovered at colonoscopy and were operated on before a malignant degeneration could ensue.

The term dysplasia is a complicated concept and not always accepted in the same way; in fact it has been calculated that even among expert pathologists (26) agreement in the evaluation of dysplasia could reach only 42% to 65% (see chapter 4). Today, it is almost universally accepted that high-grade dysplasia means inevitable evolution to cancer and warrants an immediate colectomy. Finally, it is also important to point out that dysplasia can be associated with the presence of cancer at a distance from the site of dysplasia. The real incidence of the latter situation is difficult to establish, ranging from 73% in Ransohoff series (27), 74% in

a report from the Mayo Clinic (28) and 74% of St. Mark's Hospital series (23) with a 34% to 50% rate of high-grade dysplasia (27,28).

While some disagreement exists on the real meaning of low-grade dysplasia, its presence in a single colonscopic biopsy, diagnosed by a skillful pathology, is nearly always an indication for surgical intervention (see Chapter 4 for a detailed discussion of this).

Dysplasia and Surgical Strategies and Techniques

The presence of dysplasia modifies the surgical attitude in sphincter-saving procedures such as ileorectal and ileoanal anastomosis where colonic mucosa left in situ.

Dysplasia is patchy (27), and we know that even with multiple biopsies during colonoscopy, only 0.5% to 1% of the colonic surface can be evaluated (11). These two considerations lead to the conclusion that in patients already operated on who have dysplasia in the colonic specimen, a surveillance program should be considered even for a few centimeters of residual glandular epithelium such as in IPAA. The degree of surveillance will be established according to the length of colonic mucosa left. Therefore, patients previously submitted to ileorectal anastomosis should undergo frequent and careful surveillance (every 12 months at least). Theoretically, a less strict surveillance is needed for patients with ileoanal pouch.

Ileorectal Anastomosis

Although many studies have been carried out, the cancer risk of the rectal stump is difficult to evaluate. The cumulative risk has been reported to be high in referral centers (29); in contrast, an epidemiologic study (30) in a definite group of 1274 patients in Stockholm County with diagnosis of UC from 1955 to 1979 showed a very low risk of the malignant degeneration in the remaining rectum. These differences can be explained by selection of more severe cases by referral centers. A second explanation is the higher number of patients with dysplasia or carcinoma of the colon at colectomy. In fact, in the Cleveland Clinic series (31), three out of five patients that developed cancer in the rectal stump had dysplasia or cancer at the time of colectomy. On the other hand, in the study by Löfberg (30) in a definite population, the indication for surgery was dysplasia in two patients and colonic cancer in 2 more out of 55 patients submitted to ileorectal anastomosis. None of these four patients showed any evidence of dysplasia or cancer in the rectal stump during the follow-up; whereas among the 25 patients submitted to rectal excision in the follow-up, 3 had already been operated on for dysplasia in the rectal stump and none of them had had dysplasia at the time of colectomy. Löfberg attributed this to the high proportion of rectum already excised due to relapse of symptoms before the disease could degenerate. Based on these data, the suggestion we can make is that patients with colonic dysplasia should not undergo ileorectal anastomosis even if the rectal stump does not show any evidence of dysplasia.

Ileoanal Anastomosis

One of the reasons for the worldwide popularity of this sphincter-saving procedure is the complete removal of colonic glandular mucosa that eliminates the risk of relapse of disease as well as that of malignancy. Many variants have been introduced in addition to the original technique (15). First, mucosectomy was started about 1 cm above the dentate line in order to preserve normal anal sensation (32–34). Later, the introduction of circular staplers with detachable heads made the technique of ileoanal anastomosis simpler and with a low complication rate (35). The anastomosis can be performed at about 1.5 to 2.5 cm from the dentate line; anastomoses performed lower than this measure leads to the risk of internal sphincter damage. This change however has raised the suspicion in some authors that a similar procedure could no longer be named ileal-pouch-anal anastomosis, claiming that a proper name for it could be ileal-pouch-distal rectum anastomosis (36). This definition has been proposed by the Mayo Clinic group, who found in 90% of 50 patients treated by proctocolectomy (37), the disease was present within 1 cm of the dentate line when the specimens were carefully examined histologically. Microscopically, UC was also detected by Sugerman (38) in 19 out of 20 patients after stapled IPAA; however, only three of them had symptoms. Nevertheless, the majority of surgeons considers the stapled procedure as a "true" IPAA. On the other hand, columnar epithelium and active disease can be found below the anastomosis in patients submitted to mucosectomy and hand-sewn IPAA. In our experience (39) we have found evidence of active colitis in 5.9% of patients submitted to hand-sewn ileoanal anastomosis and this was not statistically different from data concerning stapled anastomoses (9.3% of patients), although the mean distance from dentate line to the anastomosis was 0.2 cm in the hand-sewn

vs. 1.2 ± 0.7 cm in the stapled group. At confirmation of the risk of malignant degeneration of the mucosa in the few centimeters above the dentate line, King and colleagues (40) studying the specimens excised with mucosectomy, found that in 3 out of 16 patients submitted to hand-sewn ileoanal anastomosis, a colonic columnar epithelium was present lined down to the dentate line; moreover the authors found evidence of active colitis in ten cases, moderate dysplasia in four cases and a poorly differentiated adenocarcinoma in one case. Finally, two cases (41,42) of adenocarcinoma located in the mucosa below the anastomosis in patients submitted to mucosectomy and ileoanal anastomosis for ulcerative colitis as well as in one patient operated on for familial adenomatous polyposis have been reported to date (43). This leads to the conclusion that the risk of malignant degeneration may not be cancelled by a complete mucosal excision starting from the dentate line.

The above mentioned data represent, however, only an isolated confirmation of the existence of a cancer risk even in few centimeters of colonic mucosa left in place. The real risk of developing dysplasia in the anal transition zone (ATZ) after stapled IPAA is not known. Available data to answer this question come from the Cleveland Clinic (44), St. Mark's Hospital (45), and our experience. According to Ziv (44), low grade dysplasia was found in 8 out of 254 patients submitted to stapled IPAA (3.1%). In six of these patients there was no evidence of dysplasia on following examinations. Two patients were found to have dysplasia on repeated biopsies. Both of them underwent a completion transanal mucosectomy (46) with ileal pouch advancement and neoileoanal anastomosis as proposed by the same team for stenosis and anovaginal fistulas complicating stapled ileoanal pouches (47). The dysplasia in these eight patients was in 5 out of 219 cases (2.3%) not associated with premalignant or malignant degeneration in the colonic specimen, whereas in 1 out of 24 (4.2%) and in 2 out of 11 (18.2%) it was associated with high grade dysplasia and cancer in the colonic specimen, respectively. This implies that there is a significantly higher probability of developing dysplasia in the ATZ of those patients where dysplasia or cancer had previously been found at colectomy.

Similar data come from the St. Mark's series (45) where dysplasia in the mucosectomy specimen was present in two cases out of eight patients with colitis-associated cancer (25%) and in 1 out of 110 patients (0.9%) with UC without cancer. In our experience, 215 ileoanal pouches have been performed for UC with a median follow-up of 4.5 years. Out of these patients, 63 were hand sewn and 152 were stapled. Fifteen had dysplasia in the colonic specimen. Seven were submitted to hand-sewn anastomosis and eight to a stapled one. Moreover, 13 had low-grade dysplasia and 2 severe dysplasia and were submitted to hand-sewn anastomosis. Out of 215 operated patients, 182 underwent a program of histological surveillance of the mucosa below the anastomosis. This program included a double biopsy of the mucosa below the anastomosis at 6 months from operation, then once a year for 2 years and once every other year, afterwards. The presence of dysplasia below the anastomosis has been detected only in one patient (0.7%). Further biopsies showed no evidence of dysplasia. This patient had no dysplasia in the colonic specimen. On the other hand, out of the 15 patients with dysplasia in the colonic specimen none shows dysplasia to date.

In conclusion, we can state that the hand-sewn IPAA with mucosectomy reduces the risk of retained colonic mucosa below the anastomosis, but does not allow complete removal of columnar epithelium with its potential evolution to a malignant state. However, the incidence of dysplasia in the ATZ after stapled IPAA is low and it is possible to transform a stapled into a hand-sewn IPAA with mucosectomy. Dysplasia in the ATZ is significantly linked to the presence of dysplasia or cancer in the rest of the colon. In case of preoperative diagnosis of dysplasia or evidence of dysplasia in the specimen at the time of subtotal colectomy, we strongly recommend total proctocolectomy with mucosectomy starting from the dentate line and hand-sewn IPAA.

Cancer and Ulcerative Colitis

Differences in Surgical Technique

The three surgical options available today for the therapy of ulcerative colitis are total proctocolectomy with permanent ileostomy (Brooke (48) or Kock (49) type), ileorectal anastomosis, and ileoanal anastomosis. From the technical point of view, they do not substantially differ with regard to surgical technique in case of benign disease or malignant degeneration. For this reason no higher morbidity rate can be expected in patients operated on for colitis-associated carcinoma.

There are only two technical differences in patients with cancer complicating ulcerative colitis in comparison with uncomplicated ulcerative colitis and they concern the proctectomy and the mesocolon excision for extended lymphadenectomy.

The Proctectomy

Some surgeons, like Nicholls (50), have emphasized the importance in benign disease of carrying out the proctectomy within the mesorectum to reduce the incidence of urinary and sexual dysfunctions. Most surgeons, including ourselves, do not currently agree with this attitude. In fact, this goal can be reached performing the proctectomy along the presacral avascular plane; this technique is easier and there is less bleeding; however, both these techniques in expert hands bear the same low morbidity rate. The dissection along the parietal pelvic fascia has other advantages: it can also be used in malignant disease (51,52) because it allows *en bloc* resection of lymphatic tissue surrounding the mesorectum, thus guaranteeing the oncologically correct excision of the rectum. Moreover, this dissection even in neoplastic disease permits sparing of the hypogastric nerves (sympathetic) and of the truncal sacral nerves (parasympathetic).

The difference between this kind of proctectomy, whether carried out for benign or malignant disease, regards the lateral dissection. In benign diseases, in fact, the inferior hypogastric plexus running close to the mesorectum should be preserved. This leads to a very low impotence rate of 1.5% to 4% (53,54) from about 15% in neoplastic disease (51).

Extension of the Mesocolon Excision

This is the major relevant difference with regard to technique in case of colitis-associated carcinoma. In fact, the colectomy must be performed according to the principles of segmental colonic resection for malignant disease (55). In this view, the ligation at the origin of all the vascular pedicles should be performed. A particular problem for a radical procedure to be performed can be the presence of cancer in the right colon. An oncologically safe resection requires sacrifice of the ileocolic artery. Also, the same artery can be extremely useful in J-pouch anal anastomosis. In fact, salvage of the ileocolic artery allows the section of more proximal ileal branches of superior mesenteric artery without compromising the vascularization of the reservoir in the generation of satisfactory mesenteric length to reach the anus without tension (56).

The therapeutic efficacy of lymphadenectomy in the radical treatment of colonic and rectal cancer has been widely discussed (57–61). In our view extended lymphadenectomy is useful primarily for the staging of the disease, particularly in those cases in which the cancer, not suspected preoperatively, is located in the intraperitoneal colon. Under these circumstances, some advocate a subtotal colectomy with temporary ileostomy (62,63).

With the exception of the above mentioned technical details, there are no particular differences in the operative strategy concerning total proctocolectomy with permanent ileostomy and ileorectal anastomosis among the patients with or without malignant degeneration of UC. The only comparative data available are those concerning IPAA and in these cases the comparison has been made not so much because of a real difference in surgical technique as to support or not the indication for IPAA for cancer on UC. Surgeons disagree on this point. The only significant results come from the experiences of the Cleveland Clinic (64,65) and the Mayo Clinic (66). Both series show that procedure-associated morbidity is similar to control groups of patients operated on for benign disease. Even functional results do not show a statistically significant difference in the incidence of leakage and need for antidiarrheal medications in patients operated on for cancer compared to those operated on for benign disease.

Our experience includes 319 procedures for UC performed between 1981 and 1995. Fifty-six were total proctocolectomy with permanent Brooke ileostomy, 48 ileorectal anastomoses, and 215 IPAA. Cancer was found in 15 patients (4.7%). The surgical treatment of UC-associated cancer was total proctocolectomy with permanent ileostomy in six patients, ileorectal anastomosis in three, and IPAA in six. Thirty more patients were treated with IPAA for familial adenomatous polyposis. The number of cancers in these patients was 12. There were 18 of 245 patients with cancer treated with IPAA.

The morbidity rate and septic complications are not significantly different (9.4% in benign disease vs. 5.6% in cancer). Functional results such as the number of bowel movements nocturnally and in 24 hours, the incidence of leakage, the discrimination betweeen feces and flatus, the need for antidiarrheal drugs are comparable (Table 15.1). Finally, the quality of life parameters such as dietary restrictions, sexual activity, and return to work did not show any statistically significant difference.

Cancer and Type of Procedure: Feasibility of Each Procedure for Any Stage and Location of the Disease

Total proctocolectomy with permanent ileostomy is always feasible for any stage and location of the disease, provided oncological principles of resec-

tability are respected. The only choice on which debate is still alive regards ileorectal (except in case of associated cancer of the rectum) or IPAA.

A uniform view does not exist on the indications for one procedure according to the stage of disease; what follows only represents our philosophy, based on experience and common sense more than on controlled studies.

First of all, we need to say that our attitude has changed with increasing experience. In 1993 at the meeting in Versailles on IPAA (67), we had presented our experience and our opinion on the indications for IPAA for colitis-associated cancer. The main ideas that we pointed out were: In early stage cancer (Dukes' A and B) we gave the same indications as in benign disease. Therefore, total proctocolectomy with IPAA was the first choice procedure. In advanced stages of the disease (Dukes' D) there was an absolute contraindication to IPAA because such a demanding procedure with a major complication rate was not suitable for patients with a short life expectancy. In these cases, total proctocolectomy for any location or palliative ileorectal anastomosis for intraperitoneal colonic location, were warranted.

The change in our philosophy mainly regards selected cases of advanced rectal cancer. In fact, the increasing experience and the decreasing complication rate, the achievement of good functional results, and most of all, the feasibility of a single stage procedure without a protective ileostomy, make it possible today to advocate IPAA even in cases of advanced disease. In these cases we cannot improve the survival rate but we have a definitive impact on the quality of life, since the alternative is proctocolectomy with permanent ileostomy. This is valid provided that morbidity is low (68) and that this approach is carried out in centers with specific experience in pouch-anal surgery.

Beyond these extreme issues, the problem of the choice of surgical procedure is basically a problem of preoperative staging. This is particularly important in Dukes' C stage, since lymph node involvement becomes evident only after the pathologic examination of the specimen. An accurate preoperative staging will often be impossible and sometimes it is even difficult to establish a preoperative diagnosis of cancer in UC. In this regard, data coming from the Mayo Clinic are demonstrative (66): according to this report, all of the 34 patients referred to this institution with cancer in UC had a preoperative diagnosis of "nonrespondent colitis" and in 16 the diagnosis of cancer was established only at operation.

Table 15.1. Functional results and quality of life parameters.

	IPAA Ulcerative colitis 209 pts	IPAA for Ulcerative colitis- associated cancer 6 pts
Bowel movements/24 hrs	4.9%	5.7%
Nocturnal Bowel movements	0.8%	1.3%
Need of antidiarrheal drugs	9.1%	11.1%
Urgency	2.5%	—
Discrimination between feces and flatus	70.7%	77.8%
Leakage	60.6%	44.9%
Return to previous work	85.3%	77.8%
Sexual activity: Unmodified	76.6%	77.7%
Improved	9.1%	22.3%
Worsened	14.3%	—

IPAA is therefore indicated for almost any location of malignant degeneration. The absolute contraindication to this procedure arises in ours as well as in others' experience (68,69) in the face of such a low rectal tumor in which a curative resection could damage the sphincter function. In contrast, in cases of rectal cancer in the upper or middle third of the rectum, IPAA is warranted, provided the proctectomy is carried out as a radical and oncologically safe procedure with total mesorectum excision. An exception to this attitude is related to the stage of the tumor, as previously mentioned. In cases of a Dukes' C rectal cancer or without any signs of lymph node involvement but high local aggressiveness (Dukes' B2), adjuvant chemo/radiotherapy is necessary. The next section of this chapter deals specifically with this issue.

Functional Results after Adjuvant Chemo/Radiotherapy

Once again the question regards only one of the surgical options, which is IPAA. In fact, patients submitted to total proctocolectomy with permanent ileostomy and patients submitted to ileorectal anastomosis, especially with intraabdominal anastomosis with long rectal stump, are less likely to suffer from clinical sequela following adjuvant chemo/radiotherapy.

There are not many reports related to this. In 1992 Fozard (67) presented a report at the American Society of Colon and Rectal Surgeons meeting on 34 cases of IPAA in patients affected by UC-associated cancer and eleven patients with degenerated familial adenomatous polyposis. Thirty-five patients had a functioning pouch after a median follow-up of three years. Surgical complications occurred in 25% of cases after IPAA (11/45). The surgical complication rate in the 35 patients who underwent closure of the temporary ileostomy was particularly remarkable, reaching 35.3%. Twelve patients had postoperative adjuvant therapy. Eight had chemotherapy alone, three chemo/radiotherapy and one radiotherapy alone. The four patients treated with radiotherapy required ileostomy diversion. The other eight patients who underwent only chemotherapy had no related complications.

Our experience includes 18 patients with malignancy submitted to IPAA (6 for UC and 12 for FAP). All the patients affected by FAP underwent a hand-sewn IPAA with loop ileostomy that was subsequently closed in 9 cases. Of the remaining three patients, one is still awaiting his closure, one was converted to permanent ileostomy due to surgical complications and one died with his ileostomy still open from diffuse carcinomatosis. Among them six received chemotherapy (four with open ileostomy). No complications were recorded.

In the six patients with colitis-associated cancer, two had Dukes' B2, three had Dukes' C and one had an incidental carcinoid of the appendix (T1 N0 M0). The patient with carcinoid of the appendix was first submitted to subtotal colectomy and subsequently to IPAA; adjuvant therapy was not added. Among the other five patients, two underwent an IPAA without protective ileostomy. One of them (C1 stage) subsequently received adjuvant chemotherapy. The other one was a 77-year-old woman, who did not receive adjuvant chemotherapy despite a C1 carcinoma. They are both alive and well after 34 and 48 months, respectively. The remaining three patients were submitted to IPAA with protective ileostomy which was subsequently closed. Despite chemotherapy, the patient with Dukes' C2 stage died 9 months after his pouch procedure because of diffuse dis-

Table 15.2.   Cancer in ulcerative colitis surgical strategies.

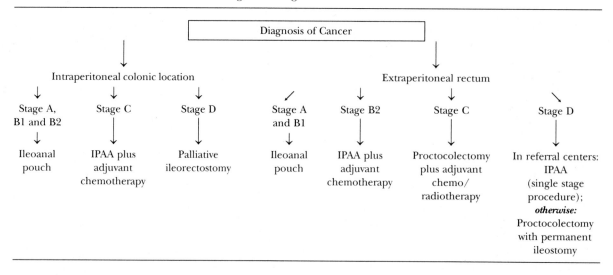

ease. The other two are alive and well after 65 and 4 months. One was found to have a B2 well differentiated carcinoma and chemotherapy was not delivered whereas the other is currently undertaking adjuvant chemotherapy for a B2 undifferentiated tumor.

Summary

Surgical treatment of ulcerative colitis complicated by cancer is based on the principles of oncologic clearance, maintenance of anorectal, sexual, and urological function, need for adjuvant therapy anal sphincter function, patient's body habitus, and choice. The influence of anal sphincter function, patient's body habitus, and choice has been discussed in other chapters when discussing the choice between an anal sphincter saving procedure and a proctocolectomy with ileostomy. The need for a complete mucosectomy and the negative effect of radiotherapy on a newly fashioned ileal pouch have been discussed in this chapter. Although a proctocolectomy with ileostomy represents a valid option in all cases of ulcerative colitis complicated by cancer, a restorative proctocolectomy with ileoanal pouch anastomosis or an abdominal colectomy with ileorectostomy may offer alternative options in selected cases. Table 15.2 summarizes all alternative options to a proctocolectomy with ileostomy according to location of cancer (colon or rectal) and stage of disease.

In case of tumor of the middle rectum (8 to 12 cm from the anal verge) with a B2 or C stage, a feasible alternative to this treatment can be a total

proctocolectomy extended to the pelvic floor with closure of the anal canal using a linear stapler and covered, if possible, with omentum along with Brooke ileostomy. This is followed by a period of chemo/radiotherapy. After 18 to 24 months a new staging of the disease is performed associated with sphincter function assessment. If advisable, an IPAA can then be carried out.

We do not have any experience of this kind of treatment in cases of cancer, but we have done this procedure in two cases of redo pouch, performed because of surgical complications (70). These patients had been treated elsewhere with IPAA complicated by anastomotic breakdown. They underwent refashioning of the ileostomy, pelvic space drainage, closure of the anal canal and its protection with omentum. Both of them underwent a subsequent redo pouch with hand-sewn IPAA after 8 and 11 months, respectively, after having a preoperative CT scan revealed the absence of significant pelvic fibrosis. This confirms that the procedure can be technically feasible, although one can surmise that the addition of postoperative radiotherapy may make it technically challenging or, at times, even impossible.

References

1. Sloan WP Jr, Bargen JA, Gage RP. Life histories of patients with chronic ulcerative colitis: a review of 2000 cases. Gastroenterology 1950;16:25–38.
2. Kewenter J, Ahlman H, Hultén L. Cancer risk in extensive ulcerative colitis. Ann Surg 1978;188:824–8.
3. Ekbom A, Hecmick C, Zack M, et al. Ulcerative colitis and colorectal cancer. N Engl J Med 1990;323:1228–33.

4. Broström O, Löfberg L, Nordenvall B, et al. The risk of colorectal cancer in ulcerative colitis. An epidemiologic study. Scand J Gastroenterol 1987;22:1 193–9.

5. Gyde SN, Prior P, Allan RN, et al. Colorectal cancer in ulcerative colitis: a cohort study of primary referrals from three centers. Gut 1988;29:206–17.

6. Langholz E, Munkholm P, Davidsen M, et al. Colorectal cancer risk and mortality in patients with ulcerative colitis. Gastroenterology 1992;10:1444–51.

7. Morson BC, Pang LS. Rectal biopsy as an aid to cancer control in ulcerative colitis. Gut 1967;8:423–34.

8. Riddel RH, Morson BC. Value of sigmoidoscopy and biopsy in the detection of carcinoma and premalignant change in ulcerative colitis. Gut 1979;20:575–80.

9. Collins RH Jr, Feldman M, Fordtran JS. Colon cancer, dysplasia, and surveillance in patients with ulcerative colitis. A critical review. N Engl J Med 1987;316:1654–8.

10. Gyde S. Screening for colorectal cancer in ulcerative colitis: dubious benefits and high costs. Gut 1990;31:1089–92.

11. Lynch DAF, Lobo AJ, Sobala GM, et al. Failure of colonoscopic surveillance in ulcerative colitis. Gut 1993;34:1075–80.

12. Axon ATR. Cancer surveillance in ulcerative colitis—a time for reappraisal. Gut 1994;35:587–9.

13. Aylett SO. Conservative surgery in the treatment of ulcerative colitis. Br Med J 1953;2:1348–51.

14. Aylett SO. Three hundred cases of diffuse ulcerative colitis treated by total colectomy and ileorectal anastomosis. Br Med J 1966;1:1001–5.

15. Parks AG, Nicholls RJ. Restorative proctocolectomy with ileostomy for ulcerative colitis. Br Med J 1978;2:85–8.

16. Pemberton JH, Kelly KA, Beart RW Jr, et al. Ileal pouch-anal anastomosis for chronic ulcerative colitis: long-term results. Ann Surg 1987;206:504–13.

17. Fleshman JW, Mc Leod RS, Cohen Z, et al. Improved results following use of an advancement technique in the treatment of ileoanal anastomotic complications. Int J Colorectal Dis 1988;3:161–5.

18. Ambroze WL Jr, Dozois RR, Pemberton JH, et al. Familial adenomatous polyposis: results following ileal pouch-anal anastomosis and ileorectostomy. Dis Colon Rectum 1992;35:12 5.

19. Jonsson B, Åhsgren L, Andersson LO, et al. Colorectal cancer surveillance in patients with ulcerative colitits. Br J Surg 1994;81:689–91.

20. Devroede GJ, Taylor WF, Sauer WG, et al. Cancer risk and life expectancy of children with ulcerative colitis. N Engl J Med 1971;285:17–21.

21. Lennard-Jones JE, Morson BC, Ritchie JK, et al. Cancer in colitis: assessment of the individual risk by clinical and histological criteria. Gastroenterology 1977;78:1280–9.

22. Medical knowledge self-assessment program VII. Part 2. Book B. Philadelphia: American College of Physicians, 1986:20–1.

23. Connel WR, Talbot IC, Harpaz N, et al. Clinicopathological characteristics of colorectal carcinoma complicating ulcerative colitis. Gut 1994;35:1419–23.

24. Biasco G, Brandi G, Paganelli GM, et al. Colorectal cancer in patients with ulcerative colitis. Cancer 1995;75:2045–50.

25. Lennard-Jones JE, Melville DM, Morson BC, et al. Precancer and cancer in extensive ulcerative colitis: findings among 401 patients over 22 years. Gut, 1990;31:800–6.

26. Melville DM, Jass JR, Morson BC, et al. Observer study on the grading of dysplasia in ulcerative colitis: comparison with clinical outcome. Hum Pathol 1990.

27. Ransohoff DF, Riddel RH, Levin B. Ulcerative colitis and colonic cancer: problems in assessing the diagnostic usefulness of mucosal dysplasia. Dis Colon Rectum 1985;28:383–8.

28. Taylor BA, Pemberton JH, Carpenter HA, et al. Dysplasia in chronic ulcerative colitis: implications for colonoscopic surveillance. Dis Colon Rectum 1992;35:950–6.

29. Baker WN, Glass RE, Ritchie JR, et al. Cancer of the rectum following colectomy and ileorectal anastomosis for ulcerative colitis. Br J Surg 1978;61:86–9.

30. Löfberg R, Leijonmarck C-E, Broström O, et al. Mucosal dysplasia and DNA content in ulcerative colitis patients with ileorectal anastomosis: follow-up study in a defined patient group. Dis Colon Rectum 1991;34:566–71.

31. Grundfest SF, Fazio VW, Weiss RA, et al. The risk of cancer following colectomy and ileorectal anastomosis for extensive mucosal ulcerative colitis. Ann Surg 1981;193:9–14.

32. Miller R, Orrom WJ, Dutjie G, et al. Ambulatory anorectal physiology in patients following restorative proctocolectomy for ulcerative colitis: comparison with normal controls. Br J Surg 1990;77:895–7.

33. Miller R, Bartolo DCC, Cervero F, et al. Does preservation of the anal transition zone influence sensation after ileoanal anastomosis for ulcerative colititts? Clinical controversies in inflammatory bowel disease. Bologna: Tipografia Negri SRL, 1987;205.

34. Holdsworth PJ, Johnston D. Anal sensation after restorative proctocolectomy for ulcerative colitis. Br J Surg 1988;75:993–6.

35. Heald AJ, Allen DR. Stapled ileoanal anastomosis: a technique to avoid mucosal proctectomy in the ileal pouch operation. Br J Surg 1986;75:571–2.

36. Kelly KA. Anal sphincter-saving operations for chronic ulcerative colitis. Am J Surg 1992;163:5–11.

37. Ambroze WL, Pemberton JH, Dozois RR, et al. Does retaining the anal transition zone (ATZ) fail to extirpate chronic ulcerative colitis (CUC) after ileal pouch-anal anastomosis (IPAA)? [abstract] Dis Colon Rectum 1991;34:20

38. Sugerman HJ, Newsome HH, Decosta G, et al. Stapled ileoanal anastomosis for ulcerative colitis and familial polyposis without a temporary diverting ileostomy. Ann Surg 1991;213:606–19.

39. Gozzetti G, Poggioli G, Marchetti F, et al. Functional outcome in hand-sewn versus stapled ileal pouch-anal anastomosis. Am J Surg 1994;168:325–9.

40. King DW, Lubowski DZ, Cook TA. Anal canal mucosa in restorative proctocolectomy for ulcerative colitis. Br J Surg 1989;76:970–2.

41. Stern H, Walfish S, Mullen B, et al. Cancer in an ileoanal reservoir: a new late complication? Gut 1990;32:473–5.

42. Puthu D, Narayanan R, Rao R, et al. Carcinoma of the rectal pouch following restorative proctocolectomy. Dis Colon Rectum 1992;35:257–60.

43. Hoehner JC, Metcalf AM. Development of invasive adenocarcinoma following colectomy with ileoanal anastomosis for familial polyposis coli. Dis Colon Rectum 1994;37:824–8.

44. Ziv Y, Fazio VW, Sirimarco MT, et al. Incidence, risk factors, and treatment of dysplasia in the anal transitional zone after ileal pouch-anal anastomosis. Dis Colon Rectum 1994;37:1281–5.

45. Tsunoda A, Talbot IC, Nicholls RJ. Incidence of dysplasia in the anorectal mucosa in patients having restorative proctocolectomy. Br J Surg 1990;77:506–8.

46. Fazio VW, Tjandra JJ. Transanal mucosectomy: ileal pouch advancement for anorectal dysplasia or inflammation after restorative proctocolectomy. Dis Colon Rectum 1994;37:1008–11.

47. Fazio VW, Tjandra JJ. Pouch advancement and neo-ileoanal anastomosis for anastomotic stricture and anovaginal fistula complicating restorative proctocolectomy. Br J Surg 1992;79:694–6.

48. Brooke BN. The management of an ileostomy including its complication. Lancet 1952;2:102.

49. Kock NG. Intra-abdominal "reservoir" in patients with permanent ileostomy: preliminary observations on a procedure resulting in feacal "continence" in five ileostomy patients. Arch Surg 1969;99:223.

50. Nicholls RJ. Restorative proctocolectomy with various type of reservoir. World J Surg 1987;11:751–62.

51. Enker WE. Potency, cure, and local control in the operative treatment of rectal cancer. Arch Surg 1992;127:1396–402.

52. Heald RJ. Rectal cancer: anterior resection and local recurrence—personal view. Perspect Colon Rectal Surg 1988;1:1–26.

53. Pemberton JH, Kelly KA, Beart RW Jr, et al. Ileal pouch-anal anastomosis for chronic ulcerative colitis. Ann Surg 1987:504–13.

54. Öresland T, Fasth S, Nordgren S, et al. The clinical and functional outcome after restorative proctocolectomy. A prospective study in 100 patients. Int J Colorect Dis 1989;4:50–6.

55. Imbembo A, Lefor AT. Cancer of the colon, rectum and anus. In Sabiston DC Jr.: Textbook of Surgery 14th ed. WB Saunders 1991.

56. Burnstein MJ, Shoetz DJ Jr, Coller JA, et al. Technique of mesenteric lengthening in ileal reservoir-anal anastomosis. Dis Colon Rectum 1987;30:863–6.

57. Rosi PA, Cahill WJ, Carey J. A 10 year study of hemicolectomy in the treatment of cancer of the left half of the colon. Surg Gynecol Obstet 1962;114:15–24.

58. Enker WE, Laffer UT, Block GE. Enhanced survival of patients with colon and rectal cancer is based upon wide anatomic resection. Ann Surg 1979;190:350–60.

59. Pollet WG, Nicholls RJ. The relationship between the extent of distal clearance and survival and local recurrence rate after curative anterior resection for carcinoma of the rectum. Ann Surg 1983;198:1559–63.

60. Pezim ME, Nicholls RJ. Survival of patients after high and low ligation of inferior mesenteric artery. Ann Surg 1984;200(6):729–33.

61. Michelassi F, Vannuci L, Ayala J, et al. Local recurrence after curative resection of colorectal adenocarcinoma. Surgery 1990;108:787–93.

62. Wiltz O, Hashmi HF, Schoetz DJ Jr, et al. Carcinoma and the ileal pouch-anal anastomosis. Dis Colon Rectum 1991;34:805–9.

63. Tjandra JJ, Fazio VW. The ileal pouch—indications for its use and results in clinical practice. Curr Pract Surg 1993;4:22–8.

64. Strong SA, Oakley JR, Fazio VW, et al. Ileal pouch-anal anastomosis: a safe option in advanced colon carcinoma. [Abstract] Dis Colon Rectum 1992;52:22.

65. Ziv Y, Fazio VW, Strong SA, et al. Ulcerative colitis and coexisting colorectal cancer: recurrence rate after restorative proctocolectomy. Ann Surg Oncol 1994;1(6):512–5.

66. Fozard JBJ, Nelson H, Pemberton JH, et al. Primary ileal pouch-anal anastomosis and colorectal cancer—results and contraindications [Abstract]. Dis Colon Rectum 1992;52:22.

67. Gozzetti G. IPAA and cancer. Lecture at "Ileal pouch-anal anastomosis. International Symposium". Versailles (France) 1992:18–9.

68. Taylor BA, Wolff BG, Dozois RR, et al. Ileal pouch-anal anastomosis for chronic ulcerative colitis and familial adenomatous polyposis coli complicated by adenocarcinoma. Dis Colon Rectum 1988;31:358–62.

69. Stelzner M, Fonkalsrud EW. The endorectal ileal pullthrough procedure in patients with ulcerative colitis and familial polyposis with carcinoma. Surg Gynecol Obstet 1989;169:187–94.

70. Poggioli G, Marchetti F, Selleri S, et al. Redo pouches: salvaging of failed ileal-pouch-anal anastomoses. Dis Colon Rectum 1993;36:492–6.

Section III
Crohn's Disease

Part I
Operative Technique

16 Strictureplasty and Mechanical Dilation in Strictured Crohn's Disease

Jeffrey W. Milsom

The appreciable morbidity and mortality associated with an unusual variant of Crohn's disease, diffuse jejunoileitis, gave rise to a search for an alternative to resection for the treatment of this severe form of small bowel Crohn's disease. Emmanoel Lee, working in Oxford in the 1970s was stimulated by the work of Katariya and others in India, who had shown that revision, *not* resection, of ileal tuberculous strictures was possible with a high rate of healing and relief of the obstruction associated with them (1,2). Lee pioneered the application of the same procedure, strictureplasty, to that form of Crohn's disease in which short fibrotic strictures of small intestine occur (2). Since that time, the techniques of intestinal strictureplasty have been adopted and used in a large number of centers specializing in inflammatory bowel disease surgery, particularly in Birmingham, UK, under the leadership of Alexander Williams, and in the department of colorectal surgery at the Cleveland Clinic, under the leadership of Victor Fazio. Although questions exist about the exact role of intestinal strictureplasty and its long-term consequences in patients with Crohn's disease, this procedure has become an accepted mode of therapy for many patients who might otherwise have developed or become vulnerable to a short bowel syndrome. Its role in the treatment of Crohn's disease is still evolving. In this chapter, we outline the principal indications and contraindications for intestinal strictureplasty, the various techniques used, and their complications. Results of various surgical series, including our own, are presented along with speculation on where strictureplasty may be applied as a therapy for Crohn's disease in the future. We also will discuss the role of mechanical dilation in the management of intestinal Crohn's disease. This technique has far less application in the treatment of Crohn's disease.

Indications and Contraindications

Most patients with Crohn's disease of the small intestine are not candidates for strictureplasty, and are best served by a simple resection of the affected segment with reanastomosis. We believe a reasonable list of indications for intestinal strictureplasty to be as follows:

1. Diffuse jejunoileitis causing significant obstruction that has failed to respond to medical management—expecially single or multiple short fibrotic strictures.
2. Patients with multiple prior intestinal resections presenting with recurrent stricturing disease, at risk for development of a short bowel syndrome.
3. Recurrence of strictures within twelve months of a previous resection.
4. Isolated and limited ileocolonic anastomotic strictures.
5. Selected duodenal strictures.

Initial concerns about a role for strictureplasty in Crohn's disease were based on traditional teaching of avoiding anastomoses in diseased bowel. Thus, the risks of suture line disruption was felt to be considerable—if not prohibitive—by most surgeons who reviewed Dr. Lee's preliminary report. Since then, the concerns have been largely put to rest by numerous reports, including a long-term outcome report from the Oxford Group—the surgical team of which the late Dr. Lee was a member and leader (3). Extrapolation of the risks of strictureplasty breakdown to other situations in which adverse healing factors are reported led to recommendation to avoid strictureplasty when certain features were present e.g., paraintestinal abscess, enteric fistula, peritonitis, severe malnutrition, or hypoalbuminemia, e.g., < 2G/dL. Other contraindications were based upon the risks of leaving an occult cancer behind, or a poor benefit-to-risk ratio e.g., multiple anastomoses in a short segment, the saving of which is not worth the risk of dehiscence from multiple anastomoses. A list of accepted contraindications follows:

Contraindications

1. Diffuse peritonitis.
2. Free perforation of the affected bowel segment.
3. Phlegmon or abscess associated with the affected bowel segment.
4. Fistulous disease with inflammatory resection of the diseased intestinal segment.
5. Multiple strictured segments within a short distance that might be better treated using a single resection.
6. Suspicion of carcinoma.
7. Hypoalbuminemia.

What Are the Surgical Options in Extensive, Stricturing Crohn's Disease?

When a patient with Crohn's disease presents with either acute or subacute obstruction, associated with multiple areas of segmental narrowing of the small bowel he or she is vulnerable to the consequences of excisional therapy and the specter of a short bowel syndrome always looms as a potential outcome. If single or multiple segmental resection is not an option, alternatives for such patients with stricturing disease include dilation, bypass, or strictureplasty.

Dilation, generally performed endoscopically with inflatable balloons, has limited applications. The difficulty in reaching the majority of strictures endoscopically, the applicability of this technique only to short techniques (4), and the short-term benefit of the treatment limit the use of dilatation. Few surgeons now advocate balloon dilatation in the management of intestinal strictures due to Crohn's disease because of the high rate of recurrencen (5). In addition, the success rate of strictureplasty has reduced the indications for balloon dilatation even further. Nowadays mechanized

dilatation with dilators is used for isolated stenosis, and pneumatic dilatation with endoscopy is reserved to selected, isolated, and short strictures of ileocolonic or ileorectal anastomosis.

Bypass operations have a limited role in Crohn's and are described in Chapter 17. Strictureplasty thus becomes the preferred option for this difficult problem, and clinical series attest to its effectiveness.

Operative Strategy

In all of Crohn's disease surgery, the underlying principle is conservatism, reserving operative intervention for complications. Surgery should preserve as much bowel, especially small bowel, as possible and it must be safe. With these principles in mind, the preoperative preparation in a patient who may require a strictureplasty operation is as follows:

1. Mechanical whole gut lavage if not obstructed.
2. In presence of significant obstruction, 48 to 72 hours clear liquid diet and preoperative enemas.
3. Correction of anemia, to achieve a hemoglobin level of at least 9 g/dL.
4. Intravenous broad spectrum antibiotics given one hour preoperatively, then one dose postoperatively (longer if significant contamination has occurred).
5. Supine position on the operating room in a way or to facilitate changing the frontier to modified lithotomy, should this become necessary in the course of the caes.
6. Calf compression stockings, placed in the operating room.
7. Rectal washout in the operating room immediately before incision if distal colonic or rectal surgery may be necessary.

Once the small bowel has been freed of adhesions, the surgeon must decide on a plan of action. Obvious signs of stricturing include narrowing of the bowel with proximal dilatation. Fat wrapping, thickening of the mesentery, palpable fibrosis, and corkscrew vessels on the serosa of the bowel all signal the possibility of stricturing being present. Once the most obvious area of bowel is transected or opened in preparation for a resection or strictureplasty, then intraluminal sounding is done by introducing a Foley catheter in the lumen: inflation of the balloon with varying amounts of water will help assessing the potential area of the stricture.

The foley catheter is particularly useful for sounding the duodenal sweep via a strictureplasty site in the proximal jejunum, if the duodenum is suspected of having a stricture. As we identify areas of stricturing, they are marked with a stitch on the antimesenteric border for later evaluation. Since most patients will require a concomitant resection along with strictureplasty, we will generally perform the resection first. This is done according to conventional methods.

The strictured sites are then isolated proximally and distally from the rest of the intestine by encircling umbilical tapes or by noncrushing intestinal clamps so as to avoid spillage of intestinal contents. Next a longitudinal incision through the strictureplasty site is made using electrosurgery. It is helpful to begin the incision about 2 or 3 cm from the stricture, in normal bowel, then insert a long forceps into the lumen of the bowel through the stricture. The forceps is then held up out of the abdomen to place the area to be incised under tension, and the electrosurgery is used to cut through the stricture and beyond it for an additional 2 or 3 cm into normal bowel. Once the bowel is opened, the stricture site is inspected and biopsied along its mesenteric border, where a characteristic ulceration usually lies. We do this to exclude an occult malignancy. We have seen one case of a malignancy occurring in a strictureplasty site 8 years after it was performed (7). This patient had adult-onset celiac disease (in which patients are also at an increased risk for the development of small bowel cancer), thus it is difficult to attribute this to one causative factor. Hemostasis of the opened bowel edges is obtained using electrosurgery, then the repair is begun.

The basic strictureplasty methods (Heineke-Mikulicz and Finney) are similar techniques to those for which they are named in upper gastrointestinal surgery. The Heineke-Mikulicz method is used in strictures less than 8 to 10 cm in length. Longer strictures than this would likely have too much tension placed on the central part of the repair, thus the Finney repair is useful for strictures greater than 10 cm and up to 20 to 25 cm in length.

The Heineke-Mikulicz Strictureplasty

After opening the bowel, carefully incising into normal bowel proximal and distal to the stricture exactly on the antimesenteric border, braided polyglycolic acid 3–0 sutures are placed at the edges of the strictured area and at the central portion of it,

distracting the edges and changing the longitudinal incision into a transverse one (Fig. 16.1). Interrupted sutures are then placed to achieve good tissue approximation. The site is marked on its mesentery with a metallic clip (Fig. 16.2) and sites are numbered from proximal to distal with progressively added clips so these areas can theoretically be evaluated radiographically in the postoperative period or at a future laparotomy.

The Finney Strictureplasty

Long strictures (over 10 cm) require this method because of the tension on the strictureplasty created by attempting to bend the bowel back on itself by the Heineke-Mikulicz method. The Finney method bends the affected segment in a U-shape, and the bowel is incised with the electrosurgery again beginning with normal bowel 2 or 3 cm from the stricture. The incision is begun in this area directly on the antimesenteric border, but as the midportion of the stricture is reached, the incision is placed slightly closer to the mesenteric border (Fig. 16.3). This helps relieve some of the tension that can occur in placing the sutures in this area, and appears to allow better apposition of the cut edges of the bowel than if the incision is kept on the mesenteric edge. Sutures are first placed between normal bowel edges at the proximal and distal ends of the enterotomy and at the apex of the strictureplasty on the posterior wall of the enterotomy, using bites that are full thickness of the wall so as to maximize hemostasis of the suture line. Size 3–0 polyglycolic acid sutures are used, and are placed in a continuous running fashion first closing the posterior wall, then the anterior one. Interrupted sutures are placed as necessary to achieve good tissue apposition (Fig. 16.4). A clip is placed on the central portion of the strictureplasty as described above.

The Combination Strictureplasty

A combination method that contains elements of both the Heineke-Mikulicz and the Finney methods has been described by Fazio (8) for two closely approximated long strictures that, if closed by separate strictureplasties could result in one or two diverticula that could predispose to stasis of the bowel contents. The combination method begins by making a long incision through both strictures, then sews up the central part of the incised segment in a Finney method (folding it outwards on both sides), thereafter closing it in a Heineke-

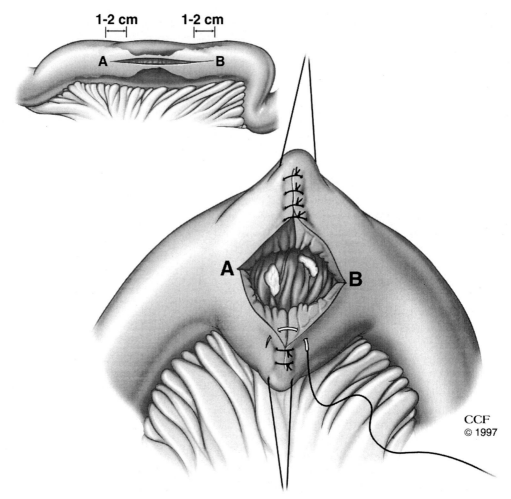

Fig. 16.1.   After incising the stricture and adjacent "normal" small bowel longitudinally, the defect is closed transversely with single layer 2–0 or 3–0 polyglycolic acid sutures. Inset shows sero muscular sutures.

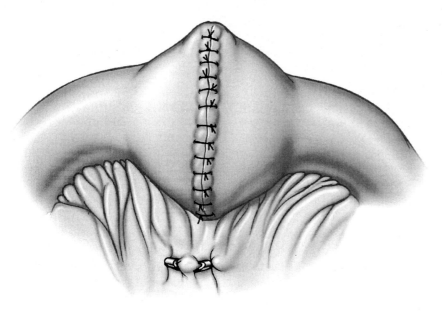

Fig. 16.2. Completed Heinecke-Mikulicz strictureplasty. Note metallic clip on mesenteric margin. This sometimes is the only evidence found at subsequent laparotomies of where a stricture once was present. It may also be helpful with future contrast studies.

Special Technical Issues and Situations

Where extensive disease is encountered, especially when this is somewhat unexpected in the malnourished or urgently operated upon patient, it is quite reasonable to consider proximal diversion (loop jejunostomy). Of course this will likely oblige the patient to a course of several months of total parenteral nutrition, but this is preferable to a disastrous outcome if poor healing ensues after multiple strictureplasties. If the patient is acutely ill, or if the tissue seems extremely fragile, then only a proximal diversion may be contemplated, with definitive therapy being reserved after 3 to 6 months, or until the patient regains a reasonable state of health. In general, we will consider diverting ostomy when serum albumin is below 2 g/dL.

Strictureplasty of all areas suspect for stenosis. Since strictureplasty has been shown to be a safe technique, even when applied to multiple areas of the bowel in the same patient, all suspicious areas should be treated at operation (10). In these situations, mild, probably asymptomatic, strictures can be operated on along with strictureplasty for even severe strictures. In these cases, when the intestinal wall at the level of the stricture is not very thick or inflamed, the strictureplasty may be performed with staples.

Duodenal Crohn's. Strictureplasty is an effective therapy for selected strictures in the duodenum. A Heineke-Mikulicz is usually performed for limited strictures of the pylorus, 2nd, 3rd, and occasionally 4th portion. A stricture of the pylorus extending proximally into the antrum may be treated with a Finney gastroduodenostomy. Alexander-Williams and Haynes reported successful in 6 patients who underwent strictureplasty for duodenal Crohn's (11). Our experience in six patients with duodenal Crohn's has similarly been met with relief of obstruction in all patients (12).

Stricture at the ileocolonic anastomosis. Certain patients who develop a stricture at the ileocolic anastomosis may be candidates for strictureplasty at this site. This may include young patients, patients who have undergone multiple previous operations for Crohn's, patients with a short stricture where strictureplasty offers an easier alternative to resection or any patient at risk for the development of a short bowel syndrome. We have reviewed a series of 22 patients who underwent strictureplasty of the ileocolonic anastomosis for stricturing disease. There were 15 Heineke-Mikulicz and 7 Finney strictureplasties, performed a median of 2 years

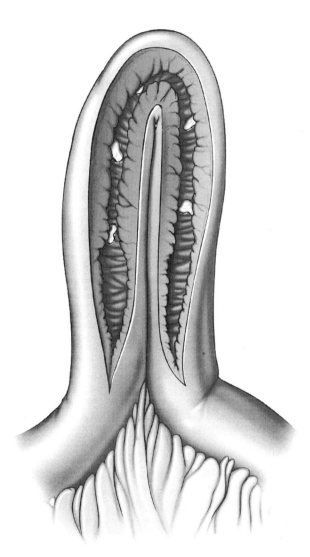

Fig. 16.3. Finney strictureplasty. The two loops are opposed and antimesenteric enterotomy is made. Biopsies are taken.

Mikulicz fashion (Fig. 6.5). This method theoretically minimizes the chances for stasis of the repaired segment (10).

The Side-to-Side Isoperistaltic Strictureplasty

Michelassi has described this method to treat long strictures and has reported its successful application in three patients with extensive Crohn's disease (9). The method entails transecting the affected segment at its midpoint, then moving the proximal loop over the distal one in a side-to-side fashion. The two loops are approximated by a layer of 3–0 sutures, closing off the ends in a tapered fashion in order to avoid any blind stumps (Fig. 16.6).

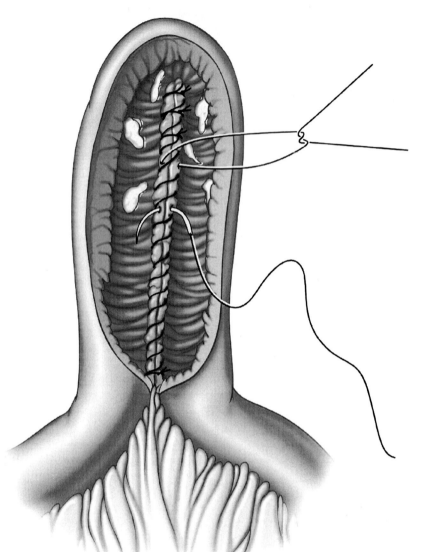

Fig. 16.4. The posterior layer is closed with continuous 2–0 polyglycolic acid. Strategically placed sutures, interrupted, help to reinforce that layer. The anterior edges are then sutured to complete the Finney strictureplasty.

after the initial operation. Postoperatively, there was no mortality and no major septic complication, with symptomatic relief in all patients (13).

Outcome of Surgery

The pattern of Crohn's disease in which small bowel strictures occur commonly involves both ileum and jejunum. Most patients with diffuse small bowel disease have had long-standing illness, in excess of 10 years. Rates of admission to hospital, steroid use, previous surgery, use of total parenteral nutrition and features of malnutrition are more common than in patients undergoing solely segmental small bowel resection. Fazio et al. (12) reviewed their experience with strictureplasty and noted that the majority of their patients had dis-

ease longer than 10 years and had preoperative weight loss. One fourth required preoperative parenteral alimentation (with 7% shared on parenteral alimentation at home). Interestingly, 61% underwent a synchronous resection (Table 16.1).

In subsequent reports from our unit (14,15) in 162 patients undergoing 698 strictureplasties during the course of 191 operations, we showed similar trends as shown in Table 16.1. No mortality was seen. With longer follow-up cumulative five year reoperative recurrences were 28%. For 52 patients who underwent strictureplasty alone, cumulative recurrence was 31% at five years compared with 27% for those with strictureplasty and synchronous resection (*n* = 100 patients). In studying complications, (15) median hospital stay was eight days, and perioperative sepsis occurred in 5% with need for

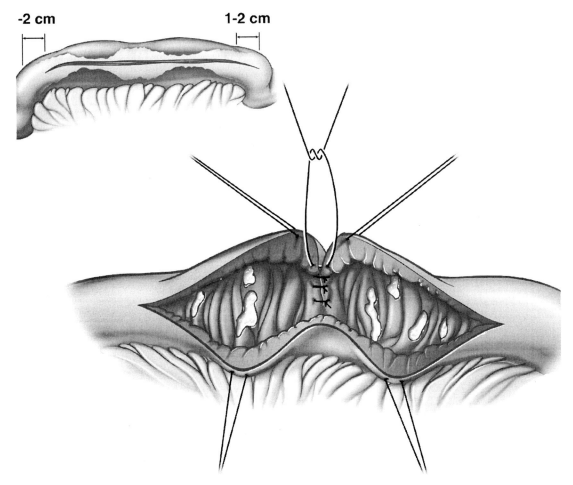

Fig. 16.5. Technique for treatment of long or multiple near—confluent strictures—the combination stricture-plasty. Antimesenteric enterotomy passes through both strictures into the normal bowel. The posterior layers of the mid point of the defect are closed by the Finney technique (i.e., a continuous closure).

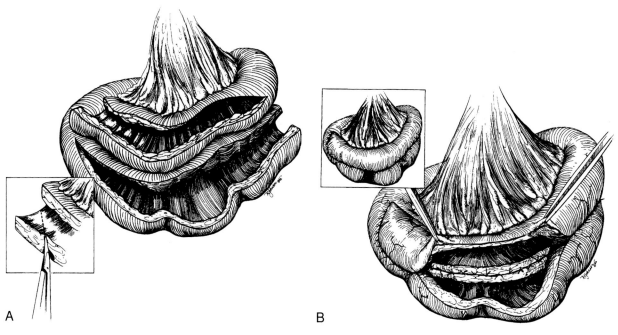

A   B

Fig. 16.6. (A) A longitudinal enterotomy is performed on both loops, and the intestinal ends are spatulated to avoid blind stumps (inset). (B) Both outer and inner suture lines are continued and finished anteriorly. The completed side-to-side isolperistaltic strictureplasty is shown in the inset.

Table 16.1. Patients' characteristics.

Patient	116
Number of strictureplasties (SXPL)	452
Heinecke Mikulicz	405
Finney	47
Median SXPL per case	3
Range	(1–15)
Synchronous resection	71 (61%)
Duration of Crohn's disease	
Median	12 year
Range	1–32 years
Preoperative weight loss	52%
	(median 7kg)
Preoperative TPN	27%
Permanent home TPN	7%
Hemoglobin (median)	10.4 g %
Albumin (median)	3.6 g %

reoperation for sepsis in only 3%. New stricture formation requiring surgery occurred in 15% with median follow-up of 42 months overall. Only 2.8% of all patients developed restricturing at the site of a previous strictureplasty. Relief of obstruction was achieved in all but 2 patients, and 50% of patients were able to be weaned off steroids.

At the time of repeat operation for recurrent stricturing, nearly all reporting centers have noted that the majority of new strictures occur at new sites, with recurrent stricturing at the previous strictureplasty sites occurring at a rate of about 3 or 4% (3,14). This is an interesting observation and one that does not have a clear explanation. Alexander-Williams has suggested that Crohn's disease at strictureplasty sites heal due to the relief of the obstruction, breaking a vicious cycle of bacterial overgrowth, ulceratious, and more scarring (16).

Although we have seen a significant association of septic complications with hypoalbuminemia, there is no association of this complication with the number of strictureplasties, strictureplasty length, use of steroids, or whether or not a resection was performed coincident with the strictureplasties (15). Yet, significant gastrointestinal hemorrhage requiring blood transfusion occurred in our series in 9% of 139 patients (523 strictureplasties) (4% had transfusions in excess of 3 units) (17). This could be a major problem if reoperation were required, since it would be difficult to ascertain which of the strictureplasty sites was bleeding. Thus far we have not had to reoperate on any patient. In two instances, patients were sent to the angiography suite and underwent selective mesenteric angiography which identified the site of hemorrhage (at a strictureplasty site). Use of intraarterial vas-

opressin was effective in controlling the hemorrhage in both patients (17). This may be a reasonable approach for significant gastrointestinal in the early postoperative period.

Strictureplasty: Present and Future

There remain many questions about how strictureplasty works, and what the long term outcome of the strictureplasty sites will be. For example, what is the risk of carcinoma developing in these areas? After healing, do the strictureplasty sites function and absorb nutrients? Can or should stricureplasty be used at all in the colon since the colon may be at an increased risk to undergo malignant change?

Despite these questions, there is little doubt that in complex Crohn's disease with jejunoileitis, strictureplasty has now been demonstrated to be a safe and effective therapy in hundreds of reported cases in the literature. The techniques involved are familiar to most gastrointestinal surgeons, and evidence suggests that strictureplasty should be applied liberally in patients with stricturing disease.

Whether it should be used in patients, especially young patients, with more limited disease, is worthy of investigation. One might argue that if a safe method exists for healing the strictured site while preserving bowel length, then this method should be applied when the Crohn's patient is at significant risk for disease recurrence. Alexander-Williams also suggests that the use of strictureplasty might also be reasonable in more patients with fistulous or localized septic complications of the disease, representing the best of poor options.

Another question worthy of future investigation is whether techniques that minimize the potential for stasis of the repaired site should be applied more liberally (i.e., the combination strictureplasty or the isoperistaltic side-to-side technique). These may minimize malabsorption and bacterial overgrowth, important considerations for patients with marginal intestinal reserve.

Other surgical therapies will likely emerge in the therapy of Crohn's disease. Strictureplasty is not ideal for the majority of patients requiring surgery for the complications of this disease, and must be utilized only if it seems to fit into the strategic plan for the individual patient over the course of his/her lifetime. Nonetheless, strictureplasty represents a major advance in the treatment of stricturing Crohn's disease affecting multiple segments or in patients at risk for the development of a short bowel syndrome who require surgery.

References

1. Katariya RN, Sood S, Rao PG, et al. Strictureplasty for tubercular strictures of the gastrointestinal tract. Br J Surg 1977; 64:496–4.

2. Lee ECG, Papaioannou N. Minimal surgery for chronic obstruction in patients with extensive or universal Crohn's disease. Ann R Coll Surg 1982; 64:229–33.

3. Stebbing JF, Jewell DP, Kettlewell MG, et al. Long-term results of recurrence and reoperation after strictureplasty for obstructive Crohn's disease. Br J Surg 1995; 82:1471–4.

4. Alexander-Williams J, Allan A, Morel P, et al. The therapeutic dilatation of enteric strictures due to Crohn's disease. Ann Coll Surg Engl 1986; 68:1–3.

5. Williams AJK, Palmer KR. Endoscopic balloon dilatation as a therapeutic option in the management of intestinal strictures resulting from Crohn's disease. Br J Surg 1991; 78:453, 454.

6. Alexander-Williams J. Surgical management of small intestinal Crohn's disease: resection or strictureplasty. Semin Colon Rectal Surg 1994; 5:193–8.

7. Marchetti F, Fazio VW, Ozuner G. Adenocarcinoma arising from a strictureplasty site in Crohn's disease. Dis Colon Rectum 1996; 39:1315–21.

8. Fazio VW, Tjandra JJ. Strictureplasty for Crohn's disease with multiple long strictures. Dis Colon Rectum 1993; 36:71, 72.

9. Michelassi, F. Side-to-side isojuestaltic strictureplasty for resection Crohn's strictures. Dis Col Rectum 1996; 39:345–7.

10. Sasaki I, Funayama Y, Naito H, et al. Extended strictureplasty for multiple short skipped strictures of Crohn's disease. Dis Colon Rectum 1996; 39: 342–4.

11. Alexander-Williams J, Haynes IG. Conservative operations for Crohn's disease of the small bowel. World J Surg 1985; 9:945–51.

12. Fazio VW, Tjandra JJ, Lavery IC, et al. Long-term follow-up for strictureplasty in Crohn's disease. Dis Colon Rectum 1993; 36:353.

13. Tjandra JJ, Fazio VW. Strictureplasty for ileocolic anastomotic strictures in Crohn's disease. Dis Colon Rectum 1993; 36:1099–104.

14. Ozuner G, Fazio VW, Lavery IC, et al. Reoperative rates for Crohn's disease following strictureplasty: long-term analysis. Dis Colon Rectum 1996; 39:1–5.

15. Ozuner G, Fazio VW, Lavery IC, et al. How safe is strictureplasty in the management of Crohn's disease? Am J Surg 1996; 171:57–61.

16. Alexander-Williams J, Fornaro M. Strictureplasty beim morbus Crohn der chirurg. Chirurg 1982; 53:799–801.

17. Ozuner G, Fazio VW. Management of gastrointestinal bleeding after strictureplasty for Crohn's disease. Dis Colon Rectum 1995; 38:297–300.

17 Bypass Procedures

Bruce G. Wolff and Denis C.N.K. Nyam

The type of operation recommended for the common form of Crohn's disease in the terminal ileum has changed several times since the disease was first described in 1932. Radical resection was initially practiced but due to the unacceptably high mortality of the procedure the operating strategy was changed to simple short-circuiting procedures. This was rapidly followed by relapse or recurrent disease and subsequently this strategy was abandoned to be replaced by bypass with exclusion to completely divert the fecal stream away from the diseased ileum. This procedure was devised at the Mt Sinai Hospital in New York and had a low mortality (the most famous recipient of this operation was President Eisenhower [1]).

With the advancement in perioperative antibiotics and fluid electrolyte management, resection regained favor and is the operation of choice in most forms of Crohn's disease today.

Gastroduodenal Crohn's disease may be the only exception to this in which the principle of nonexclusion bypass has been used with success. This is because the magnitude of a duodenal resection is excessive in an ill patient with a chronic relapsing disease like Crohn's. In addition, the indication for surgery is usually to relieve obstruction rather than for acute inflammatory complications. Bypass surgery in other parts of the gastrointestinal tract is only done under very special circumstances.

Indications for Surgery

The choice of the operative procedure best suited for a particular patient depends upon the type of disease, the presence of any complications, the metabolic state of the patient and life style considerations. In addition the operative findings and the patient's intraoperative condition may modify the choice. Specific indications for bypass include the following.

Gastroduodenal Crohn's

The duodenum is involved in only 1% to 2% of patients with Crohn's disease. One third of these patients requires surgical treatment (2,3) indicated by obstruction or, much less frequently, by hemorrhage. Obstruction of the first and second portion of the duodenum can be treated with a gastrojejunostomy and vagotomy; if the obstruction is in the third or fourth position, a duodenojejunal bypass is sufficient.

Duodenal Involvement by Adjacent Segments

Duodenal involvement is most commonly a result of inflammation from surrounding segments of diseased bowel. Recurrence at an ileocolic anastomosis can often lead to duodenal involvement with or without an enteroduodenal fistula. After resection of the diseased ileocolonic segment, the duodenum may be left with a full thickness defect. Such defect can be treated either by an onlay patch or a bypass.

Complex Small Bowel or Ileocolonic Crohn's

The rare instance where the inflammation is so severe that the inflammatory mass cannot be safely mobilized without danger to important structures like the ureter. Under such circumstances it is more prudent to bypass the diseased segment.

Pitfalls and Danger Points

Resection of the diseased segment is preferable to an exclusion bypass, because the excluded segment is associated with a worrisome set of late complications. These include the presence or subsequent development of carcinoma (4,5), reactivation of disease, and free perforation with further sepsis. These must be borne in mind when weighing the possibilities of a resection vs. bypass in a very sick patient with Crohn's disease deemed "not suitable for a resection." With modern surgical techniques and perioperative care, a resection can be carried out with equal safety as a bypass in nearly all situations. Moreover, when the severe inflammatory reaction surrounding an abnormal terminal ileum has caused an obstructive uropathy, the bypass is not likely to relieve the ureteral obstruction.

Operative Strategy

Any surgical procedure in Crohn's disease must be tailored to the anatomic location and to the severity of the problem at hand.

Bypass surgery is most commonly chosen in the gastroduodenal region. As the magnitude of a pancreatoduodenectomy seems excessive in a patient with Crohn's disease of the duodenum, this is the only area in which a bypass in continuity is considered the preferred treatment. The best results have been achieved with gastrojejunostomy (6,7). Since the jejunal segment is known to be particularly susceptible to ulceration, and since patients who have extensive small bowel resection may have secondary gastric hypersecretion, it is suggested that a vagotomy be added to decrease the risk of stomal ulceration.

Selective or highly selective vagotomy has the theoretical advantage of being less likely to induce troublesome diarrhea. It is convenient to perform the vagotomy before the gastrojejunostomy to avoid potential tension on a freshly fashioned anastomosis during attempts at gaining exposure at the level of the esophageal hiatus.

Bypass surgery is an infrequently indicated option in the surgical treatment of small bowel or ileocolic disease. The main aim in bypass surgery is palliation of immediate danger to life with the ileoileo or ileotransverse bypass. Patients considered for such an option are usually too ill to withstand a resection, even one without an anastomosis.

Operative Technique

Gastrojejunostomy and Vagotomy

An upper gastrointestinal bypass and vagotomy are best performed through a midline incision. After the vagotomy is performed, the gastrojejunostomy is fashioned either in an anticolic or retrocolic position. In general, we prefer an antecolic anastomosis in order to keep any further inflammation due to anastomotic problems or recurrent Crohn's away from the retroperitoneum. The anastomosis can be hand-sewn or stapled. Due to the similarity of these techniques in all segments of the gastrointestinal tract, we will describe one technique stapled and one hand-sewn.

Antecolic Stapled Gastrojejunostomy

The most dependent part of the stomach on the greater curve is used. The most proximal loop of jejunum that comes out to lie comfortably next to the greater curve is selected. Two stay sutures that hold the small bowel and stomach together are placed, taking care to allow room for a 5 cm anastomosis to be made. An enterotomy and a gastrotomy are then made (Fig. 17.1A) allowing the blades of the linear cutter to be inserted (Fig. 17.1B) and fired (Fig. 17.1C). The enterotomy is then closed using two layers of interrupted 3–0 absorbable suture (Fig. 17.1D).

Retrocolic Hand-sewn Gastrojejunostomy

There is no functional difference in having the anastomosis ante or retrocolic. Its description here is to outline different possibilities. A window is made in an avascular area of the transverse mesocolon (Fig. 17.2A) and the posterior wall of the stomach is then exposed. To facilitate this maneuver, the middle colic artery must be identified to avoid injuring it and the adhesions of the transverse mesocolon to the posterior wall of the stomach are best taken down to gain adequate exposure. A posterior layer of interrupted 3–0 silk sutures is used to approximate the stomach and the small bowel. After the gastrotomy and the enterotomy are completed (Fig. 17.2B) a continuous inner suture layer is done with 3–0 absorbable suture (Fig. 17.2C). The anastomosis is completed with an outer anterior layer of interrupted 3–0 silk (Fig. 17.2D) and closure of the mesocolon defect.

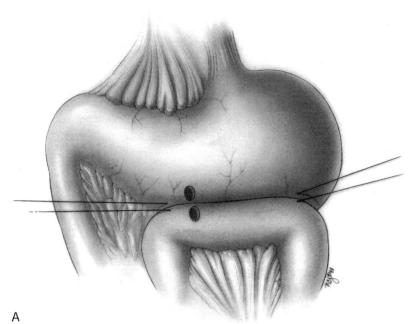

A

Fig. 17.1. Antecolic stapled gastrojejunostomy. (A) Stay sutures inserted, enterotomy and gastrotomy made for insertion of staplers. (B) Linear stapler inserted into enterotomy and gastrotomy. (C) Stapler gun approximated and fired. (D) Enterotomy and gastrotomy closed with interrupted 3–0 sutures.

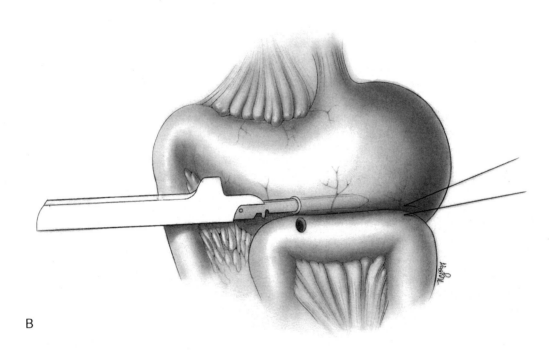

B

Fig. 17.1. (*Continued*).

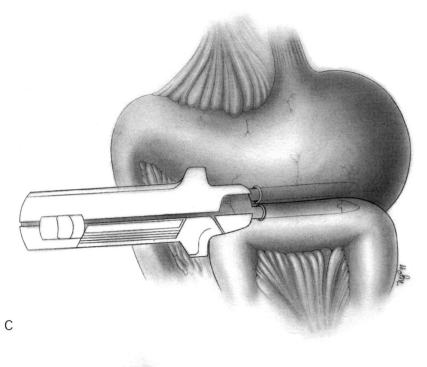

C

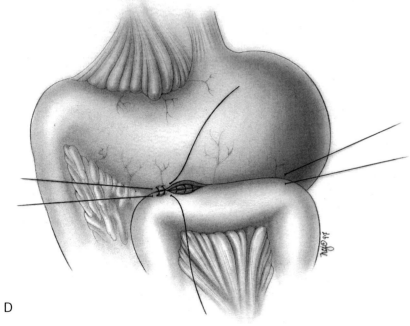

D

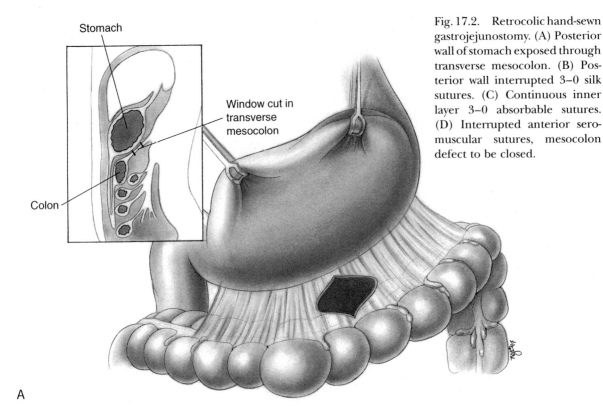

Fig. 17.2.   Retrocolic hand-sewn gastrojejunostomy. (A) Posterior wall of stomach exposed through transverse mesocolon. (B) Posterior wall interrupted 3–0 silk sutures. (C) Continuous inner layer 3–0 absorbable sutures. (D) Interrupted anterior sero-muscular sutures, mesocolon defect to be closed.

Stomach

Window cut in transverse mesocolon

Colon

A

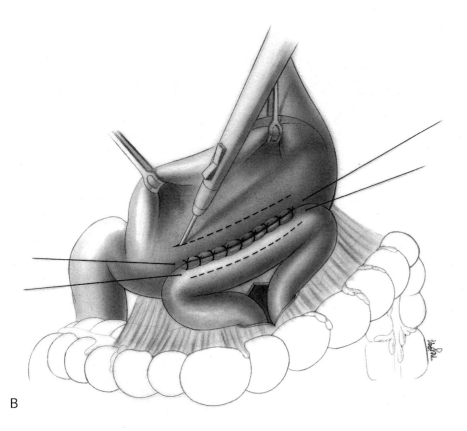

B

Fig. 17.2. (*Continued*).

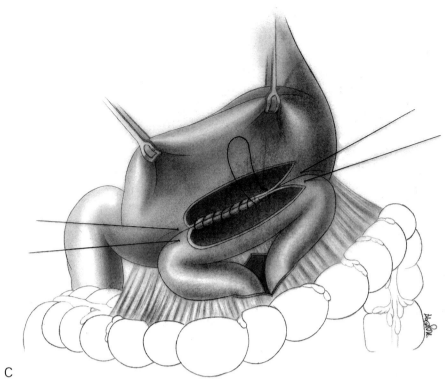

C

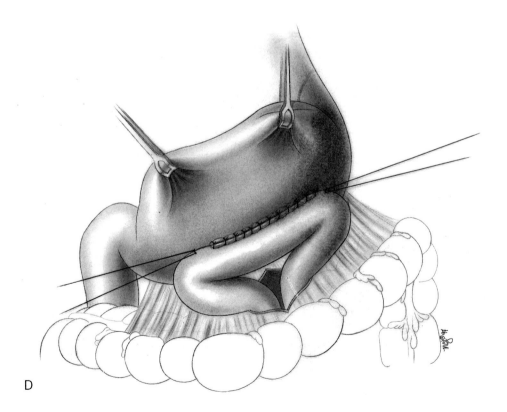

D

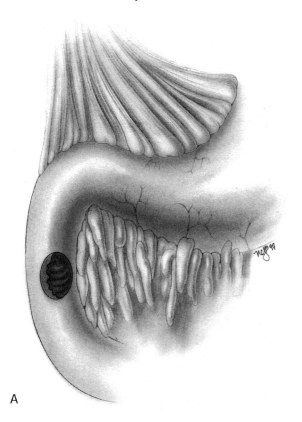

Fig. 17.3.   Duodenal jejunal bypass. (A) Defect left after excising a duodenal colic fistula. (B) Posterior layer with seromuscular interrupted sutures with 3–0 silk. (C) Inner layer with continuous 3–0 absorbable suture. (D) Anterior layer of interrupted seromuscular 3–0 silk.

A

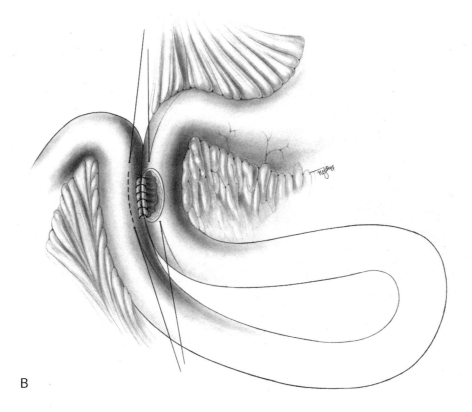

B

Fig. 17.3. (*Continued*).

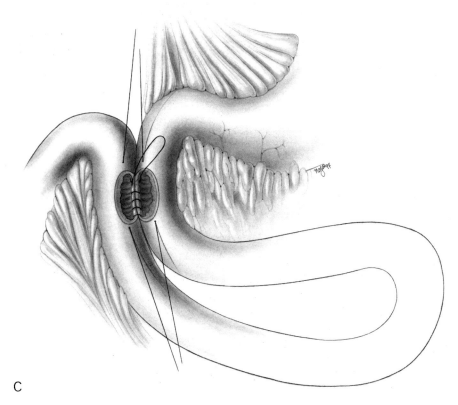

C

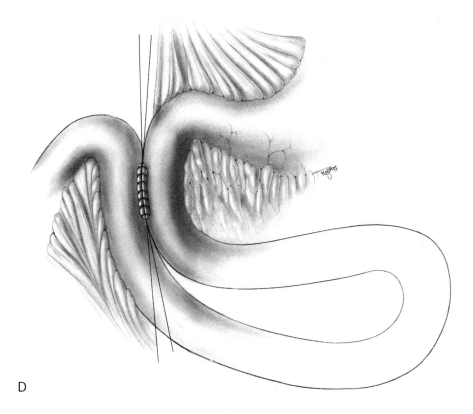

D

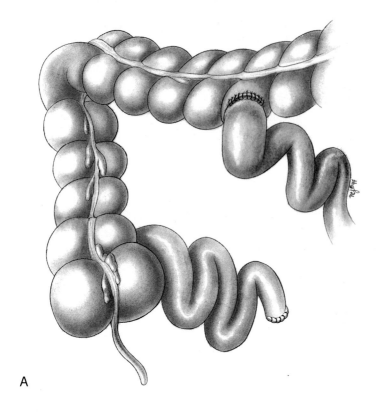

A

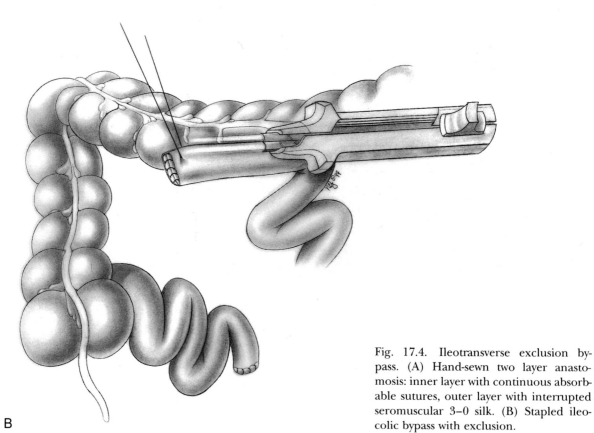

B

Fig. 17.4. Ileotransverse exclusion by-pass. (A) Hand-sewn two layer anastomosis: inner layer with continuous absorbable sutures, outer layer with interrupted seromuscular 3–0 silk. (B) Stapled ileocolic bypass with exclusion.

Duodenojejunal Bypass

This procedure does not need a complementing vagotomy. The anastomosis is performed in similar fashion as for a hand-sewn gastrojejunostomy, securing a posterior layer of interrupted 3–0 silk (Fig. 17.3A, 17.3.B) followed by a continuous inner layer of 3–0 absorbable sutures (Fig. 17.3C) and finally an anterior layer of seromuscular 3–0 silk (Fig. 17.3D). Occasionally the duodenum may need to be mobilized off the retroperitoneum in order to get adequate exposure.

Ileotransverse Bypass

This anastomosis can be fashioned using either staplers (Fig. 17.4A) or a hand-sewn technique (Fig. 17.4B). The technique is similar to the one described for the gastrojejunostomy, with the difference that the hand-sewn technique is preferred in the end-to-side anostomosis.

Complications

The complications encountered after bypass for Crohn's disease can be related to the diseased bypassed segment (Table 17.1) and general complications. The general complications are similar to all intraabdominal surgery with an anastomosis, with none specific to the procedure.

Long-Term Results

Gastroduodenal Crohn's

In a series of 70 patients followed up for 30 years, a third of patients who underwent a surgical procedure required a second operation (2). The Cleveland Clinic experience showed that 20% of patients require reoperation at 5 years and almost 70% at 11 years. The majority of reoperations are due to profession of Crohn's disease.

Small Bowel or Ileocolonic Bypass

Although many reports (10,11,12) have analyzed results obtained with nonexclusion and exclusion bypass without attempting a separate analysis nonexclusional bypass is notoriously known for higher recurrence rates, as high as 90% (13,14).

The perception that the excluded segment would heal while defunctioned and then be available for subsequent use has been realized only on rare occasions (15). At one time it was even claimed that exclusion bypass had a lower rate of recurrence than resection (16,17) but these impressions have not been confirmed by others and now resec-

Table 17.1. Complications of the bypassed segment.

1. Reactivation of disease.
2. Perforation (9,10). In most of these cases there is distal obstruction in the bypass loop which contributes to the perforation.
3. Persistent sepsis.
4. Development of carcinoma (4,5).

tion has become the treatment of choice by the majority (11,13,18). The cumulative risk of recurrence and of requiring an additional major operation each year after bypass is approximately twice the risk after resection (11). This is due to complications (Table 17.1) of the bypassed segment requiring resection (19–21).

The majority of surgical opinion currently favors exclusion bypass in the rare instance in which bypass is indicated. Almost nothing can be gained by a nonexclusion bypass since the fecal stream continues to flow to the diseased segment to a greater or lesser degree. In addition, in the majority of the time the bypass is now the first of a two stage procedure with the aim of resecting the involved segment once the patient's general condition improves.

References

1. Heaton LD, et al. President Eisenhower's operation for regional enteritis. A footnote to history. Ann Surg 1965;159:661
2. Murray JJ, Schoetz DJ Jr, Nugent FW. Surgical management of Crohn's disease involving the duodenum. Am J Surg 1984;147:58.
3. Nugent FW, Roy MA. Duodenal Crohn's disease. An analysis of 89 cases. Am J Gasteroenterol 1989;84:249.
4. Greenstein AJ, Sachar D, Pucillo A, et al. Cancer in Crohn's disease after diversionary surgery. A report of seven carcinomas occurring in occluded bowel. Am J Surg 1978;135:86–90.
5. Senay E, Sachar DB, Keohane M, et al. Small bowel carcinoma in Crohn's disease. Cancer 1989;63:360–3.
6. Colcock BP. Regional enteritis: a surgical enigma. Surg Clin North Am 1964;44:779–84.
7. Fielding JF, Toye DK, Deton DC, et al. Crohn's disease of the stomach and duodenum. Gut 1970;11:1101–6.
8. Ross TM, Fazio VW, Farmer RG. Long term results of surgical treatment for Crohn's disease of the duodenum. Ann Surg 1983;197:399.
9. Farmer RG, Hawk WA, Turnbull RB, Jr. Crohn's disease of the duodenum (transmural duodenitis) Clinical manifestations. Report of 11 cases. Am J Dig Dis 1972;17:191.

10. Alexander-Williams J. Progress report: the place of surgery in Crohn's disease. Gut 1971;12:739.

11. Alexander-Williams J, Fielding JF. Crooke WT. A comparison of results of excision and bypass for ileal Crohn's disease. Gut 1972;13:973.

12. Atwell JK, Duthie JL, Goligher JC. The outcome of Crohn's disease. Br J Surg 1965;52:966.

13. Homan WP, Dineen P. Comparison of the results of resection, bypass and bypass with exclusion for ileocecal Crohn's disease. Ann Surg 1978;187:530.

14. Young S, et al. Results of surgery for Crohn's disease in the Glasgow region, 1961–1970. Br J Surg 1975; 52:528.

15. Ferguson LK. Concepts in the surgical treatment of regional enteritis. N Engl J Med 1961;264:748.

16. Garlock JH, Crohn BB, Klein SH, et al. An appraisal of the long-term results of surgical treatment of regional enteritis. Gastroenterology 1951;19:414.

17. Garlock JH, Crohn BB. An appraisal of the results of surgery in the treatment of regional enteritis. J Am Med Assoc 1945;127:205.

18. Crohn BB. Panel Discussion. Regional enteritis. Gasteroenterology 1959;36:398.

19. Trnka YM, et al. The long-term outcome of restorative operation in Crohn's disease. Influence of location, prognostic factors and surgical guidelines. Ann Surg 1982;196:345.

20. Colcock BP. Operative technique in surgery for Crohn's disease and its relationship to recurrence. Surg Clin North Am 1973;53:375.

21. Nesbit RR Jr, Elbadawi NA, Morton J, et al. Carcinoma of the bowel: a complication of regional enteritis. Cancer 1976;37:2959.

18 Small Bowel Resection

Sergio Casillas and Jeffrey W. Milsom

Surgical intervention in patients with Crohn's disease is limited to the treatment of acute and chronic complications for which medical therapy is not effective. At the Cleveland Clinic, rates of surgery with disease of 10 years' duration were 90% of patients with ileocolitis and 70% of those with only ileal involvement (1). Thus, for the vast majority of patients with Crohn's disease involving the small bowel, surgery is unavoidable. The surgeon treating these patients must be familiar with the spectrum of complications that may require specific surgical interventions. Resection of the diseased small bowel, the subject of this chapter, is a very effective short-term treatment for most complications.

Conservative, limited resections are nearly always recommended since the vast majority of patients will require two or more surgical interventions during their life time and the short bowel syndrome looms as a haunting outcome that both patient and surgeon attempt to avoid. This conservative approach has recently been strongly supported by the prospective randomized study by Fazio et al. in 131 patients with small bowel Crohn's disease showing that recurrence is not affected by the length of the margins utilized at the time of small bowel resection (2). In rare urgent or emergency circumstances, small bowel diversion or bypass procedures may be indicated provided that subsequent resection of the diseased segment be performed during a second stage operation. This is due to the high risk of subsequent complications occurring in the bypassed segment, including the long term risk of cancer.

Especially difficult to define may be how severe, disabling or morbidity-producing the particular complication has to be before recommending surgery. This may impact upon the timing and staging of an operation. We will attempt to clarify these indications below.

Indications

There are a number of situations generally regarded as indications for operation in Crohn's disease of the small bowel: obstruction, sepsis, fistula, free perforation, obstructive uropathy, major hemorrhage, carcinoma, and failure to thrive (including extra intestinal manifestations). Each of these indications will be discussed before specific operation therapy is outlined.

Small Bowel Obstruction

Some degree of small bowel obstruction is the most common complication requiring surgical intervention, reportedly affecting up to 54% of patients with Crohn's disease (1,3). Most patients present to the surgeon with a history of several episodes of subacute obstruction partially alleviated by reducing oral intake and increasing steroid medication. In addition to the obstructive symptoms, candidates for surgical intervention may also have episodic fever with or without documented leukocytosis; abdominal mass; obstructive bouts occurring at frequent intervals and with longer recovery period between bouts; hypoalbuminemia; anemia; internal or external fistula; and failure to tolerate medication (4). Acute bowel obstruction is an unusual complication leading to surgery, and patients with known small bowel Crohn's disease presenting with acute bowel obstruction should undergo a trial of supportive therapy in the hospital prior to considering operative intervention, which may hopefully be postponed to an elective setting.

Sepsis

Intraabdominal abscess occurs in 12% to 28% of patients with Crohn's disease (5). Most abscesses arise secondary to the penetrating ulceration of the Crohn's disease completely through the bowel wall. Adjacent viscera and omentum are commonly attached to this phlegmous mass providing a partial or complete walling off of the perforated bowel loop. At early stages, abscesses may respond to medical therapy. In addition, computerized tomography (CT)-guided drainage of selective enteroparietal, retroperitoneal, and psoas abscesses, may allow elective bowel resection 4 to 6 weeks later (6). Immediate surgical drainage and resection may be indicated in the presence of an intramesenteric abscess, especially if it is inadequately drained or not accessible to CT-guided drainage (7). Intraperitoneal rupture of the abscess is an indication for immediate surgical drainage after medical resuscitation of the patient, although this is an unusual event because the chronicity of the pathological process as described above usually leads to a walling off of the inflammatory process.

Fistula

Fistulas are a likely sequel to abscess formation and also are secondary to transmural penetrating ulceration. They may be internal or external. Although with the drainage of an associated abscess the septic condition may subside and the obstructive symptoms, if present, may transiently improve, surgery is usually required.

Enterocutaneous fistulas are not a common finding in primary perforating Crohn's disease and are more often present in the patient with recurrent disease. Those fistulas arising soon after resective surgery are probably not due to residual disease, but rather emanate from the anastomotic site and usually heal by bowel rest and total parenteral nutrition (TPN). On the other hand, late fistulas caused by recurrent Crohn's disease will usually require surgical resection (8). *Enteroperineal fistulas* after proctocolectomy can be mistaken early on for the more common complication of delayed or non-healing perineal wound. Laparotomy with resection of the diseased small bowel is likely to be needed, with curettage of the perineal wound (9). Nonetheless, a period of several months of bowel rest and TPN may be warranted in order to permit healing of the fistula spontaneously if it occurs early after surgery. If the treating surgeon antici-

pates that the inflammatory process may be great after the initial operation, proximal diversion (jejunostomy) with TPN may be warranted.

Enteroenteric fistulas occur in 30% of patients with Crohn's disease and require resection of the fistula source (it is usually ileal), freshening of the defect in the adjacent bowel loop by wedge excision (unless the fistula is to the cecum in ileal Crohn's disease, in which an ileocecectomy is performed), and suture closure of the defect (10,11). Primary bowel anastomosis after excision of the diseased segment is usually performed. Sound judgement is required before deciding on operative intervention solely for an enteroenteric fistula. If it causes no symptoms, it may be reasonable to leave it alone unless another complication intervenes.

Patients with *enterovesical fistulas* also generally require surgical intervention and usually present with other complications such as bowel obstruction, severe urinary tract infection, or other fistulas (12). *Enterovaginal* and *enterogenital fistulas* are other complications that are recognized as indications for surgery.

Free Perforation

Free perforation is a rare complication of small bowel Crohn's disease (2% incidence), affecting mostly patients with chronic obstructive disease (13). In the majority of cases perforation occurs at or just proximal to a strictured site in a relatively normal bowel segment. The safest procedure is resection of perforated segment with formation of a proximal enterostomy. The distal end is generally closed and implanted in the operative incision so it heals in the subcutaneous tissues. Bowel continuity is then restored 3 to 6 months later when a reasonable state of health is restored. If the perforation is discovered early after onset, and contamination is minimal, it may be reasonable to consider a limited resection with primary anastomosis. This should only be considered if the resection can be safely limited to a short segment.

Obstructive Uropathy

Ureteral obstruction in Crohn's small intestinal disease is a rare but well recognized complication of the disease. The reported incidence of some degree (partial or complete) of ureteral obstruction varies from 5% to 25% (14). Several etiologic factors play a role in the development of this condition, including ureteral akinesia secondary to inflammation, ureteral compression by an intestinal localized abscess or phlegmon, and retroperitoneal and periureteral scarring with fibrosis. Gastrointestinal symptoms usually predominate. Drainage of the abscess is followed by elective resection. If there is no abscess or one that is not amenable to CT drainage, drainage via laparotomy is performed with resective surgery of the compromised segment of small bowel. Although some authors recommend ureterolysis, the experience in our institution is that it is not necessary because in almost every case the obstructive uropathy resolves spontaneously after adequate treatment of the affected bowel segment and associated infection (14).

Hemorrhage

Hemorrhage is another uncommon acute complication (about 1%) of patients with small bowel Crohn's disease (15). Immediate laparotomy and small bowel resection has been associated with high postoperative morbidity and mortality. If the bleeding is massive, localization of the bleeding site by angiography and concomitant infusion of Pitressin through the superior mesenteric artery, has resulted in high success rates in controlling the bleeding (16). If this approach is not successful, the catheter is left in the superior mesenteric artery, Pitressin infusion is continued, and laparotomy is performed coincident with a plan for intraoperative upper and lower endoscopy. Resection of a segment is contemplated only if the site can be localized.

Malignancy

Patients with Crohn's disease are at a significantly higher risk of developing gastrointestinal malignancies than the general population. The observed-to-expected ratio for small bowel cancer has been reported in 114:5 in one series (17). In a review of 61 cases of carcinoma of the small intestine in patients with Crohn's disease, Hawker et al. found that 67% of the cancers occurred in the ileum (18). This is in contrast with the 20.5% to 30.5% of small bowel cancers occurring in the ileum in the general population (18). Frequently, small bowel cancer has been an incidental finding during surgery and its relatively lower incidence, compared to colorectal cancers, has been attributed to the multiple resections that a Crohn's disease patient requires during the course of this illness. Patients in which small bowel bypass has been performed are at higher risk of developing malignancy in the blind loop (19). Thus, patients who previously have undergone small bowel bypass must be considered candidates

for resection unless other medical or surgical problems contraindicate this.

Failure to Thrive

Failure to thrive occurs as an isolated symptom in about 8% of patients with ileal involvement or ileocolitis (1). It includes a number of clinical entities namely: poor response to medical therapy, excessive side effects of medication, inability to withdraw the patient from high doses of steroid treatment, growth retardation, chronic anemia unresponsive to medication, debilitating diarrhea and incontinence, and extraintestinal manifestations of Crohn's disease. Patients requiring large doses of prednisone (i.e., more than 20 mg per day) to maintain remission over 6 to 12 months, are probably candidates for surgery. Another indication for surgery is the inability of medical therapy to induce disease remission in a patient with therapeutic doses of steroids administered for more than 3 to 6 months.

Most of the extraintestinal manifestations of Crohn's disease are colitis-related and rarely are present in patients with small bowel disease. Most extraintestinal manifestations (i.e., arthritis, erythema nodosum, pyoderma gangrenosum, iritis, uveitis, and glomerulonephritis) may improve after resection of the diseased bowel. Primary sclerosing cholangitis and ankylosing spondylitis are not likely to improve after surgery (20).

Preoperative Preparation

Since patients with Crohn's disease of the small bowel are generally compromised in some way before surgery, they usually require a number of preoperative measures that will provide them with a better outcome after surgery.

Correction of Electrolyte Imbalance, Anemia, and Hypoproteinemia; Nasogastric Suction

Severe electrolyte imbalances may be present in patients with Crohn's disease: dehydratation, hypokalemia, hypomagnesemia, and hypophosphatemia (21). Anemia is associated with acute or chronic bleeding and with Vitamin B_{12} deficiency. Transfusion of packed red blood cells are given for chronic anemia to achieve a hemoglobin level of 9 g/dL or above. Severe hypoproteinemia (i.e., albumin <2.5 g/dL) is a reliable indicator of poor healing, and should prompt the surgeon to consider avoiding formation of a primary anastomosis (22). Nasogastric suction may be necessary to relieve symptoms associated with bowel obstruction and frequently converts an urgent situation to a more elective one that may require surgery.

Steroids

Avoidance of acute adrenal insufficiency is particularly important in patients who have been taking steroids in a 6 to 12 month period prior to surgery. Stress doses of steroids are required (intravenous hydrocortisone 100 mg every 8 hours is a standard dose). A gradual tapering program is then given when resective surgery has been completed and the patient has recovered from the operation.

Total Parenteral Nutrition (TPN)

Although preoperative TPN in Crohn's disease can lead to some measurable improvements in nutritional parameters, this has not lead to a demonstrable reduction in postoperative complications unless severe malnutrition is present. With severe nutritional deficits (serum albumin <2.5 g/dL and transferrin levels <150 mg/dL) prior to surgical resection (22), an improved outcome is seen after TPN is administered for a period of 5 to 7 days before surgery.

Preoperative Bowel Preparation

Conventional mechanical bowel preparation is frequently not possible in patients with obstructing Crohn's disease. Dietary restriction of solids with use of a modified elemental liquid diet several days before surgery may be required to prepare the bowel of these patients. In addition, moderate catharsis with small amounts of polyethylene glycol or with magnesium citrate solution may achieve a mechanical washout of the small bowel prior to surgery.

Antibiotic Preparation

We give intravenous cefotaxime 1.0 g and metronidazole 500 mg 1 hour before operation and every 8 hours thereafter for the first postoperative day. If major contamination occurs, antibiotic may be prolonged for 3 to 5 days. Additionally, we consider oral antibiotic administration preoperatively in patients with partial obstruction since luminal bacterial levels are likely to be elevated. Neomycin and erythromycin base are given in three doses of one gram per dose the evening before surgery (we do not give these if there is no element of obstruction).

Stoma Marking

Patients who are acutely ill or debilitated should be mentally and physically prepared for a stoma creation. A mark on the skin is made using permanent ink or a scratch with a hypodermic needle. Visibility of the stoma site to the patient is extremely important. Other principles include: leaving a zone of 5 cm of undisturbed skin around the stoma site for proper adherence of the appliance; locating the site over the rectus abdominus muscle; and locating the site far from skin creases, scars, or bony prominences. Achieving all of these principles may be challenging in a complex Crohn's disease patient, thus collaboration with a well-trained enterostomal therapy nurse may be extremely helpful.

Pitfalls and Danger Points

Incidental Appendectomy in Patients with Crohn's Disease

There are conflicting reports in the surgical literature regarding the safety of incidental appendectomy performed during laparotomy when Crohn's disease is discovered (23). This issue is even more problematic in patients with classical acute appendicitis in whom, on laparotomy, the appendix is found to be normal and Crohn's disease of the terminal ileum and/or cecum is diagnosed. In such cases it is recommended not to perform an appendectomy whenever the appendix looks normal and the cecum is inflamed (24). If appendectomy is performed under these circumstances, fistula from the diseased bowel is a common complication, occurring in about one third of patients (24–26).

Crohn's disease limited to the appendix is extremely unusual. In such cases, the average duration of symptoms is uncharacteristically long for diagnosis of appendicitis. Blood tests may also suggest a chronic inflammatory process. Appendectomy or a limited ileocolectomy is the treatment of choice. Some authors also recommend postoperative TPN to minimize the possibility of fistula formation (25). We would not advocate this unless severe malnutrition exists.

Nongranulomatous appendicitis does occur in the course of regional enteritis. Appendectomy is the treatment of choice in those cases, and confers the advantage of simplifying evaluation of abdominal pain in the future (26).

Ileoduodenal Fistula Complicating Crohn's Disease

Although a rare circumstance, patients who have previously had resection of the terminal ileum and right colon for Crohn's disease are at particular risk for the development of a duodenal fistula because the ileocolic anastomosis may lie directly over the second portion of the duodenum. Diarrhea, weight loss and occasionally feculent vomiting are the most important clinical features of patients having this complication (27). Intraoperatively, the surgeon should suspect a duodenal fistula whenever he/she encounters a right upper quadrant mass involving ileum, colon, and duodenum (28). The mass will be densely adherent to the duodenum and head of the pancreas, but must be carefully dissected away from the head of the pancreas (10). Details of the operative management are discussed below in the section on Operative Techniques, Technique of Anastomosis.

Ileosigmoid Fistula Complicating Crohn's Disease

When an ileosigmoid fistula is present, typically there is a large inflammatory mass involving the ileocecal region to which the sigmoid is attached. The mass may be densely adherent to the right pelvis wall as well (29). The base of the bladder may also be involved. The surgeon must decide whether Crohn's disease is present and, if so, to what extent. In the differential diagnosis, in a previously undiagnosed patient, is a sealed perforation due to carcinoma of the sigmoid involving the small intestine especially in an older person. Ileosigmoid fistula due to diverticulitis is also in the differential diagnosis in these types of cases. When the inflammatory mass is entirely within the sigmoid mesentery the possibility of a fistula is less likely. However, when this inflammatory nest involves any part of the surface of the sigmoid colon, it should be presumed that a macroscopic or microscopic fistula is present. An en bloc resection is then recommended resecting the ileocecal area involved with Crohn's disease in continuity with a segment of sigmoid involved with the fistula (11). The resection lines on the sigmoid colon are chosen where the colon wall feels soft and pliable, where no serositis or thickening is present. A conservative sigmoid resection is usually performed with reanastomosis unless there is peritonitis, sepsis, or severe malnutrition (11,30). If there is minimal involvement of the sigmoid, it is acceptable to consider excising only the fistula tract itself with trimming of the edges so soft pliable bowel can be sutured closed primarily.

Free Perforation in Small Bowel Crohn's Disease

This is an unusual complication, but most patients present with sudden acute abdominal pains and/or distention that may radiate to the shoulders and may be associated with unstable vital signs. Patients on steroids are extremely worrisome because they may manifest few systemic signs until they are seriously ill. The ileum is the most common site of perforation (65%), followed by the colon (22%), and the jejunum (12%) (13). At surgery, patients with several stricture sites or with diffuse Crohn's disease may be difficult to assess. Salvage operations in these patients usually include resection of the perforated segment and proximal diversion. In the very seriously ill patient, simple exteriorization of the perforated segment with proximal diversion (usually loop jejunostomy) may be the treatment associated with the least morbidity and mortality. In such circumstances, TPN will be necessary until restoring the bowel continuity during a second stage operation (31).

Crohn's Disease Associated with Occult Chronic Bleeding

Most patients with Crohn's disease will eventually develop some degree of bleeding during the course of their illness. Patients with chronic bleeding can have a severe anemia based on blood loss plus the anemic syndrome of vitamin B_{12} and folate deficiency commonly present in Crohn's disease. Even in circumstances of acute gastrointestinal hemorrhage, it may be difficult to establish the exact source of the bleeding. Angiography and technetium-labeled red blood cell scintigraphy can only detect bleeding at a rate of 0.2 to 0.5 cc/min. When these methods fail to demonstrate the location of the bleeding and surgical therapy is needed, intraoperative enteroscopy is performed (32). This method has been shown to be highly accurate in detecting the bleeding site, although it requires some level of expertise, team work, and a number of manual maneuvers to avoid damage to the small bowel or its mesentery, or excessive air insufflation (33).

Malignancy Complicating Small Bowel Crohn's Disease

Malignancy should be suspected in patients who relapse after a long period of inactive disease. Patients with bypassed segments are at a significantly higher risk of developing small bowel cancer compared to other Crohn's patients (19). A careful inspection of the mucosa at strictureplasty sites and resection margins should be commonly carried out and frozen sections are imperative if there is any suspicion of malignancy. If a malignancy is found, resection of the diseased segment with intraoperative histologic inspection of the resection margins is mandatory (34). Assessment of lymph node metastases is also important. Small bowel cancer in patients with Crohn's disease is usually associated with a bad prognosis (19).

Crohn's Disease of the Small Bowel and Pregnancy

Many patients with small bowel Crohn's disease are ill during their reproductive years. Active disease during pregnancy, although relatively uncommon, may be a particularly complex situation for the surgeon. Although inactive disease is not associated with a higher rate of complications during pregnancy compared to the normal population, patients with active disease are at significantly higher risk of having spontaneous abortion and preterm delivery (35,36). Furthermore, if the disease is active at the onset of the pregnancy, it is likely to remain so or to worsen. Exacerbation or worsening of Crohn's disease is most likely to occur during the third trimester (37). Surgeons should bear the following in mind in treating pregnant Crohn's patients: (a) Medical therapy is maintained as long as the patient's clinical condition does not deteriorate and, preferably until the third trimester of pregnancy, when there is a lower risk of fetal death. (b) There is little evidence that the use of sulfasalazine or steroids is harmful to the mother or baby when used in pregnant patients with Crohn's disease, although with patients on sulfasalazine there is a theoretical risk of kernicterus. Both of these drugs have also been shown to be safe during the nursing period (35). (c) Immunosuppressive agents (i.e., azathioprine and 6-mercaptopurine) are avoided because of their teratogenic and tumorigenic effects (37). (d) Elemental diets and TPN during pregnancy have shown some promise in the treatment of patients with active Crohn's disease of the small bowel (38,39). (e) Surgery is an appropriate treatment when other measures are either inadequate or unsuccessful to control complications of the active disease and the mother's life is at stake.

Operative Strategy

General Principles

The strategy for surgery of small bowel Crohn's follows certain definite principles.

Incision

We prefer a midline incision, since this represents the most versatile type of incision. It permits exploration of all quadrants and extension superiorly or inferiorly as necessary. The infraumbilical right and left lower quadrants should be preserved for potential stoma siting either at the current or future operations.

Recognition of the Extent of the Disease

The surgeon should attempt to assess the entire abdomen and particularly the entire length of the small bowel. Common gross findings are serositis, a corkscrew appearance of the serosal vessels, mesenteric lymphadenopathy, and partial or complete fat "wrapping" of the intestine. In more complicated cases a phlegmon or periintestinal abscess may be present (40). Presence of adherent loops of small bowel may be indicators of enteroenteric fistulas. About 15% of patients will show evidence of skip lesions ranging from slight thickening of the bowel, to tight strictures associated with gross proximal small bowel dilatation (41).

Bowel Conservation

Conservation without leaving significant disease behind is a fundamental principle of small bowel Crohn's surgery. We favor conservative resection margins with proximal clearances of 2 cm above the macroscopic disease, and distal margins of generally the same. A randomized controlled trial performed in 152 patients with Crohn's diseases at our institution, demonstrated that recurrence of Crohn's disease is unaffected by the width of the margin of resection (2 cm versus 12 cm) from macroscopically involved bowel (2). Recurrence rates also do not increase when microscopic disease is left at the resection margins. Aphthous ulcerations discovered even at the margin of resection does not mandate further resection. The bowel ends to be anastomosed should be soft, pliable, and without signs of gross ulcerations.

Temporary Ostomies

Indications for temporary diverting ostomies are: incompletely removed sepsis (i.e., a phlegmonous area of inflammation or pyogenic membrane in the surrounding tissues adjacent to an anastomosis); excessive blood loss during a long operation, especially when several anastomosis have been made; and serum albumin levels less than 2.5 g/dL (42,43).

Early Reoperative Surgery

If reoperative surgery becomes necessary immediately after surgery, the following should be kept in mind: there is a special window 7 to 10 days after laparotomy when reoperation may be technically possible (31). Indications that may require early surgical reintervention are major enterocutaneous fistulas, significant postoperative hemorrhage, and adhesive complete bowel obstruction. Operative interventions after this window may lead to serious complications like sepsis, fistula, and persistent obstruction. For the obstructed patient or for the patient with a postoperative enterocutaneous fistula 7 to 10 days after surgery, a better alternative to surgery is long-term administration of TPN and percutaneous gastrostomy. In Crohn's disease it is important to allow a minimum interval of 3 to 6 months from the patient's last operation before an elective reoperation because of the formidable number of dense adhesions formed during this period of time.

Management of Specific Clinical Entities

Sepsis. Abscess are drained percutaneously whenever possible to minimize the spreading of septic contents into the abdominal cavity during laparotomy. Some collections, however, are best drained at laparotomy such as enteroparietal abscess that can be palpated abdominally or interloop abscess found at the time of operation (40). Bowel resection may be risky if an extensive intramesenteric abscess with associated retroperitoneal inflammation is present. Because division of the major vascular pedicle is potentially hazardous in this situation,

exclusion bypass of the particular segment with counterdrainage of the cavity is a useful alternative (Fig. 18.1). Few psoas abscesses will be recognized until the time of laparotomy. Exploration of the deep-lying cavity after mobilizing the adherent terminal ileum will reveal extent of the abscess. Unroofing of the abscess, placement of 1-in. latex rubber drains, and resection of the affected small bowel is done in such cases. In other instances, psoas abscesses can be very difficult to find even at laparotomy, especially if they are small or have been incompletely drained by CT scan. In those cases, needle stick/aspiration with a 14-gauge needle might be valuable in localizing the abscess after mobilizing the diseased intestine. Septic symptoms may persist if the collection is not localized and well drained. Finally, the drained site is usually covered by suturing omentum over the cavity, if this is available.

Malignancy. The risk of small bowel malignancy in patients with Crohn's disease is well documented. There are several principles that have to be considered regarding this issue: (1) excluded segments of small bowel are at higher risk of developing malignancy and therefore, usually are resected (19). (2) If dysplasia or adenoma in an area of definite Crohn's disease is identified, resection is also recommended. The dysplasia-cancer sequence is not clear-cut in small bowel Crohn's disease. (3) Patient with long-standing Crohn's disease (i.e., 20 years), are at particular risk of ma-

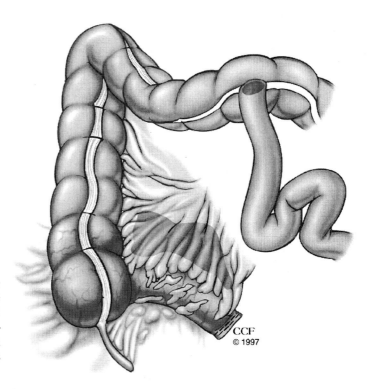

Fig. 18.1. The exclusion bypass operation for severe ileocolonic Crohn's disease: it is rarely used, but may be useful in the situation where the patient is critically ill with an intramesenteric/retroperitoneal abscess present and where division of the ileocolic mesentery and removal of the acutely inflamed bowel segment is hazardous.

lignancy. A strong consideration for resectional surgery has to be given for individual strictured segments of long duration, providing there is no risk for developing short bowel syndrome. Frozen section biopsies of all structures should be done is strictureplasty is a consideration. (4) Strictureplasty is avoided if there is any possible consideration of malignancy at the time of resection.

Staging Procedures

Following percutaneous abscess drainage of retroperitoneal or pelvic origin, elective resection is usually performed 2 to 4 weeks later. When a bypassed segment is left intact, resection is recommended because of the risk of malignancy. Elective resection about 3 to 6 months after the bypass procedure is usually preferred depending on the severity of the disease.

Operative Technique

Once the primary pathology has been identified, the entire bowel is inspected for evidence of coexisting Crohn's disease. When this preliminary assessment is complete, it is advisable to mobilize or isolate the diseased segment as well as the adjacent normal intestine. It is critical to minimize the possibility of contamination, especially in the patient with partial or total bowel obstruction in whom the proximal bowel will potentially be filled with fecal material. To minimize this risk, contents of the small bowel are milked in a proximal or distal direction, beyond the margins of the potential anastomosis and, using a linen tape, the proximal bowel segment is occluded. It is also recommended to pack off the operative area to minimize the possibility of any spill into the abdominal cavity. It is common, especially in patients with terminal ileal disease, to find adjacent matted loops of small bowel or omentum (Fig. 18.2). Mobilization of the ileocecal region by division of the peritoneum over the lateral margin of the caecum and over the inferior aspect of the terminal ileum is necessary to allow the delivery of those matted loops outside the abdominal cavity. Care must be taken not to damage the ureter or right-sided ovarian or testicular vessels when the mass is being delivered into the operative field. After this mobilization, separation of the loops is possible by a combination of sharp and gentle blunt dissection. This also allows a more precise examination of bowel segments to be resected and areas to be preserved. The limit of the macroscopic disease is marked on the bowel with stay sutures (Fig. 18.3). In most cases, a conserva-

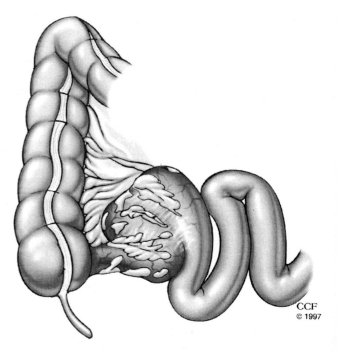

Fig. 18.2.   Matted loops of ileum are commonly encountered in terminal ileal Crohn's disease. Ileoileal or ileocolonic fistulas may be present between loops.

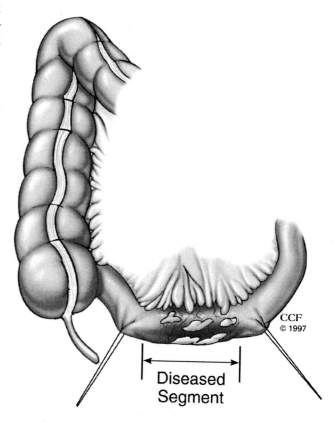

Fig. 18.3.   A useful maneuver to delineate the limits of ileal resection for Crohn's disease is to place small sutures on the antimesenteric side at the bowel margins.

Fig. 18.4. Placing overlapping Kocher-type clamps across the bowel, sequentially suture ligating them, is the best way to safely transect and attain hemostasis of a thickened Crohn's mesentery

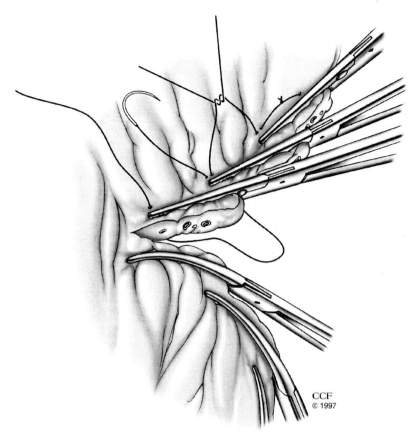

CCF
© 1997

tive margin of 2 cm of intestine can be taken proximally and distally. The method of palpating the mesenteric-bowel edge and seeking and area where the transition from abnormal to normal is a reliable one (see Chapter 19).

The trickiest part of the operation often involves handling the mesenteric margin when transecting the bowel and its mesentery. The ileal mesentery is commonly thickened due to fat deposition and enlarged mesenteric nodes following the course of the ileocolic and sometimes of the superior mesenteric vessels in a cephalad direction towards the duodenum and head of the pancreas. Conventional ligation carries the risk of injuring the vessels and thus, the development of an intramesenteric hematoma. Fazio et al. have described a technique of overlapping Kocher clamps to control the thick mesentery (Fig. 18.4). Using this technique, the vascular pedicules are sutured-ligated using size 0 or 1-0 absorbable sutures so the pedicles are serially underrun, minimizing the risk of vessel injury and hematoma. Resection of adjacent lymph nodes is considered, if feasible, without extending the limit of bowel resection.

If the ileal disease is complicated by enteroenteric fistula, the associated loops of bowel (usually the ileum or sigmoid) are pinched off the ileal segment if the inflammatory response is confined to the ileum. Once the adherent loops of bowel have been dissected from the diseased segment of small bowel, the primary affected loop is resected and the ends anastomosed, leaving the secondary loop connected to the fistula to be either closed by primary repair, by strictureplasty, or resected as indicated.

Not all of the obstructing disease can be identified from examination of the serosal surface of the bowel. In those cases when additional areas of stenosis are suspected, a Foley catheter with a balloon inflated to produce a diameter of 2 to 2.5 cm (6 to 8 mL of water), can be used to assess such regions (45). Slow traction of the inflated catheter will identify any stenotic lesion which then is marked by a suture on the serosal surface of the bowel. These lesions may be treated by strictureplasty (see Chapter 16).

Technique of Anastomosis

General principles of bowel anastomosis must be scrupulously adhered to when operating on patients with Crohn's disease, namely good blood

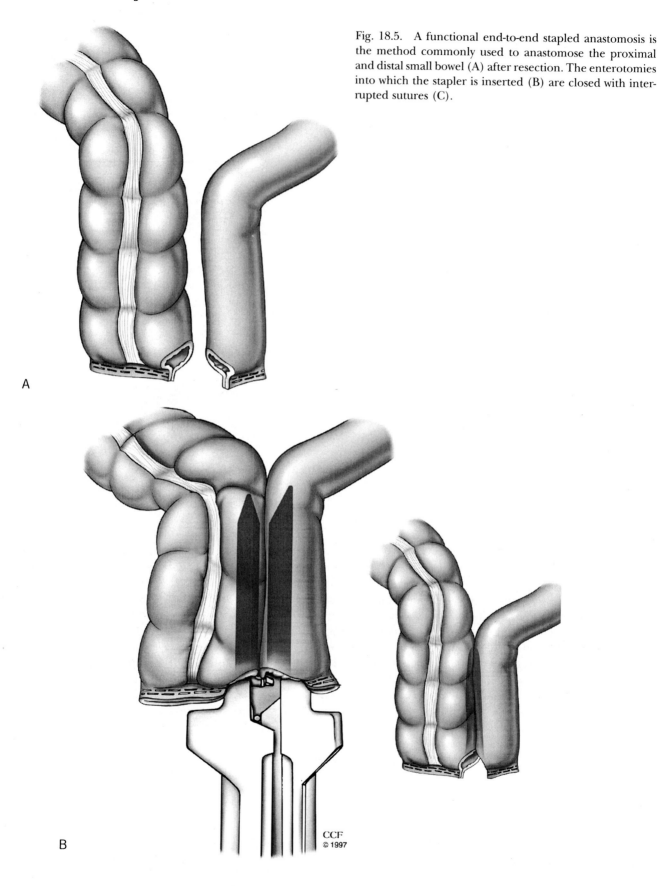

Fig. 18.5.   A functional end-to-end stapled anastomosis is the method commonly used to anastomose the proximal and distal small bowel (A) after resection. The enterotomies into which the stapler is inserted (B) are closed with interrupted sutures (C).

A

B

CCF
© 1997

Fig. 18.5. (*Continued*).

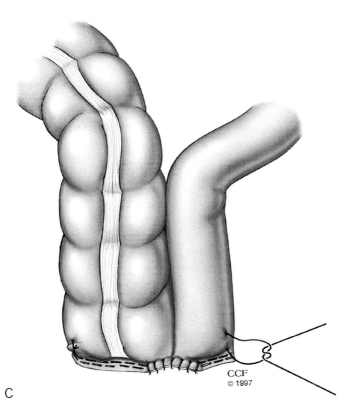

C

supply to the bowel ends, anastomosis conducted in a tension-free manner, equilibration of the lumen caliber for both proximal and distal sides, avoidance of any twisting of the bowel, and closure of the mesenteric defect. A variety of techniques currently exist, but it always is mandatory to examine the lumen on both sides of the anastomosis. The presence of aphthoid ulcers at the anastomotic site are not a contraindication for a primary anastomosis. Large longitudinal ulcers, on the other hand, are not incorporated into the anastomotic margins whenever possible, although this may be unavoidable in patients at risk of developing short bowel syndrome. As mentioned previously, there is no circumstance under which suturing of a stricture to another portion of the bowel is justified. Strictureplasty, another consideration, are discussed in detail in Chapter 16.

Assessing the distal margins of resection may not always be feasible, as in midtransverse or distal colon anastomosis where the bowel is transected and closed with a mechanical stapler prior to anastomosis. In such cases, careful examination of the distal bowel is necessary, with consideration of intraoperative colonoscopy.

Our preference for small bowel Crohn's disease has been to perform a side-to-side stapled anastomosis with a GIA-60 stapler (United States Surgical Corporation, Norwalk, CT) (Fig. 18.5). The defect into which the limbs of the stapler have been intro-

duced is closed with two layers of 3-0 polyglycolic acid suture or using a linear stapler.

In the case of duodenal fistula, the duodenal wall should be excised so that edges of the wall to be closed are grossly free of inflammation or thickening. The resulting defect can be up to 1 to 3 cm in diameter. If small, it can be closed primarily. Otherwise, it is advisable to create a primary duodenojejunal anastomosis using a short loop of jejunum brought directly into apposition with the duodenal defect. A cross-cut of the jejunum is made and anastomosed in a transverse fashion to the duodenal opening (11) (Fig. 18.6). When ileocolonic anastomosis is performed, it is placed as far away as possible from the duodenojejunostomy. If possible, the omentum should be placed between the duodenum and the ileocolic anastomosis to minimize the chance of refistulization (44).

Finally, integrity of the anastomosis can be assessed by introducing carbon dioxide into the small bowel through a nasogastric tube. The abdomen is filled with saline so any air leak from the anastomosis can be detected. We do not routinely perform this, but it has been described as a method to check anastomoses by Keighley and Alexander-Williams.

Bypass Procedures

Bypass procedures were originally developed in response to the high mortality for resections per-

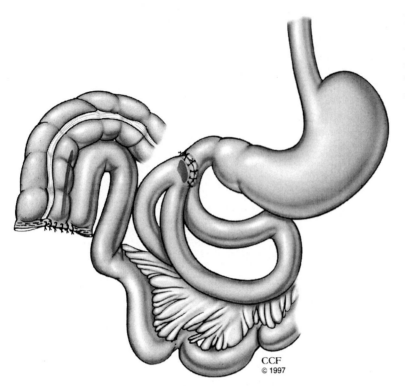

Fig. 18.6.   Closure of a duodenal defect after take down of an ileo or coloduodenal fistula is usually effected with an onlay jejunoduodenal anastomosis using one or two layers. A segment well upstream of the ileocolonic anastomosis should be used.

formed in the 1940s and 1950s (46). However, disease recurrence and risk of malignancy were significantly higher in patients who underwent bypass operations. There currently are very few indications for this kind of operation. The main indication occurs when a patient can be managed more safely during an acute situation with a bypass procedure, particularly when associated with an abscess or a phlegmon densely adherent to the retroperitoneum associated with signs of systemic sepsis. Unilateral exclusion bypass is generally favored over bilateral exclusion bypass because there is one less mucous fistula for the patient to dress. An incontinuity bypass cannot be recommended for ileocecal Crohn's disease because any septic component of the disease will tend to persist. A bypass incontinuity, on the other hand, is preferred for gastroduodenal Crohn's disease and for the majority of patients with multiple obstructing skip lesions when strictureplasty is not feasible (31). Resection of the excluded segment must be considered at a second stage operation because of the risk of malignancy. If the bypassed segment is not resected, frequent screening for cancer with annual colonoscopy or even enteroscopy must be considered.

Another type of bypass procedure that may be performed is a temporary ileostomy or even jejunostomy. Particularly in the emergency situation, local conditions may preclude the formation of a safe resection and anastomosis. Patients at risk of

developing anastomotic leak include those presenting with peritonitis, abscess collection, fecal contamination, free perforation of the small bowel, and patients with severe hemorrhage who require more than 3 units of blood to be stabilized hemodynamically before surgery. Ileostomies, both of the end and loop variety, may be helpful and occasionally life saving in these situations. Resection of the diseased segment, ileostomy and mucous fistula is the treatment of choice in most of those cases. There are other circumstances in which a "protective" ileostomy must also be considered: multiple resections or strictureplasties, and patients who are severely debilitated or have fulminating disease.

Drains

A septic pyogenic membrane may remain at the completion of resection, or an infected retroperitoneal space may be identified. In such cases closed suction silastic sump drains are sutured over the phlegmon or into the cavity. These drains are usually left for 2 weeks, at which time they are replaced by a small catheter for 3 to 6 weeks to prevent premature closure of the external skin opening. A contrast study with water soluble contrast through the catheter may be used to confirm no communication with the bowel or anastomosis.

In the presence of a presacral abscess due to an ileorectal fistula, the presacral space is widely drained after mobilization and resection of the diseased segment. Drains are usually left for a minimum of 5 to 7 days.

Postoperative Care

Postoperative care of these patients include standard procedures applied after bowel resection. Nasogastric suction until evidence of normal bowel function is important particularly in patients operated on for obstructive symptoms. Intravenous antibiotics are desirable during the 24 hours following operation and may be prolonged in patients with incompletely resolved sepsis.

A standard program to taper steroid therapy is initiated particularly in patients who have been taking medication during the last 6 months. Particularly important is to monitor for any sign of sepsis, including care of the abdominal wound, examination and quantification of fluid collected by drains, and observation of any sign of fistula formation. Urinary catheter is left for 7 to 10 days after resection of enterovesical fistulas. Finally, standard measures for the care of ostomies in patients diverted are required, enlisting the help of an enterostomal therapy nurse in all cases.

Complications

Postoperative death, a rare occurrence after small bowel resection for Crohn's disease, is mainly due to intraabdominal sepsis and bacteremia, although vascular thrombotic disease may occasionally be a cause. At the Cleveland Clinic mortality in patients undergoing operation for Crohn's disease has been estimated in 1.9% (46). The principal complications after small bowel resection for Crohn's disease include wound sepsis, intraabdominal abscess, adhesive obstruction, urinary tract infection, septicemia, postoperative peritonitis and fistula from anastomotic breakdown.

Postoperative abscesses occur in 11% of patients and may arise from intraperitoneal contamination during surgery, or from anastomotic leaks (40). Postoperative abscesses account for 20 to 25% of intraabdominal abscesses occurring during the course of Crohn's disease (7,40). Percutaneous drainage (usually CT-guided) is usually considered before any attempt at reoperation.

Enterocutaneous fistulas occurring shortly after surgery are treated by bowel rest, TPN, and adequate drainage of sepsis. Fistulas are commonly related to technical aspects of anastomosis construction or to faulty judgement in the construction of an anastomosis where there is a high risk of leakage (free perforation, malnutrition).

Enteroperineal fistulas following proctocolectomy for Crohn's disease may arise secondary to disease recurrence. The perineal drainage may be mistaken for the commoner complication of delayed or nonhealing perineal wound. Management involves radiographic demonstration of the communication by fistulogram or small-bowel series. In case of gastrointestinal communication, laparotomy is required to correct the problem.

Hemorrhage during the early postoperative period may be related to the anastomosis or strictureplasties. Conservative management is required with ruling out an upper gastrointestinal source, restoration of any coagulation defect, blood transfusion, and angiography if there is evidence of continued bleeding from a site in the small bowel. In this situation, intraarterial Pitressin infusion has been proven to be of great value (47). If these measures fail to stop the bleeding and the patient is hemodynamically unstable, relaparotomy with resection of the bleeding site may be necessary. This can be a very difficult clinical problem.

Adhesive obstruction is a relatively uncommon complication in the early postoperative period after small bowel resection for Crohn's disease. It may be related to the original process that mandated operation on the patient (i.e., septic collections or multiple adhesions). Nearly always the surgeon should utilize nonoperative methods (nasogastric suction, intravenous fluid replacement, and, if necessary, nutritional support in anticipation that this will resolve spontaneously. Small bowel instruction occuring remate from the surgery (3 > 6 months) likewise should usually be handled with supportive measures, and the possibility that recurrent disease is causing the situation should be considered.

Metabolic complications may result from multiple small bowel resections. Deficiencies of vitamin B$_{12}$, iron, and folate may result from ileal resection (48). Disturbances in the enterohepatic circulation may be manifested by an increased incidence of cholelithiasis and urolithiasis (49). Malabsorption and short bowel syndrome are serious complications after repetitive jejunum resections. Elemental diets and TPN may be required in those patients for long periods of time.

Long-term *disease recurrence* requiring reoperation is unavoidable for a considerable number of patients with Crohn's disease. Farmer et al. reported in a series of 391 patients who underwent surgery for Crohn's disease at the Cleveland Clinic, a risk of recurrence of 35% at a mean follow-up of 11.5 years (46). The cumulative recurrence rate in patients with ileocolic disease was greater than in others, with 50% requiring reoperation after 14 years. For patients with small bowel involvement alone, this risk was estimated at 39%, whereas patients with only colonic involvement, the risk was 33% during the same period of time. Other factors reported to influence disease recurrence include the age of the patient (younger patients are at higher risk), the use of bypass surgery, the extent of the disease in the small bowel, and preservation of residual disease (bowel and/or lymph nodes). Careful consideration, before surgery is decided upon, should be given to patients at high risk of developing short-bowel syndrome.

Conclusion

Small bowel resection in Crohn's disease is reserved for patients manifesting complications of the disease that have failed to be resolved by conservative (medical) therapy. The surgeon must be familiar with this spectrum of complications and individualize the best timing of operation for each particular patient. Removal of the diseased segment and of any septic collection is effective in most cases. Conservative resections are preferred to avoid metabolic complications of small bowel resection and short bowel syndrome. Bypass procedures are rarely recommended and are related with considerable risk of malignancy and disease recurrence. Strictureplasty has a promising role in treating small bowel Crohn's and will be discussed in Chapter 16.

References

1. Farmer R, Hawk W, Turnbull R. Indications for surgery in Crohn's disease. Gastroenterology 1976;71:245–50.
2. Fazio V, Marchetti F, Church J, et al. Effects of resection margins of the recurrence of Crohn's disease in the small bowel. A randomized controlled trial. Ann Surg 1996;224:563–73.
3. Platell C, Mackay J, Collopy B, et al. Crohn's disease: a colon and rectal department experience. Aust N Z J Surg 1995;65:570–5.
4. Bergman L, Krause U. Crohn's disease: a long-term study of the clinical course. Scand J Gastroenterology 1977;12:937–44.
5. Nagler S, Poticha S. Intraabdominal abscess in regional enteritis. Am J Surg 1979;137:350–4.
6. Doemeny J, Burke D, Meranze S. Percutaneous drainage of abscesses in patients with Crohn's disease. Gastrointest Radiol 1988;13:237–41.
7. Ayuk P, Williams N, Scott N, et al. Management of intra-abdominal abscesses in Crohn's disease. Ann R Coll Surg Engl 1996;78:5–10.
8. Pettit S, Irving M. The operative management of fistulous Crohn's disease. Surg Gyn Obst 1988;167:223–8.
9. Irving M. Assessment and management of external fistulas in Crohn's disease. Br J Surg 1983;70:233–6.
10. Fazio V, Wilk P, Turnbull R, et al. Ileosigmoidal fistula complicating Crohn's disease. Dis Colon Rectum 1977;20:381–6.
11. Wilk P, Fazio V, Turnbull R. Ileoduodenal fistula complicating Crohn's disease. Dis Colon Rectum 1977;20:387–92.
12. McNamara M, Fazio V, Lavery I, et al. Surgical treatment of enterovesical fistulas in Crohn's disease. Dis Colon Rectum 1990;33:271–6.
13. Greenstein A, Mann B, Aufses A. Free perforation in Crohn's disease: a survey of 99 cases. Am J Gastroenterol 1985;80:682–9.
14. Siminovitch J, Fazio V. Ureteral obstruction secondary to Crohn's disease: a need for ureterolysis? Am J Surg 1980;139:95–8.
15. Homan W, Tang C, Thorbjarnarson B, et al. Acute massive hemorrhage from intestinal Crohn's disease: report of seven cases and review of the literature. Arch Surg 1976;111:901–5.
16. Fazio V, Zelas P, Weakley F. Intraoperative angiography and the localization of bleeding from the small intestine. Surg Gyn Obst 1980;151:637–40.
17. Greenstein A, Sachar D, Smith H, et al. A comparison of cancer risk in Crohn's disease and ulcerative colitis. Cancer 1981;48:2742–5.
18. Hawker P, Gyde S, Thompson H, et al. Adenocarcinoma of the small intestine complicating Crohn's disease. Gut 1982;23:188–93.
19. Greenstein A, Sachar D, Smith H, et al. Patterns of neoplasia in Crohn's disease and ulcerative colitis. Cancer 1980;46:403–7.
20. Greenstein A, Janowitz A, Sachar D. The extraintestinal manifestations of Crohn's disease and ulcerative colitis: a study of 700 patients. Medicine 1976;55:401–12.
21. Lindor K, Fleming R, Ilstrup D. Preoperative nutritional status and other factors that influence surgical outcome in patients with Crohn's disease. Mayo Clin Proc 1985;60:393–6.
22. Rombeau J, Barot L, Williamson C, et al. Preoperative total parenteral nutrition and surgical outcome in patients with inflammatory bowel disease. Am J Surg 1982;143:139–43.
23. Fisher K, Ross D. Guidelines for therapeutic decision in incidental appendectomy. Surg Gyn Obst 1990;171:95–8.
24. Kovalcik P, Simstein L, Weiss M, et al. Crohn's disease and appendectomy. Dis Colon Rectum 1977;20:377–80.
25. Ruiz V, Unger S, Morgan J. Crohn's disease of the appendix. Surgery 1990;107:113–7.

26. Oren R, Rachmilewitz D. Preoperative clues to Crohn's disease in suspected, acute appendicitis. J Clin Gastroenterol 1992;15:306–10.

27. Klein S, Greenstein A, Sachar D. Duodenal fistulas in Crohn's disease. J Clin Gastroenterol 1987;9:46–9.

28. Pichney L, Fantry G, Graham S. Gastrocolic and duodenocolic fistulas in Crohn's disease. J Clin Gastroenterol 1992;15:205–11.

29. Saint-Marc O, Vaillant J, Frileux P, et al. Surgical management of ileosigmoid fistulas in Crohn's disease: role of preoperative colonoscopy. Dis Colon Rectum 1995;38:1084–87.

30. Saint-Marc O, Tiret E, Vaillant J, et al. Surgical management of internal fistulas in Crohn's disease. J Am Coll Surg 1996;183:97–100.

31. Fazio V. Crohn's disease of the small bowel-operative techniques and tactics. Hepato-gastroenterology 1990;37:56–62.

32. Smedh K, Olaison G, Nystrom P, et al. Intraoperative enteroscopy in Crohn's disease. Br J Surg 1993;80:897–900.

33. Lopez M, Cooley J, Petros J, et al. Complete intraoperative small bowel endoscopy in the evaluation of occult gastrointestinal bleeding using the sonde enteroscope. Arch Surg 1996;131:272–7.

34. Michelassi F, Testa G, Pomidor W, et al. Adenocarcinoma complicating Crohn's disease. Dis Colon Rectum 1993;36:654–61.

35. Baird D, Narendranathan M, Sandler R. Increased risk of preterm birth for women with inflammatory bowel disease. Gastroenterology 1990;99:987–94.

36. Moeller D. Crohn's disease beginning during pregnancy. S Med J 1988;81:1067.

37. Woolfon K, Cohen Z, McLeod R. Crohn's disease and pregnancy. Dis Colon Rectum 1990;33:869–73.

38. Teahon K, Pearson M, Levi A, et al. Elemental diet in the management of Crohn's disease during pregnancy. Gut 1991;32:1079–81.

39. Nugent W, Rajala M, O'Shea R, et al. Total parenteral nutrition in pregnancy: conception to delivery. J Parent Enter Nutr 1987;11:424–7.

40. Ribeiro M, Greenstein A, Yamazaki Y, et al. Intraabdominal abscess in regional enteritis. Ann Surg 1991;213:32–6.

41. Fazio V. Regional enteritis (Crohn's disease): indications for surgery and operative strategy. Surg Clin North Am 1983;63:27–47.

42. Post S, Betzler M, Ditfurth B, et al. Risks of intestinal anastomoses in Crohn's disease. Ann Surg 1991;213:37–42.

43. Post S, Herfarth Ch, Schumacher H, et al. Experience with ileostomy and colostomy in Crohn's disease. Br J Surg 1995;82:1629–33.

44. Fazio V, Strong S. 1995. The surgical management of Crohn's disease. In: Kirsner J, Shorter R. eds. Inflammatory bowel disease. 4th ed. Baltimore: Williams & Wilkins, 1995;830–87.

45. Keighley M. Surgical treatment of small bowel Crohn's disease. In: Keighley M, and Williams N, eds. Surgery of the Anus, Rectum, and Colon. W.B. Saunders 1993;1710–57.

46. Lock R, Farmer R, Fazio V, et al. Recurrence and reoperation for Crohn's disease. The role of disease location in prognosis. N Engl J Med 1981;304:1586–8.

47. Leitman I, Paul D, Shires G. Evaluation and management of massive lower gastrointestinal hemorrhage. Ann Surg 1989;209:175–80.

48. Fernandez-Banares F, Abad-Lacruz A, Xiol X, et al. Vitamin status in patients with inflammatory bowel disease. Am J Gastroenterol 1989;84:744–8.

49. Andersson H, Bosaeus I, Fasth S, et al. Cholelithiasis and urolithiasis in Crohn's disease. Scand J Gastroenterology 1987;22:253–6.

19 Ileocecectomy

Ciaran J. Walsh and Ian C. Lavery

Indication

Ileocecectomy is indicated for ileocecal Crohn's disease complicated by obstruction, fistula formation or perforation with or without abscess formation.

Preoperative Preparation

Patients with ileocecal Crohn's disease may be malnourished, anemic, and dehydrated. As a result they may require preoperative nutritional support, rehydration and blood transfusion. Severely malnourished patients will benefit from preoperative total parenteral nutrition (TPN) that can be continued in the peri- and postoperative periods. The vast majority of patients will be able to have an ileocecal resection and primary ileocolic anastomosis without a proximal stoma. If there are clinical or radiological findings that raise the possibility of a need for a stoma, these patients are seen preoperatively by a stoma therapist. They are marked for an ileostomy and are educated about the possibility of a temporary stoma and its implications. Recently many of these patients are being treated with immunosuppressive drugs such as imuran or 6-mercaptopurine. Our preference is to stop these for as long a time as possible before surgery. If the patient is taking oral steroids we continue these up to the day before surgery, and administer 100 mg hydrocortisone intravenous (IV) immediately before surgery. In the absence of obstructive symptoms we use polyethylene glycol to prepare the bowel the evening before surgery. Patients with obstructive symptoms are instructed to take only clear liquids by mouth for two days before surgery. On the evening before surgery they take 12 ounces of magnesium citrate by mouth. If there is a large palpable mass or other reason to suspect that the right ureter might be involved in the inflammatory process [such as evidence of a retroperitoneal perforation or abscess on computerized tomography (CT) scan], it is prudent to place a ureteric stent at the beginning of the procedure. This should be discussed with the patient as part of their informed consent. We routinely use prophylactic antibiotics. Our preference is intravenous ceftizoxime 1 g and metronidazole 500 mg, given at the time of induction of anesthesia and twice postoperatively at eight hourly intervals. In patients with genuine penicillin allergies we use ciprofloxacin and metronidazole. We routinely place the patient supine on the operating table, but will use Lloyd Davies stirrups in selected cases. In particular ileocecal Crohn's may be complicated by an ileosigmoid fistula that may, albeit uncommonly, require sigmoid resection. If suspected preoperatively Lloyd Davies stirrups would be used in this instance to support the legs, in case a circular stapler might need to be passed transanally for the colorectal anastomosis.

Pitfalls and Danger Points

1. Damage to right ureter.
2. Development of a mesenteric hematoma.
3. Damage to duodenum.
4. Placement of ileocolic anastomosis adjacent to duodenum.
5. Failure to recognize a proximal small bowel stricture.
6. Failure to recognize an ileosigmoid or vesical fistula.

7. Failure to recognize a psoas abscess or failing to drain it properly.
8. Failure of anastomosis.

Operative Strategy

Abdominal operations for Crohn's disease should be performed via midline incisions. Adhering to this basic principle will lessen difficulties with stoma placement at this or subsequent operations. As in all cases of Crohn's disease the operative strategy is based on the premise of only operating on the complications of Crohn's, preserving as much bowel as possible and anticipating the propensity for the disease to recur. Crohn's disease is a benign disease. There is no need to perform a wide or extensive mesenteric excision. There is a balance with regard to how much mesentery is resected. Attempts at resection very close to the bowel result in difficulty with controlling the mesentery due to mesenteric thickening from fat wrapping and adenopathy. More proximal resection results in the need to resect more bowel than is necessary. Ileocecal Crohn's is often associated with marked mesenteric adenopathy particularly along the ileocolic vessels and although removal of these nodes is not a primary objective of surgery we tend to remove them if this can be done without requiring further small bowel resection as a result of vascular compromise. It should be stressed that this is not a right hemicolectomy. Only the diseased colon, most often the cecum, need be removed with the terminal ileum. The anastomosis is made to the proximal ascending colon. In this way the minimum amount of bowel is removed. This helps maintain the facility for water absorption from the right colon and thus decrease the diarrhea that may result from resection of the ileocecal valve. Furthermore the anastomosis is away from the duodenum, thus reducing the risk of a duodenal fistula should there be a preanastomotic recurrence. Another way in which this operation differs from right hemicolectomy for cancer is the manner in which the mesentery is managed. As mentioned earlier the mesentery is often markedly thickened in Crohn's disease and requires particular care and attention to prevent mesenteric hematoma formation. The mesenteric vessels are not divided at their origin as they are in an operation for a malignancy.

Operative Technique

The incision is made in the midline. A laparotomy is performed and the extent of disease is assessed, including the presence of any complications such as localized perforations, abscesses, or fistulous communications. The sigmoid colon and bladder in particular need to be inspected carefully to see that they are free of any secondary involvement. The three main objectives in examining the small bowel are: (1) to assess the extent of small bowel disease including the proximal resection site (2) to look for strictures remote from the ileocecal disease and (3) to measure the length of small bowel proximal to the proposed ileal resection margin.

Mobilization

The surgeon stands on the patient's left side. A Balfour retractor is placed in the wound and the surgeon retracts the cecum and ascending colon towards himself in order to identify the plane of dissection along the peritoneal reflection lateral to the cecum. After developing the plane the surgeons left index finger can then be insinuated under the peritoneal reflection and the dissection continued cephalad (Fig. 19.1). This technique is continued towards the hepatic flexure as far as needed to have adequate mobilization to perform bowel transection and subsequent anastomosis. Following full mobilization, the inflammatory ileocecal mass can be delivered into the wound, facilitating resection.

Choosing Levels of Resection

The proximal extent of the disease is first assessed by noting the presence of fat wrapping, curlicue vessels, or a point of obstruction (Fig. 19.2). The best guide to the proximal extent of disease is palpation along the enteric/mesenteric margin. Nondiseased bowel proximal to the affected ileocecal segment may be dilated but there is no mesenteric thickening. One is able to palpate a step between the edge of the bowel wall and the mesentery. A segment with significant mucosal disease will be associated with mesenteric thickening and there is no palpable step between the edge of the bowel and the mesentery (Fig. 19.3). Lymph node enlargement in the mesentery corresponds well to the limits of ulceration of the mucosa. Having chosen the proposed site of transection it is important to inspect the bowel when it is divided. Deep longitudinal ulcers at the cut edge will require further resection, whereas small aphthous ulcers in otherwise soft pliable bowel will not. A margin of two centimeters of macroscopically normal bowel proximal and distal to the diseased segment is adequate. Recurrence rates do not increase when there is microscopic disease at the resection margins. Having

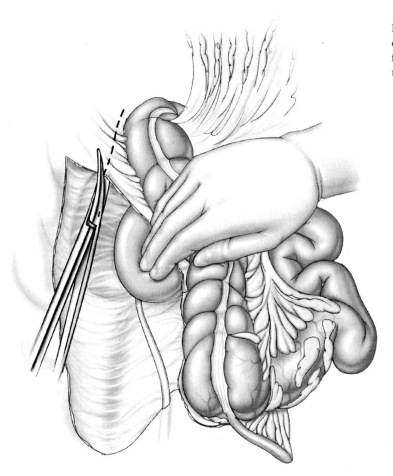

Fig. 19.1. Mobilization of the right colon. The dissection is carried around the hepatic flexure to facilitate delivery of the inflammatory ileocecal mass into the wound.

identified the proximal and distal lines of resection, hernia tapes are placed beyond the resection lines to prevent spillage of the lumenal contents. We prefer this technique to the use of noncrushing bowel clamps as it is less traumatic, and tapes do not get in the way or get sutures hooked on them.

Bowel Resection

Resection is begun by division of the mesentery. The mesentery of the affected bowel is thick and sclerotic making it very difficult or impossible to identify blood vessels in order that they may be controlled individually. If the mesentery is divided without control the vessels retract and are difficult to find and control. This leads to the development of a hematoma. To avoid this, we use a technique where the mesentery is clamped between overlapping Kocher clamps and suture ligated (Fig. 19.4). Dissection begins at the mesenteric margin of the small bowel. A small window is made with electrocautery and the ileal mesentery clamped between Kocher clamps. The mesentery is divided between the clamps, up to, but not past their tips. A second pair of clamps is placed on the next segment of

mesentery to be divided ensuring that these overlap the tips of the previous pair. The mesentery is divided in a likewise fashion to the preselected site at the mesenteric border of the colon. The colon and ileum are divided between clamps and the specimen removed. The vessels in the mesentery are controlled with suture ligatures of heavy absorbable suture material. By placing interlocking sutures no segment of small bowel mesentery escapes suture ligation (Fig. 19.5). When dividing the mesentery a short cuff is left distal to the suture ligature to facilitate later safe closure of the mesenteric defect.

Anastomosis

Our preference is an end to side stapled anastomosis, using as large a staple gun as the cut end of the ileum will accommodate. A 2-0 proline purse string suture is placed in the cut end of the ileum. It is important to include all layers of the bowel without placing more tissue in the instrument than its capacity allows. Small seromuscular bites and even smaller mucosal bites are taken 1.5 cm apart. If too much tissue is inverted, as the instrument is

Fig. 19.2. Planned site of mesenteric division is outlined as are proximal and distal lines of resection.

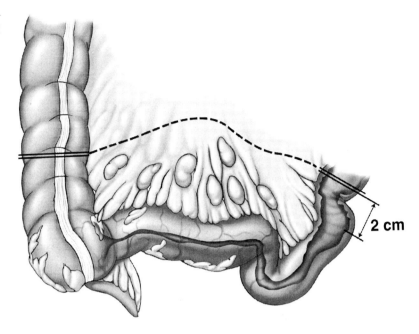

2 cm

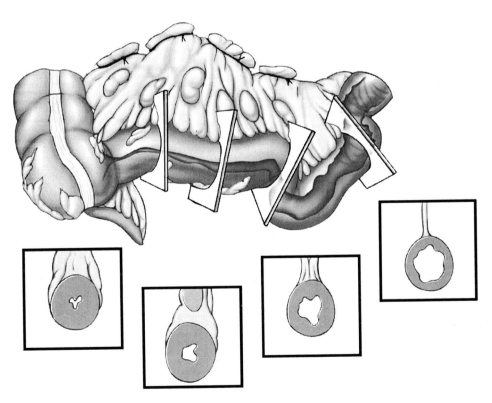

Fig. 19.3. Cross sections through the distal ileum and mesentery. The gradual change in bowel wall and mesenteric thickness is shown. At the proposed level of resection a definite step should be palpable between finger and thumb at the mesenteric margin of the bowel.

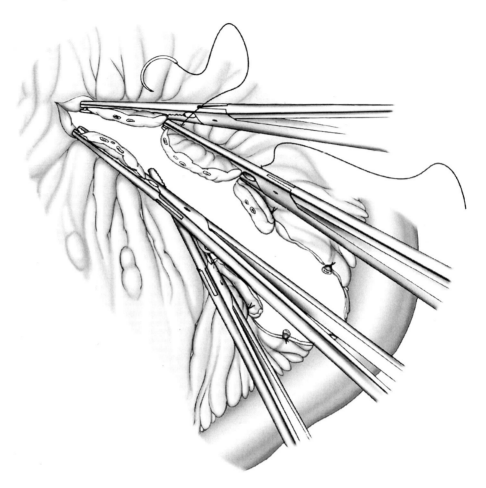

Fig. 19.4.   Technique for division of small bowel mesentery using overlapping Kocher clamps and suture ligation.

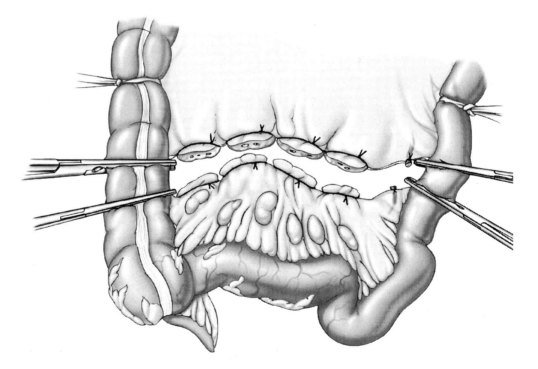

Fig. 19.5.   The mesentery is divided. Hernia tapes have been placed to isolate the resection specimen and the bowel is ready to be divided between clamps. Note how the transfixion sutures in the mesentery overlap.

closed tissue is squeezed out and results in a defect in the anastomosis. The clamp from the cut end of the colon is removed. While holding the colon up to prevent contamination the stapling instrument is inserted through the end of the colon. The instrument is then opened so the spike comes through the bowel wall 4 to 5 cm from the cut edge at an appropriate part of the wall. The anvil in the ileum is then attached (Fig. 19.6A) and the anastomosis is fashioned. The integrity of the tissue donuts is checked. Having established the end to side anastomosis, a linear stapler is used to close the end of the colon (Fig. 19.6B). If the integrity of this staple line is in doubt if it is oversewn with 3-0 vicryl. The anastomosis is supported with two seromuscular stitches in the angles thus taking the weight off the staple line. If the small bowel is very thickened and dilated secondary to obstruction, it is preferable to hand sew the anastomosis as the thickened bowel will be crushed and possibly rendered ischemic by squeezing it into the firing zone of an automatic stapler. An end to end hand-sewn anastomosis is easily performed with or without a short Cheadle slit in the ileum.

Closure

Closing the mesenteric defect may be important to prevent an internal hernia (Fig. 19.7). Technique is critical as it is possible to damage vessels and therefore blood supply in the free edge of the cut mesentery. When the mesentery is divided a cuff of tissue is left distal to the suture ligature. By doing this the interrupted sutures used to close the defect can be placed through these tufts and not risk injuring a mesenteric vessel. Following closure of the mesenteric defect the peritoneal cavity is liberally lavaged with warm saline. Hemostasis is checked and secured. The anastomosis is placed in the abdomen away from the duodenum, and if appropriate, is wrapped in greater omentum to further protect against a duodenal fistula in the future. No drains are used unless there was an associated inflammatory nest in which case a suction drain is placed in the region of the cavity. The wound is closed using a mass closure technique with looped size #1 polydioxanone suture (PDS) and the skin closed with staples.

Special Circumstances:

1. Mass involving right ureter.
   Retroperitoneal inflammation may involve the ureter. In our experience, ureteric obstruction is uncommon, and ureterolysis is rarely indicated. The ileocolic resection will lead to successful resolution of the obstruction in the majority of cases. Careful dissection of the ureter from the inflammatory mass is usually possible without a formal ureterolysis that may devascularize the ureter. This procedure is facilitated by the use of a ureteric stent which also helps identify and lessen a ureteric injury should it occur.

2. Localized perforation and abscess.
   Usually an abscess or perforation is diagnosed preoperatively by a combination of the patient's signs and symptoms and radiological investigations. If there is CT scan evidence of an abscess our preference is to drain this percutaneously under CT control and place the patient on IV antibiotics (ceftizoxime and metronidazole until culture results are available). If there is no improvement surgery needs to be brought forward. After the inflammation has resolved an operation can be performed under more favorable conditions about two weeks later. One will not always have this luxury and occasionally a previously unrecognized perforation and abscess is identified during the course of the operation. A mesenteric abscess is aspirated. The pus is sent for culture and sensitivity and the abscess cavity opened and curettaged if it is not to be included in the resection specimen. If there is an interloop abscess abutting the sigmoid colon with or without an associated inflammatory mass a careful search for a fistula must be made. Psoas abscesses deserve special mention. Ileocecal Crohn's disease is now the commonest cause of psoas abscess in our practice. A high index of suspicion is required as they may be missed. They may have a collar stud configuration with pus emanating from a small breach in the psoas fascia associated with a large subfascial abscess cavity (Fig. 19.8). Extensive unroofing of the abscess and placement of drains is required (Fig. 19.9). Care should be taken not to damage the retroperitoneal nerves lying deep to the iliopsoas fascia when laying open these abscesses. In the absence of generalized peritonitis an ileocecectomy and primary anastomosis is the procedure of choice. If there is gross peritoneal soiling or a large inflammatory nest in the region of the anastomosis a loop ileostomy is constructed proximal to the anastomosis, or an end ileostomy and mucus fistula is constructed. Intestinal continuity is restored when the inflammatory changes have resolved and the patient is healthy and off

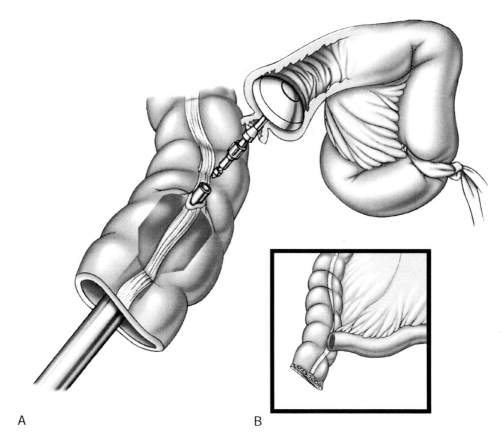

Fig. 19.6.   (A) Stapled end to side anastomosis using a circular stapler. (B) The completed anastomosis with the distal colon closed with a linear stapler.

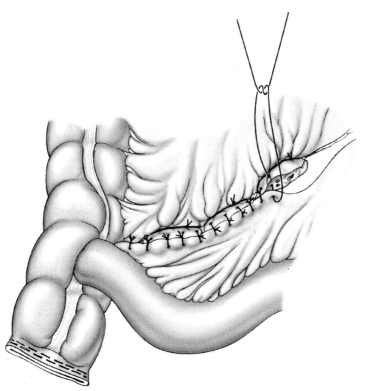

Fig. 19.7.   Closure of the mesenteric defect. Place sutures through the tufts of mesentery distal to the transfixion sutures to avoid bleeding from the edge of the mesentery.

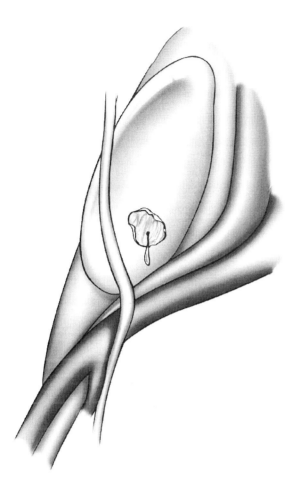

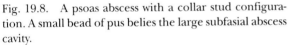

Fig. 19.8. A psoas abscess with a collar stud configuration. A small bead of pus belies the large subfasial abscess cavity.

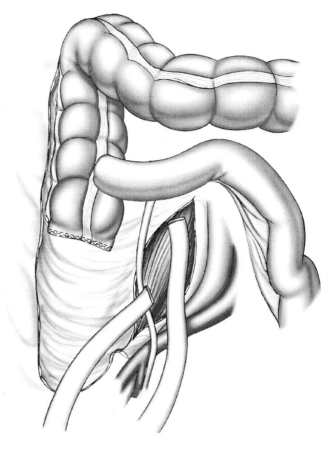

Fig. 19.9. Extensive deroofing of the right psoas abscess and placement of multiple drains. Prolonged drainage and antibiotic therapy may be required. Tucking some mentrum into the cavity (if available) will help isolate the area from the anastomosis.

medication. This usually takes three to six months.

3. Internal fistulae.

In our experience internal fistulae occur in about one third of patients with ileocecal Crohn's disease. In the majority of cases the target organ is secondarily involved. An ileosigmoid fistula is the most common enteroenteral fistula encountered. In these cases an ileocecal phlegmon is found adherent to the antimesenteric aspect of the sigmoid colon or the sigmoid colon may form one of the walls of an abscess cavity associated with the ileocecal disease. Occasionally it can be difficult to demonstrate the fistulous communication despite provocative measures to demonstrate it. Such measures may include probing and air insufflation during intraoperative colonoscopy. In the majority of cases the sigmoid is secondarily involved and the fistula can be

"pinched off" and the sigmoid colotomy sutured closed after excision back to normal tissue. On occasion this may require excision of the sigmoid colon with subsequent anastomosis. If there is induration and granulation tissue in the wall the safest thing to do is a wedge excision back to normal bowel with closure of the colotomy. If the fistula is more complex (e.g., an ileovesicosigmoid fistula or there are multiple fistulous communications or evidence of Crohn's disease of the sigmoid), then a separate segmental resection of the sigmoid colon with a colocolonic anastomosis is performed. A proximal loop ileostomy is recommended if there is evidence of pelvic sepsis or small bowel obstruction. Ileotransverse and ileo-ileal fistulae are the next most common enteroenteral fistulae. The same principles apply (i.e., the target organ is secondarily affected and the fistula can be pinched off and the enterotomy closed after trimming back) to healthy bowel. It is not enough to just close the fistula. As previously if there are multiple fistulous communications or the target organ is also diseased then a segmental resection is preferable. Ileosigmoid fistulae are frequently associated with a vesical fistula and these need to be identified. An enterovesical fistula may be suspected preoperatively by a history of pneumaturia, fecaluria, or urinary tract infections. In patients with Crohn's disease the ileum is the most common site of origin of a vesical fistula. They may occur alone or as part of a complex inflammatory nest including an ileosigmoid fistula. The fistula is pinched off. The fistulous tract into the bladder is curettaged. The cystotomy may be left open or closed. A suction drain is placed in the pelvis and a Foley catheter left in the bladder for at least 5 to 7 days postoperatively. Provided there is good intraperitoneal pelvic drainage and a bladder catheter, the bladder will nearly always heal regardless of whether it is closed or not.

4. Proximal small bowel strictures.

It is important to carefully examine the proximal small bowel for strictures. If present and close to the terminal ileum it is reasonable to resect the stricture with the longer segment. However if the stricture is more proximal this strategy would lead to an unacceptable loss of small bowel length and therefore it is better to do a stricturoplasty on the proximal stricture (see Chapter 16).

Postoperative Care

The nasogastric tube is removed the first postoperative day. The patient is kept on IV fluids and sips of fluid by mouth until they pass flatus, after which their diet is advanced. Intravenous hydrocortisone is tapered from 100 mg IV every 8 hours on the first postoperative day to 25 mg IV every 8 hours on the fourth postoperative day. Oral prednisone is begun and hydrocortisone discontinued when the patient has resumed eating. We usually aim to discharge the patient on 15 mg prednisone per day and then taper by 5 mg per week thereafter. The urinary catheter is removed three days after surgery unless there was an enterovesical fistula in which case it is left in for 5 to 7 days. We do not routinely order a cystogram in such cases. Patients are usually ready to be discharged from hospital on the fifth postoperative day in uncomplicated cases. In the case of a psoas abscess prolonged drainage is important as is correct antibiotic coverage for the chronically infected muscle. Antibiotic treatment may need to be prolonged in these cases.

Complications

Early complications specific to this type of operation include delayed gastric emptying, ileus, small bowel obstruction, ureteric injury, and sepsis. Potential sources of sepsis after ileocecectomy include anastomotic leak, an unrecognized psoas abscess or sigmoid fistula and urosepsis.

20 Segmental Colectomy

Denis C.N.K. Nyam and John H. Pemberton

It has been reported that only 20% of patients with Crohn's colitis remain well without surgery 5 and 10 years after diagnosis (1). In contrast to surgery for ulcerative colitis, surgery for Crohn's disease will not result in a cure. Although the use of limited resection for small bowel Crohn's is widely accepted, the value of segmental resection in colonic Crohn's disease is more controversial. The role of the colon in water and electrolyte conservation and protection against volume depletion becomes increasingly important as the amount of small bowel resected increases. Therefore, although largely an expendable organ, colonic preservation may be justified in segmental Crohn's disease.

This chapter will not discuss ileocolonic disease or rectal and perineal disease which are covered in other chapters.

The arguments for and against segmental resection center around two crucial issues; recurrence and operative risks. Although there is a higher risk of anastomotic recurrence after segmental colectomy than if all the colon is removed, reoperation is generally safe in terms of morbidity and mortality (2,3). In addition, the patient can often be palliated for a number of years before total colectomy or ileostomy is ultimately required.

Indications for Surgery

The indications for surgery in Crohn's colitis are usually relative such as complications of the disease or outright failure of medical treatment (Table 20.1). Absolute indications for operations, such as bleeding, perforation, toxic dilatation, or acute obstruction, occur rarely. Failure to respond to medical therapy is more common in patients with Crohn's colitis than in those with small bowel Crohn's disease (4).

The symptoms, prognosis, and risk of recurrence vary depending on the presence of concurrent small bowel involvement (5,6). In turn, the choice of surgical procedure is dependent on the presence and severity of rectal involvement (7–9). Resection of the diseased segment should be considered if obstructive symptoms are present, if inflammation is severe and perforation imminent or if surveillance of the proximal colon is impossible due to a stricture (2). There is little question that in patients with a fistula, abscess, or stricture of a localized segment of colon, that segmental resection and anastomosis is a reasonable option (10).

Operative Strategy

Crohn's disease of the right colon requires resection of a portion of the terminal ileum, cecum, ascending and transverse colon and an ileal-transverse colostomy. The anastomosis can be wrapped with omentum to reduce the risk of fistulation.

Crohn's disease of the transverse, descending, and sigmoid colon can be treated by segmental resection and end-to-end anastomosis of the colon; however, recurrence of Crohn's disease in the remaining colon is so common that most have been reluctant to use it. Segmental colectomy facilitates maximal preservation of the colon for water absorption and may thus be the procedure of choice in the older patient with little small bowel remaining or in adolescent patients who have a high livelihood of further disease involving the small intestine. The occasional patient with an isolated area of symptomatic Crohn's colitis is a candidate for segmental resection, provided no anorectal disease is present. The rationale is that although there is a higher recurrence rate after a segmental resection

Table 20.1. Indications for surgery in colonic Crohn's disease.

1. Internal fistulae and abscess
2. Perianal disease
3. Severe disease with poor response to medical therapy
4. Toxic megacolon
5. Intestinal obstruction

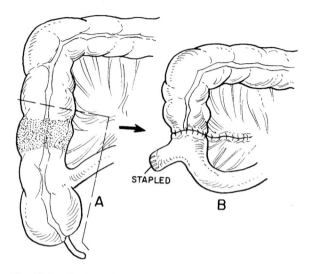

Fig. 20.1. Right sided Crohn's colitis (A) treated with a limited segmental right hemicolectomy (B).

for Crohn's colitis, the patient may have several years of "more normal" function requiring further resection. In the younger patient (<50 years) with minimal or no previous small bowel resection, the preferred procedure probably remains an ileal-sigmoid or ilealrectal anastomosis. The patient with Crohn's disease in several colonic segments is not a candidate for segmental resection unless the small bowel is critically short.

The margins of resection should be grossly free of disease. Although controversial, the Mayo Clinic practice has strived to achieve microscopically free margins. If the margin is grossly free of disease but microscopically involved, we resect another 2 to 3 cm of bowel. If the margin is still involved microscopically, no further resection is performed and an anastomosis is made. It is important to remember that Crohn's disease is panintestinal and incurable by surgical means. Lymphadenectomy is not routinely performed. The mesenteric vessels do not need to be taken near their origins. Keeping close to the bowel wall is more tedious but prevents injury to the retroperitoneal structures.

Colonoscopic dilatation of colonic Crohn's strictures has been performed, but reports are anecdotal and the procedure seems dangerous. Stricturoplasty is generally not performed in the colon.

Operative Technique

Limited Segmental Right Hemicolectomy (Fig. 20.1)

All segmental colectomies are performed using a midline incision. Other types of incisions such as Pfannenstiel, transverse, or subcostal incisions are inappropriate for an operative strategy that is fluid from the beginning; the portion of the bowel that needs to be excised in patients with Crohn's disease is often uncertain preoperatively, an inappropriately placed incision can thus be a disaster. Midline incisions are simple, heal well, and allow unhindered access to the entire abdomen.

Procedure

The cecum is grasped and elevated tenting the retroperitoneal attachments. These are incised,

taking care to identify the ureter medially. The retroperitoneal attachments are swept away up to the hepatic flexure. The retroperitoneal attachments of the distal ileal mesentery are also swept away at this point elevating the terminal ileum and cecum nicely out of the abdomen. The involved segment then resected and a side-to-side stapled functional end-to-end anastomosis is performed and is our preferred approach (4). This is done using the GIA and the TA stapler instruments (United States Surgical Corp, Norwalk, CT). Figure 20.2 details a side-to-side stapled functional end-to-end ileocolonic anastomosis. The 6 cm GIA is used to staple over ends of the ileum and colon and to establish the anastomosis. The anterior and posterior staple lines are distracted from each other and the TIA instrument used to close the resulting defect. The apex is bolstered with a silk suture and the mesenteric defect closed. Stapling of anastomoses should be done only when the bowel being stapled is normal. If there has been chronic obstruction of the terminal ileum and the bowel is dilated and thickened, then a hand-sewn anastomosis is indicated. The mesenteric defect is closed with a running absorbable suture. Our hand-sewn anastomosis is usually a side-to-end ileal ascending colostomy, in two layers. The trick to a rapid error free operation is to be sure that the cecum and terminal ileum are well mobilized, thus, allowing easy visualization of the operation you wish to perform.

Extended Right Hemicolectomy (Fig. 20.3)

An extended right hemicolectomy and ileal transverse colostomy is the operation of choice for pa-

Fig. 20.2. A stapled functional end-to-end ileo-colic anastomosis. (A) The terminal ileum is divided; (B) the anastomosis is started by inserting the linear-cutter staples into a small enterotomy of such bowel end; (C) the staples are fixed creating the anastomosis; (D) the enterotomies are closed with other linear staples.

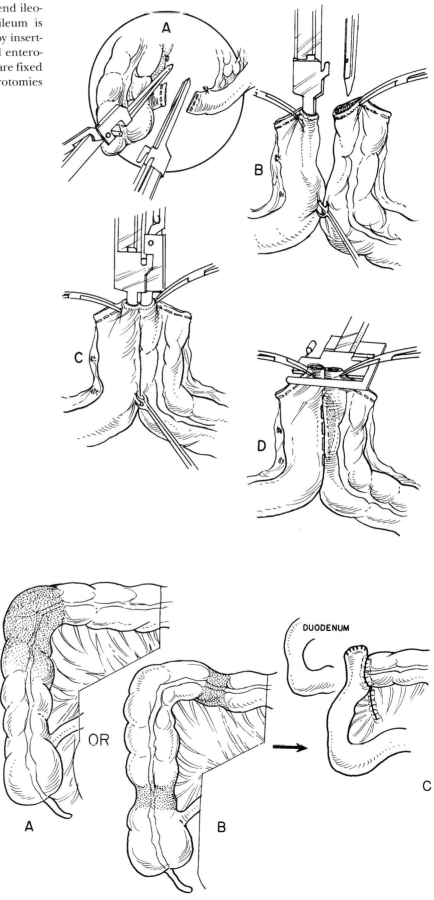

Fig. 20.3. Hepatic flexure Crohn's disease (A) or multiple skipped lesions limited to the proximal transverse colon (B) treated with an extended right hemicolectomy and ileodistal transverse anastomosis (C). The anastomosis is fashioned away from the duodenum.

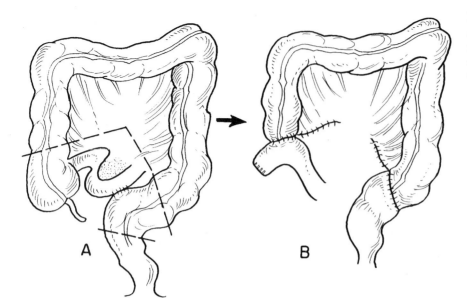

Fig. 20.4. Ileocolonic Crohn's disease with involvement of the sigmoid colon. A limited right ileocolonic and segmental resection of the sigmoid is done.

tients with terminal, ileal, and right sided colonic Crohn's disease (ileocolonic Crohn's). Here the operation is performed exactly in the manner just described, but now the dissection is carried around the hepatic flexure, separating the omental structures from the mesentery, all the way into the lesser sac. Very rarely is it necessary to sacrifice the middle colic artery; we usually take the colon up to the right branch of the middle colic artery and perform a side-to-side stapled functional end-to-end or side-to-end ileocolostomy (hand-sewn in two layers). Once again the mesentery is closed with a running absorbable suture.

Ileocolonic/Sigmoid Resection

If the terminal ileum or cecum has fistulized into the sigmoid colon and the sigmoid colon is endoscopically free of Crohn's disease, a right hemicolectomy, and oversewing of the ileosigmoid fistula is performed. The fistula is pinched off of the colon, the sigmoid edges freshened and oversewn in two layers. Leaks from the pinched off ileal sigmoid fistulae are very rare indeed. Segmental resection of sigmoid colon is reserved only in those instances when Crohn's disease is proven endoscopically (Fig. 20.4). Because the overriding goal of the surgeon is to preserve bowel, a double suture line (ileo-ascending colostomy and sigmoid colocolostomy) is a reasonable operation to do; the leak rates are no higher than if a single suture line is present.

Hand-sewn Anastomosis (Fig. 20.5)

Figure 20.5 illustrates a hand-sewn side of ileum to end of colon anastomosis that is used for nearly all

right hemicolectomies and ileorectostomies. I find the colon invariably huge so that end-to-end ileocolostomy seems impracticable; side-to-end anastomoses function well and complications are few.

Segmental Colectomy (Transverse Colon, Left Colon, and Sigmoid Colon)

Segmental colectomy for Crohn's disease in other areas of the colon is a straightforward procedure. The offending area is removed, the extent of resection determined, if necessary, by intraoperative colonoscopy. The ends of the colon should be free of gross disease. A two layer hand-sewn anastomosis is almost invariably used in these situations.

Complications

As with all operations on patients with Crohn's disease, the main complications are unexpected bleeding and infection. These include infections which can be acute, in the form of an anastomotic leak and abscess or late and take the form of a fistula. In a series of 29 patients having segmental resection and primary anastomosis, no patient had an anastomotic leak, suggesting the procedure is safe (2). Fistulas can occur internally or to the skin. One special fistula is a duodenocolic fistula which is a rare complication after an ileocolic anastomosis.

Long-Term Results

There are few reports of segmental colectomy for Crohn's disease in the literature, typically in small series (2,3,10,11). De Dombal (12) reported a

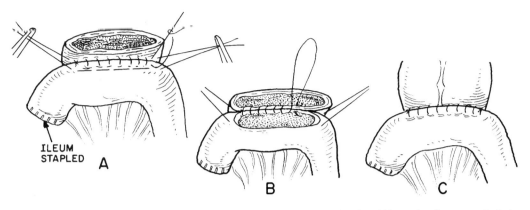

Fig. 20.5. Hand-sewn anastomosis—end colon (A) to side ileum (B). The distal ileum has been stapled closed (C).

crude recurrence rate after right and left hemi-colectomy of 39 and 29% respectively whereas it was 46% after total abdominal colectomy and ileorectal anastomosis. Allan (2) on the other hand reported a reoperative rate of 66% for segmental colectomy and 53% for segmental/ileorectal anastomosis after 10 years.

Preservation of macroscopically normal colon may have some functional advantage especially in the proximal colon where sodium absorption is much greater compared with the distal colon (13). It therefore seems reasonable to consider segmental colectomy in patients with skip areas of Crohn's disease in the colon, especially if the patient has previously undergone multiple small bowel resections and is at risk for the development of a short-bowel syndrome. Any length of intestine, even large, may be helpful in avoiding intractable diarrhea or water-electrolyte disturbances.

References

1. Allan R, Steinberg DM, Alexander-Williams J, Cooke WT. Crohn's disease involving the colon: an audit of clinical management. Gasteroenterology 1977;73: 723–32.
2. Allan A, Andrews MB, Hilton CJ, Keighley MRB, Allan RN, Alexander-Williams J. Segmental colonic resection is an appropriate operation for short skip lesions due to Crohn's disease of the colon. World J Surg 1989;13:611–6.
3. Longo WE, Ballantyne GH, Cahow E. Treatment of Crohn's colitis. Segmental or total colectomy? Arch Surg 1988;123:588–90.
4. Farmer RG, Hawker WA, Turnbull RB. Clinical patterns in Crohn's disease: a statistical study of 615 cases. Gasteroenterology 1975;68:627–35.
5. Goligher JC. The long-term results of excisional surgery for primary and recurrent Crohn's disease of the large intestine. Dis Colon Rectum 1985;28:52–5.
6. Scammell BE, Andrews H, Allan RN, Alexander-William J, Keighley MRB. Results of proctocolectomy for Crohn's disease. Br J Surg 1987;74:671–4.
7. Kodner IJ, Fry RD. Inflammatory bowel disease. CIBA Found Symp 1982;32.
8. Block GE. Current concepts: Surgical management of Crohn's colitis. N Engl J Med 1980;302:1068–70.
9. Goligher JC. Surgical treatment of Crohn's disease affecting mainly or entirely the large bowel. World J Surg 1988;12:186–90.
10. Sanfey H, Bayless TM, Cameron JL. Crohn's disease of the colon. Is there a role for limited resection? Ann J Surg 1984;147:38–42.
11. Stern HS, Goldberg SM, Rothenberger DA, Nivatvongs S, Schottler J, Christenson C, et al. Segmental versus total colectomy for large bowel Crohn's disease. World J Surg 1984;8:118–22.
12. De Dombal FT, Burton I, Goligher JC. Recurrence of Crohn's disease after primary excisional surgery. Gut 1971;12:519–27.
13. Roediger WEW, Rigol G, Rae D. Sodium absorption with bacterial fatty acids and bile salts in the proximal and distal colon as a guide to colonic resection. Dis Colon Rectum 1984;27:1–5.

21 Total Abdominal Colectomy: Indications and Technique

Walter E. Longo and Anthony M. Vernava

Indications

A surgical approach is chosen for Crohn's colitis when either medical therapy has been initiated and failed, medication has significant side effects, or because of the development of complications of the disease such as perforation, abscess, fistula, obstruction, hemorrhage, toxicity, poor bowel function, malnutrition, or extra intestinal manifestations. The decision for surgery should be unanimous between patient, gastroenterologist, and surgeon. Timing of the procedure is importance since this involves having the patient in both an optimal nutritional and emotional state and not delaying resection when it is inevitable. Basic principles regarding the surgery of Crohn's disease such as bowel conservation, margins of resection and timing of surgery have been discussed in earlier chapters.

The primary goals of surgery in Crohn's colitis are to eradicate disease, preserve bowel function, and minimize the need for future pharmacological intervention. A restorative procedure will be the first choice for most patients with large-bowel Crohn's disease in an effort to accomplish these goals. When Crohn's disease involves the entire colon with relative rectal sparing, total abdominal colectomy with ileorectal or ileosigmoid anastomosis is the natural choice procedure. Optimal surgical treatment of patients with involvement limited to only a segment of the colon exclusive of ileocecal disease is often debated as to whether a segmental colectomy or an abdominal colectomy is required. This is also discussed in Chapter 20.

Total colectomy with ileorectal anastomosis may be performed as a one or two-stage procedure. A one-stage procedure is performed and preferred when optimal conditions exist such as good nutritional state and no intraabdominal infection. If integrity of the anastomosis is of concern, a protective loop ileostomy is added. The alternative method of colectomy and ileostomy with delayed ileorectal anastomosis, is usually done for fulminant disease. The downside of this approach is that a second laparotomy is required to reestablish intestinal continuity, but this is the preferable option in an unstable or malnourished patient, and it still permits restoration.

Preoperative Preparation

All patients undergoing surgery, whether elective or emergent, should have their medical conditions optimized. Most patients with Crohn's disease are young and the need for assessment of medical risks will be minimal. If however, the patient is elderly or has preexisting medical diseases, an assessment should be performed. Patients who are smokers and those with dyspnea should have pulmonary function tests. Carotid duplex may be warranted for symptoms suggestive of cerebrovascular disease. Standard preoperative laboratory testing including complete blood count, serum chemistries, and coagulation profile are essential. Any abnormalities should be corrected including anemia by red blood cell transfusion as well as correction of any electrolyte abnormalities. Patients with cachexia will benefit from preoperative total parenteral nutrition (TPN). Intravenous steroids are given prior to induction of general anesthesia if the patients has been taking prior enteral steroids over the preceding 12 months. A full mechanical and oral antibiotic preparation is given unless obstruction is present. Stomal marking in both lower quadrants is performed by a trained enterostomal therapist. Intravenous antibiotics are given 30 minutes prior to the incision and for 24 hours after the procedure.

Pitfalls and Danger Points

There are a number of pitfalls and danger points during an abdominal colectomy for Crohn's colitis. In patients with fulminant colitis, massive colonic distention could put the colon at risk for injury during entry. If this is a reoperative abdomen, the risk of enterotomies is a concern. Repair of any enterotomies should be performed in two layers. Resection and primary anastomosis may be required if repair is impossible. During mobilization of the abdominal colon, previous colonic inflammation may cause the colon to be adherent to other intrabdominal organs. Any injury to the ureters, biliary tree, duodenum, stomach, or spleen that occur must be dealt with appropriately. The major pitfall is the risk of contamination of the peritoneal cavity by inadvertent colotomy, leading to sepsis. Loss of anastomotic integrity is the most feared complication following ileorectal anastomosis. Outcome is not affected by anastomotic technique as long as there is an adequate blood supply, no tension, and minimal sepsis. Finally, in those patients not undergoing a restorative procedure, improper construction of the ileostomy may lead to the need for reoperative surgery either acutely or later in the course of the ensuing postoperative course.

There are certain circumstances when a primary anastomosis after colonic resection is dangerous and when colectomy, rectal preservation and ileostomy are indicated. These circumstances include emergency colectomy for fulminating colitis, and colectomy in the presence of severe anorectal disease or abdominal sepsis. There are other patients, however, in whom temporary sphincter preservation is likely to be indicated because the patient cannot accept a permanent stoma. In some of these patients a stoma proximal to an anastomosis may be desirable. The advantage of this approach is the rapid improvement in general health achieved by resecting diseased bowel while preserving the possibility for restoration of intestinal continuity.

Perioperative Strategy

The main indications for surgical treatment have been chronic ill health, intractable diarrhea, acute or chronic colitis, or complications of low-grade

persistent sepsis. A number of patients have either continuous colonic Crohn's disease with relative rectal sparing, or multiple strictures in the large bowel with a normal rectum. The advantage of abdominal colectomy and a primary anastomosis is that the colitis or sepsis is eliminated without the need for a stoma or a perineal wound. Anorectal physiological assessment may aid patient selection. A good functional result is dependent upon the degree of rectal distensibility, compliance, and absence of proctitis. Nevertheless, successful long-term results are jeopardized by the risk of ileal and rectal recurrence as well as the development of perianal disease.

Other issues specific to Crohn's disease are present. These include abscesses, fistulas, fulminant disease, and strictures. Abscesses in the paracolic gutter, behind the psoas or in the pelvis may require preoperative percutaneous drainage because at surgery, gross contamination of the peritoneal cavity is inevitable. Fistulas to the skin or adjacent bowel must be either separated carefully or resected in continuity. When one is operating for fulminant disease, care must be taken in handling what may be a very fragile colon to avoid rupture. Also no attempt should be made to dissect an adherent to omentum off the transverse colon, unsealing a contained perforation. Whenever intraabdominal spillage has occurred, prolonged antibiotic therapy is warranted (at least 3–5 days).

Although sphincter preservation with restoration of intestinal continuity is the most desirable option, it carries the highest reoperation rate for recurrence (see section on Complications). Frequently the sigmoid colon is not obviously involved, or the disease affects segments of the right transverse and descending colon only. Under these circumstances there are functional advantages in preserving the sigmoid colon and performing an ileosigmoid anastomosis. In operations for fistula, abscess or toxic megacolon, intensive preoperative treatment with antibiotics, nutrition and even (rarely) fecal diversion alone may be warranted prior to resection. During colectomy, dividing the mesentery at a point of convenience nearer to the colon is advised, since excessive mesenteric excision is not required. Postoperative ileostomy complications are lessened by proper placement, proper construction, and immediate maturation.

Operative Technique

The day prior to surgery, preoperative marking with a face plate from an ileostomy appliance will allow for proper stoma marking. This should occur away from creases and scars as well as in perspective of the patients belt line. We have been impressed with the benefits of epidural anesthesia for postoperative pain control. In the operating room, we prefer to position the patient in Lloyd-Davies leg rests. Venadyne boots are applied. The rectum is washed out with 1000 cc of saline and 250 cc of a 50% betadine solution. A large Foley catheter is left in the rectum and allowed to drain into a plastic bag during the case. Laparoscopic approaches for the treatment of Crohn's colitis are currently being assessed. This topic is discussed in detail in Chapter 23. The abdomen is entered through a midline incision that may be extended as needed. This type of incision will not interfere with the ileostomy appliance. A meticulous examination of both the abdominal and the pelvic viscera is done. A Balfour retractor is placed. The surgeon chooses his option of either mobilizing the colon from the junction of the small intestine and cecum or from the peritoneal reflection at the distal sigmoid. We prefer all mobilization with electrocautery except at the level of the duodenum where scissor dissection is preferred. If the former is chosen, the surgeon, standing on the left side of the patient makes an incision in the peritoneal reflection just lateral to the cecum. He introduces his left index finger into this retroperitoneal plane and gently elevates the peritoneum close to the cecum and ascending colon. Furthermore, the small intestinal mesentery is incised and the distal six inches of ileum mobilized. The surgeon continues the mobilization of the right colon up to the hepatic flexure, keeping close to the colon. Care is maintained to preserve and protect the ureter and gonadal vessels. At the hepatic flexure, the gastrocolic ligament is encountered and usually ligation of vessels within is required. The omentum is preserved by retracting it cephalad and, using electrocautery, raising it as a flap from the transverse colon and mesocolon. The omentum is further raised distally from the transverse colon approaching the splenic flexure. The approach to mobilization of the splenic flexure is best accomplished by mobilization of the left colon.

The descending colon is retracted medially, and the lateral peritoneal gutter is incised over the white line. The left ureter and gonadal vessels are again visualized and protected. Care must be taken to avoid developing a plane posterior to Gerota's fascia. The descending colon and sigmoid colon are easily mobilized by dividing any previously fused parietes. As the splenic flexure is approached, the incision is carried about one centimeter away from the left side of the colon. The

posterior surface of the splenic flexure or descending colon is gently pulled downward and medially with its mesocolon until safe ligation of the blood supply of the colon can be accomplished. After the peritoneal attachments of the splenic flexure have been divided, the renocolic ligament is divided. The distal descending colon and sigmoid colon are further mobilized by incision along the white line. The vascular pedicles of the mesocolon are divided from the cecum distally by doubly clamping, dividing and ligation with O silk. This includes the ileocolic branches and right colic branches, the middle colic, two branches of the left colic and each sigmoidal branch. All vessels are ligated close to the intestine unless there is suspicion of carcinoma. The terminal ileum is transected as close to the ileocecal value as possible. The exception is when there is obvious Crohn's involvement of the terminal ileum. A surgical stapler is applied to the ileum. The distal line of rectal resection is usually located at the sacral promontory, which obviates the need for any presacral space dissection.

The technique of anastomosis may be either end to end or side to end; hand sutured or stapled. The blood supply of the intestinal ends is checked for adequacy by trimming the ends until arterial bleeding is seen. The ends of the ileum and rectum are usually of different caliber. One accommodates this discrepancy by making an antimesenteric (Cheadle) slit in the small intestine. We prefer the method popularized by Fazio. A 000 silk suture is placed through all layers in a vertical mattress fashion and tied, the mesenteric side being anastomosed first. The mattress suture is formed by returning the needle through the mucosa only. The posterior layer is then completed. Having completed the mesenteric half of the anastomosis, the surgeon begins the anterior half. This is done with 000 silk in a seromuscular fashion. The end-to-end anastomosis with the surgical stapler is an alternative to the hand-sewn technique. The stapler creates an inverting double-layered anastomosis. The largest diameter cartridge is recommended, but is often limited by the ability to introduce the instrument into the lumen.

The surgeon may wish to protect the anastomosis with a loop ileostomy. At the operation, a circumferential skin incision 3.5 cm in diameter is made around the previously placed stoma mark. A vertical incision is made in the subcutaneous fat, Scarpa's fascia, and anterior rectus sheath, splitting the rectus fibers. The posterior fascia and peritoneum are incised. A cotton tape is placed around a loop of ileum approximately 15 cm above the anastomosis and is used to bring the loop through the abdominal wall aperture. A plastic rod is then used to replace the tape. An enterotomy is made through four fifths of the circumference of the ileal loop on its downstream end 1 cm above skin level. Sutures of 000 vicryl are placed through the full thickness of the cut edge of the ileum and the subcuticular layer of skin. These sutures are tied down, and the proximal functional limb becomes dominant. The rod is removed 7 days after the operation, and the ileostomy is closed 2 to 3 months later.

Postoperative Care

The patient is transferred back to his or her room, unless either an untoward intraoperative event or prior comorbidity require intensive care unit monitoring. Nasogastric suction is used until return of active bowel sounds occur. Intravenous balanced salt solution is continuously administered until a regular diet is tolerated. Intravenous antibiotics are used prophylactically for 24 hours. Operative contamination requires a longer course depending upon the clinical postoperative course. Intravenous steroids are maintained until diet is resumed when oral steroids are begun. Serum hemoglobin is checked daily until stable, serum electrolytes and renal function followed until diet is resumed. If a stoma is present, stoma education is begun on the first or second postoperative day.

Diarrhea occurs almost invariably after ileorectal anastomosis. It begins around the fourth to seventh day, and when it does the clinician may be inclined to prescribe antidiarrheal medications. Early use of these medications could result in an ileus. It is preferable to allow the patient to have diarrhea for several days, withholding antidiarrheal drugs until about the tenth postoperative day.

Complications

The operative mortality of ileorectal anastomosis for Crohn's colitis usually reportedly ranges from 0% to 7%, but may be as high as 10% (1–8). Aside from those complications that may occur with any operations involving general anesthesia (stroke, myocardial infarction, or death), specific complications occur following total abdominal colectomy and are either major complications or minor morbidity. Major complications involve either loss of anastomotic integrity, intraabdominal abscesses unrelated to the anastomosis, intestinal obstruction and complications related to the stoma, when applicable.

Anastomotic dehiscence is the most important source of morbidity and has an incidence of 5% to 30% (1,4,6,9). A covering loop ileostomy will reduce the consequences of this complication and may even reduce the incidence of leakage. Anastomotic leak seems to be closely related to malnutrition, steroid medication, and particularly to preexisting abdominal sepsis. Under any of these three circumstances we would advise a protecting stoma. Anastomotic leaks are suspected clinically in the presence of fever, leukocytosis, abdominal pain and tenderness, and prolonged ileus. Radiographic studies using water soluble contrast media in the rectum or an examination under anesthesia with endoscopy are used to ascertain if a leak has occurred. Minor leaks without abscess or only a small one (<2 cm) are managed by bowel rest and intravenous antibiotics. Minor leaks with abscess are managed by drainage (either percutaneous, transrectal or transvaginal) along with systemic antibiotics. Occasionally, diversion and drainage will permit satisfactory healing of a minor anastomotic leak. In the case of a major leak, immediate laparotomy with dismantling of the anastomosis, pelvic drainage, and end ileostomy is warranted.

Between 59% and 65% of patients have a satisfactory result without needing further surgery over 10 years (1,5,6,10). The recurrence rate after ileorectal anastomosis is approximately twice that after proctocolectomy (9,10–18). Results from St Mark's Hospital indicated that the cumulative recurrence rate was 38% ± 8% at 5 years and 56% ± 9% at 10 years, which compared with a 10-year recurrence rate of 10% after proctocolectomy (6,15). The recurrence rate is partly related to concomitant ileal disease (6,10–12). Some recurrences are confined to the ileum, and can sometimes be managed by local ileal resection and a further ileorectal anastomosis (1,13–18). Not all recurrences require reoperation.

Ileorectal anastomosis when compared with colectomy and ileostomy or proctocolectomy remains the treatment of choice in the majority of patients with rectal sparing in Crohn's colitis, since it can restore health without the need for a permanent stoma or a perineal wound. In the experience of the Cleveland Clinic group, 131 patients underwent ileorectal anastomosis for Crohn's colitis. After a mean follow-up of 9.5 years, 61% retained a functioning anastomosis, with 61% being free of disease. The mean stool frequency was 4.7 per day. With the passage of time, approximately one third developed symptoms severe enough to require either proctectomy or diversion (1). Even those individuals who must undergo a second procedure can still be relatively well served by temporarily avoiding an ileostomy. Those who are troubled by frequent bowel movements can often be helped by the addition of a bulk agent containing psyllium, as well as "slowing" medications such as codeine, deodorized tincture of opium, and Lomotil or Imodium. If resection of the distal ileum is performed, cholestyramine (Questran) may be helpful in controlling diarrhea because of its binding to bile salts.

References

1. Longo WE, Oakley JR, Lavery IC, et al. Outcome of ileorectal anastomosis for Crohn's colitis. Dis Colon Rectum 1992;35:1066–71.

2. Ambrose NS, Keighley MRB, Alexander-Williams J, et al. Clinical impact of colectomy and ileorectal anastomosis in the management of Crohn's disease. Gut 1984;25:223–7.

3. Baker WNW. Ileorectal anastomosis for Crohn's disease of the colon. Gut 1971;12:427–31.

4. Buchman P, Weterman IT, Keighley MRB, et al. The prognosis of ileorectal anastomosis in Crohn's disease. Br J Surg 1981;68:7–10.

5. Burman JH, Cooke WT, Alexander-Williams J. The fate of ileorectal anastomosis in Crohn's disease. Gut 1971;12:432–6.

6. Cooper JC, Jones D, Williams NS. Outcome of colectomy and ileorectal anastomosis in Crohn's disease. Ann R Coll Surg Engl 1986;68:279–82.

7. Fazio V, Turnbull RB, Goldsmith MG. Ileorectal anastomosis: a safe surgical technique. Dis Colon Rectum 1975;18:107–14.

8. Flint G, Strauss R, Platt N, et al. Ileorectal anastomosis in patients with Crohn's disease of the colon. Gut 1977;18:236–9.

9. Goligher JC. The long term results of excisional surgery for primary and recurrence Crohn's disease of the large intestine. Dis Colon Rectum 1985;28:51–5.

10. Goligher JC. Surgical treatment of Crohn's disease affecting mainly or entirely the large bowel. World J Surg 1988;12:186–90.

11. Greenstein AJ, Sachar DB, Pasternack BS, et al. Reoperation and recurrence in Crohn's colitis and ileocolitis. Crude and cumulative recurrence rates. New Engl J Med 1975;293:685–90.

12. Hughes ESR, McDermott FT, Masterson JP. Ileorectal anastomosis for inflammatory bowel disease. 15 year followup. Dis Colon Rectum 1980;23:399–400.

13. Lefton HB, Farmer RG, Fazio V. Ileorectal anastomosis for Crohn's disease of the colon. Gastroenterology 1975;69:612–7.

14. Nugent FW, Veidenheimer MC, Meissner WA, et al. Prognosis after colonic resection for Crohn's disease of the colon. Gastroenterology 1973;65:398.

15. Baker WN. The results of ileorectal anastomosis at St. Mark's Hospital from 1953 to 1968. Gut 1970;11:235.

16. Watts J, Hughes ESR. Ulcerative colitis and Crohn's disease; results after colectomy and ileorectal anastomosis. Br J Surg 1977;64:77.

17. Williams JA, Buchman P. Criteria of assessment for suitability and results of ileorectal anastomosis. Clin Gastroenterol 1980;9:409.

18. Weterman IT, Pena AS. The long term prognosis of ileorectal anastomosis and proctocolectomy in Crohn's disease. Scand J Gastroenterol 1976;11:185–91.

19. Lavery IC, Michener WM, Jagelman DG. Ileorectal anastomosis for inflammatory bowel disease in children and adolescents. Surg Gynecol Obstet 1983;157:553–6.

20. Keighley MR, Buchman P, Lee JR. Assessment of anorectal function in selection of patients for ileorectal anastomosis in Crohn's Colitis. Gut 1982;23:102–7.

21. Veidenheimer MC, Dailey TH, Meissner WA. Ileorectal anastomosis for inflammatory bowel disease of the large bowel. Am J Surg 1970;119:375–8.

22 Abdominal-Perineal Resection

Roger Hurst

The indications for abdominal-perineal resection for Crohn's disease are (1) Crohn's proctitis unresponsive to medical management, (2) severe debilitating perianal Crohn's disease, (3) any other medical reason for which the patient is unsuitable for ileorectal anastomosis.

Crohn's proctitis that is unresponsive to either medical management or lesser surgical treatment such as fecal diversion is the most common indication for proctectomy in Crohn's disease. Uncontrollable symptoms such as diarrhea, bleeding, stricture, supralevator fistulas, abscess formation, incontinence, or tenesmus often necessitate an aggressive surgical approach (1).

Persistent perianal Crohn's disease in many instances can only be managed with proctectomy. In severe cases patients may suffer from continuous perianal sepsis and drainage that cannot be controlled with local surgical procedures such as incision and drainage, fistulotomy, seton application, or even fecal diversion. This is particularly true if the rectum itself is primarily involved with active Crohn's disease. Under these conditions patients are best treated by removal of the rectum (2). Perianal disease may also result in permanent anal incontinence requiring proctectomy.

Some patients with Crohn's colitis without involvement of the rectum will require a proctocolectomy with ileostomy instead of an ileorectal anastomosis. Candidates for proctocolectomy include elderly patients and patients with poor sphincter tone or previous ileal resection, as these patients are at high risk for failure of ileorectal anastomosis due to postoperative anal incontinence or debilitating diarrhea (3). Due to the risk of adenocarcinoma and the potential damage from progressive disease, the rectum should not be left in situ as a permanently defunctionalized pouch except under special circumstances (e.g., extremes of age, severe intraabdominal adhesions).

Preoperative Preparation

Prior to operation the surgeon should confer with the patient and family so that they understand the nature and magnitude of the operation, the necessity for surgery, the treatment options including alternative therapies, operative hazards, possible complications, and potential benefits. Most importantly, the patient should have a thorough understanding of the nature of an abdominal stoma and be aware of the possibility of impairment of sexual function. All appropriate candidates are given the opportunity for autologous blood donation. Additionally, male patients who may desire to father children in the future are given the option to cryopreserve a sample of their sperm prior to operation.

Selection of the optimal placement of the stoma should be determined preoperatively. Proper stoma location is a critical step in the performance of proctectomy as it will have a profound effect on the patient's postoperative adjustment (4). Consultation with an enterostomal therapist should be made to assist in the placement of the proposed stoma. Ideally the site should be located over the rectus muscle on a flat area away from deep skin folds and bony prominences. The surface of the abdomen should be evaluated in the supine, sitting, and standing positions as this will often demonstrate skin folds and creases not evident in the

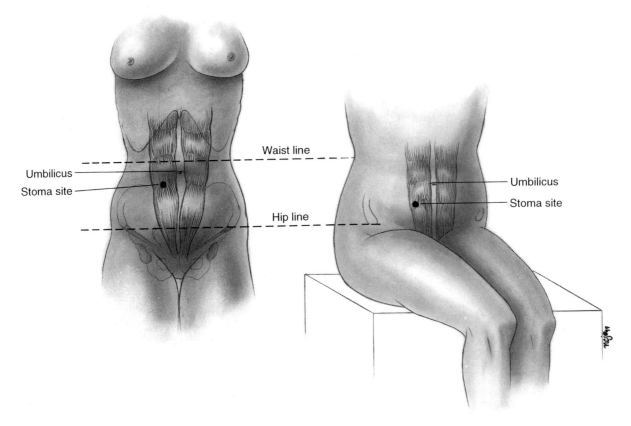

Fig. 22.1.   The stoma site is marked prior to surgery. The stoma should be located over the rectus abdominus muscle on a flat area away from skin folds and bony promi- nences. The drawing depicts the ideal location for an ileostomy. A descending colostomy would be located at the same level through the left rectus abdominus.

other positions (Fig. 22.1). Finally, the patient's belt line is determined and every effort is made to place the stoma below it. Once the optimal posi- tion of the stoma has been identified it is marked with an intradermal injection of methylene blue or india ink. This results in a "tattoo" that remains visible for approximately two weeks (methylene blue) or permanently (india ink).

Specific medical problems such as anemia, hy- perglycemia and electrolyte abnormalities should be discovered and remedied prior to operation.

The bowel is mechanically cleansed with a com- bination of a clear liquid diet beginning 48 hours prior to operation and oral polyethylene glycol so- lution the evening before surgery. Patients recently treated with corticosteroids should be given intra- venous stress dose hydrocortisone prior to induc- tion of anesthesia and continued through the post- operative course (5). Intravenous prophylactic antibiotics should be administered one hour prior to surgery so that maximal tissue antibiotic levels are achieved at the time of the skin incision (6).

Pitfalls and Danger Points

Although abdominal perineal resection for Crohn's disease entails potential pitfalls and danger points, most are, however, readily avoidable with proper technique. They include:

1. Injury to pelvic autonomic nerves with resul- tant sexual and urinary dysfunction.
2. Ureteral injuries.
3. Fecal contamination with resultant risk of in- traabdominal sepsis and wound infections.
4. Improper plane of dissection along the sacrum resulting in excessive blood loss.
5. Improper stoma placement and construction.

Operative Strategies

Unless the rectum is known to harbor an invasive adenocarcinoma, the dissection should remain close to the rectal wall. Wide surgical dissection, particularly in the lateral aspects of the mid-rectum, is unnecessary and can result in autonomic nerve injury with resultant sexual and bladder dysfunction.

If severe perianal disease with active infection is present, fecal diversion with drainage of perineal sepsis is advisable prior to proctectomy. This will usually allow for some degree of healing of the perineum and lessen the likelihood of perineal wound infection and chronic perineal sinus formation.

The extent of proximal resection is a controversial issue. After resection for distal proctocolitis, recurrence of Crohn's disease in the remaining colon is high (7). It is possible that overall recurrence rates for Crohn's disease may be lessened when total proctocolectomy with end-ileostomy is performed compared to a resection that only encompasses the active disease within the distal colon and rectum (8,9). Patients with no active Crohn's disease in the rectum or colon who require proctectomy for management of severe perianal disease or for management of incontinence do not require colectomy and are probably best managed with an end-sigmoid colostomy. Patients with proctocolitis extending proximally to the splenic flexure or beyond are best treated with total proctocolectomy with ileostomy. For patients with proctocolitis limited to the rectum and sigmoid the appropriate extent of proximal resection remains a difficult clinical decision. The risk of possible rapid recurrence following partial colectomy must be weighed against the physiologic consequences a total proctocolectomy (7). For these patients the decision to preserve the unaffected colon must be individualized, taking into account the patient's age, ability to tolerate additional surgeries, and the patient's history of previous small bowel resections. Young patients or patients with complicated medical conditions who have not had a previous ileal resection are probably best treated with total proctocolectomy with end-ileostomy, whereas elderly patients or patients who have had a previous extensive ileal resection may require preservation of whatever colon possible in hopes of avoiding the sequella of a high output stoma.

With Crohn's disease, inflammation and scarring may extend well beyond the wall of the rectum to involve perirectal tissues. Great care must be exercised to ensure that the dissection is carried out along the appropriate plans to avoid excessive bleeding and injury to pelvic autonomic nerves. Abscesses and fistulas may be encountered during mobilization of the rectum and they should be fully drained and inflamed tissue debrided.

Perineal dissection is best performed along the plane between the internal and external sphincters. Dissection along this intrasphincteric plane is less likely to result in bladder or sexual dysfunction and allows for easy and effective closure of the perineal floor. For patients with severe perirectal disease wide excision of the affected perineal skin and complete removal of the anal sphincter mechanism may be required. This wider dissection is performed rarely and not so much to cure disease as to excise tissue that has largely been destroyed by chronic inflammation and infection. In rare instances, the extent of perineal resection is so great that local tissue transfer flaps are required for adequate perineal closure (see Chapter 36). An alternative to wide excision is to lay open the fistula tracks and allow them to heal in by secondary intention while preserving the pelvic floor and external sphincters.

Operative Technique

Position

The abdominal portion of the procedure is performed with the patient supine. Once the abdominal and pelvic dissections are complete, the patient is placed in the modified lithotomy position for the perineal dissection. It is therefore advantageous to position the patient with the buttocks at the break of the table prior to induction of anesthesia. While in the lithotomy position the legs are supported with Allen stirrups (Allen Manufacturing Company, Cleveland, OH). With ample padding, the patient's heel should rest flat in the well of the stirrups with a majority of the extremity's weight being placed on the sole of the foot. The thighs are flexed 45° and abducted to expose the perineum. To avoid pressure on the peroneal nerve the legs should be internally rotated. The proper position is reached when the lower leg points in a direction overlying the contralateral shoulder (Fig. 22.2).

Incision

The abdominal portion of the procedure is best performed through either a vertical midline incision or an infraumbilical transverse incision. Both of these incisions provide adequate access to the recesses of the abdomen and pelvis. The transverse incision has the advantages of excellent protection against fascial dehiscence and superior cosmetic healing, whereas the vertical midline incision is less time consuming. If a transverse incision is selected, it should be made so as to avoid interference with the planed stoma site. If interference with the planned stoma site is not avoidable, a midline incision should be selected. A midline incision is neces-

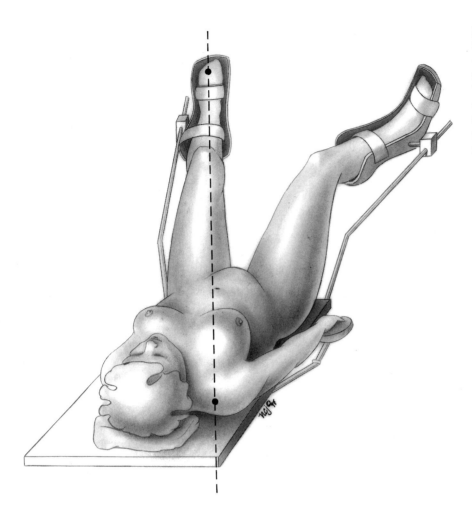

Fig. 22.2.   In the lithotomy position the thighs are abducted and flexed 45°. The tip of the coccyx should be accessible from the end of the table. To avoid lateral pressure on the peroneal nerve, the legs are internally rotated and the bower legs are aligned in a direction that points to the contralateral shoulder.

sary if the operative plan includes rectus abdominus muscle flaps to fill the pelvic dead space or to reinforce the posterior vaginal wall after repair of a rectovaginal fistula (10).

Exploration

Upon entering the abdomen it is important to fully examine the viscera to accurately assess the extent of Crohn's disease and synchronous pathology.

Mobilization of the Left Colon

Adhesions of the sigmoid colon to the left posterior lateral abdominal and pelvic walls are divided. The peritoneum is then incised along the lateral reflection (line of Toldt) (Fig. 22.3). This is best accomplished by lifting the peritoneum with a right angle clamp while the first assistant divides the peritoneum with the electrocautery using the coagulation current. When encountered, small vessels are grasped with forceps and cauterized using a coaptive technique prior to their division. A layer of connective tissue referred to as the "fusion fascia" lies just underneath the peritoneum. This thin layer of tissue should be divided parallel to the inci-

sion in the peritoneal reflection. With this, the proper surgical plane is entered and the mesentery of the colon can be fully mobilized while the left ureter and gonadal vessels remain in their normal retroperitoneal position. Incising the lateral peritoneum without dividing the fusion fascia results in a dissection that is too posterior, causing the ureter to remain attached to the posterior surface of the mesentery of the colon. Incision of the peritoneum and fusion fascia is carried superiorly towards the splenic flexure.

Division of the Mesentery

Before the sigmoid mesentery is divided, the left ureter is identified to ensure its safety. Normal colon proximal to the disease is divided between bowel clamps or with a gastrointestinal anastomotic (GIA) stapling device and the mesentery is divided. To keep a safe distance from the sympathetic neural plexus the division of the sigmoid mesentery is carried out close to the bowel, between the first and second vascular arcades. Larger vessels are doubly ligated while avascular portions of the mesocolon can be incised with electrocautery. Once the division of the sigmoid mesentery

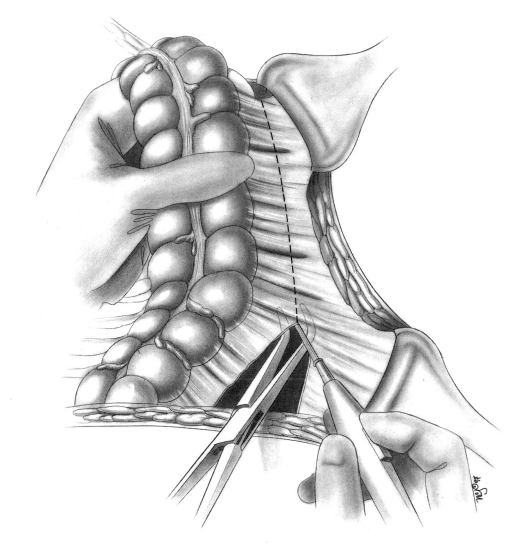

Fig. 22.3.   The left colon is mobilized by incising the lateral peritoneal reflection.

has reached a level below the sacral promontory the superior rectal vessels are ligated and divided. Since the sympathetic neural plexus lies directly behind the inferior mesenteric artery at the pelvic brim, the nerves are clearly identified at this point, dissected free of the vessels then the terminal branches of the inferior mesenteric artery and vein (superior rectal vessels) are divided with the undisturbed neural plexus in full view (Fig. 22.4).

Pelvic Dissection

The pelvic dissection of the rectum is greatly simplified if undertaken in an orderly and step wise fashion. The dissection begins with complete posterior mobilization of the rectum. Initial posterior mobilization allows for clear definition of the lateral rectal ligaments that are divided as the second step of the pelvic dissection. Division of the lateral ligaments in turn results in forward mobilization of

the rectum and unravels the deep recess of the rectovaginal or rectovesicle pouch. This unraveling provides better exposure for the final anterior dissection.

After division of the superior rectal vessels at the level of the sacral promontory the parietal peritoneum is incised from the point of ligation of the superior rectal vessels inferior and laterally for a distance just sufficient to gain full access to the presacral space. The left and right ureters should again be clearly identified as they course laterally across the true pelvis. The rectum is retracted anteriorly and the loose areolar tissue along the presacral space is divided under direct vision using electrocautery (Fig. 22.5). Care must be used to ensure that the dissection continues in the proper plane between the fascia propria of the rectum and the presacral fascia. The presacral venous plexus should remain covered by the presacral fascia, otherwise bleeding that is often difficult to control will

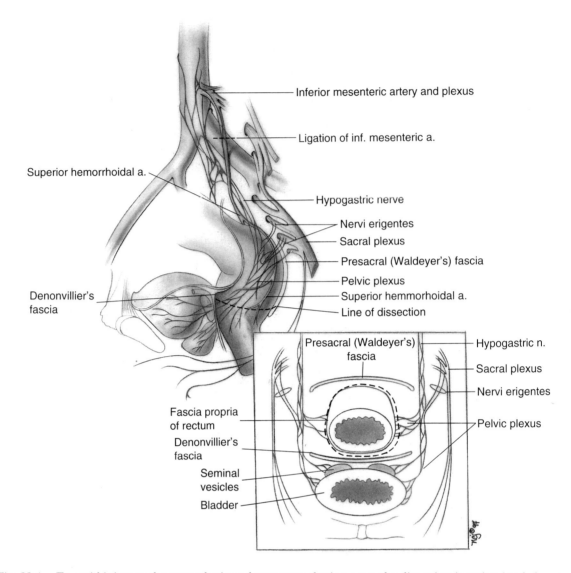

Fig. 22.4.   To avoid injury to the sympathetic and parasympathetic nerves, the dissection is maintained close to the rectum.

occur. If the uncovered veins of the presacral venous plexus are seen, then the approach is too deep and the dissection should be carried closer to the rectum. Even when in the proper plane, small communicating vessels between the rectum and the presacral plexus can occur and for this reason, mobilization of the rectum blindly with blunt hand dissection is to be avoided. Posterior mobilization should extend beyond the level of the coccyx with Waldeyer's fascia being incised with electrocautery. The resultant posterior mobilization of the rectum defines the posterior surface of the lateral ligaments (Fig. 22.6).

The previously identified preaortic sympathetic nerves divide into two major trunks in the upper sacral area and continue laterally to the right and left walls of the pelvis, passing through the tissue of the lateral rectal ligaments. The sympathetic nerves are gently dissected off the posterolateral aspect of the rectum and the lateral rectal ligaments are then divided as close as possible to the rectal wall. Division of the lateral ligaments close to the rectum also avoids injury to the more caudad sacral parasympathetic nerves. A majority of this pelvic dissection can be accomplished with electrocautery with larger vessels being ligated prior to division. To facilitate the division of the lateral rectal ligaments, anterior and superior traction is placed on the rectum with the aid of a sturdy right angle bowel clamp (Wertheim Cullen pedicle clamp). This upward retraction places tension on the lateral ligaments, further defining their attachment to the rectal wall (Fig. 22.7).

Following the posterior and lateral mobilization,

Fig. 22.5. After division of the superior rectal vessels, the rectum is retracted forward and anteriorly by dissecting along the presacral space under direct vision.

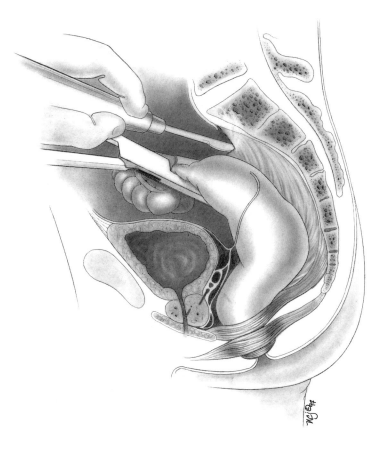

superior traction of the rectum will result in the unfolding of the recesses of the rectovaginal or rectovesicle pouch. This unfolding greatly facilitates the anterior dissection by providing better exposure and allowing for the efficient application of tension and countertension at the point of dissection. The anterior peritoneum and underlying fatty tissue is incised to expose the longitudinal muscle fibers of the anterior wall of the rectum. At this level (posterior to Denonvilliers' fascia) the anterior dissection is undertaken in an inferior direction. The anterior dissection is greatly facilitated by sturdy traction on the rectum directed towards the sacral promontory. In the male the anterior dissection is continued to the level of the inferior border of the prostate. Completion of the anterior dissection can be determined by palpating the Foley catheter as it passes through the membranous urethra. In the female patient the anterior dissection is continued until the thickening of the peritoneal body and anal sphincter mechanisms can be palpated. After the anterior dissection is complete additional lateral dissection may be necessary so that the rectum is circumferentialy mobilized to the level of the levator ani muscles.

If a rectovaginal fistula is encountered, it is divided and the vaginal defect is debrided and closed with interrupted absorbable suture. In these cases it may be advisable to reinforce the repair of the posterior vaginal wall with a rectus muscle flap based on the inferior epigastric vessels (see Chapter 36). With very large or multiple fistulas the resultant defect in the vaginal wall may be large. In order to close large defects in the vagina while insuring an adequate vaginal lumen a myocutaneous rectus abdominus flap can be used (11). With this reconstruction the rectus muscle is rotated to fill the pelvis and obliterate dead space and the overlying skin and subcutaineous tissue is used to reconstruct the posterior wall of the vagina.

With completion of the pelvic dissection the mobilized rectum is examined. If the wall is pliable and relatively free of disease then it can be closed with a TA stapling device. The rectum is divided above the staple line leaving behind a short rectal stump (Fig. 22.8). A soft closed suction drain is placed deep into the pelvis over the remaining rectal stump and is brought out through a separate stab incision in the lower abdominal wall far from the planned stoma position. Alternatively if the wall

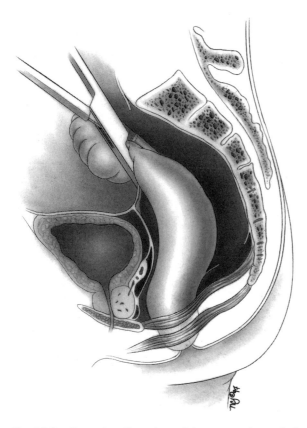

Fig. 22.6.   Posterior dissection of the rectum is carried through Waldeyer's fascia to lift the rectum from both the sacrum and the posterior aspect of the levator sling. With further mobilization, superior traction draws the rectovesical recesses cephalad to facilitate the anterior dissection.

of the distal rectum is thickened and diseased, as is often the case with active Crohn's proctitis, transection and safe closure of the rectal stump may not be feasible and removal of the specimen may have to wait for completion of the perineal phase of the procedure.

Creation of the Stoma

Over the marked ostomy site a circular incision is made two centimeters in diameter. The subcutaneous fat is divided transversely and the anterior rectus sheath is opened with a cruciate incision. The fibers of the rectus abdominus muscle are bluntly separated with the aid of hand-held retractors. The posterior rectus sheath is then incised. The cut end of the colon is delivered through the ostomy incision so that approximately four centimeters of colon extends above the surface of the skin. To prevent stomal prolapse the mesentery of the colon is sutured to the inner surface of the anterior abdominal wall. The abdominal cavity is then irrigated and the celiotomy incision is closed.

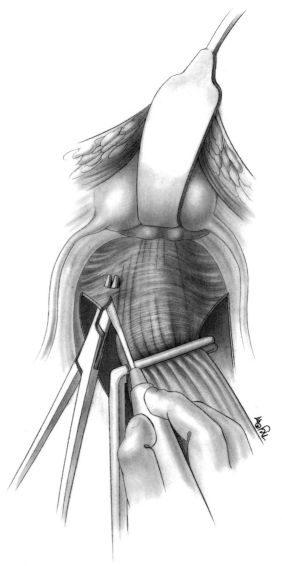

Fig. 22.7.   The lateral ligaments are divided close to the rectal wall so as to avoid injury to the autonomic nerves. A majority of this dissection can be accomplished with electrocautery.

The colostomy is matured using interrupted 3-0 chromic suture. Protrusion of the colostomy is not as critical as for an ileostomy, yet the management of the colostomy is enhanced by a slight degree of eversion. To accomplish this an everting seromuscular suture is first placed at the antimesenteric edge of the colon Everting sutures are also placed at ninety degrees to the antimesenteric stitch (Fig. 22.9). These three sutures are placed with a full thickness bite of the open end of the colon, a seromuscular bite of the ileum at the skin level, and a subcuticular bite of the skin. Once all three everting sutures have been placed, they are then tied. The resultant stoma should protrude ap-

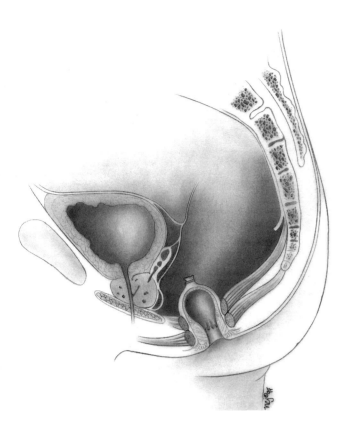

Fig. 22.8. With completion of the abdominal and pelvic dissections, a short rectal stump remains.

proximately one to two centimeters above the abdominal wall (Fig. 22.10). Simple sutures between the cut edge of the colon and the dermis are then placed circumferentially to allow complete approximation of the mucocutaneous junction.

Perineal Dissection

The patient is placed in a lithotomy position using Allen stirrups and the rectal stump is gently irrigated with a povidine-iodine solution. A povidine-iodine soaked gauze is then placed into the rectal stump and the anus is sutured closed with a pursestring suture placed at the level of the anal verge. The perineum is then shaved and sterilely prepped. In the female patient the vagina is also prepped.

Removal of the rectal stump is best carried out along the plane between the internal and external sphincters (Fig. 22.11). With a needlepoint electrocautery, a circular incision is made over the palpable groove between the internal and external sphincters. If the patient suffers from perineal scarring for perianal Crohn's disease, the incision should be adjusted to allow for the excision of damaged and diseased tissue near the anal canal. The intersphincteric plane is easiest to identify laterally, thus, the dissection should commence on the left and right sides and then proceed to connect posteriorly and anteriorly. The dissection is carried upward until the pelvic cavity is entered and the rectal stump is completely excised (Fig. 22.12). Through the perineal wound the closed

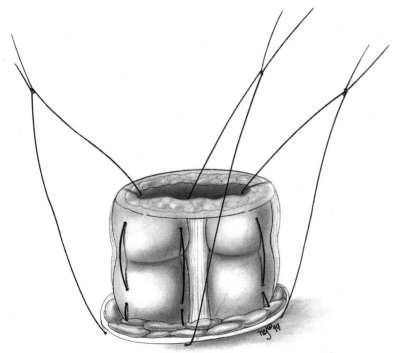

Fig. 22.9. Four centimeters of colon is delivered through the stoma incision and everting sutures are placed on the antimesenteric edge of the colon and at 90° on either side of this stitch.

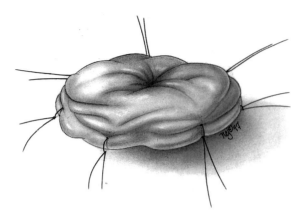

Fig. 22.10. The three everting sutures are tied and simple sutures are placed between the cut edge of the colon and the dermis.

suction drain can be identified and its proper position at the level of the levator-ani should be ensured. The perineal wound is closed by approximately the external sphincter mechanism in layers using absorbable suture. The skin edges are trimmed with a scalpel and the skin closed with several nylon interrupted vertical mattress sutures (Fig. 22.13). If a significant amount of perineal sepsis was present, the skin edges and the subcutaneous tissue are left open.

Postoperative Care

The nasogastric tube can almost always be removed in the operating room. In the absence of intra-

operative contamination perioperative antibiotics are discontinued within twenty-four hours. Sequential compression stockings are continued until the patient is fully ambulatory. The Foley catheter is removed on the fourth postoperative day. The diet is advanced once output from the colostomy has begun.

Complications

Perineal Wound Infection

Perineal wound infection often manifests with fever, perineal pain, erythema, and purulent drainage. This complication is best avoided by proper bowel preparation, prophylactic antibiotics, avoidance of fecal soilage, and avoidance of primary wound closure in the presence of extensive perineal sepsis. Intersphincteric perineal dissection as described above allows for effective closure of the perineal dead space and thus may also reduce the likelihood of this complication (12). When perineal wound infection occurs, the skin sutures are removed, purulent fluid is completely drained, necrotic tissue debrided and the wound packed. Perineal wound infection may result in a persistent perineal sinus.

Persistent Perineal Sinus

A persistent perineal sinus is defined as a perineal wound that fails to heal properly resulting in an open infected sinus that persists for six months or

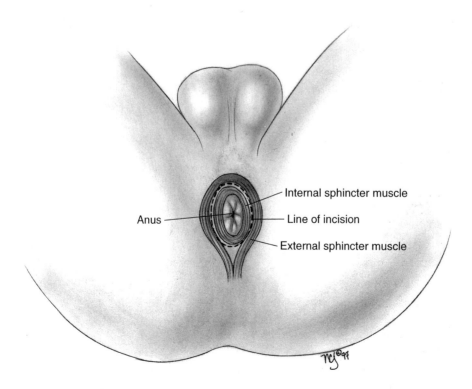

Fig. 22.11. Line of incision for the perineal dissection.

Fig. 22.12. The line of dissection is carried out between the internal and external anal sphincters.

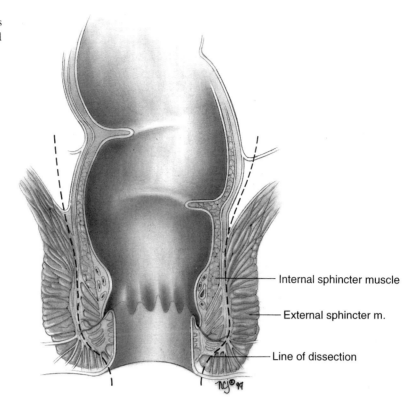

— Internal sphincter muscle

— External sphincter m.

— Line of dissection

longer. The incidence of persistent perineal sinus after proctectomy for Crohn's disease is reported to be as high as 40% (13). Although many of these wounds are minor cutaneous sinuses and are merely a nuisance to the patient, others are large, purulent cavities that interfere with the patient's health, rehabilitation and social acceptance. Avoidance of pelvic sepsis is the best prevention of this complication. Additionally, ligatures made of permanent material and metal clips are to be avoided during the pelvic dissection as foreign material can often be the nidus for persistent perineal sepsis. When a large, infected persistent perineal wound occurs, it is important to verify that no fistula, foreign body or unrecognized abscess is to blame. If these are present they are treated appropriately.

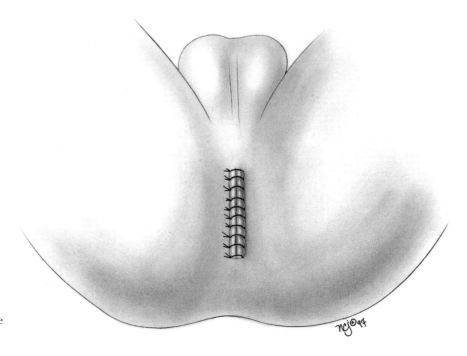

Fig. 22.13. Closure of the perineal wound.

Large perineal wounds typically develop a chronic, thick-walled fibrous cavity bearing infected granulation tissue. Under anesthesia the entire thick fibrous wall of the cavity must be excised. Simple curettage is inadequate treatment for this problem. During excision of the fibrous wall the surgeon must exercise care not to injure the bladder and urethra anteriorly, or the small bowel that may be in close proximity to the superior portion of the cavity. After excision of the cavity wall, spontaneous healing will occur within a few weeks in a majority of cases. However, in certain individuals with very large cavities, reexcision alone will not suffice and closure with myocutaneous flaps is required (13).

Urinary Retention

Postoperative urinary retention may result from the use of opiates, anticholinergic medication, pre-existing mechanical urinary obstruction, such as benign prostatic hypertrophy, or from intraoperative autonomic nerve injury. Overuse of opiates and the administration of anticholinergic medication should be avoided if the patient experiences difficulty voiding after urinary catheter removal. Patients with a history of symptoms consistent with urinary obstruction should be investigated prior to proctocolectomy.

Urinary retention due to autonomic nerve injury is best avoided by conducting the pelvic dissection as close to the rectum as possible. This is particularly true for the division of the lateral ligaments and the anterior rectal dissection. Urinary retention related to autonomic nerve injury is best managed with intermittent catheterization. In most instances this is required for only a limited time as bladder function tends to recover. Long term intermittent self catheterization is rarely necessary.

Sexual Dysfunction

Impotence is an uncommon complication following total proctocolectomy and occurs in approximately 1% to 2% of male patients (14). Retrograde ejaculation, however, is more common and occurs in up to 5% of males. Sexual dysfunction in the female is for the most part limited to dyspareunia and is seen in 30% of cases. Female fertility is maintained following total proctocolectomy and this procedure does not preclude full term pregnancy with normal vaginal delivery (15).

Stomal Complications

Complications related to the abdominal stoma are common and include stomal necrosis, peristomal hernia, prolapse, and stricture. Up to 25% of patients will require surgical revision of their stoma to deal with one or more of these complications (13,16).

Long-Term Results

The long-term results for any surgical treatment of Crohn's disease is mainly dependent upon the risk of recurrent disease. Attempts have been made to determine those patients at highest risk for recurrence, but this has been proven to be a difficult task (17). To date the most powerful independent predictor of postsurgical recurrence is the presence of multiple sites of disease (18). It also appears that Crohn's colitis can rapidly recur in the remaining colon whereas recurrence in the ileum after total proctocolectomy may be less likely to recur.

References

1. Tjandra JJ, Fazio VW. Surgery for Crohn's colitis. Int Surg 1992;77:9–14.
2. Block GE, Michelassi F. Crohn's disease. Curr Probl Surg 1993;30:173–265.
3. Ambrose NS, Keighley MR, Alexander-Williams J, et al. Clinical impact of colectomy and ileorectal anastomosis in the management of Crohn's disease. Gut 1984;25:223–7.
4. Tomaselli N, Jenks J, Morin KH. Body image in patients with stomas: a critical review of the literature. J Enterostom Ther 1991;18:95–9.
5. Salem M, Tainsh RE, Bromberg J, et al. Perioperative glucocorticoid coverage. A reassessment 42 years after emergence of a problem. Ann Surg 1994;219:416–25.
6. Kaiser AB. Antibiotic prophylaxis in surgery. N Engl J Med 1996;315:1129–38.
7. Mekhjian HS, Switz DM, Watts HD, et al. National cooperative Crohn's disease study: factors determining recurrence of Crohn's disease after surgery. Gastroenterology 1979;77:907–13.
8. Heimann TM, Greenstein AJ, Lewis B, et al. Prediction of early symptomatic recurrence after intestinal resection in Crohn's disease. Ann Surg 1993;218:294–8.
9. Ritchie JK, Lockhart-Mummery HE. Non-restorative surgery in the treatment of Crohn's disease of the colon. Gut 1973;14:263–9.
10. Kluger Y, Townsend RN, Paul DB, et al. Rectus muscle flap for the reconstruction of disrupted pelvic floor. J Am Coll Surg 1994;179:344–6.
11. Erdmann MW, Waterhouse N. The transpelvic rectus abdominis flap: its use in the reconstruction of extensive perineal defects. Ann Royal Coll Surg 1995;77:229–32.

12. Berry AR, Campos RDE, Lee ECG. Perineal and pelvic morbidity following perimuscular excision of the rectum for inflammatory bowel disease. Br J Surg 1986;73:675.

13. Block GE, Hurst RD. Complications of the surgical treatment of ulcerative colitis and Crohn's disease. In: Kirshner JB, Shorter RG, eds. Inflammatory Bowel Disease. 4th ed. Baltimore: Williams & Wilkins, 1995:898–922.

14. Bauer JJ, Gelernt IM, Salky B, et al. Sexual dysfunction following proctocolectomy for benign disease of the colon and rectum. Ann Surg 1983;197:363–7.

15. Metcalf AM, Dozois RR, Kelly KA. Sexual function in women after proctocolectomy. Ann Surg 1986;204:624–7.

16. Post S, Herfarth C, Schumacher H, et al. Experience with ileostomy and colostomy in Crohn's disease. Br J Surg 1995;82:1629–33.

17. Bayless TM, Harris ML. Prognostic considerations in idiopathic inflammatory bowel disease. In: Kirshner JB, Shorter RG, eds. Inflammatory Bowel Disease. 4th ed. Baltimore: Williams & Wilkins, 1995:961–84.

18. Michelassi F, Balestracci T, Chappel R, et al. Primary and recurrent Crohn's disease. Experience with 1379 patients. Ann Surg 1991;214:230–8.

23 Laparoscopy in Inflammatory Bowel Disease

Seon-Hahn Kim and Jeffrey W. Milsom

Over the past several years, laparoscopic techniques have been applied to the surgical management of almost all abdominal disorders, including both benign and malignant intestinal diseases. Although laparoscopic cholecystectomy has clearly gained acceptance as a major advance in abdominal surgery, having readily apparent benefits over conventional surgery (1), the role of laparoscopic techniques in managing intestinal disorders remains unclear.

The use of laparoscopic techniques to diagnose and treat intestinal diseases has developed slowly because of inadequate technology, a steep learning curve for interested surgeons, and because of the major differences between laparoscopic bowel resection and removal of end organs such as the gall bladder (Table 23.1). Nonetheless, the theoretical advantages of this minimally invasive technology—less postoperative pain, short hospitalization time, early return to work, less adhesion formation, and superior cosmesis—are compelling reasons to consider application of laparoscopic techniques to the management of intestinal diseases, especially for the commonly afflicted young patients with a chronic, stressful disease who are likely to undergo multiple operations over time. The potential advantages of minimal invasive surgery are summarized in Table 23.2.

Since the inflammation of the bowel and its mesentery in inflammatory bowel disease may lead to increased bleeding and friability of the tissues being manipulated, the technical feasibility of a laparoscopic approach was the first and most basic issue to be addressed in this field. A chronic inflammatory process may also obliterate avascular surgical planes, making proper dissection difficult, increasing the risk of inadvertent injury to retroperitoneal structures, such as gonadal and iliac vessels or ureters. In fact, despite several series reporting a large number of laparoscopic intestinal resections for a variety of indications, relatively few cases of Crohn's or ulcerative colitis have been reported in these series (2–6). Nonetheless, in recent years, a possible role for laparoscopic techniques in the management of inflammatory bowel disease has begun to emerge (7–11). In our experience at the Cleveland Clinic, we have performed 49 of 303 laparoscopic colorectal operations up until November of 1996 for Crohn's disease, nearly all for ileocolitis. Thirty-five of the patients are entered on a prospective randomized protocol comparing laparoscopic to conventional ileocolic resections (Cleveland Clinic Foundation Research Procedures Committee Protocol #4189).

In this chapter, the current indications and techniques for laparoscopy in inflammatory bowel diseases will be described, and its role in the future management of these patients will be discussed.

Laparoscopy in Crohn's Disease

Despite the obvious technical challenges of performing laparoscopic intestinal surgery, the proposed advantages of laparoscopic surgery make it particularly attractive for patients with Crohn's disease (10).

Patients with complete or near-complete obstruction, intraabdominal abscess, perforation or signs of peritonitis, and the presence of extensive intestinal fistulas are not considered for laparoscopic surgery. Exceptions to this might be the ileal-to-ileal or ileal-to-right colon fistula that would

Table 23.1. Major differences between laparoscopic bowel resection and cholecystectomy.

	Laparoscopic bowel resection	Laparoscopic cholecystectomy
Target organ	Mobile	Fixed
Need for repositioning of instruments	Frequent	Rare
Dissection	In multiple quadrants	In a single quadrant
Blood supply	Complex and variable	Single and constant (relatively)
Anastomosis	Necessary	Not necessary
Content in organ	Feces	Bile
Major indication(s)	Inflammation and cancer	Cholelithiasis

be removed in continuity with an ileal resection. To date, there has been no reported experience with laparoscopic intestinal surgery to manage acute toxic manifestations of inflammatory bowel disease (fever, abdominal distension, or other signs of toxicity). We do not recommend laparoscopic intestinal surgery in acutely ill patients mainly because the intestinal tissues are likely to be fragile and prone to injury using current laparoscopic instruments.

Laparoscopy has proven useful in several clinical circumstances in Crohn's disease (8–10). Laparoscopy as a diagnostic tool alone should be considered in instances where the diagnosis may be uncertain despite an extensive preoperative evaluation (endoscopy, contrast small bowel series, and computerized tomography). In unusual instances, a biopsy can be performed laparoscopically to differentiate between an unusual appearance of Crohn's disease and other pathological processes, such as intestinal lymphoma or intestinal tuberculosis. Diagnostic laparoscopy will not likely become a common indication in Crohn's disease, but has probably been underutilized in the past.

In instances of uncontrolled perineal sepsis or complex perianal fistula related to Crohn's disease, we have found laparoscopic fecal diversion, coupled with adequate drainage of any anal infection, to be a valuable and simple procedure (10) (Fig. 23.1; see color plate). We have now performed

Table 23.2. Potential advantages of minimal invasive surgery.

Less pain
Blood loss
Length of stay
Postoperative ileus
Morbidity
Detriment on immune system?
Stress
Wound infection?
Intestinal adhesions?

approximately thirty ileostomies or colostomies for Crohn's disease. This allows for fecal diversion (usually ileostomy) without a major laparotomy, with a diagnostic laparoscopy at the same time (Figs. 23.2 and 23.3; see color plates). The simplicity of this procedure, usually requiring only two small puncture incisions, allows for a rapid recovery of the patients along with resolution of the acute septic process. This procedure has been safe, with no complications noted, and all stomas have functioned well. We believe that laparoscopic stoma creation is an extremely valuable technique that can provide all expected benefits of a minimal invasive procedure, and it has been now our preferred approach in patients requiring fecal diversion (12).

Elective laparoscopic-assisted ileocolic resections for Crohn's ileocolitis or terminal ileitis are also feasible at the present time (Fig. 23.4; see color plate). We use the term "assisted" because we perform all of the mobilization and division of the major vascular pedicle inside the abdomen, then bring the diseased segment out through a 3 to 6 cm incision in the midline or right lower quadrant cannula and perform the remainder of the mesenteric ligation and the bowel resection plus anastomosis at that site using conventional techniques. Since the laparoscopic procedure should not compromise any fundamental surgical principles in managing Crohn's disease, the initial step is a thorough abdominal exploration. The small bowel must be examined over its entire length to detect any foci of inflammation and to document the approximate length of the disease-free bowel. A general inspection of all intraabdominal organs must be undertaken, and the feasibility of performing a safe and effective laparoscopic resection must be determined. The surgeon must anticipate that unexpected abscesses, fistulae, or dense adhesions may require conversion to an open procedure. Adhesiolysis can be safely performed during a laparoscopic procedure, but multiple small bowel loops that are matted together, or extensive adhesions throughout multiple quadrants are clear signs that

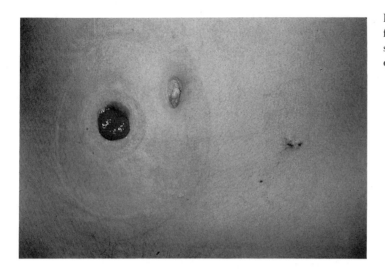

Fig. 23.1. A diverting loop ileostomy may be performed laparoscopically using only two puncture sites, one for the stoma and one in the left lower quadrant. (See color plate.)

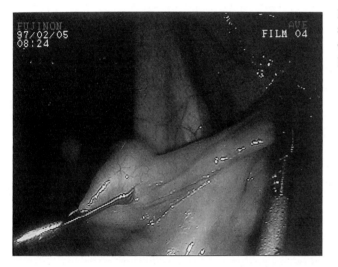

Fig. 23.2. The entire length of the small bowel may be examined laparoscopically by carefully grasping it in a "hand over hand" fashion using laparoscopic graspers. (See color plate.)

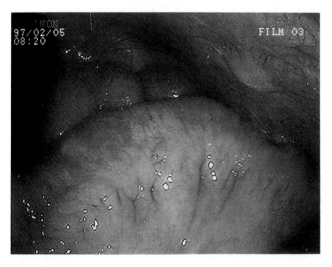

Fig. 23.3. An isolated segment of jejunal Crohn's disease is detected laparoscopically. (See color plate.)

Fig. 23.4. An ileal stricture with proximal dilation is seen laparoscopically. (See color plate.)

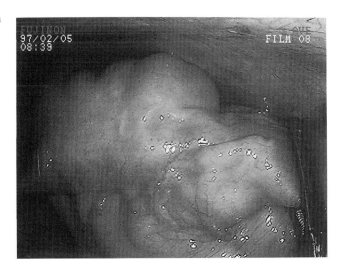

a conversion is necessary. The decrease in tactile sensation during laparoscopy (since some palpation is possible with laparoscopic instrument tips) is a concern about the use of the laparoscopic approach in inflammatory bowel disease. With the combination of careful preoperative evaluation (all patients should have a preoperative small bowel series) and thorough intraoperative exploration, we believe the chances of missing skip lesions that require surgical treatment are minimal. The palpation that is possible with laparoscopic instruments becomes more refined with experience, and suspicious areas can be tagged with a stitch and later exteriorized when the specimen is removed. Resection or stricturoplasty can be performed through this incision (we have done this in several instances). It is not yet clearly defined whether this assessment is valid, but we are studying the question in a prospective randomized comparative trial of laparoscopic versus conventional surgery in our institution.

If a laparoscopic procedure is considered feasible based on the initial exploration, resection proceeds. The division of ileocolic vascular pedicle can be performed intracorporeally as the first step of ileocolic resection in most cases. If the mesentery is remarkably thickened or inflamed, the pedicle is left alone and divided after exteriorization. The disadvantage of this is a definite loss of bowel mobility, leading to a probable need for a longer incision to extract the specimen. The pertinent bowel segment is then mobilized from the surrounding tissues. One port site (usually umbilical port) is enlarged adequately (4 to 6 cm) to deliver the thick, inflamed specimen. Ileal and colonic mesenteric divisions and anastomosis of both transected intestinal ends are performed extracorporeally

using standard techniques (typically a stapled functional end-to-end anastomosis). Most of the time, colonic mesenteric division and transection of the colon can be performed intracorporeally, then the specimen can be brought out. This will facilitate specimen removal. The preliminary results of our prospective randomized trial are encouraging (10).

Isolated stenosis of the small intestine might be an indication for a laparoscopic-assisted stricturoplasty. The affected segment can be mobilized using a laparoscopic technique, and a conventional stricturoplasty can then be performed through a small abdominal wall incision. In a recent experience, a suspicious area was identified and tagged during intraoperative exploration, which was not seen in preoperative radiographic investigation. Closer observation after exteriorization of the tagged segment through the extraction incision demonstrated the stenosis, and a stricturoplasty was performed.

Laparoscopic techniques may offer benefits to patients who undergo a restoration of intestinal continuity after Hartmann's procedure or end ileostomy. Recently, in three patients of Crohn's colitis (one with Hartmann's procedure, two with total abdominal colectomy and end ileostomy), their stomas were closed successfully using laparoscopic techniques. In brief, the stoma was freed from the abdominal wall, then an anvil of a circular stapler was inserted into the bowel end. After gas insufflation through this incision, proximal bowel and rectal stump were mobilized, then ileo- or colorectal anastomosis was performed laparoscopically via a transanal stapled approach. Our experience with over 12 patients shows laparoscopic reversal of Hartmann's procedure may be a good surgical alternative to conventional colostomy closure, be-

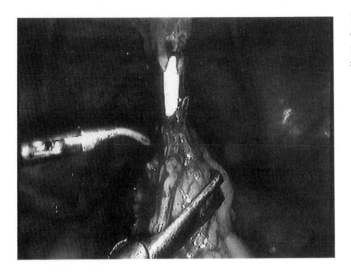

Fig. 23.5. Crohn's disease patients requiring prior percutaneous drainage of a mesenteric abscess may still be approached laparoscopically, carefully dissecting down adhesions with laparoscopic instruments. (See color plate.)

cause of a short recovery time (median time to discharge, 5 days), a high success rate (conversion to open in one patient) and its safety (no intraoperative complications) (13).

Although total abdominal colectomy with completely intracorporeal ileorectal anastomosis or end ileostomy has been performed laparoscopically in several patients, this extensive procedure is still under investigation at our institution and elsewhere in the management of colonic Crohn's disease. Segmental colectomy could also reasonably be performed in rare instances, but we have no experience with this operation yet by laparoscopy. In addition, feeding jejunostomy placed by laparoscopic techniques may be helpful for some malnourished patients with obstructive duodenal Crohn's disease. Bypass surgery (gastrojejunostomy) may be also applicable using laparoscopy in these patients.

Results of Laparoscopic Surgery in Crohn's Disease

Our preliminary report on an experience with 31 patients with Crohn's disease who underwent laparoscopic intestinal surgery over a 2-year period demonstrated that laparoscopic intestinal surgery, both for resection and diversion, is feasible and safe for the management of selected patients (10). All data were collected perspectively. There were 18 women and 13 men, with a median age of 39 years (range 22 to 79). Indications for operation included 13 patients with primary terminal ileitis, 2 with recurrent ileitis, 3 with Crohn's colitis, 6 with rectovaginal fistula, and 7 with severe perianal disease. Twenty-five of 31 procedures (81%) were completed laparoscopically: loop ileostomy (ten),

loop colostomy (two); ileocecectomy (ten); segmental colon resection (two); and total abdominal colectomy with ileorectal anastomosis (one). Six cases were converted to conventional surgery secondary to extensive adhesions from prior surgery (two) or severe inflammation (four). No cases were converted because of intraoperative complications (Fig. 23.5; see color plate). Median operative time for diversion procedure was 53 minutes (range, 20–90) and for resections 195 minutes (range, 90–380). Median blood loss was 100 mL (range, 10–500), and there were no intraoperative complications. Only one postoperative complication occurred (myocardial infarction), although this occurred 5 days after the surgical procedure. Median times to passage of flatus and bowel movement were both 3 days (range, 1–6). Median time to discharge was 6 days (range, 2–21) for diversion patients, and 6 days (range, 3–7) for resected patients. Previous intraabdominal surgery should not be considered a contraindication to laparoscopic surgery, as 10 of our patients had undergone previous abdominal operation and 8 underwent a successful laparoscopic procedure. Only two of six conversions were a result of dense adhesions from previous operation. Operation times seem to be falling as experience is gained. The average operative time for our first eight resections was 4.1 hours, for the second eight patients 2.8 hours, and for the last five completed resections 2.2 hours. We believe that with better instrumentation, especially better laparoscopes and intestinal retractors, operative times will continue to decrease.

Thibault and Poulin (11) reported three cases of total laparoscopic proctocolectomy with end ileostomy for intractable Crohn's proctocolitis. Average operating time was over 7 hours, and blood loss

Table 23.3. Laparoscopic procedures used in the management of Crohn's disease.

Three main procedures
   Diagnostic with/without biopsy
   Creation of stoma: ileostomy, colostomy
   Ileocolectomy or isolated small bowel resection
Other applicable procedures
   Total abdominal colectomy
   Left colectomy
   Hartmann's procedure
   Reversal of Hartmann's procedure
   Proctectomy
   Adhesiolysis
   Stricturoplasty
   Feeding jejunostomy
   Intestinal bypass surgery
   Total proctocolectomy?

Table 23.4. Potential indications for laparoscopic surgery in Crohn's disease.

Diagnostic when preoperative tests are indeterminate
Severe perineal sepsis
Complex perineal fistulas
Terminal ileitis
Segmental colitis
Pancolitis with rectal sparing?
Duodenal Crohn's disease with obstruction

Table 23.5. Contraindications to laparoscopic surgery in Crohn's disease.

Peritonitis/perforation
Acute osbruction
Dense adhesions
Intraabdominal abscess
All but the most simple of intestinal fistulas
Multiple previous operations?

was 500 to 800 mL. One patient had urinary retention postoperatively. Average postoperative stay in hospital was 10 days. They found the procedure offered few, if any, advantages. We have no experience in this procedure for Crohn's disease. It needs to be evaluated further.

Laparoscopic procedures currently used or possibly applicable in the future in the management of Crohn's disease are summarized in Table 23.3. Indications and contraindications to laparoscopic procedures in Crohn's disease are also summarized in Table 23.4 and Table 23.5.

Laparoscopy in Mucosal Ulcerative Colitis

Since laparoscopic techniques have not been used extensively in the management of ulcerative colitis, there is as yet no defined role for laparoscopy in this disease (Table 23.6). Reissman et al. (9) described laparoscopic total proctocolectomy with ileal-pouch/anal anastomosis in 22 patients with mucosal ulcerative colitis. They found the procedure was associated with a much greater operative time and a higher morbidity including three cases of postoperative pelvic abscess in patients who received high doses of preoperative steroids. We have some concern that their technique really is not comparable to other laparoscopic procedures, since careful scrutiny of their technique reveals that the laparoscopic portion is really only mobilization of the left and right colic gutters and the flexures, thereafter performing all of the resection (including proctectomy) and ileal pouch formation through a generous Pfannenstiel-type incision (14). Peters (7) reported successful results with laparoscopic total proctocolectomy and end ileostomy in two patients with severe ulcerative colitis. One patient was discharged on the third postoperative day. We have not yet performed any laparoscopic colectomies for ulcerative colitis. In theory, laparoscopic techniques should not be specifically contraindicated in the management of ulcerative colitis, except in critically ill patients with fulminant colitis, toxic megacolon, or massive hemorrhage. If malignancy has developed or is a consideration, laparoscopic techniques based on oncologic principles in accordance with intraoperative laparoscopic ultrasonography (15), will be needed. However, in our opinion, the laparoscopic approach to total abdominal colectomy or total proctocolectomy must still be evaluated further before recommending this for ulcerative colitis.

We have demonstrated laparoscopic total abdominal colectomy with ileorectal anastomosis to be a feasible and acceptable operation in selected patients with familial adenomatous polyposis (16). In 16 patients with familial adenomatous polyposis, the entire procedure was performed intracor-

Table 23.6. Laparoscopic procedures that may theoretically be used for the management of mucosal ulcerative colitis.

Total proctocolectomy with ileal reservoir
Total proctocolectomy with ileostomy
Urgent subtotal colectomy with ileostomy (most immediately
   possible)

poreally with a 3 to 6 cm specimen extraction incision. Median operative time was 232 minutes (range, 156 to 285) and blood loss 175 mL (range, 50 to 675). The only intraoperative complication, a twisted ileorectal anastomosis, was noted intraoperatively and revised immediately. There were no conversions to open procedure. Median time to passage of flatus and bowel movement were both 3 days (range, 1 to 4). Median time to discharge was 5 days (range, 3 to 11). Thus total abdominal colectomy may be a reasonable consideration in ulcerative colitis patients in the future.

Recently, we have developed a new laparoscopic retractor in concert with a major instrument manufacturer in the United States (Endo Paddle Retract, United States Surgical Corporation, Norwalk, CT) that permits effective and safe retraction of the small or large intestines. It helps almost all laparoscopic procedures to be performed more easily and safely, and is especially helpful in taking down the hepatic and splenic flexures, and in dissecting the mesorectum (17). New technologies, improved surgical techniques, and a skilled teamwork may soon make a laparoscopic subtotal colectomy with ileostomy a feasible and safe procedure even under urgent circumstances.

Other Inflammatory Conditions

Elective resection of diverticular disease may be one of the more reasonable indications for laparoscopic resection because it is usually a localized and benign inflammatory process. We have performed over 40 cases of sigmoid colectomy laparoscopically for sigmoid diverticulitis, and we believe it is a safe procedure that significantly shortens recovery. A detailed description is outside the scope of this book, except that a similar concept applies to localized Crohn's disease.

Anecdotally, we have also used laparoscopic techniques to divert three patients with sepsis related to overwhelming infectious (pseudomembranous) colitides, with good result. Again, the "minimally-invasive" approach may offer some advantages in critically ill patients who are poor candidates for a major laparotomy.

Surgical Techniques

We describe herein in detail only stoma creation and ileocolectomy because of their more common indications for laparoscopic management of inflammatory bowel disease. The laparoscopic total abdominal colectomy procedure will also be described briefly, and should be considered as a technique still very much in evolution.

Stoma Procedures

Orally ingested polyethylene glycol 4L (Golytely, Braintree, Massachusetts, USA) was formerly used for a standard preoperative bowel preparation, but now sodium phosphate 120 mL (Fleet's Phospho-Soda, Lynchburg, Virginia, USA) is used the night before surgery because it produces less fluids in the bowel loops. Intravenous prophylactic antibiotics are administered at induction. The patient is placed on a molded bean bag support (providing lateral support during left and right tilting) on the operating table in the supine position. Padded shoulder braces are put in place to prevent the patient from sliding on the operating table during periods of deep Trendelenburg positioning. At the premarked stoma site (for ileostomy, this is usually in the right lower quadrant over the rectus sheath), a 2- to 3-cm disk of skin is excised, and subcutaneous fat and anterior rectus sheath are incised vertically. The rectus muscle is spread open in the direction of its fibers, and then the posterior rectus sheath is exposed and incised 1.5 to 2 cm. A heavy purse-string suture is placed around the opening in the posterior sheath, a 10-mm cannula is inserted into the peritoneal cavity without the trocar, and the purse-string suture is tightened and secured with a Rumel tourniquet. Carbon dioxide insufflator tubing is attached to the cannula and pneumoperitoneum is established, then the laparoscope is inserted.

First, the abdominal and pelvic cavities are thoroughly inspected to ensure that stoma procedure can be performed laparoscopically. Next the patient is tilted stoma side down, then the second 10-mm cannula is inserted lateral to the rectus sheath in the lower quadrant contralateral to the stoma site under laparoscopic vision. If the small bowel must be completely inspected (the detailed method on how to run the small bowel will be described in the next section on ileocolectomy) or if two handed manipulation is necessary (e.g., for adhesiolysis), then a third 5-mm cannula should be inserted. The surgeon should judge the best location for this cannula so he/she can work easily with both hands, but usually this third cannula is inserted in the suprapubic area. Once the diagnostic laparoscopy has been completed, the scope is placed in the cannula opposite the stoma site and a laparoscopic Babcock-type clamp is inserted through the stoma site cannula.

For loop ileostomy, the patient is next tilted left side down, and the surgeon operates from the siding opposite the stoma site, using the Babcock clamp to identify the appropriate loop of bowel

Fig. 23.6. In performing a laparoscopic ileostomy procedure, the ileum is grasped with a Babcock clamp through the cannula at the ileostomy site. Special care is needed to avoid twisting the bowel.

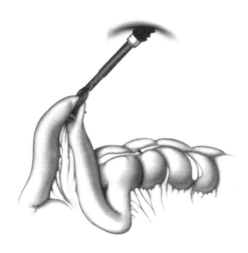

and lift it up to the stoma site (Fig. 23.6). The terminal ileum may not be immediately apparent, but by grasping and elevating the cecum it comes into view and can be traced back proximally from the cecum until an appropriate ileal loop is chosen to easily reach up to the anterior abdominal wall, usually 15 to 20 cm proximal to the ileocecal valve.

The bowel is then brought up to the abdominal wall. Special care is taken to avoid twisting the bowel. Orienting the bowel properly to the abdominal wall may require placing the afferent limb in either an inferior or superior position (most commonly it is placed superiorly). A small bore spinal needle can be passed through the abdominal wall medial to the stoma to tattoo the afferent and efferent limbs with methylene blue for easy identification (one dot proximal and two dots distal). Releasing pneumoperitoneum somewhat may be necessary to fully evaluate the amount of tension needed to bring the loop comfortably up to the skin. Once the bowel is oriented, the endoscopic Babcock clamp should be held on its shaft, not its handles, in a fixed position to prevent rotation. Pneumoperitoneum is fully released, and the Babcock clamp is left with its tip positioned just below the fascia. The cannula at the stoma site is pulled out of the abdominal wall (this will require cutting the purse-string suture), then the posterior sheath incision is enlarged to approximately two finger widths using finger dilation or blunt-tipped scissors so the intestinal loop can be easily delivered out. As soon as the ileal loop is seen, two conventional Babcock clamps are placed on the bowel to hold it in place. The intestinal loop is delivered to skin level while maintaining proper orientation.

With the bowel loop occluding the stoma site, pneumoperitoneum is reestablished through the remaining cannula, and the laparoscope is reinserted. The loop is confirmed for proper orientation, as is the mesentery for proper tension. The surgeon may insert a small finger alongside the loop to check the orientation, if needed. A plastic stoma rod is passed beneath the loop, then the ostomy is matured using standard techniques. Because a symptomatic hernia through a 10-mm incision can be possible, closure of the cannula site opposite the stoma requires special mention. We place a stitch at the beginning of the operation using a laparoscopic fascial closure device, leaving the stitch loose, to be tied at the end of the procedure. More recently, we have used a 5 mm diameter laparoscope, throughout the case, then used a 5 mm cannula at the secondary abdominal port site. This site does not then require a fascial stitch.

For sigmoid colostomy, the same techniques are used, with mirror image instrument positioning compared to the ileostomy formation and the patient being tilted right side down. An additional 5-mm suprapubic cannula should be placed to insert endoscopic scissors when the lateral retroperitoneal attachments along the white line of Toldt need to be incised to further mobilize the sigmoid colon. If the sigmoid colon needs to be divided for end colostomy, division is most easily and rapidly done by bringing the loop through the stoma, placing bowel clamps, and dividing it between the clamps with a conventional linear cutting stapler. The distal limb is then oversewn and dropped back into the peritoneal cavity. The proximal limb is matured to the skin in a routine manner.

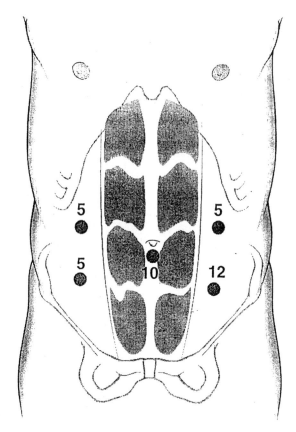

Fig. 23.7. Positions of cannulas for a laparoscopic ileocolic resection. Numbers refer to the size of each cannula in millimeters.

Ileocolectomy

The patient is placed in a modified lithotomy position using padded stirrups (Dan Allen Medical, Bedford Heights, Ohio, USA) in a steep Trendelenburg position. Carbon dioxide pneumoperitoneum is established through a Veress needle at an infraumbilical site. A 10-mm cannula is inserted at the same site for an endoscopic camera. One 10-mm (recently, 12-mm for using an endoscopic retractor) and three 5-mm cannulas are placed as shown in Fig. 23.7. The surgeon stands on the patient's left side.

The operation begins with a thorough inspection of the peritoneal cavity to confirm the preoperative diagnosis and feasibility of the procedure. The patient is tilted right side down, then the small bowel should be completely run from the terminal ileum to the ligament of Treitz using a laparoscopic "hand-over-hand," or sometimes "hand-to-hand" technique (Fig. 23.8; see color plate). It is important to keep the patient's position in the steep Trendelenburg position with right side down to move the small intestine toward the right

upper quadrant, especially during examination of the proximal half of the small intestine, because the small intestine moves away from the surgeon's instruments in this way, being protected from injury caused by frequent back-and-forth instrumental movements to run the bowel.

If a laparoscopic procedure is considered feasible, resection proceeds. The patient is tilted left side down. The mesentery of the right colon is grasped dorsally with a Babcock-type grasper by an assistant. With adequate traction of right colonic mesentery towards the right side of the patient by the first assistant (standing between the patient's legs), the ileocolic pedicle is easily identified in most cases. The peritoneum over the ileocolic pedicle is incised near its origin from the superior mesenteric vessels. The ileocolic vessels are further isolated from the surrounding mesentery and the retroperitoneum (Fig. 23.9, see color plate). The duodenum is especially protected and swept clear of the vessels, which are then divided at a safe distance from the superior mesenteric vessels using a 30-mm laparoscopic linear stapler. If the mesentery is remarkably thickened or inflamed, the pedicle is left alone and divided after exteriorization. The mesentery of the cecum and ascending colon is then dissected retroperitoneally from a medial to lateral direction, so a tunnel is created beneath the mesentery in this avascular plane. This tunnel can be created almost entirely to the lateral gutter by blunt dissection, with only an occasional need for sharp dissection. Using this maneuver, the duodenum and Gerota's fascia can be readily swept away from the dorsal aspect of the right colonic mesentery (Fig. 23.10, see color plate). The lateral peritoneal attachments of the diseased segment are then divided under tension, taking care once again to identify the ureter and gonadal vessels and protect them (Fig. 23.11).

Next, a small incision (3 to 6 cm) is made at the umbilical cannula site, and the specimen is delivered through the wound. Ileal and colonic mesenteric divisions, plus anastomosis of both transected intestinal ends, are performed extracorporeally using standard techniques (typically a stapled functional end-to-end anastomosis). Sometimes, colonic mesenteric division and transection of the colon can be performed more easily intracorporeally, then the specimen can possibly be brought out more easily.

Total Abdominal Colectomy

The dissection commences with an incision of the peritoneum at the sacral promontory just to the right of the inferior mesenteric artery. The inferior

Fig. 23.8. Friability of affected segments of small bowel Crohn's disease mean special care must be taken when grasping with laparoscopic instruments. (See color plate.)

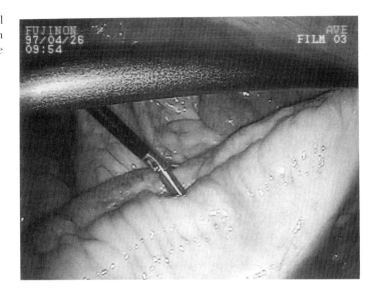

Fig. 23.9. The mesentery of the cecum and ascending colon is dissected retroperitoneally, so a tunnel is created beneath the mesentery in this avascular plane. Using this maneuver, the duodenum, ureter, gonadal vessels, and Gerota's fascia can be readily swept away from the dorsal aspect of the right colonic mesentery. (See color plate.)

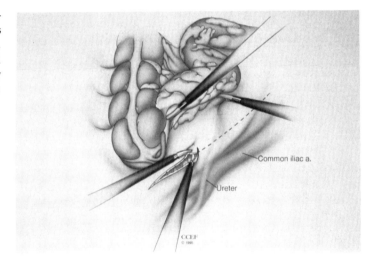

Fig. 23.10. The ileocolic pedicle is isolated from the retroperitoneum. The duodenum and ureter are especially protected and swept clear of the ileocolic vessels. (See color plate.)

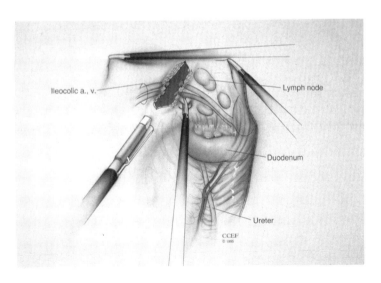

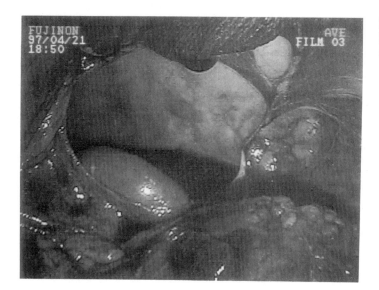

Fig. 23.11. A laparoscopic paddle retractor (at top) holds the intestine anteriorly so dissection of posterior and lateral attachments may be expedited. (See color plate.)

mesenteric pedicle is then isolated and divided. The sigmoid colon and rectum are mobilized, and the rectum is divided. Rigid proctoscopy is used to identify an appropriate distal resection line in the upper rectum (approximately 15 cm from the anal verge, typically) based on location of inflammation and ease of reach with the proctoscope. A retroperitoneal approach is utilized for dissection proceeding from medial to lateral, separating the mesentery of the descending colon, splenic flexure, and distal transverse colon from the retroperitoneum.

The ileum, right colon, and hepatic flexure, along with the proximal transverse colon are mobilized, again using a retroperitoneal approach with early ligation of the vascular pedicles and late division of the lateral attachments. When dissection of the terminal ileal mesentery is complete, the specimen is extracted through the transversely enlarged (3 to 6 cm) suprapubic or right lower quadrant cannula site. The bowel is then divided near the ileocecal junction, the anvil and center rod of a circular stapler are secured in position with a purse-string suture, and the ileum is returned to the abdomen.

The abdomen is irrigated through the incision, then closed. Pneumoperitoneum is reestablished and a 28 or 31-mm circular stapler (Premium CEEA, US Surgical Corp., Norwalk, CT) is placed transanally to perform the double stapled ileorectal anastomosis. Great care is taken not to twist the ileal mesentery. After the tissue rings are examined for defects, the anastomosis is tested for leaks by filling the pelvis with saline and air insufflating the rectum.

Pitfalls in Laparoscopic Techniques

For resection these are:

1. Need to adequately assess (to "run") the entire length of small bowel.
2. Safe division of thickened mesentery intracorporeally.
3. Need for identification of retroperitoneal structures (ureters, gonadal vessels).
4. Adequate wound opening for thick, inflamed specimen removal.
5. Handling of fistulas and bowel loops stuck together.
6. Safe management of intraabdominal sepsis.

For stoma creation these are:

1. Avoidance of twisting or misorienting the bowel.
2. Achieving adequate mesenteric length.

The Future

It is extremely likely that the use of laparoscopic techniques in inflammatory bowel disease will increase in the next 3 to 5 years. If the theoretical advantages of minimally invasive techniques, such as less postoperative pain, short hospitalization time, less operative stress, early return to work, less adhesion formation, and superior cosmesis, are proven to be true by sound scientific studies, then laparoscopic surgery for Crohn's disease may become the optimal mode of resection. New technologies including improved optical equipment, laparoscopic retractors, and improved stapling/suturing devices will allow for many procedures to be readily performed by laparoscopy.

References

1. Soper NJ, B runt LM, Kerbl K. Laparoscopic general surgery. N Engl J Med 1994;330:409–19.

2. Phillips EH, Franklin M, Carroll BJ, et al. Laparoscopic colectomy. Ann Surg 1992;216:703–7.

3. Falk PM, Beart RW, Wexner SD, et al. Laparoscopic colectomy: a critical appraisal. Dis Colon Rectum 1993;36:24–34.

4. Franklin ME, Ramos R, Rosenthal D, et al. Laparoscopic colonic procedures. World J Surg 1993;17:51–6.

5. Scoggin SD, Frazee RC, Snyder SK, et al. Laparoscopic-assisted bowel surgery. Dis Colon Rectum 1993;36:747–50.

6. Hoffmann GC, Baker JW, Fitchell CW, et al. Laparoscopic assisted-colectomy. Initial experience. Ann Surg 1994;219:732–43.

7. Peters WR. Laparoscopic total proctocolectomy with creation of ileostomy for ulcerative colitis: report of two cases. J Laparoendosc Surg 1992;2:175–8.

8. Kreissler-Haag D, Hildebrandt U, Pistorius G, et al. Laparoscopic surgery in Crohn's disease. Surg Endos 1994;8:1002 (abstract).

9. Reissman P, Salky BA, Pfeifer J, et al. Laparoscopic surgery in the management of inflammatory bowel disease. Am J Surg 1996;171:47–51.

10. Ludwig KA, Milsom JW, Church JM, et al. Prelimi-nary experience with laparoscopic intestinal surgery for Crohn's disease. Am J Surg 1996;171:52–6.

11. Thibault C, Poulin EC. Total laparoscopic proctocolectomy and laparoscopy-assisted proctocolectomy for inflammatory bowel disease: operative technique and preliminary report. Surg Laparosc Endosc 1995;5:472–6.

12. Ludwig KA, Milsom JW, Garcia-Ruiz A, et al. Laparoscopic techniques for fecal diversion. Dis Colon Rectum 1996;39:285–8.

13. Kim SH, Milsom JW, Shore GI, et al. Laparoscopic reversal of Hartmann's procedure. Presented at the 96th ASCRS annual convention, June 22–26, 1997, Philadelphia, Pennsylvania.

14. Wexner SD, Johansen OB, Nogueeras JJ, et al. Laparoscopic total abdominal colectomy: a prospective trial. Dis Colon Rectum 1992;35:651–5.

15. Marchesa P, Milsom JW, Hale JC, et al. Intraoperative laparoscopic liver ultrasonography for staging of colorectal cancer: initial experience. Dis Colon Rectum 1996;39:S73–S78.

16. Milsom JW, Ludwig KA, Church JM, et al. Laparoscopic total abdominal colectomy with ileorectal anastomosis for familial adenomatous polyposis. Dis Colon Rectum 1997;40:675–8.

17. Milsom JW, Okuda J, Kim SH, et al. Atraumatic and expeditious laparoscopic bowel handling using a new endoscopic device. Dis Colon Rectum 1997;40:1394–5.

24 Perineal Proctectomy

Fabrizio Michelassi and Roger Hurst

Indications

Perineal proctectomy is indicated:

1. In the patient, usually elderly, who has undergone an abdominal colectomy for ulcerative colitis and has decided to opt for a completion proctectomy rather than a reconstructive procedure. In these cases, if the transection of the rectum was carried out near the plane of the levators, the completion proctectomy can be performed exclusively through a perineal approach.
2. In the patient with severe and extensive septic perineal complications of Crohn's disease, who has undergone an abdominal proctocolectomy with proximal closure of the rectal stump and drainage of the perineal sepsis. In these cases, the completion proctectomy is delayed to a later time, when the patient has recovered from the initial procedure and the perineum has healed by secondary intention.
3. In the patient with Crohn's proctitis unresponsive to fecal diversion and medical management.
4. In the patient with a rectal stump which has developed an invasive adenocarcinoma.

Pitfalls and Danger Points

1. Inadequate management of the perineal wound, resulting in a chronic perineal draining sinus.
2. Faulty dissection of the rectal stump resulting in inadvertent proctotomies, or injury to the posterior wall of the vagina in the female patient or the urethra in the male patient; injury to small bowel loops located in the pelvis.

Preoperative Preparation

Patients should be kept NPO (nil per os) from midnight prior to the scheduled surgical procedure. Patients recently treated with corticosteroids should be given intravenous hydrocortisone at stress doses prior to induction of anesthesia and continued through the postoperative course. Intravenous prophylactic antibiotics should be administered one hour prior to surgery so that maximum tissue antibiotic levels are achieved by the time of the skin incision.

Operative Strategy

Unless the rectum is known to harbor an invasive adenocarcinoma, the dissection should remain close to the rectal wall. The perineal dissection is started with an incision at the right or left of the anus where the intersphincteric groove can easily be palpated. The dissection is continued in this plane and then carried out circumferentially around the anal canal. A proctectomy done in this manner, leaves the entire levator diaphragm intact resulting in less operative trauma and ease of closure of the pelvic floor (1). This translates into a reduction of the incidence of chronic perineal draining sinuses.

For patients with severe perineal scarring from previous drainage procedures, wide excision of the affected skin is required to remove tissue that lacks the pliability necessary to allow for satisfactory and tension-free perineal closure.

If the patient is known to have an invasive adenocarcinoma in the rectal stump or a squamocellular carcinoma originating from a chronic fistula-in-

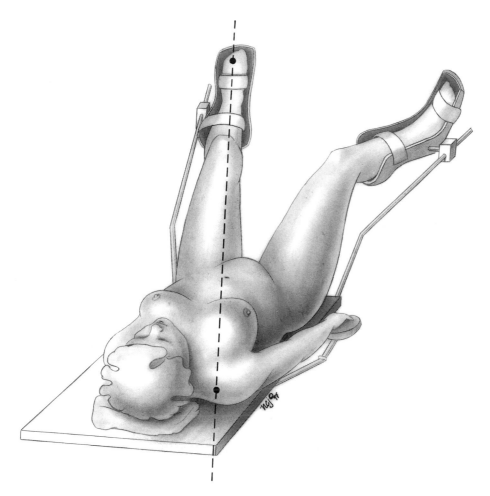

Fig. 24.1. Modified lithotomy, position with legs supported by Allen stirrups.

Operative Technique

ano, the proctectomy needs to include the levators and whatever remains of the rectal mesentery. The initial incision is much wider encompassing a wide skin margin and the entire external sphincter mechanism. In rare instances, the extent of perineal resection is so great that local tissue transfer flaps are required for adequate perineal closure.

Operative Technique

The patient is placed in the modified lithotomy position with the legs supported by Allen stirrups (Allen Manufacturing Company, Cleveland, OH). With ample padding, the patient's heels should rest flat in the well of the stirrup with the majority of the extremity's weight being placed on the sole of the foot. Thighs are flexed 45° and abducted to expose the perineum. To avoid pressure on the perineal nerve, the leg should be internally rotated (Fig. 24.1). The rectal stump is gently irrigated with a povidine-iodine solution. A dry gauze is then placed into the rectal stump to absorb any rectal

secretion and avoid a potential source of contamination. In addition, the anus is closed with a pursestring suture placed at the level of the anal verge. The perineum is then shaved and sterilely prepped. In the female patient the vagina is also prepped.

Removal of the rectal stump is best carried out along the plane between the internal and external sphincters. With a needle-point electrocautery, the skin incision is made over the palpable groove between the internal and external sphincter (Fig. 24.2). If the patient suffers from perineal scarring from perianal Crohn's disease, the incision should be adjusted to allow for excision of scarred tissue.

The intersphincteric plane is easiest to identify laterally, thus, the dissection should commence on the left and right side of the anus and then proceed to connect posteriorly and anteriorly. The dissection is carried in a craniad direction until the rectal stump is completely excised.

The pelvic space is thoroughly irrigated and drained with a closed-suction drain placed through

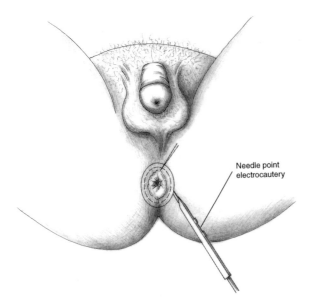

Fig. 24.2. Skin incision over the palpable groove between the internal and external sphincter.

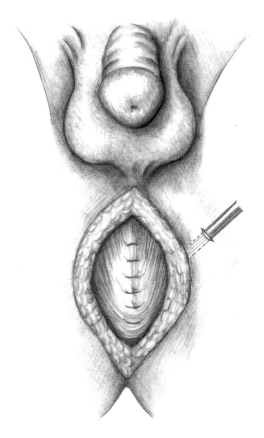

Fig. 24.3. Closure of the pelvic floor.

a separate incision. The perineal wound is closed by approximating the external sphincter mechanism in layers using absorbable sutures (Fig. 24.3). The skin edges are trimmed with a scalpel and the skin closed with a nylon interrupted vertical mattress suture.

Postoperative Care

In the absence of intraoperative contamination, perioperative antibiotics are discontinued within 24 hours. The Foley catheter is removed but attention must be paid to acute urinary retention, especially in the male.

Complications

Perineal Wound Infection

Perineal wound infection often manifests with fever, perineal pain, erythema, and purulent drainage. This complication is best avoided by prophylactic antibiotics and avoidance of inadvertent proctotomies. Intersphincteric perineal dissection as described above allows for effective closure of the perineal dead space and thus also reduces the likelihood of this complication (2). When perineal wound infection occurs, the skin sutures are removed, purulent fluid is completely drained, necrotic tissue debrided and the wound packed. Perineal wound infection often results in a persistent perineal sinus.

Persistent Perineal Sinus

A persistent perineal sinus is defined as a perineal wound that fails to heal properly resulting in an open infected sinus that persists for six months or longer. The incidence of persistent perineal sinus after proctectomy for Crohn's disease is reported to be as high as 40% (3). Although many of these wounds are minor cutaneous sinuses and are merely a nuisance to the patient, others are large, purulent cavities that interfere with the patient's health, rehabilitation, and social acceptance. Avoidance of pelvic sepsis is the best prevention of this complication. Additionally, ligatures made of permanent material and metal clips are to be avoided during the pelvic dissection as foreign material can often be the nidus for persistent perineal sepsis. When a large, infected perineal wound fails to heal, it is important to verify that no fistula, foreign body, or unrecognized abscess cavity is to blame for its persistence. If these are present, they must be treated appropriately for closure to be achieved.

Large perineal wounds typically develop a chronic, thick-walled fibrous cavity bearing infected granulation tissue. Under anesthesia the entire thick fibrous wall must be excised. Simple curettage is inadequate. During excision of the fibrous wall the surgeon must exercise care not to injure the vagina or the bladder and urethra anteriorly, or the small bowel that may be in close proximity to the craniad portion of the cavity. After excision of the cavity wall, spontaneous healing will occur within a few weeks in the majority of cases. However, in certain individuals with very large cavities, reexcision alone will not suffice and closure with myocutaneous flaps is required (3). An in-depth discussion of the etiology and management of persistent perineal sinus is to be found in Chapter 36.

Urinary Retention

Postoperative urinary retention may result from the use of opiates, anticholinergic medication or preexisting mechanical urinary obstruction, such as benign prostatic hypertrophy. Overuse of opiates and the administration of anticholinergic medication should be avoided if the patient experiences difficulty voiding after urinary catheter removal.

References

1. Lyttle JA, Parks AG. Intrasphincteric incision of the rectum. Br J Surg 1977;413:64–7.

2. Berry AR, Campos RDE, Lee ECG. Perineal and pelvic morbidity following perimuscular excision of the rectum for inflammatory bowel disease. Br J Surg 1986; 73:675.

3. Block GE, Hurst RD. Complications of the surgical treatment of ulcerative colitis and Crohn's disease. In: Kirsner JB, Shorter RG, eds. Inflammatory Bowel Disease. 4th ed. Baltimore: Williams & Wilkins, 1995: 898–922.

25 Construction of Intestinal Stomas

James M. Becker and Diane Bryant

Intestinal Stomas

Despite intense medical treatment, for most patients with Crohn's disease surgery will eventually become necessary. It has been shown that 75% of all patients with Crohn's disease will eventually undergo an operation on some area of their intestinal tract (1–5). A major concern of the surgeon is to preserve as much of the intestinal tract as possible since intestinal resection is palliative for patients with Crohn's disease. Therefore, the goal of surgery is to perform targeted and limited resections to alleviate the clinical symptoms and complications of Crohn's disease (4). In this context, it frequently becomes necessary to create a temporary or permanent intestinal stoma. The creation and management of end and loop intestinal stomas requires special attention by the surgeon and other members of the healthcare team to avoid complications and to allow patients to return to an active lifestyle. Pieper (6) and others report that people with newly constructed intestinal stomas have many concerns about resuming their previous lifestyle, including household activities, sexual function, and leisure activities. In this chapter the indications, surgical techniques, management and complications of end and loop stomas in patients with Crohn's disease will be reviewed.

Indications

Intestinal stomas performed for Crohn's disease become necessary for patients who fail traditional medical therapy to relieve clinical signs and symptoms, and where primary anastomosis is technically impossible or dangerous. Failed medical therapy is defined as the persistence of clinical manifestations despite a variety of pharmacological agents or the inability of the patient to tolerate the drug therapy. Clinical signs and symptoms may include fever, abdominal pain, malaise, anorexia, nausea, vomiting, weight loss, and malnutrition. Other indications may include obstruction, abscess formation, perianal fistula formation, hemorrhage, or if there is a need to divert the fecal stream (4). For many patients experiencing such debilitating symptoms, surgery with an intestinal stoma is considered an improvement in their quality of life.

The literature supports the need for a total proctocolectomy with end ileostomy when the disease is confined to the colon and rectum because of the low rate of recurrence compared with segmental or subtotal resection (4,5,7–9). The reasons for this are not well understood, but researchers are examining the site of the anastomosis and the extent of the margins during resection (4). It has been shown, however that if recurrence of the disease occurs it will be at the peristomal ileum and the ileostomy will frequently not be affected.

The surgeon may consider a "temporary" loop stoma if there is hope of reestablishing the fecal stream or if the patient is toxic and unable to tolerate an extensive surgical procedure. The loop stoma has surgical advantages discussed below.

Emergency Surgical Options

Several types of operations have been used in Crohn's colitis in need of emergent surgery (10). Some surgeons have advocated simple loop ileostomy without resection of diseased colon. The other end of the spectrum is the use of emergency total proctocolectomy and permanent ileostomy. The former option may relieve toxic dilatation but has no impact on the acute inflammatory process. Total proctocolectomy is associated with a high morbidity in the acute setting and may be overly aggressive in eliminating any option for restoration of continence. Most surgeons feel that the most satisfactory operation in the emergency setting for Crohn's colitis is a subtotal colectomy with ileostomy and Hartmann closure of the rectum. This allows removal of the majority of disease-bearing tissue, the establishment of a firm histologic diagnosis, and does not preclude subsequent restorative procedures. Likewise, in an urgent/emergent operation for perforated or obstructed small bowel, a proximal loop jejunostomy may be an excellent temporizing measure. This may permit resolution of the inflammation around many loops of non-diseased segments and the salvage of as much length of the intestinal tract as possible. We always advocate this approach in the emergency situation, even if it means prolonged parenteral nutrition, rather than resection of multiple inflamed segments of bowel in the acute situation. The technical aspects of this procedure are discussed below.

Elective Surgical Options

For patients requiring operative intervention for the elective treatment of colorectal Crohn's disease, a number of operative alternatives are available (7–9). These range from the use of a temporary defunctioning ileostomy to resection of segments of diseased colon or even the entire colon and rectum.

Temporary defunctioning ileostomy was originally advocated by Truelove at Oxford in 1965 and Oberhelman at Stanford in 1968. It was argued that this might provide temporary improvement of systemic, colonic, or anorectal symptoms. A number of studies have demonstrated that in patients in whom a defunctioning ileostomy was performed as an elective surgical treatment for Crohn's colitis, only 15% had intestinal continuity restored. Others have advocated the use of an ileostomy as a staged procedure in preparation for later resection. With currently available perioperative care, a preliminary diverting loop ileostomy prior to colectomy is rarely necessary.

As suggested above, subtotal colectomy with ileostomy and Hartmann closure of the rectum may be the operation of choice when an urgent operation is necessary in a critically ill patient with Crohn's colitis (10). This is also an acceptable alternative in the elective setting, particularly in patients in whom there is uncertainty about the inflammatory status of the rectum, in those in whom perianal abscess precludes proctectomy, and finally in those patients in whom there is uncertainty about the diagnosis of Crohn's disease vs. ulcerative colitis. It may be necessary in 15% to 20% of patients. The mortality and morbidity of elective subtotal colectomy is quite low. Following subtotal colectomy there are three potential outcomes: staged proctectomy in patients with severe Crohn's proctitis, ileorectal anastomosis if the rectum remains spared, or maintenance of the status quo. In this latter group of patients one must consider the risk of the development of rectal carcinoma and monitor the rectal segment with yearly biopsies checking for dysplasia or consider proctectomy.

The most aggressive approach for the management of diffuse Crohn's proctocolitis is total proctocolectomy and Brooke ileostomy (11). This may be necessary in 55% to 60% of all patients. In the elective setting, the operation is associated with a mortality of 2% to 4%. The literature would suggest that it also has the lowest clinical recurrence rate, ranging from 3% to 46% with an average of 20%. Goligher (8) has suggested that while there is a linear increase in recurrence during the first 10 years after proctocolectomy, thereafter it tends to plateau at the 20% range. The operation is, however, associated with significant complications including chronic perineal wound problems that may develop in 10% to 30% of patients. It should also be emphasized that these patients tend to have a higher incidence of ileostomy complications including fluid and electrolyte problems, vitamin B_{12} malabsorption, and bile acid malabsorption.

Preoperative Preparation

Physicians should involve other members of the healthcare team to assist them in the preoperative preparation and rehabilitation of the patient undergoing a newly constructed stoma. Many patients require extensive preoperative preparation that includes intravenous hydration, antibiotics, a nutritional consult and parenteral steroids (12). In addition, in the elective situation the bowel requires mechanical preparation with an electrolyte and polyglycol solution.

The surgical team must also prepare the patient psychologically for the effect of having an intestinal stoma. Patients need to be counseled individually by an enterostomal therapy (ET) nurse or a knowledgeable healthcare provider that can address individual needs and concerns. This visit should be arranged preoperatively in elective procedures and as soon as possible for patients facing urgent surgery. When the decision is made that the patient will have a temporary or permanent stoma, the patient and family should receive written and oral teachings about intestinal stomas.

Information covered during the preoperative teaching session should include the impact of an ostomy on lifestyle, occupational roles, social activity, and sexual function. The surgeon and ET nurse review with the patient and significant others basic anatomy and physiology, the surgical procedure, the concept of an ostomy, characteristics of the stoma, type of effluent, pouching systems, dietary concerns, clothing, activities of daily living, intimacy issues, and options for management of the intestinal stoma. This should be done regardless of whether the stoma is temporary or permanent.

Critically important, a stoma site must be selected preoperatively by the ET nurse and/or physician. In selecting the site, the ET nurse or physician identifies the rectus muscle, avoids creases and folds, chooses a flat surface, avoids the belt line and, most importantly, ensures that it is visible to the patient. Ideally, ileostomies should protrude at least 2 cm. The stoma site is marked with an indelible mark, such as a surgical marker, methylene blue injected intradermally, or a scratch to the epidermis in a cruciate fashion. Colostomy sites are usually located in the left mid or lower part of the abdomen. Stoma sites for end and loop ileostomies are usually located in the right lower quadrant unless other factors preclude this site placement, including old incisions or scars, supportive equipment, if the patient is confined to a wheelchair and other criteria mentioned above. A loop jejunostomy, usually fashioned emergently after small bowel perforation, abscess, or obstruction necessitates such a stoma, and is generally located in the left upper abdomen. It is important that the stoma lie within the rectus muscle in order to reduce the subsequent development of peristomal hernias. A faceplate should be placed on the abdomen to ensure that the site chosen will make for a properly fitting appliance. The site must lie on a flat area of the skin in the supine, sitting, and standing positions. The faceplate must not impinge on any bony prominences, previous skin incisions, skin creases, or the umbilicus. As a rule, this point is a line drawn between the lowest point of the costal margin to the pubic tubercle and where it intersects a line drawn between the umbilicus and the anterior superior iliac spine. Allowances must be made for abdominal distention.

Physicians and other healthcare providers have additional resources to assist the patient in coping with a new stoma, such as the United Ostomy Association; Wound, Ostomy and Continence Nurses Society (a society for enterostomal therapy nurses) and the Crohn's and Colitis Foundation of America. These societies are fantastic resources for written, video, personal, and moral support for the patient. The goal of preoperative teaching and postoperative support is to inform, support, and encourage the patient to resume their previous lifestyle.

Operative Technique

End Ileostomy

The importance of providing the patients with a well-functioning, trouble-free ileostomy cannot be overemphasized. Most surgeons have accepted the technique described by Sir Brian Brooke in the 1950's (Fig. 25.1). The principles include passing the end of the ileum through an opening in the mid-aspect of the right rectus muscle at a point below the umbilicus that allows convenient placement of the adhesive appliance of an ileostomy bag. Placement that is too low or too lateral may lead to serious problems in ileostomy care and function. The site should be located such that the ileum will traverse the anterior and posterior rectus sheath and the rectus muscle. A circular incision of skin is excised that will approximate the transverse diameter of the terminal ileum. The anterior rectus sheath is incised in a cruciate manner. It is important to make the opening in the fascia no larger than needed to accommodate the ileum and its mesentery. If the incision is too large, parastomal hernia is more likely to occur. Likewise, if the incision is made too laterally, the inferior epigastric vessels may be lacerated.

The terminal ileal arcades are identified. The arcade closest to the mesenteric surface of the ileal wall is left intact for as long a distance as possible. The mesentery can be transilluminated so that the blood vessels supplying the terminal ileum can be visualized. It is not necessary to dissect all the mesentery from the ileum for a distance of 3 to 4 cm; rather, it is better to taper the mesentery as it approaches the terminal ileum to be divided. The ileum is divided with a gastrointestinal stapling device. Using a Babcock clamp, the ileum is brought out through the abdominal wall with the mesenteric aspect oriented superiorly. It is important to prevent axial twisting of the ileum. The ileum is brought through the abdominal wall defect for a

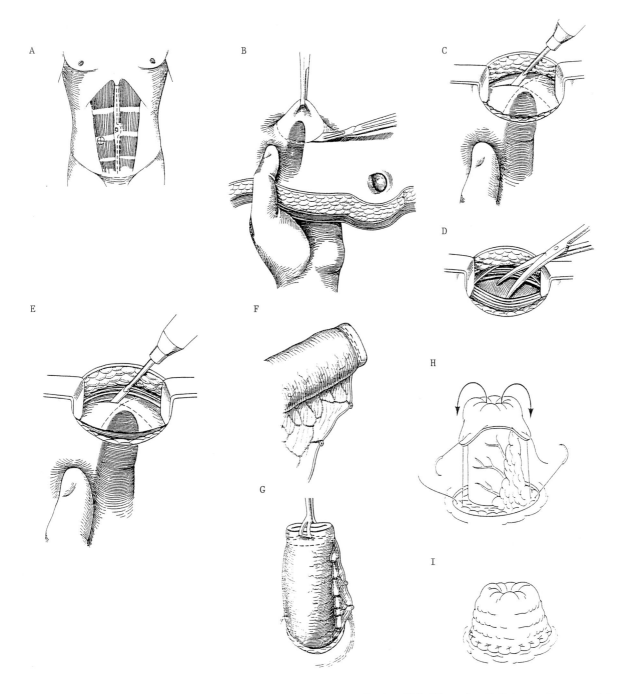

Fig. 25.1.   Construction of an end ileostomy. The terminal ileum is brought 5 cm through an abdominal wall defect in the right lower abdomen (A–G), everted (H), and sutured to the more proximal ileal seromuscularis and then dermis to mature the ileostomy (I).

(From Becker JM. Ulcerative Colitis. In: Surgery: Scientific Principles and Practice. Edited by Greenfield LJ, Mulholland MW, Oldham KT, Zelenock GB, JB Lippincott Company, Philadelphia, PA, 1993;995; with permission)

distance of 5 cm above the skin so that when the ileostomy is matured by folding it upon itself, 2 to 3 cm will protrude from the surface. The incisions through the various layers of the abdominal wall should allow the terminal ileum to take a direct and perpendicular path through it. The ileal wall is

sutured in four quadrants to the peritoneum with 3-0 polyglycolic acid sutures. The ileostomy is matured after closure of the abdominal wound. The wound is protected with a towel and the stoma is matured in a Brooke-type eversion method as demonstrated in the diagram. The staple line is excised with electrocautery. Four-0 polyglycolic acid sutures are first placed through the full thickness of the cut edge of the ileum, then into the seromusculari where the ileum emerges from the abdominal wall, and finally brought out at the subcuticular level of the skin.

The folding back or "maturing" prevents the development of an inflammatory response in the serosa and provides more substance to the protruding ileal nipple. Every attempt should be made not to place sutures through epidermis of the skin because the occasional hypertrophic scar that may form will make it difficult for the appliance to adhere. A groomed stoma plate is then secured around the stoma and a bag snapped into place. Simply and easily applied receptacles are now available.

Loop Ileostomy

A loop ileostomy is usually designed as a temporary diverting stoma. As with an end ileostomy, it is essential to select an appropriate stoma site preoperatively. At the time of operation, a mobile loop of ileum, as close as possible to the distal ileum or colon is identified, and a Penrose drain passed through a small mesenteric window made at the site of the proposed loop. A stomal opening is constructed in the abdominal wall in the right lower quadrant, and a Penrose drain is used to direct the ileal loop through this defect. The ileal loop should be oriented so that the ileal mesentery is not twisted. This sometimes means the afferent limb is located inferiorly, but more often superiorly. These same principles may be applied to the loop jejunostomy in the left upper quadrant. The ileal loop is then suspended over an ileostomy rod (Fig. 25.2). The ileum is not tacked to the peritoneum or fascia. This facilitates subsequent ileostomy closure. The abdominal wound is closed, and the loop ileostomy is then matured. This is done by opening the ileum transversely with electrocautery. The ileal wall is folded back onto itself and sutured to the surrounding seromuscular layer and dermis using interrupted 4-0 polyglycolic acid sutures. The stoma is matured asymmetrically with the afferent or superior component protruding more than the efferent or inferior component. This technique creates a diverting ileostomy that functions well and can be readily closed.

Closure of Loop Ileostomy

To close the loop ileostomy a transverse elliptical incision is made around the stoma (Fig. 25.3). Elec-

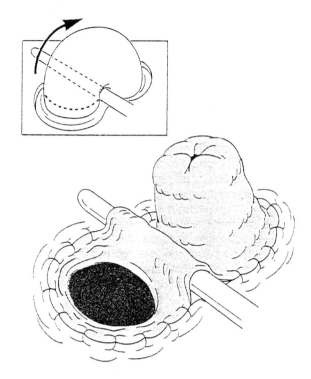

Fig. 25.2. A loop ileostomy is constructed proximal to the bowel to be diverted and is matured over a rod. (From Becker JM. Ulcerative Colitis. In: Surgery: Scientific Principles and Practice. Edited by Greenfield LJ, Mulholland MW, Oldham KT, Zelenock GB, JB Lippincott Company, Philadelphia, PA, 1993;1000; with permission)

trocautery is used to dissect through the subcutaneous fat to the limbs of the intestine, and at that point, sharp dissection is begun. The dissection is continued down through the muscle and the peritoneum until the peritoneal cavity is entered. At this point, the limbs of intestine are freed from any intraabdominal adhesions and allowed to extend from the abdominal wall for 5 to 7 cm.

The antimesenteric surfaces of the limbs are identified and tacked together with several 3-0 sutures. This assures that the subsequent staple line is placed from the antimesenteric surface of one limb to the antimesenteric surface of the other, without stapling across the mesentery. Electrocautery is then used to create enterotomies in both limbs. This is done as close to the previous stoma site as possible so as not to sacrifice important ileal length.

The forks of the intestinal anastomosing stapler are passed through the enterotomies and carefully down into the lumen of each of the intestinal limbs. It is important that the stapler be angled anteriorly such that the mesentery falls away posteriorly

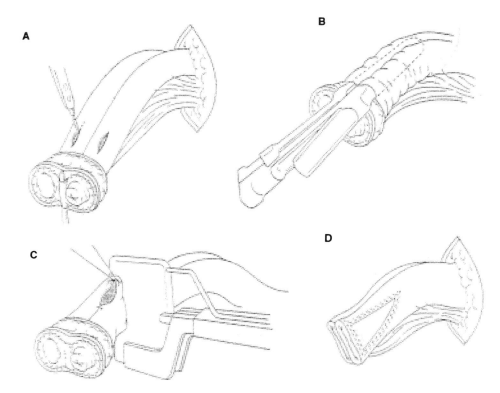

Fig. 25.3. Closure of loop ileostomy after it has been freed from the abdominal wall. (A) A transverse elliptical incision is made around the stoma and the limbs are dissected free. (B) The antimesenteric surfaces of the limbs are tacked together and the jaws of an anastomosing stapler are passed through enterotomies and down into the lumen of each of the intestinal limbs, and fired to create a side-to-side anastomosis between the afferent and efferent ileal limb. (C) A linear stapler is placed and fired below the former stoma and below the edges of the enterotomies. The stoma and distal limbs are amputated and the stapler is released. The anastomosis is dropped back into the peritoneal cavity and the peritoneum, fascia, and skin are closed. (From Becker JM. Ulcerative Colitis. In: Surgery: Scientific Principles and Practice. Edited by Greenfield LJ, Mulholland MW, Oldham KT, Zelenock GB, JB Lippincott Company, Philadelphia, PA, 1993;1000; with permission)

and is not stapled. The stapler is closed and fired to create a side-to-side anastomosis between the afferent and efferent ileal limbs. The stapler is removed, and the staple lines are inspected to ensure that there is adequate hemostasis.

The staple lines are distracted. A linear stapler is placed below the former stoma and below the edges of the enterotomy, crossing both anastomotic staple lines and is fired. The stoma is amputated, the stapler is released slowly, and any areas of bleeding are selectively electrocauterized. The anastomosis is digitally examined. The apex of the staple line is reinforced with a 3-0 polyglycolic acid suture. Alternatively, a handsewn closure may be carried out by trimming the edges of the desuscepted ileum back to soft bowel, then closing the lumen with interrupted or running absorbable suture. The anastomosis is then dropped back into the peritoneal cavity. The peritoneum, fascia, and skin are closed.

Colostomy

As for an ileostomy or a jejunostomy, it is imperative that the surgeon and an enterostomal therapy nurse see the the patient before the operation to choose an adequate colostomy site. Important factors to consider in choosing the ostomy site are the proposed location of the abdominal incision; the anatomy of the patient's abdomen (e.g., skin folds and previous scars); bony prominences, including the anterior superior iliac spine; and the location of the patient's natural belt line. An effort should be made to locate the colostomy several inches above or below the belt line in an accessible site.

In constructing the colostomy the adequacy of blood supply to the terminal end of the colon must be established. If the distal colon appears dusky, further resection should be carried out until active bleeding from the cut edge of the colon is seen. It is

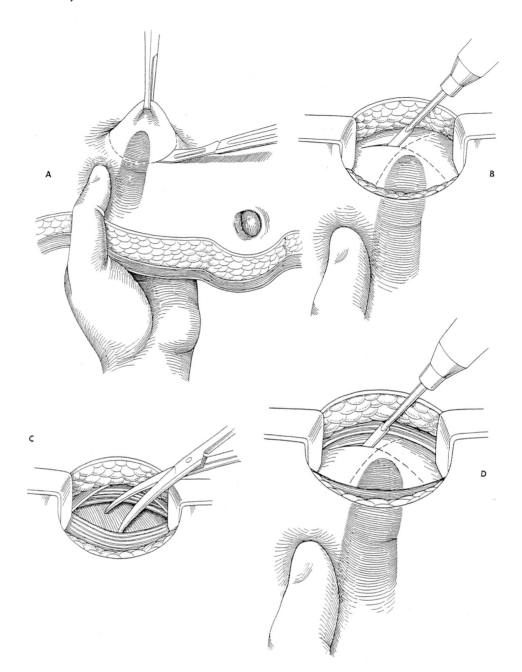

Fig. 25.4A. Colostomy Construction. (A) A scalpel is used to remove a button of skin approximately 2 cm in diameter. A core of subcutaneous tissue is removed down to the anterior fascia with electrocautery. (B) A cruciate incision is made in the anterior fascia with electrocautery or scalpel. (C) Muscle fibers are split, and (D) electro-cautery is used to open the posterior layers, including the peritoneum. (From Becker JM. Abdominoperineal Resection for Cancer of the Rectum. In: Colorectal Surgery Illustrated: A Focused Approach, Edited by Bauer JJ, Mosby Year Book, Inc., St. Louis, MO, 1992;151; with permission).

important that the left colon be adequately mobilized; in some cases this may require incising the peritoneal reflection up to or around the splenic flexure. At the site marked before surgery for the stoma, a Kocher clamp is placed on the skin. A scalpel is used to remove a button of skin approxi-mately 2 cm in diameter (Fig. 25.4). A core of subcutaneous tissue is removed down to the anterior fascia with electrocautery. A cruciate incision is made in the anterior fascia with electrocautery or scalpel. Muscle fibers are split, and electrocautery is used to open the posterior layers, including the

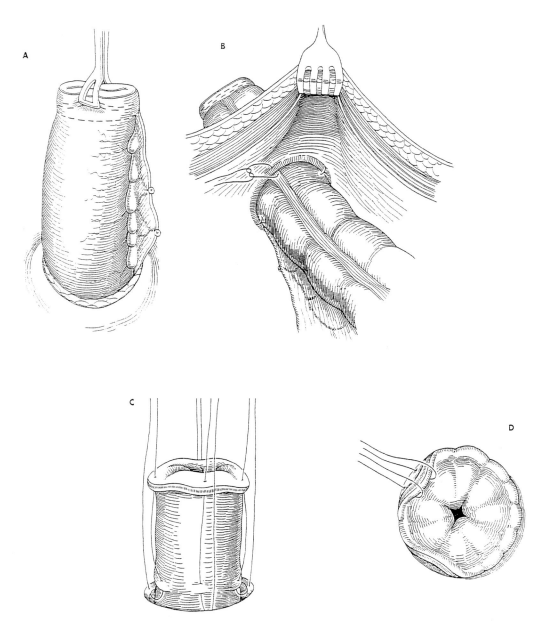

Fig. 25.4B. Colostomy construction. (A) The colon is delivered through the abdominal wall so that it extends approximately 2 to 3 cm beyond the surface of the skin. (B) The bowel is tacked internally to the peritoneal defect with several circumferentially placed interrupted sutures. Before maturing the colostomy, the midline fascia and skin are closed. A sterile towel is then placed over the wound to protect it from the colostomy. The staple line on the terminus of the colon is excised with electrocautery to open the colon. (C) The colostomy is matured us-ing interrupted 4-0 polyglycolic acid sutures. Four stitches are placed in each quadrant, incorporating the full-thickness cut end of the colon, the seromuscular surface of the colon approximately 1 to 2 cm below the cut end, and then up to the dermis. (D) Several additional simple sutures are placed in each quadrant to complete the stoma. (From Becker JM. Abdominoperineal Resection for Cancer of the Rectum. In: Colorectal Surgery Illustrated: A Focused Approach, Edited by Bauer JJ, Mosby Year Book, Inc., St. Louis, MO, 1992;152–53; with permission)

peritoneum. Two digits are passed through the defect, which is gently dilated to allow free passage of the digits. A Babcock clamp is passed through the stoma site, and the distal end of the colon is grasped.

The colon is delivered through the abdominal wall so that it extends approximately 2 to 3 cm beyond the surface of the skin. The bowel is tacked internally to the peritoneal defect with several interrupted sutures. Before maturing the colostomy, the midline fascia and skin are closed. A sterile towel is then placed over the wound to protect it from the colostomy.

The staple line on the terminus of the colon is excised with electrocautery to open the lumen and completely remove the staples. The colostomy is matured using interrupted 4-0 polyglycolic acid sutures. Approximately four stitches are placed in each quadrant, incorporating the full-thickness cut end of the colon, the seromuscular surface of the colon approximately 1 to 2 cm below the cut end, and then up to the dermis. Several additional simple sutures are placed in each quadrant to complete the stoma. A Karaya plate is groomed to closely accommodate the diameter of the colostomy, and a bag is snapped into place.

Complications

During the past several decades attention has been paid by many surgeons and enterostomal therapists to the construction, management, and care of intestinal stomas. This current practice has led to the ease of patients in caring for newly constructed stomas thus influencing their ability to return to their previous lifestyle. It is important to remember, however, that at the same time that improvements were made in the construction of intestinal stomas attention was also paid to the long-term management of ileostomies. The pioneer in the area of ostomy care was Norma Gill. Ms. Gill practiced at the Cleveland Clinic and devoted her time and energy in caring for patients with newly constructed ostomies. Her contributions to ostomy care are recognized by her peers and is the basis for current practice (13).

The construction and location of the stoma determines the type of appliance, the frequency of appliance changes and the need for additional accessory products. Despite this current practice, many complications still occur with intestinal stomas. Complications with ileostomies are related to technique, recurrent disease, and peristomal skin breakdown. The literature reveals that 20% to 40% of patients with end ileostomies will experience some type of complication and up to one half of these patients will require operative revision (14). Therefore, it is necessary for surgeons to adhere to the basic principles of stoma construction and for the patient to receive in-depth individualized teaching related to stoma care.

During the postoperative phase, the stoma is carefully assessed for viability, color, location, and the status of the mucocutaneous border and peristomal skin. Complications seen during the immediate postoperative period include ischemia, mucocutaneous separation, peristomal abscess, fistulas, and retraction of the stoma. Later complications may be related to peristomal skin breakdown, intraluminal obstruction and peristomal hernia or prolapse (14) (see Chapter 37).

Summary

The construction and management of end and loop ostomies for patients with inflammatory bowel disease involves extensive preoperative preparation of the patient, an experienced surgeon and enterostomal therapist and close follow-up of the patient. Problems with most intestinal stomas can be avoided if close attention is paid preoperatively and during the operation. In the majority of cases, patients with inflammatory bowel disease do not choose to have an intestinal stoma, but for many patients it can not only be a life-saving procedure, but also significantly improve quality of life. Therefore, surgeons, ET nurses, and other healthcare providers have a responsibility to teach and inform their patients about intestinal stomas.

References

1. Strong SA, Fazio FW. Crohn's disease of the colon, rectum, and anus. Surg Clin North Am 1993;73(5):933–59.
2. Bryant RA, Buls JG. Pathophysiology and diagnostic studies of gastrointestinal tract disorders. In: Hampton BG, Bryant RA, eds. Ostomies and Continent Diversions Nursing Management. St. Louis, MO; Mosby Year Book, 1992:299–348.
3. Hanauer SB. Diagnosis and medical management of inflammatory bowel disease in adults. Problems Gen Surg 1993;10(1):1–13.
4. Nogueras JJ, Wexner SD. Surgical management of primary and recurrent Crohn's disease. Problems Gen Surg 1993;10(1):123–35.
5. Glotzer DJ. Surgical therapy for Crohn's disease. Gastro Clin North Amer 1995;24(3)577–96.
6. Pieper B, Mikols C. Predischarge and postdischarge concerns of persons with an ostomy. J Wound Ost Cont Nurs 1996;23(2):105–9.
7. Schrock TR. Surgery for Crohn's Colitis. Cur Mngt Inflam Bowel Dis 1989;290–4.
8. Goligher JC. Surgical treatment of Crohn's disease affecting mainly or entirely the large bowel. World J Surg 1988;12(2):186–90.
9. Shorb PE. Surgical therapy for Crohn's disease. Gastroenterol Clin North Am 1989;18(1):111–28.

10. Zenilman ME, Becker JM. Emergencies in inflammatory bowel disease. Gastroenterol Clin North Am 1988;17(2):387–405.

11. Scammel B, Ambrose NS, Williams JA, et al. Recurrent small bowel Crohn's disease is more frequent after subtotal colectomy and ileorectal anastomosis than proctocolectomy. Dis Colon Rect 1985;28:770–1.

12. Nelson RL. Diagnostic techniques in inflammatory bowel disease. Surg Clin North Am 1993;73(5):879–89.

13. Weakley FL. A historical perspective of stomal construction. J Wound Ostom Cont Nur 1994;21(3):59–75.

14. Fazio VW. Prevention and management of ileostomy complications. J ET Nurs 1992;19:48–53.

Section III
Crohn's Disease

Part II
Surgical Treatment of Specific Complications

26 Surgical Treatment of Fistulas

Fabrizio Michelassi

Fistulas are common complications of Crohn's disease occurring in about one third of all patients (1). Recognized early by Crohn (2), they result from full-thickness disease rupturing into an adjacent hollow viscus or through the abdominal wall. The disease is usually confined to the site of origin and does not involve the nearby viscus or organ.

When a fistula connects a diseased segment of intestine with another intestinal segment or another hollow viscus lined by adenomatous or transitional epithelium, the fistula is defined as internal. Internal fistulas may affect any part of the intestinal tract, genitourinary tract, pancreatobiliary tract, or even the bronchopulmonary system. External fistulas connect diseased segments of intestine with organs lined by squamous epithelium, such as the skin (enterocutaneous or colocutaneous fistulas, fistula-in-ano) or the vagina (enterovaginal fistulas).

Diagnosis of internal fistulas is often problematic. Enterovesical fistulas are the only internal fistulas with manifestations that are distinctive enough to suggest the diagnosis as two thirds of patients experience pneumaturia and/or fecaluria (1). Yet, as many as one third of all patients with internal fistulas are asymptomatic and their fistulas are discovered incidentally during surgical exploration. Conversely, external fistulas are easily recognized by their drainage.

Despite the prevalence of fistulas in Crohn's disease, surgical treatment is infrequently indicated solely for their repair. In a series of 331 patients with Crohn's disease of the terminal ileum, 285 intraabdominal fistulas were detected in 227 patients (65.5%) (1). However, fistulas were the primary indication for surgery in only 6% of these patients.

Contrast studies of the upper and lower gastrointestinal tract, fistulograms, and endoscopic examinations are helpful to determine the extent of gastrointestinal involvement by Crohn's disease and the need for surgical treatment. In addition, they help to delineate the anatomy of the fistula.

This chapter will review treatment options for different types of intraabdominal fistulas. After an initial section on general considerations, the material is divided into sections according to the organ into which the fistula drains. Treatment of fistula-in-ano and anovaginal fistula is discussed in Chapter 32.

General Considerations

Although fistulas are common in patients with Crohn's disease, they represent the single indication to surgical treatment in only a few cases. In our experience, we consider the presence of a fistula to be an indication to surgery only when (1) the fistula has produced a functional or anatomic bypass of a major segment of intestine with consequent malabsorption and/or profuse diarrhea; (2) the fistula communicates with the genito-urinary, biliopancreatic or bronchopulmonary system; or (3) the drainage is a matter of personal embarrassment. In all the other cases, the indication for surgical treatment is more commonly represented by the presence of an inflammatory mass or abscess, by a partial or complete intestinal obstruction, or by failure of medical treatment.

The appropriate surgical management of Crohn's intraabdominal fistulas follows the principle of resection of the primary disease with extirpation of the fistula. In internal fistulas, closure of the defect in the organ where the disease has fistulized to is also necessary. Closure of the defect may pose a technical challenge when the organ involved is the duodenum or the rectum. In both situations, when (1) the intestinal wall is inflamed, thickened, friable, and rigid; (2) the debridement of the edges of the fistula has resulted in a large defect; and (3) the opening of the fistula is on the mesenteric side, primary closure may be difficult. Different surgical strategies apply due to the very proximal and very distal location in the gastrointestinal tract of the duodenum and rectum, respectively, and are discussed under the appropriate section.

A temporary stoma may be necessary in the surgical treatment of intraabdominal fistulas in the presence of sepsis, inadequate bowel preparation or malnutrition. Yet, the presence of an intraabdominal fistula is never the only reason for a permanent stoma.

Despite preoperative malnutrition and high doses of exogenous steroids, morbidity and mortality can be limited. The incidence of postoperative wound infection and abdominal abscesses can be minimized by routinely adhering to steps to contain contamination of the abdominal wound and peritoneal cavity. Early on during the course of the operative procedure, the edges of the abdominal incision should be protected with impermeable, impervious wound protection. The uncontaminated peritoneal cavity should be walled off with laparotomy pads and, where possible, the intestinal lumen should be occluded proximally and distally to a fistula with noncrushing intestinal clamps before severing the fistulous tract. Finally, at the time of severance of the fistula, the surgeon must be ready to contain spillage by proper use of the suction.

Gastroduodenal-Enteric Fistulas

Although the stomach and duodenum are rarely primarily affected by Crohn's disease, they may be involved in fistula formation owing to their proximity to the terminal ileum and colon. In primary Crohn's disease, fistulas originating from a diseased terminal ileum or ascending colon drain into the duodenum and fistulas originating from a diseased transverse colon drain into the stomach. In recurrent Crohn's disease, fistulas forming from a previous ileocolonic anastomosis may drain into either the duodenum or the stomach, depending on the location of the anastomosis in the abdomen.

Gastroduodenal-enteric fistulas are rare, with fewer than 100 of these complications reported in the English literature (3–7).

Gastroduodenal-enteric fistulas are treated with resection of the primary disease, extirpation of the fistula, and closure of the gastroduodenal defect (8–10). Although this can usually be accomplished when the stomach is involved, it may prove a challenge if the fistula drains into the duodenum. When the duodenal defect is close to the pancreatic border, the surgeon must perform meticulous dissection to mobilize healthy duodenal wall away from the pancreas. In these cases, to reinforce a difficult primary closure, an omental patch or a peritoneal patch can be used. Additionally, to protect the duodenal closure, a decompressing tube with multiple holes may be inserted through the stomach all the way to the fourth portion of the duodenum and left to intermittent low suction in the immediate postoperative period (Fig. 26.1). Conversely, when the duodenal wall is edematous and friable, or when the duodenal defect is large, a primary closure cannot be safely performed. In these cases, a side-to-side or Roux-en-Y duodeno-jejunostomy is recommended (Fig. 26.2A and B).

Enteroenteric Fistulas

Since enteroenteric fistula often cause no symptoms, up to two thirds of these are discovered only during surgical exploration or examination of the resected specimen (1). The mere presence of such a fistula does not necessitate surgery (11). Surgical intervention should be reserved for fistulas causing massive diarrhea and/or malabsorption due to bypass of a large intestinal segment, or associated with sepsis or intestinal obstruction.

Surgical treatment of enteroenteric fistulas usually comprises en-bloc resection of the fistula along with the diseased segment of intestine. If this procedure would remove too long a segment of healthy intestine, the surgeon should try to separate the normal-appearing loops from the diseased area. After separation of the fistula, the edges of the defect are debrided to healthy intestinal wall in preparation for closure of the defect.

Ileocolonic Fistulas

The most common ileocolonic fistulas are those that connect the terminal ileum with the cecum or the right colon. Although a surgical procedure is never indicated simply to resect ileocecal and ileo-right colonic fistulas, these fistulas are usually

Fig. 26.1. Use of a transduodenal decompressing drain after primary closure of a duodenal defect.

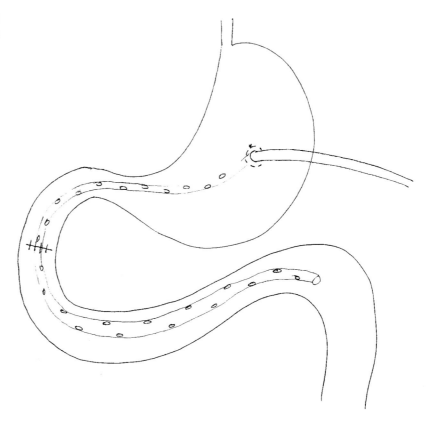

markers of severe Crohn's disease that may require surgical treatment. These fistulas are best removed *en bloc* with the involved segment of intestine.

Ileosigmoid-Rectal Fistulas

Ileosigmoid-rectal fistulas usually originate from a diseased terminal ileum and drain into the sigmoid, or less often, into the rectum. The rectosigmoid is typically not affected with Crohn's disease. Although resection of both terminal ileum and sigmoid has been recommended (12), the edges of the fistula can be debrided and the defect in the sigmoid wall usually closed primarily. Resection of the rectosigmoid is needed if the colon is affected by primary Crohn's disease or if there are technical difficulties in accomplishing a primary closure due to inflammation, thickening and rigidity of the intestinal wall, presence of a large defect after debridement, or due to the location of the fistulous opening near the mesenteric side of the rectosigmoid. If a stoma is necessary to divert the fecal stream away from the rectosigmoid closure, the neoterminal ileum can be exteriorized as an end-ileostomy rather than anastomosed to the colon after resection of the diseased segment. The colonic end can be safely closed and repositioned intraabdominally. Closure of the ileostomy is usually performed two to six months later depending on the amount of pelvic inflammation, the recovery of the patient and the radiologic confirmation of a healed rectosigmoid closure via retrograde contrast enema. In the cases when the rectosigmoid closure is so tenuous as to dictate the need for a temporary diverting stoma, closed-suction drains should be placed near the closure to allow for drainage of fecal spillage from a possible dehiscence.

Enterocutaneous Fistula

Enterocutaneous fistulas result from drainage of intraabdominal disease through the abdominal wall. Fistulas may drain spontaneously (usually through old scars, such as previous incisions or the umbilicus (13,14) or may be formed when an intraabdominal abscess is drained percutaneously.

Many enterocutaneous fistulas do not need to be treated surgically if the drainage is minor and the disease is well controlled. In some cases, the cutaneous drainage site is near an established stoma and can be incorporated into the ostomy appliance. Yet, surgical repair is needed when the underlying Crohn's disease is severe and unresponsive to medical treatment, and when the drainage is cause of social embarrassment, poor hygiene, se-

358 F. Michelassi

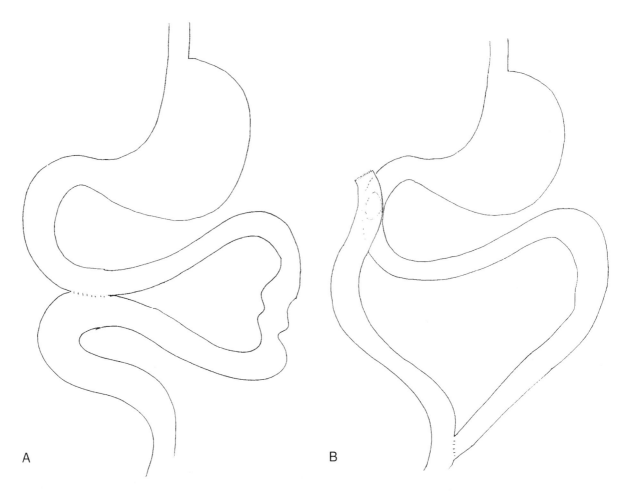

Fig. 26.2. Side-to-side (A) or Roux-en-Y (B) duodenojejunostomy in the closure of a large duodenal defect.

vere skin excoriation or recurrent painful sub-cutaneous abscesses.

An enterocutaneous fistula is treated by resect-ing the diseased intestinal segment, removing the fistula, and debriding the fistulous tract through the abdominal wall and subcutaneous tissue. Several subcutaneous fistulotomies may be needed to effect complete drainage and they should be left to heal by secondary intention. If the fistula origi-nated from recurrent disease in a permanent end ileostomy, resiting of the stoma to a different ab-dominal quadrant may be necessary to avoid inter-ference of the subcutaneous fistulotomies with the stoma appliance.

Enterogenital Fistulas

Women with enterovaginal fistulas experience va-ginal discharge and discomfort that contribute to social and sexual embarrassment and personal hygiene problems. Rare complications of Crohn's disease (15), enterovaginal fistulas typically de-velop after hysterectomy. Because they suffer con-siderable distress, many women with enterovaginal fistula not only agree to operation but often ac-tively request surgical intervention.

An enterovaginal fistula is managed surgically by resection of the diseased portion of bowel, extirpa-tion or debridement of the fistulous tract, and drainage of any intervening abscess. Since the opening into the vaginal cuff is typically small and located in the center of an area of induration and inflammation, it does not need to be sutured and invariably closes by secondary intention.

Enterosalpingeal and enterouterine fistulas are extremely rare. In these cases, the affected tube or the uterus is removed along with the fistula and the diseased intestinal segment. The uterus may be left in place in the female operated on during childbearing years.

Enterovesical Fistulas

Fistulas develop between the gut and the urinary tract in 2% to 5% of patients with Crohn's disease

(16–18). Enterovesical fistulas predispose to recurrent urinary tract infections, which cause urgency, frequency, dysuria, suprapubic discomfort, stranguray, and occasionally bloody urine. Symptoms may include recurrent urinary tract infections, pneumaturia and less frequently, fecaluria.

The potential for severe renal dysfunction secondary to chronic urinary tract infections makes surgical intervention essential even when the symptoms of urinary tract infections are controlled by antibiotics and urinary antiseptics. Surgical correction for enterovesical fistulas is based on similar principles as for other types of fistulas. The diseased bowel segment is removed along with the fistulous tract. The fistula usually opens in the dome of the bladder; this location facilitates debridement and primary closure of the bladder without risking injury to the trigone. Intraoperatively, a closed suction drain is placed near the bladder closure to drain any urine that may extravasate and an indwelling catheter is left in the bladder for urinary drainage. The bladder catheter and the closed-suction drain are removed 5 to 7 days postoperatively after radiographic confirmation of suture line healing via a retrograde cystogram. If a dehiscence is present, the drain and the urinary catheter are left in place to facilitate the healing of the dehiscence and the drainage of any extravasated urine. Careful monitoring of the daily amount of drainage from the closed-suction drain helps in assessing the progress of healing of the dehiscence. In addition, blood urea, nitrogen, and creatinine levels in the fluid off the drain are elevated if a dehiscence is present, but return to normal (i.e., equal to serum's) when the dehiscence heals. These tests, easily obtained in the outpatient setting, help determine the optimal timing for a repeated retrograde cystogram to confirm complete healing of the bladder repair before removal of the closed-suction drain and the urinary catheter.

Conclusions

Fistulas arc common complications of Crohn's disease but they are rarely the primary indication for surgical intervention. The appropriate surgical management of intraabdominal fistulas follows the principle of resection of the primary disease with extirpation of the fistula. Adherence to important steps designed to contain contamination of the abdominal wound and peritoneal cavity minimizes postoperative septic complications.

References

1. Michelassi F, Stella M, Balestracci T, et al. Incidence, diagnosis and treatment of enteric and colorectal fistulas in patients with Crohn's disease. Ann Surg 1993;218:660.

2. Crohn BB. Regional ileitis. New York, Grune & Stratton, 1949.

3. Spirt M, Sachar DB, Greenstein AJ. Symptomatic differentiation of duodenal from gastric fistulas in Crohn's disease. Am J Gastroenterol 1990;84:455.

4. Lee KKW, Schraut WH. Diagnosis and treatment of duodenoenteric fistulas complicating Crohn's disease. Arch Surg 1989;124:712.

5. Thompson WM, Cockrill H Jr, Rick RP. Regional enteritis of the duodenum. AJR 1975;123:252.

6. Fitzgibbons TJ, Green G, Silberman H, et al. Management of Crohn's disease involving the duodenum, including duodenal cutaneous fistula. Arch Surg 1980;115:1022.

7. Glass RE, Ritchie JK, Lennard-Jones JE, et al. Internal fistulas in Crohn's disease. Dis Colon Rectum 1985;28:557.

8. Goldwasser B, Mazor A, Wiznitzer T. Enteroduodenal fistula in Crohn's disease. Dis Colon Rectum 1981;24:485.

9. Wilk PJ, Fazio V, Turnbull RB Jr. The dilemma of Crohn's disease: ileoduodenal fistula complicating Crohn's disease. Dis Colon Rectum 1977;20:387.

10. Smith TR, Goldin RR. Radiographic and clinic sequelae of the duodenocolic anatomic relationship: two cases of Crohn's disease with fistulization to the duodenum. Dis Colon Rectum 1997;20:257.

11. Broe PH, Bayless TM, Cameron JL. Crohn's disease: are enteroenteral fistulas an indication for surgery? Surgery 1982;91:249.

12. Fazio VW, Wilk P, Turnbull RB Jr, et al. The dilemma of Crohn's disease: ileosigmoid fistula complicating Crohn's disease. Dis Colon Rectum 1977;20:381.

13. Jensen JA, McClenathan JH. Umbilical fistulas in Crohn's disease. Surg Gynecol Obstet 1987;164:445.

14. Veloso FT, Bardoso V, Fraga J, et al. Spontaneous umbilical fistula in Crohn's disease. J Clin Gastroenterol 1989;11:197.

15. Heyen F, Winslet MC, Andrews J, et al. Vaginal fistulas in Crohn's disease. Dis Colon Rectum 1989;32:379.

16. Crohn BB, Yarnis H. Regional enteritis. 2nd ed. New York, Grune & Stratton, 1958.

17. Talamini MA, Broe TJ, Cameron JL. Urinary fistulas in Crohn's disease. Surg Gynecol Obstet 1982;154:553.

18. Kyle J, Murray CM. Ileovesical fistula in Crohn's disease. Surgery 1969;66;497.

27 Intraabdominal Mass and/or Abscess

Ronald J. Nicholls

Intraabdominal Mass

The majority of patients suffering from Crohn's disease undergo surgery for complications of their disease. Failure of medical management to resolve a persisting abdominal mass is a common indication for surgery (1). More than 25% of all patients undergoing surgery for Crohn's disease will have either an intraabdominal mass or abscess (2). An abdominal mass may be the main indication for surgery but it often accompanies other complications of the disease such as obstruction or fistula formation. Approximately 40% of patients with an intraabdominal mass have a fistula associated with the mass, usually originating from small bowel disease. The decision to perform surgery is often made after prolonged medical treatment. It is undertaken to relieve symptoms of obstruction and sepsis to rid the patient of malaise and malnutrition.

An intraabdominal mass may be due to loops of dilated bowel proximal to a stricture, a length of bowel thickened by active disease, a phlegmon of inflamed bowel with associated enteric fistula, and lastly a frank abscess. Omentum adherent to diseased bowel or the walls of an abscess may be responsible for the bulk of the mass. Clinical assessment of the degree of intraabdominal sepsis or obstruction will direct initial investigations.

Investigation

In the presence of unresolving obstruction or sepsis, plain abdominal radiography may demonstrate signs of complete intestinal obstruction. Gastrointestinal contrast radiology may demonstrate partial obstruction, diseased bowel, or fistulation at the site of the mass. Ultrasound examination may show an intraabdominal abscess. It may also delineate a single length of diseased or obstructed bowel. CT scanning and MRI may be useful in elucidating masses not readily identifiable by ultrasound. However, these expensive investigations should be used only in the light of the clinical picture and information from ultrasound and usually are superfluous to decision taking. The use of a radiolabeled leukocyte scan may distinguish matted loops of inflamed bowel from an abscess by the earlier uptake and clearance of white cells from inflamed bowel compared with late uptake by an abscess (Fig. 27.1).

Contrast radiology may indicate the presence of an enteroenteric fistula. These are not in themselves an indication for surgery but in the presence of other complications such as obstruction or sepsis, surgery is indicated. Where a mass is due to a phlegmon of diseased bowel the amount of pus is usually small; this will not generally diminish the need for eventual surgery.

Clinical Pathology

An intraabdominal mass caused by a substantial abscess is relatively uncommon compared with a mass due to a phlegmon or loops of adherent or obstructed bowel (Fig. 27.2). Abscesses result from local perforation due to progression of transmural inflammation and fissuring through the serosa. The characteristic deep fissuring leading to penetration of the bowel wall very occasionally leads to acute perforation. Usually, however, the process of transmural inflammation is gradual, leading to adhesion formation between the adjacent serosa and

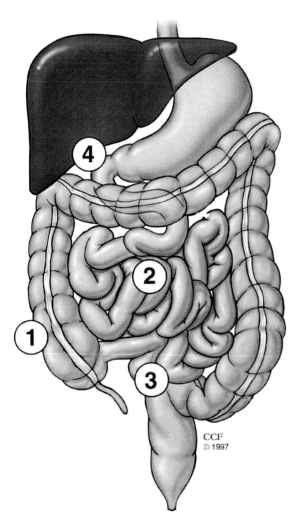

Fig. 27.1. Most common sites for intraabdominal abscesses in Crohn's disease (1) Paracaecal/right iliac fossa (2) interloop abscess (3) pelvic (4) subhepatic.

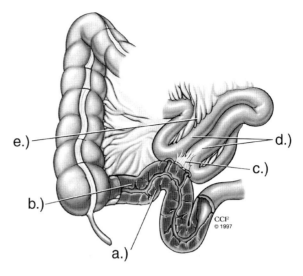

Fig. 27.2. Complex abdominal mass demonstrating (a) thickened ileal wall with (b) fissuring and (c) interloop abscess. Other loops of ileum (d) are drawn into the mass. Note fat wrapping (e).

surrounding structures. Perforation is thus contained, leading to the development of a localized abscess. This may subsequently penetrate the adjacent organ, including the skin, leading to a fistula. Abscesses in Crohn's disease were once thought to be small and contain much granulation tissue and rarely with caseating material rather than large amounts of free pus (3). However, it is now clear that they may be substantial and contain large amounts of pus.

The presence of fever, chills, and a leukocytois may be masked by medical treatment with steroids and antibiotics and this should be borne in mind when the surgeon is presented with an acutely unwell patient with established Crohn's disease. The presence of an abscess should be considered in patients with a severe symptomatic relapse of

Crohn's disease, especially those not responsive to steroid therapy. Up to 30% of such patients may have abscesses (4).

Although medical treatment of partial obstruction or phlegmon may be justified if symptoms are thought to be due to an acute exacerbation, any associated abscess must be treated surgically to prevent the development of more widespread sepsis by local extension into other tissue planes or rarely by perforation into the peritoneal cavity. Once an abscess is established symptoms will not resolve until pus is drained.

Retroperitoneal Abscess

Crohn's disease developing in parts of the intestine not fully invested in peritoneal covering may give rise to a retroperitoneal abscess. Thus, local perforation of the ascending and descending colon and, rarely, the retroperitoneal part of the duodenum may result in a retroperitoneal abscess. Anorectal abscess related to Crohn's disease is considered in Chapter 32.

Psoas abscess from the local perforation of ileocecal Crohn's disease is the most common example of retroperitoneal abscess and is now the most common cause of psoas abscess in the developed world (5). Most of these cases are due to terminal ileal disease. Retroperitoneal abscesses may present in a wide variety of ways depending on the progression of sepsis and anatomical site of perforation. Pointing or spontaneous rupture may occur in the groin, the flank, or lumbar region. In the case of psoas abscess, a septic arthritis of the hip can develop. Symptoms often precede signs, with pain in the hip or sacrum occurring before obvious sepsis or other clinical findings. Pus tracking down the obturator fascia may lead to a gluteal abscess (6) and upper abdominal abscesses may arise from duodenal disease.

Intraperitoneal Abscess

Reports of the incidence of intraabdominal abscess in Crohn's disease vary from 9% to 28% (2,7). In a prospective study by Weldon et al. of patients undergoing investigation for abdominal abscess, 50% of patients had inflammatory bowel disease and 38% of patients developed abdominal abscesses spontaneously, secondary to their Crohn's disease. This is similar to the finding of Ayuk et al. (8) who identified 21% of Crohn's patients who developed spontaneous intraabdominal abscesses. The presenting clinical features of such an abscess are pain, fever, and a palpable mass. The abscess may have loops of bowel adherent to it that can lead to obstruction. The location of the abscess is determined by the site of intestinal disease. The commonest is the right iliac fossa due to the chronic perforation of terminal ileal disease (Fig. 27.3). An abscess, however, may occur at any site in the abdomen but is more common where enteric fistulae arise such as those between loops of terminal ileum, between terminal ileum and sigmoid colon, or where the ileum has fistulized into the sig-

Table 27.1. Abscess site in patients with Crohn's disease.*

Abscess site	Spontaneous	Postoperative
Right lower quadrant	21	3
Pelvis	8	4
Left lower quadrant	3	1
Left upper quadrant	2	0
Subhepatic	0	1
Subphrenic	1	1
Psoas	2	0
Other	3	4
Total	40	14

*From Ayuk et al. 1996 (8).

moid or upper rectum. Collections may develop in any of the potential spaces of the peritoneal cavity but tend to be localized by the adjacent inflamed structures. Rarely, they may develop between the leaves of the mesentery. The abscess may rupture into adjacent organs or into the retroperitoneum or pelvis, resulting in fistula between the bowel and structures such as bladder or vagina. Other fistulae are reported from abscesses arising adjacent to spleen and ureter. In addition, unexplained sterile abscesses are sometimes found in Crohn's disease not obviously related to adjacent inflamed bowel (9).

Extraintestinal air seen on plain abdominal film is diagnostic of an intraabdominal abscess. Perforation with free peritoneal air is seen in 2% to 3% of cases (10) that may occur as direct penetration of the bowel wall from ulceration, fissuring or necrosis, or the rupture of a chronic intraabdominal abscess. Perforation may also occur in otherwise normal bowel proximal to an obstructed segment. Perforation of the colon is very rare, except in toxic megacolon when perforations tend to be small and multiple. Pericolic abscesses are seen in the elderly in whom a second peak incidence of Crohn's disease coincides with preexisting diverticular disease (11,12).

Abscesses may also occur as a postoperative complication. Preoperative contamination or subsequent anastomotic leakage into the peritoneal cavity may result in peritonitis, the development of an enterocutaneous fistula or collections in the pelvis or subphrenic space. Large collections may be surrounded by loops of small bowel that are bound together by dense adhesions though perhaps surprisingly, fistulating Crohn's disease leading to anastomotic leakage tends to present as an early enterocutaneous fistula through the abdominal wound rather than as an intraperitoneal abscess.

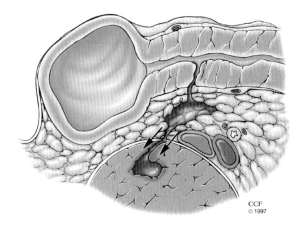

Fig. 27.3. Cross-section of right iliac fossa to demonstrate paracaecal abscess and psoas abscess. Note close proximity of ureter which may be involved in the inflammatory mass. (After Keighley & Williams, eds. Surgery of the Anus, Rectum, and Colon. WB Saunders, London, 1993).

Ultrasound is an extremely useful method of screening patients in whom an abscess is suspected clinically. It is a quick, cheap tool for the identification of collections of intraabdominal fluid and may be performed at the bedside of critically ill patients if they are too ill to be transported safely to the radiology department. Ultrasound may be more difficult in the postoperative patient owing to the site of abdominal wounds and intraabdominal air. When localization is possible, it may be technically difficult to distinguish abscesses from other fluid filled collections such as hematoma.

In a retrospective study of 220 patients, Taylor et al. (13) demonstrated that it is possible to locate collections in the pelvis or abdomen in over 90% of cases with a specificity of over 98%. More recently, in a prospective study of 50 patients comparing ultrasound with radioisotope scans in the detection of intraabdominal abscesses, Weldon et al. (14) demonstrated ultrasound to have a 71% sensitivity and 87% specificity. Radiolabeled leukocyte scans were more accurate (76% sensitive and 100% specific). Both studies emphasize that ultrasound should be the first investigation of choice in a patient in whom intraabdominal sepsis is suspected. If the results are equivocal or inconsistent with clinical findings the further investigation with CT or radiolabeled leukocyte scans should be performed. Leukocyte scans are not useful if a significant white cell infiltrate is not suspected, and is particularly appropriate to identify the source of chronic, low-grade infection.

Computerized tomography (CT) is more accurate than ustrasound (US) in the early detection of intraabdominal abscesses and is the investigation of choice for retroperitoneal lesions (15). A retrospective study of 170 patients using US, CT, and radiolabeled leukocyte scans (LS) by Knochel et al. (16) demonstrated a diagnostic accuracy of 96% for CT, 90% for ultrasound, and 92% for Indium labelled LS. CT offers an advantage over ultrasound in the retroperitoneum, the diagnosis of fluid collections lying between loops of bowel or in a patient with an ileus. Both CT and US may have difficulty in determining the fluid nature of suspected collections and in these circumstances a diagnostic fluid aspiration may be performed to identify the nature of the collection.

Percutaneous Drainage

Antibiotic therapy may have been employed as part of medical treatment of an inflammatory mass but if a significant collection is demonstrated this should be drained. Traditionally, the majority of abscesses associated with Crohn's disease have been drained surgically. However, improved radiological techniques have resulted in the increased use of percutaneous drainage. This approach allows the patient to recover from acute sepsis and is a useful temporizing measure, facilitating an improvement in the general condition before definitive surgery is undertaken at a later date to remove the diseased bowel. Initial percutaneous drainage (PD) may reduce or eliminate the need for a two or three stage procedure to be performed at subsequent surgery, allowing instead definitive surgery and reanastomosis. A percutaneous approach may avoid the morbidity and mortality of surgical drainage that may be as high as 15% and 4% respectively (17,18).

Diagnostic Fluid Aspiration

The procedure of percutaneous diagnostic aspiration requires only a small sterile needle and local anesthesia. It is most conveniently performed under ultrasound guidance. Selection of the appropriate access route is a critical issue. In contrast to the biopsy of a solid tumor, it is imperative not to transgress the bowel lumen, even with a narrow gauge needle, en route to a collection of unknown fluid collection. An uninfected collection such as hematoma may thus become infected and result in an abscess. Aspiration may yield enough fluid for analysis and if pus is thick or fluid cannot be withdrawn then a larger needle or catheter may be inserted.

Technique of Percutaneous Abscess Drainage

To achieve optimum drainage, a guide wire is inserted via the needle into the abscess cavity under radiological guidance. The track is then progressively dilated until a suitably large drain can be inserted. Catheters may be introduced either by the Seldinger technique or by a single puncture technique by which a catheter is advanced over a trocar.

Obtaining adequate access for drainage of abscesses in the true pelvis can be difficult; only a minority can be drained using the anterior approach. For those patients in whom an anterior approach is not possible, drainage may be achieved per rectum or vagina, or via a transgluteal approach (Fig. 27.4).

The procedure is carried out by the radiologist with local anesthesia under US or CT guidance and is particularly appropriate in the very sick patient. Once the diagnosis of an intraabdominal abscess has been made the patient can be started on

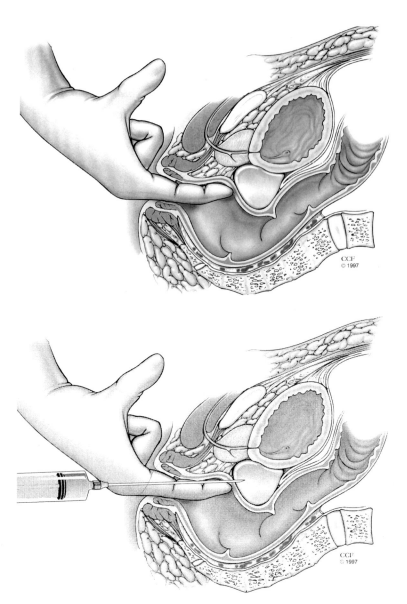

Fig. 27.4. Pelvic abscess may be palpable per rectum and drained per rectum or per vaginam using a large bore needle. If necessary, ultrasound imaging allows deeper less accessible abscesses to be drained, either directly with a needle or by inserting a catheter.

intravenous (IV) antibiotics and intravenous fluids. Antibiotic therapy should cover gram negative and anaerobic bacteria and should be continued for 24 hours after the procedure.

Pelvic abscesses may be drained transrectally, if amenable via, transrectal US control (19). Transrectal, transvaginal, or transgluteal routes may be used, with up to eighty-five percent success rates.

Pitfalls and Danger Points

Although percutaneous drainage of large collections may be technically possible in the majority of cases, accurate localization of the collection may be difficult. Ultrasound may fail to diagnose abscesses because of overlying gas filled bowel and small col-

lections may not be visible on CT. The success of drainage is limited by the anatomic site of the abscess. Adequate drainage cannot be achieved if access to the abscess is limited by adjacent structures such as overlying bowel or retroperitoneal organs (Fig. 27.5). Enterocutaneous fistulae may develop from the site of drainage. This is particularly likely if drainage is achieved by the insertion of a drain into the cavity and if the abscess is associated with an enteric fistula.

Despite apparent adequate percutaneous drainage abscesses may re-collect, especially if the abscess is associated with an enteric fistula. Further attempts at drainage are feasible but if permanent drainage is not achieved or sepsis inadequately controlled, operative drainage is indicated.

Fig. 27.5. CT scan of a pelvic abscess surrounded by loops of bowel in a woman of 23 years. Cross-section of pelvis showing mass of thickened small bowel loops surrounding abscess. Calcified material in center of abscess.

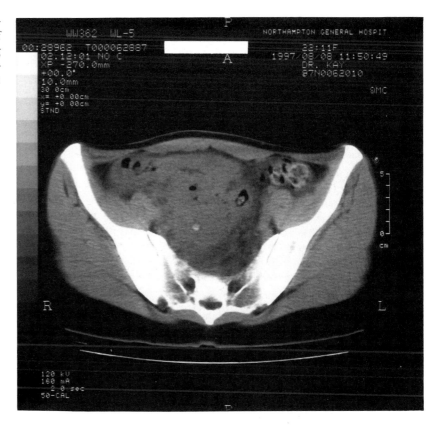

In the acutely septic patient with an intraabdominal abscess, aspiration is likely to offer only temporary relief. If immediate improvement does not occur surgery is indicated to eradicate sepsis. A percutaneous tube placed to facilitate further drainage is likely to result in a fistula, requiring definitive surgical treatment at a later date. Not using a drain may avoid this complication but may also compromise the amount of pus drained from the cavity and may make sepsis harder to control. Crohn's abscesses may contain little frank pus and adequate drainage of infected granulation tissue and caseous material may not be possible without the insertion of a drain.

Surgical Drainage

Although percutaneous drainage may give useful time for a patient to recover from acute illness and sepsis, definitive treatment of a diseased bowel segment is only possible by surgery. The aim of surgery is to eradicate sepsis, to resect the minimum length of diseased bowel consistent with effecting a satisfactory outcome, and to restore intestinal continuity where possible (Fig. 27.6). Ideally, drainage of the abscess and resection of the involved intestine should be undertaken in one stage because it may be technically easier than a two stage pro-

cedure and hopefully a definitive solution will be achieved in one operation. Surgical drainage of an abscess cavity may be a life-saving maneuver in the desperately sick patient but is likely to result in fistula formation. Definitive surgery will need to be performed subsequently to resect the diseased segment of bowel associated with the abscess. This second surgery can be impaired by dense adhesions and the risk of causing further fistulae from enterotomies incurred during the laparotomy.

A phlegmon of diseased intestine may consist of several segments of bowel densely adherent to an abscess wall. Multiple fistulae from various segments of bowel entering the abscess may be encountered, the whole forming the intraabdominal mass. Resection of this mass is likely to be treated by the resection en bloc of the diseased segments of bowel. When this approach might lead to excessive sacrifice of healthy, uninvolved intestine, the normal loops of bowel need to be carefully dissected free from diseased segments, being careful to minimize contamination of the operative field from transected fistulae or interloop abscesses that often form part of the inflammatory mass. This may be particularly difficult if thickened mesentery is involved in the abscess. As in all cases of surgery for Crohn's disease, the utmost care must be taken to preserve the maximum length of bowel, without

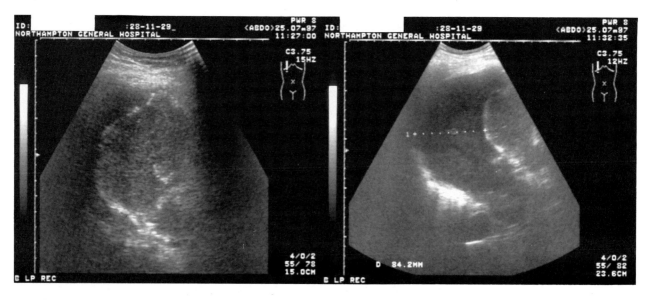

Fig. 27.6.   Postoperative subhepatic collection in a 68-year-old man following surgical resection of small bowel. This was drained successfully percutaneously without need for further treatment.

compromising blood supply. The abscess cavity should be curetted and the cavity packed with omentum if this is technically feasible.

In the presence of substantial intraabdominal sepsis or if multiple segments of gut have to be resected, a protective stoma above the anastomoses should be considered (Fig. 27.7). A stoma may be appropriate if surgery has to be performed on unprepared bowel, or if obstruction makes bowel preparation impossible.

Drainage of the peritoneal cavity is controversial, since the drain may predispose to fistulation itself. However, if extensive debridement has been performed or there is any residual site of sepsis e.g., an abscess cavity in the pelvis, a soft drain for 48 hours may be appropriate, brought out through a separate incision and with as short an intraabdominal course as possible. The use of parenteral feeding is also controversial; patients who are nutritionally compromised and in whom it is thought

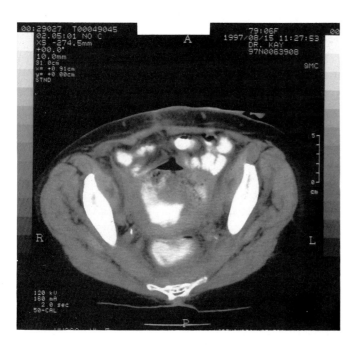

Fig. 27.7.   Abscess in lower abdomen surrounding loops of thickened bowel. This complex mass of bowel and abscess was surgically resected and a primary anastomosis performed from ileum to ascending colon.

are unlikely to resume enteral feeding soon after surgery will benefit from IV nutrition. There is no evidence for the benefit of routine parenteral nutrition malnourished patients undergoing surgery.

Pitfalls and Danger Points

The aim of preserving as great a length of normal intestine as possible has already been alluded to. The anatomy is likely to be distorted by an extensive abscess cavity and care has to be taken not to damage adjacent structures. The ureters are especially vulnerable by being drawn up into dense fibrous tissue associated with a phlegmon; indeed the ureter may be found to be obstructed by the mass and will need to be carefully dissected out where it is impinged upon by the abscess. Gonadal vessels and fallopian tubes may also be drawn into the mass. The use of ureteric stents or preoperative intravenous urography (IVU) to help define anatomy is advocated by some but it is our view that these measures do not substantially reduce the risk of injury provided careful surgical technique is employed.

Results

Various studies over the last decade have compared the drainage of intraabdominal abscesses by percutaneous and open surgical techniques.

In a retrospective review Ayuk et al. (8), reviewed 192 patients with Crohn's disease presenting over 5 years in whom 54 abscesses were identified in 40 patients. Six abscesses arose as postoperative complications and of these three were managed successfully by percutaneous drainage PD. A further eight abscesses that arose spontaneously were treated with PD of which three had a successful outcome; success was rigorously defined as no further sepsis or fistula formation for at least six months. In two cases a temporizing effect was achieved, downgrading the degree of sepsis and subsequently allowing a definitive one-stage surgical procedure to be undertaken. The remaining cases required surgical treatment in two or three stage procedures. No enterocutaneous fistulae developed in the percutaneously drained patients. A retrospective case-controlled study by Olak et al. (20) compared the outcome of 27 patients with intraabdominal abscesses of various etiology treated with PD versus those treated with surgical drainage. The majority of these patients (*n* = 22) suffered postoperative abscesses (82%) and only two (7%) had Crohn's disease. Age, acute physiology score, site of abscess and etiology was carefully

matched between groups. Nineteen patients (70%) were treated successfully with PD, needing no further intervention. There were eight (30%) failures with failure to control sepsis requiring further surgery. In addition, three (11%) developed enterocutaneous fistulae that required further surgery. The patients in the surgically drained group (*n* = 27) had no significantly different morbidity from the percutaneously treated group, with four patients (14%) developing early recurrence of sepsis and one who developed a fistula requiring surgical treatment. Surgery was restricted to simple drainage of the abscess. In a very similar study by Hemming et al. (21) the same findings were made with no difference in mortality or morbidity between patients treated with percutaneous or surgical drainage. In a subgroup of patients with spontaneous abscess arising in diverticular disease, which perhaps most closely resembles the etiology of abscess in Crohn's disease, the authors found that percutaneous drainage allowed later definitive surgery and primary anastomosis.

Doemeny (22) describes a series of nine patients with intraabdominal abscesses arising in patients suffering from Crohn's disease who were treated by percutaneous drainage. Patients presented with sepsis from abscesses in the right paracolic gutter, the pelvis, between loops of small bowel and the subhepatic space. In seven patients abscesses had risen following surgery to resect affected bowel and percutaneous drainage was successful in five, who required no further surgery. Two patients required further surgery to excise a persistent enteric fistula. The two patients who presented with a spontaneous abscess had their sepsis successfully controlled initially by PD but both required subsequent surgery. Percutaneous drainage was not curative in patients in whom a fistula was demonstrated radiologically.

In Ayuk's study (8), the surgical drainage alone of spontaneous intraabdominal abscesses resulted in enterocutaneous fistulae in all cases (*n* = 5). These later went on to have definitive surgery. Fifteen patients underwent surgical drainage and definitive surgery as a one stage procedure of which 14 cases (93%) were successful. A further 15 cases were managed as two stage procedures that were successful in nine (60%). The remaining patients suffered recurrent sepsis. It is not clear in this retrospective study which factors determined a single stage or two stage approach.

The successful treatment of postoperative abscesses by percutaneous drainage is well described and it is logical to adopt this approach initially as further laparotomy may be avoided. The use of PD as a primary treatment of abscesses arising spontaneously in patients with Crohn's disease is less likely to be successful, especially if there is an associated enteric fistula. However, the use of a technique that requires only local anaesthesia may be beneficial in controlling sepsis and improving the patients general condition before undertaking definitive surgery.

References

1. Michelassi F, Stella M. Balestracci T, Giulante F, Marogna P, Block G. Incidence, diagnosis and treatment of enteric and colorectal fistulae in patients with Crohn's disease. Ann Surg 1993;218:660–6.

2. Nagler and Poticha. Intraabdominal abscess in Crohn's disease. Am J Surg 1979;137:350–4.

3. Crohn BB, Ginzburg L, Oppenheimer GD. Regional ileitis. JAMA 1932; 99: 1325.

4. Wheller JG, Slack NF, Duncan A, Whitehead PJ, et al. The diagnosis of intraabdominal abscesses in patients with severe Crohn's disease. Quart J Med 1992;82:159–67.

5. Walsh TR, Reilly JR, Hanley E, Webster M, Peitzman A, Steed DL. Changing etiology of psoas abscess. Am J Surg 1995;163:413–6.

6. Mayer DA, Zingale RG. Gluteal abscess due to Crohn's disease. Ostomy Manag 1994;39:30–4.

7. Steinberg DM. Abscesses and fistulae in Crohn's disease. Gut 1973;14:865.

8. Ayuk P, Williams N, Scott NA, Nicholson DA, Irving MH. Management of intra-abdominal abscesses in Crohn's disease. Ann Roy Coll Surg Engl 1996;78:5–10.

9. Andre M, Amaitre O, Marchez JC, Piette JC. Unexplained sterile abscesses in Crohn's disease. Am J Gastroenterol 1995;90:1183–4.

10. Kyle J, Cardin T, Dungan T, Ewen SWB. Free perforation in regional enteritis. Am J Dig Dis 1968;13:275.

11. Meyers MA, Alonso DR, Morson BC. Pathogenesis of diverticulitis complicating granulomatous colitis. Gastroenterology 1978;74:24.

12. Schmidt GT, Lennard Jones, JE, Morson BC et al. Crohn's disease of the colon and its distinction from diverticulitis. Gut 1968;9:7.

13. Taylor KJW, Sullivan DC, Watson JF, Rosenfield HT. Ultrasonography and gallium scanning for the presence of abdominal and pelvic abscesses. Gastrointestinal Radiol 1978;3:281–6.

14. Weldon MJ, Joseph AE, French A, Saverymuttu SH. Comparison of technecium labelled leucocyte with ultrasound in the diagnosis of intraabdominal abscess. Gut 1995;37:557–64.

15. Halbe MD, Daffner RH, Morgan CL. Intraabdominal abscesses: current concepts in radiological evaluation. Am J Roenterol 1979;133:9.

16. Knochel JQ, Koehlner R, Lee TG, Welch DM. Diagnosis of abdominal abcesses with computer tomography, ultrasound and 111-leucocyte scans. Radiology 1980;137:25–31.

17. Bensoussan A, Letourneau JN, Morin CC. Surgical treatment of Crohn's disease. Can J Surg 1982; 25: 515–7.

18. Greenstein AJ, Meyers S, Sher L, Heimann T, Aufses AH. Surgery and its sequelae for Crohn's colitis and ileocolitis. Arch Surg 1981;116:285–8.

19. Kuligowska E, Keller E, Ferrucci JT. The treatment of pelvic abscesses: value of sonographically guided transrectal needle aspiration and lavage. Am J Roentgenol 1995;164:201.

20. Olak J, Christou NV, Stein LA, Casola G, Meakins JL. Operative vs percutaneous drainage of intra-abdominal abscess. Arch Surg 1986;121:141–6.

21. Hemming A, Davis NL, Robins RE. Surgical versus percutaneous drainage of intra-abdominal abscesses. Am J Surg 1991;161:593–5.

22. Doemeny JM, Burke DR, Meranze SG. Percutaneous drainage of abscesses in patients with Crohn's disease. Gastrointestinal Radiol 1988;13:237–41.

28 Free Perforation

Bernard Nordlinger and Olivier Saint-Marc

Free perforation in the case of Crohn's disease is an uncommon but severe complication. The first case of free perforation was reported in 1935 by Arnheim (1), describing the case of a 47 year-old woman with chronic diarrhea and abdominal pain, who suffered an acute exacerbation of symptoms and died. Autopsy revealed regional ileitis complicated by a perforated abscess with peritonitis. Hallingen et al. (2) described in 1937 the first case of a spontaneous perforation that was the initial symptom of Crohn's disease. Despite these early reports, free perforation appeared to be a rare condition, as by 1957 Crohn had not seen any at the Mount Sinai Hospital (3). Greenstein, in a recent review of the available literature and personal series (4), collected 99 cases of free perforation. In 1986, Katz (5) reported 33 personal cases. Altogether, the precise incidence of peritonitis in Crohn's disease remains unknown, but appears to be between 1% and 2% in surgical series (5). In a series of 650 patients treated for a complicated Crohn's disease at our institution, 22 (3.4%) suffered free perforation.

Etiology

The pathologic features of Crohn's disease predispose to the risk of abscess and fistula: transmural inflammation, ulceration, and fissuration, together with adjacent viscus adhesions form the histologic basis for the occurence of internal and external fistulas, and intraabdominal abscess, but not for free diffusion of infection to the whole peritoneal cavity (6). In 1965, Crohn reported six cases of free perforation and suggested a pathogenetic mechanism: "acute perforation can and does occur in the presence of diffuse suppurative infiltration of the mucosa, submucosa, and muscularis because the protective granulomatous reaction has not yet taken place" (7).

Site of Perforation

Most perforations occur in the diseased distal ileum. Gastroduodenal and jejunal perforations can also occur, but appear to be much less frequent. Colonic perforations appeared first to be rare, but are now thought to be responsible for almost 20% of all cases (4), and in our experience represent 50% of spontaneous perforations. Perforation can occur at any site affected by the disease, i.e., in a bypassed intestinal loop (8), or near an anastomotic site after previous surgical resection (9). Multiple synchronous perforations may also be found, especially in the case of severe pancolitis.

Mechanism of Perforation

Many theories have been proposed to explain the phenomenon of spontaneous perforation:

Stage of the disease: for Crohn (7), free perforation seemed only possible at an early stage of the disease, when the lack of parietal fibrosis, scarring, serosal involvement and adhesions facilitate its event. For some other authors, chronicity is essential to the pathogenesis of the perforation (8). Fisher advocated the role of single ulcers or fissures that do not penetrate close enough to the serosal surface to produce adhesive peritoneal inflammatory reaction (10). Free perforation was the initial symptom of Crohn's disease in about 30% of reported cases of the literature (4), 21% in our experience. The mean disease duration of 3.3 years in the Greenstein's series (11), and 5.3 years in our personal experience do not support Crohn's original theory. It is then likely that both the acute and the chronic forms of the disease can cause free perforation.

Intestinal obstruction may lead to an increased intraluminal pressure close to the stenotic lesion. This can cause perforation during an acute exacerbation of the disease (8). Independent of obstruction, when dilatation does occur, colonic distension can lead to mucosal ischemia, necrosis, and multiple perforations. Free perforation is one of the factors that increases mortality in patients with toxic megacolon (12).

Infarction and perforation could be the final result of the obliterative inflammation of intramural vessels, as suggested by Kyle (9).

Corticosteroids and immunosuppressive agents do not seem to increase the risk of free perforation and have even been advocated in the treatment of fistulous Crohn's disease (13). However, it has been suggested that steroids might promote generalized peritonitis by preventing the sealing of a perforation (14).

Perforation may also be secondary to rupture of an intraabdominal abscess, perforation of an adenocarcinoma, anastomotic olehisceuce or endoscopy.

Rupture of an intraabdominal abscess: there is a high incidence of abscess in Crohn's disease (21.2% in a recent series (11)). Free diffusion into the peritoneal cavity may occur if the abscess is not drained spontaneously into an adjacent organ or to the skin, or surgically.

Perforated adenocarcinoma (11): adenocarcinoma is a late complication in the course of Crohn's disease and can be occasionally complicated by perforation, as reported by Greenstein (4).

Postoperative peritonitis (4) may follow an anastomotic leakage, or be the consequence of a perforation distant from the anastomosis. In our experience of six patients with postoperative peritonitis, there was only one anastomotic breakdown, whereas five perforations occured far away from the anastomosis in a segment affected by Crohn's disease (one in the duodenum, four in the ileum). This can be the consequence of a surgical trauma suffered during the dissection of an inflamed intestine, of liberation of previous adhesions with a sealed microperforation, and of postoperative ileus that increases intraluminal pressure.

Iatrogenic perforation after endoscopy: the risk is low when colonoscopy is performed with a normal bowel, but appears to be increased in inflammatory bowel disease (15). Greenstein reported three patients who suffered perforation during endoscopy in a series of 1415 patients admitted to the Mount Sinai Hospital (4). Perforation usually occurs in a segment affected by the disease. We have had two cases of postcolonoscopic perforation due to the rupture of an ileosigmoid fistula and to a sigmoid perforation in a diseased segment.

Clinical Presentation and Preoperative Strategy

Intestinal perforation may be clinically difficult to distinguish from an acute exacerbation of the disease or from the formation of an intraabdominal abscess. Diffuse abdominal pain, generalized abdominal tenderness and guarding, fever, intestinal obstruction, or diarrhea are frequently observed, but remain nonspecific. Steroids and immunosuppressive agents may mask the clinical symptoms of an early diagnosis of perforation. Pneumoperitoneum is a relatively uncommon feature (20% in the Greenstein's series (16), 18% in our experience), whereas intestinal obstruction can be found more often (32% in our experience). Pneumoperitoneum appears to be more frequent in colonic perforation than in perforations of the small bowel, probably due to the larger amount of air in the large bowel lumen. When diagnosis of peritonitis remains uncertain, CT scanning and/or ultrasonography can be of value in distinguishing it from an intraabdominal abscess, and can furthermore permit percutaneous drainage. In selected cases of colonic Crohn's disease, water-soluble contrast enema can demonstrate liquid extravasation from the lumen. However, these radiological explorations should never delay explorative laparotomy, which has a place when doubt is still present, as it is essential for the effectiveness of the treatment of peritonitis to proceed with an early surgical procedure. We have no experience with laparoscopy in this indication; it should be used with caution not to precipitate general toxemia or the rupture of a localized abscess.

Surgical Procedure

Timing of Operation

Rapid resuscitation should be achieved with intravenous fluid and antibiotic administration. A stoma site must be selected preoperatively according to the proposed location of the abdominal incision and the configuration of the patient's abdomen. (See Chapter 25 for details on how to select a stoma site.) In Greenstein's series (16), surgical procedure was performed within 24 hours of perforation in all patients. In our experience, mean delay was 16 hours.

Incision

A midline incision permits the surgeon to deal safely with the generalized peritonitis. It furthermore allows a complete abdominal exploration to determine the extent of the disease and associated lesions, and to perform irrigation of the whole peritoneal cavity, and adequate drainage.

Dealing with the Perforated Intestine

In early reports, free intestinal perforations were treated by simple suture, with or without drainage, which gave poor results. Among 13 patients reported before 1970 who were so treated, four died after operation, one died after reperforation, and five needed early reoperation (8). Since the seventies, a general consensus has developed regarding surgical management of the perforation. Resection of grossly affected bowel or at least exteriorization of the perforated site has become the cornerstone of treatment (4). However, gastroduodenal perforations will be best treated without resection. Perforated gastric and duodenal Crohn's disease can be handled by suture, with or without a wedge resection of the perforated site. Jejunal perforations should be treated with a short resection. In the case of perforation of localized ileal or ileocecal disease, ileal or ileocecal resection will be performed. In the case of extensive jejunoileitis or ileocolitis, a limited intestinal resection or simple exteriorization of the perforation is preferable to extensive resection in order to avoid postoperative malabsorption. If necessary, this perforation may also be treated by diversion using a loop jejunostomy with drainage or exteriorization of the perforated intestinal segment.

When perforation is the consequence of toxic megacolon, subtotal colectomy with preservation of the distal sigmoid colon and rectum is the procedure of choice (17). There is no indication for an emergency total proctocolectomy, which has been proved to expose the patient to a higher mortality rate. In the case of postcolonoscopic perforation, the surgical procedure depends on the localization of the perforation, the extent of the underlying Crohn's disease, and on the adequacy of the bowel preparation. A suture, with or without protection, can be performed safely in selected cases, i.e., when there is minimal peritoneal contamination and the bowel is found free of inflam-

mation and appears pliable and suturable. In other cases, resection of the diseased segment or simple exteriorization when feasible should be preferred. In the case of perforated carcinoma, a resection according to oncologic principles should be carried out. Postoperative peritonitis caused by an anastomotic fistula is generally treated by resection of both anastomotic ends and exteriorization. After breakdown of an ileorectal anastomosis, Hartmann's procedure should be considered instead of simple proximal diversion, which does not completely eradicate intraabdominal sepsis. When peritonitis originates from a different site than the anastomosis, diversion of the perforated site after short resection should be done. If there is no anastomotic fistula, there is no reason to proceed with its exteriorization.

Intestinal Reconstruction: Immediate or Late?

If there is a consensus regarding the way to deal with the perforated intestine, the opportunity to restore intestinal continuity in the same operative procedure is still a matter of debate. Some authors advocate immediate anastomosis in selected cases, with or without proximal diversion, whereas others prefer delayed reconstruction (16,18). Both procedures seem to have shown good results in published cases, but immediate anastomosis cannot be generalized without risk, mainly in the case of colonic perforation, or when there is a ruptured abscess with inflamed peritoneal tissue (16). It is only in selected cases of free perforation of the jejunum or ileum, with no associated abscess, with an early surgical procedure, and when general condition is suitable, that primary reconstruction can be proposed (18). In all other cases, intestinal diversion following resection remains the "gold-standard" of the surgical procedure, as the risk of postoperative fistula or peritoneal sepsis is high after immediate anastomosis (19). After an ileal or ileocecal resection has been performed, one or both intestinal ends may be exteriorized. After subtotal colectomy, an everting Brooke terminal ileostomy will be performed in the right iliac fossa, with establishment of a sigmoid mucous fistula in the left iliac fossa or at the bottom of the midline incision; we have no experience with immediate ileorectal anastomosis protected by proximal diversion, which could be advocated in selected cases of early procedure after perforation, with minimal peritoneal contamination.

In the particular case of unsuturable gastric or duodenal perforation, the site of perforation can safely be treated by continuous intraluminal infusion and aspiration. The same procedure can be applied with perforation of the proximal jejunum, when it is not found suitable for immediate anastomosis, or when it cannot be exteriorized (19).

Wound Closure

There is now a consensus about immediate closure of the laparotomy wound. Open laparostomy used to lead to high postoperative rates of fistulas and intraabdominal abscess and has been progressively abandoned (20). The combined use of intraabdominal resorbable prostetic material, of lateral cutaneo-aponeurotic counter-incisions, and correct placement of stomas allows to close the abdomen without tension in nearly every case (21).

Postoperative Care

Intensive nutritional support and broad spectrum antibiotics should be administered in the postoperative period. Total parenteral nutrition can first be used, but intraoperative placement of a feeding jejunal tube can achieve rapid and efficient enteral nutrition in severely ill patients. Ileostomy output will be well-controlled (and noted on the patient's record) and should not exceed 800 cc per day. A high output from the stoma can rapidly lead to an acute dehydration if not recognized and treatly. It can furthermore increase difficulties in stomal care due to leakage and soreness of the peristomal skin.

Results

Overall mortality has markly decreased since simple suture of the perforation has been abandoned in favor of resection and/or exteriorization. Recent series have achieved high survival rates (5,16), whereas morbidity remains considerable, consisting mainly of wound infections, intraabdominal abscess, pulmonary embolism, acute renal failure, or intestinal fistula. The site of the perforation does not seem to have a major influence on mortality rates, although it could be speculated that higher anaerobic bacterial counts in colonic perforations could lead to increased risk. Although multiperforated Crohn's pancolitis can lead to death (5), low mortality rates contrast with those observed with perforation in ulcerative colitis (22). Delayed intestinal reconstruction is almost always possible in patients who were treated with a diversionary procedure. Time of reconstruction depends on the patient's general condition after recovery, and on the residual active Crohn's disease lesions in the distal colon, rectum and perineum. This duration in our experience is never less than 3 months, which allows complete clearance of peritoneal inflammation and therefore a safe intestinal suture. If there are residual active Crohn's disease lesions, one should consider treating them medically before reoperation.

Controversy exists regarding the existence of two different types of Crohn's disease lesions: the perforating (fistula, abscess, perforation) and the nonperforating type (23–24). The perforating type would lead to earlier perforating type recurrence and more frequent reoperation (24). One patient in the Katz's series (5) was reoperated on 6 years after the initial peritonitis for reperforation. In 14 consecutive patients with spontaneous perforation treated at our institution, 5 patients were reoperated on with a mean follow-up of 7 years, all with a perforating complication (2 enterocutaneous fistulas, 2 intraperitonal abscess, 1 peritonitis).

Conclusion

Although progress has been made in the management of free perforation (early recognition, early operation, adequate surgical procedure, postoperative intensive medical care), generalized peritonitis remains a grave event in the course of Crohn's disease. It often occurs early in the course of the disease and can even be the initial symptom. It can affect any site of the intestinal tract. It can be the evidence for a particularly aggressive form of the disease, although it is treatable with a high success rate if suspected whenever severe sudden abdominal pain occurs in a patient with Crohn's disease.

References

1. Arnheim EE. Regional ileitis with perforation abscess and peritonitis. J Mount Sinai Hosp 1935;2:61–3.
2. Halligan EJ, Halligan HJ. Acute free perforation as first sign of regional enteritis. Am J Surg 1937;37:493–7.
3. Crohn BB. Indication for surgical intervention in regional enteritis. Arch Surg 1957;74:305–11.
4. Greenstein AJ, Mann D, Sachar DB. Free perforation in Crohn's disease: I. A survey of 99 cases. Am J Gastroenterol 1985;80:682–9.
5. Katz S, Schulman N, Levin L. Free perforation in Crohn's disease: a report of 33 cases and review of literature. Am J Gastroenterol 1986;81:38–43.
6. Morson BC, Dawson IMP, Day DW, et al. Morson and Dawson's gastrointestinal pathology. 3rd ed. Oxford: Blackwell Scientific Publications, 1990:261–9.
7. Crohn BB. The pathology of acute regional ileitis. Am J Dig Dis (New Series) 1965;10:565–72.

8. Steinberg DM, Cooke WT, Alexander-Williams J. Free perforation in Crohn's disease. Gut 1973;14:187–90.

9. Kyle J, Caridis T, Duncan T, et al. Perforation in regional enteritis. Am J Dig Dis 1968;13:275–83.

10. Fisher J, Mantz F, Calkins WG. Colonic perforation in Crohn's disease. Gastroenterology 1976;71:835–8.

11. Ribeiro MB, Greenstein AJ, Yamazaki Y, et al. Intra-abdominal abscess in regional enteritis. Ann Surg 1991;213:32–6.

12. Greenstein AJ, Sachar DB, Gibas A, et al. Outcome of toxic dilatation in ulcerative and Crohn's colitis. J Clin Gastroenterol 1985;7:137–44.

13. Korelitz BI, Present DH. Favorable effect of 6-mercapto-purine on fistulae of Crohn's disease. Dig Dis Sci 1985;30:58–64.

14. Sparberg M, Kirsner JB. Long term corticosteroid therapy for regional enteritis. Am J Dig Dis 1966;11:865–80.

15. Kozarek RA, Earnest DL, Silverstein ME, et al. Air-pressure-induced colon injury during diagnostic colonoscopy. Gastroenterology 1980;78:7–14.

16. Greenstein AJ, Mann D, Heimann T, et al. Spontaneous free perforation and perforated abscess in 30 patients with Crohn's disease. Ann Surg 1987;20772–6.

17. Block GE, Moosa AR, Simonowitz D, et al. Emergency colectomy for infammatory bowel disease. Surgery 1982;91:249–53.

18. Menguy R. Surgical management of free perforation of the small intestine complicating regional enteritis. Ann Surg 1972;175:178–89.

19. Post S, Betzler M, Von Ditfurth B, et al. Risk of intestinal anastomoses in Crohn's disease. Ann Surg 1991;213:37–42.

20. Maetani S, Tobe T. Open peritoneal drainage as effective treatment of advanced peritonitis. Surgery 1981;90:805–9.

21. Levy E, Palmer DL, Frileux P, et al. Septic necrosis in the middle wound in the postoperative peritonitis. Successfull management by debridement myocutaneous advancement and primary skin closure. Ann Surg 1988;207:470–9.

22. Strauss RJ, Flint GW, Platt N, et al. The surgical management of toxic dilatation of the colon. Ann Surg 1976;184:682–8.

23. Greenstein AJ, Lachman P, Sacher DB, et al. Perforating and nonperforating indications for repeated operations in Crohn's disease: evidence for two clinical forms. Gut 1988;29:588–92.

24. McDonnald PJ, Fazio VW, Farmer RG, et al. Perforating and nonperforating Crohn's disease Dis Colon Rectum 1989;32:117–20.

29 Intestinal Hemorrhage

Adrian J. Greenstein and Tomas M. Heimann

In the seminal manuscript by Crohn, Ginsburg, and Oppenheimer in 1932 hemorrhage was not emphasized as a manifestation of "regional enteritis." The authors noted, however, that "the stools constantly contain occult blood," and "anemia which ordinarily is moderate may progress to a severe degree" (1). The following year a sequel entitled "Non-specific Granulomata of the intestine" was coauthored by Ginzburg and Oppenheimer (2). In a section on "Hypertrophic Colitis" they described 12 patients with segmental colonic disease; 5 in the cecum and ascending colon, and 7 in the region of the sigmoid, in whom overt bleeding was a prominent feature. These lesions were characterized by "large irregular ulcerated areas (geographic ulcers), bullous polypoid mucosa, thickened and edematous submucosa, and hypertrophy of serosal fat both in the colon and mesocolon," all classic features of "Crohn's disease."

Subsequent studies of larger series of patients reported incidences ranging from 7% to 60% for overt hemorrhage in Crohn's colitis (3–6). In a reexamination of the incidence of hemorrhage in Crohn's enteritis, ileocolitis, and colitis at this institution in 1975 (7) the presence of overt bleeding was found to be highly correlated with colonic and rectal involvement (Fig. 29.1). The increased incidence of overt hemorrhage in colonic disease, ten times that in small bowel disease, confirmed the original clinical impression, and explains some of the discrepancies in incidence reported in the literature.

Classification

Hemorrhage in Crohn's disease may be classified as occult or overt according to the detection of visible blood per rectum.

Occult Hemorrhage

This form of hemorrhage, detected with the hemoccult test, originates from mucosal ulcers and it occurs twice as commonly in Crohn's colitis as in ileocolitis (Fig. 29.2) (7). Rarely its source is from ulcers in the small bowel, at locations where chronic strictures have caused dilatation, stasis, and in some instances enterolithiasis. The enteroliths are usually seen in saccular dilatations proximal to or between two strictures (Fig. 29.3) where prolonged stasis promotes stone formation. The anemia associated with enteroliths appears to be more severe and refractory to iron therapy than anemia seen in patients with chronic blood loss without enteroliths. Enteroliths may induce bleeding from the already ulcerated mucosa by producing a more extensive lesion and preventing healing. This result is continuous enteric blood loss that, in turn, produces iron deficiency anemia. Because of continuous bleeding, the anemia may not be responsive to iron replacement, and in severe cases, may require transfusions. This triad of stricture, enterolith, and anemia requires surgical correction of the strictures by either strictureplasty or resection, and removal of enteroliths (8).

Fig. 29.1. This figure shows the relationship between gastrointestinal bleeding and distal colonic disease in Crohn's disease and ulcerative colitis. The incidence of hemorrhage correlates with distal disease, and is present in almost all cases of ulcerative colitis. (Modified from Greenstein AJ, Kark AE, Dreiling DA (7)).

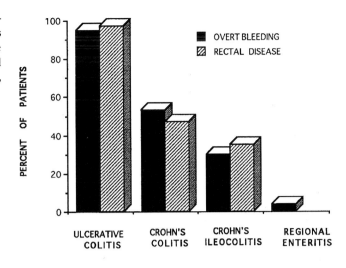

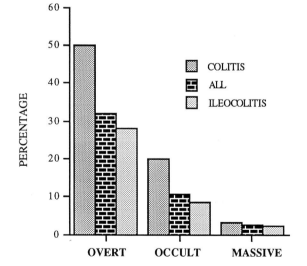

Fig. 29.2. Incidence of occult, overt, and massive hemorrhage in Crohn's disease involving the colon. Each form is more common in colitis that in ileocolitis. (Derived from data (Table 1) in Greenstein AJ, Kark AE, Dreiling DA (7)).

Overt Hemorrhage

Severe gastrointestinal hemorrhage in Crohn's disease occurs infrequently ranging from 0% to 6% in reported series (7, 9–14). It must always be born in mind that Crohn's patients may have other causes of severe hemorrhage such as peptic ulcers, diverticular disease, vascular ectasias, ischemic bowel disease, benign colonic polyps, and large bowel carcinoma. Most of these conditions may be difficult to differentiate preoperatively from Crohn's disease. Diverticular disease and ischemic colitis can be mistaken for left sided Crohn's colitis and benign colonic polyps and carcinoma may be interpreted as pseudopolyps or deep geographic ulcers in Crohn's colitis.

Avoidance of urgent surgery, with supportive therapy, has been advocated by some (15,16) because of the possibility of spontaneous cessation of bleeding (17). In our recent review (9) of 1526 patients with Crohn's disease admitted to the Mount Sinai Hospital between 1960 and 1985, 21 patients (1.3%) required treatment for acute severe gastrointestinal hemorrhage. Severe hemorrhage was defined as a lower gastrointestinal hemorrhage originating in diseased bowel and requiring at least four units of blood over an interval not exceeding two weeks. There were 4 patients with severe hemorrhage among 597 (0.7%) with regional enteritis (RE), 14 among 650 (2.2%) with ileocolitis (IC), and 3 among 279 (1.1%) with Crohn's colitis (CC). Thus the incidence of severe hemorrhage was significantly higher in patients with colonic involvement (1.9% of 929 patients), than in those with disease limited to the small bowel (0.7%), ($p < 0.001$).

The mean age of these patients was 28 years (range 18 to 48) and the mean duration of symptoms was 6 years (range seven weeks to 26 years). Severe bleeding was never the first manifestation of disease although in three patients the duration of symptoms was less than 2 months. Seventeen patients had only one bleeding episode, three had two episodes of severe hemorrhage, and one had three episodes. Although spontaneous cessation occurred in 10 of 21 patients, 3 patients (30%) had recurrent massive hemorrhage at a mean of 22 months and 2 died. This outcome contrasts both with the low frequency of recurrent hemorrhage, 1 of 11 patients (9%), and with the high survival rate, 10 of 10 patients, following primary surgical resection. These differences favor removal of diseased bowel at the time of the first episode of massive bleeding.

Making the Diagnosis

First of all, as mentioned earlier, it must be remembered that Crohn's patients may have other causes of severe hemorrhage. Nearly 30% of patients with Crohn's disease who were treated for massive intestinal hemorrhage were found to be bleeding from a peptic ulcer (9). Furthermore, even when bleeding originates in the diseased bowel, the precise source of bleeding is rarely recognized pathologically even when the diseased segment is resected and the patient does not bleed again (9). Therefore, it behooves the treating physician to attempt preoperative localization of intestinal hemorrhage to tailor the treatment to the source of hemorrhage. In all instances of acute gastrointestinal hemorrhage, a nasogastric tube is placed, and upper endoscopy is planned unless only bilious, nonbloody fluid is aspirated from the masogastric tube. Two large bore intravenous lines are placed, and a complete blood count, coagulation studies, and a blood sample for cross matching of six units of blood are sent.

If lower gastrointestinal hemorrhage is a consideration, then proctoscopy and possible colonoscopy should be performed. Often, the patient can be prepared by nasogastric or oral administration of four liters of polyethylene glycol as soon as they are admitted to the hospital. Colonoscopy can be done within two or three hours, even if plans are being made for visceral angiography or tagged red cell scan (17).

Visceral angiography has become an important tool in localizing the bleeding site in massive gastrointestinal tract hemorrhage (18–20). If four or more units of blood were administered during the first few hours of hospitalization, the bleeding site was identified in 72% of patients (21). The same study found that the most significant factor associated with a failure to identify a colonic bleeding source on angiography was a delay of six hours prior to angiography. In patients with massive gastrointestinal hemorrhage, angiography should be the first diagnostic test following resuscitation because it can be both diagnostic and therapeutic. Vasopressin infusion, either intravenously or directly infused intraarterially through a mesenteric vessel may be used to control hemorrhage temporarily and allow one to perform surgery on a semielective basis.

When the rate of hemorrhage is slow, nuclear scans with technetium-99m sulfur colloid or tagged red blood cells can be employed to localize the hemorrhage. Orecchia showed that a tagged red cell scan may localize the bleeding in up to 94% of patients who required emergency surgery and in 18% of patients who are managed conservatively (22) for colonic sites of hemorrhage.

Szold, Lewis, and others (23–25), utilizing Sonde and push enteroscopy, found that Crohn's disease was an uncommon cause of small intestinal hemorrhage. After determination by endoscopy that the upper gastrointestinal tract and the colon are not the source of bleeding, small bowel enteroscopy is the most accurate diagnostic modality for occult hemorrhage from the small intestine. Although the source of bleeding can be correctly identified by preoperative small bowel enteroscopy in 70 percent of patients, the necessary expertise and equipment may not be available. In addition, small bowel Crohn's strictures may severely limit the examination.

In cases where surgical treatment is necessary and preoperative studies have failed to localize the source of hemorrhage, intraoperative endoscopy may be successful to localize the bleeding site at laparotomy in 50% of patients.

Surgical Therapy

Management of severe gastrointestinal hemorrhage in Crohn's disease is similar to any other gastrointestinal hemorrhage. It is based on prompt and full resuscitation, with monitoring of hemodynamic parameters, urine output and peripheral perfusion, and correction of electrolyte abnormality.

During the phases of resuscitation, every effort should be made to localize the source of hemorrhage. Precise localization of the source of gastrointestinal hemorrhage is particularly important as a Crohn's lesion may not be the source of the hemorrhage. In addition, if hemorrhage is originating from a Crohn's lesion, preoperative localization avoids being confronted with the dilemma of which site of disease is responsible for the gastrointestinal hemorrhage when multiple sites are present at abdominal exploration. If preoperative tests have failed to demonstrate the source of hemorrhage and surgical treatment becomes necessary, operative strategy will be based on intraoperative findings at inspection and endoscopy.

For gastrointestinal hemorrhage originating from a jejunoileal or terminal ileal location, a resection with primary anastomosis will suffice to stop the bleeding and resect the diseased segment. In the instance of severe gastrointestinal hemorrhage from Crohn's colitis, an abdominal colectomy is necessary to treat the bleeding and remove the diseased segment. If the rectum is free of disease, a primary or delayed ileorectal anastomosis is feasible. If the rectum is severely diseased, the abdominal colectomy and terminal ileostomy should be followed by a completion proctectomy at a later stage. Finally, in the rare case of severe hemorrhage from a diseased rectum, a proctectomy may be necessary urgently with the proximal extent of the resection dictated by the extent of the disease.

References

1. Crohn BB, Ginzburg L, Oppenheimer GD. Regional ileitis. JAMA 1932;99:1323–8.
2. Ginzburg L, Oppenheimer GD. Non-specific granulomata of the intestines (inflammatory tumors and strictures of the intestines). Ann Surg 1933;98:1046–62.
3. Janowitz HD, Linder AE, Marshak RH. Granulomatous colitis. JAMA 1965;191:825–8.
4. Schofield PF, Fox H. The diagnosis of Crohn's disease of the colon. A clinicopathological study. Br J Surgery 1969;54:307–11.
5. Lockhart-Mummery HE, Morson BC. Crohn's disease of the large intestine. Gut 1964;5:439–509.
6. Farmer RG, Hawk WA, Turnbull RB. Regional enteritis of the colon: a clinical study pathological comparison with ulcerative colitis. Am J Dig Dis 1968;13:501–51.
7. Greenstein AJ, Kark AE, Dreiling DA. Crohn's disease of the colon. II. Controversial aspect of hemorrhage, anemia and rectal involvement in granulomatous disease involving the colon. Am J Gastroenterol 1975;63:40–8.
8. Yuan JG, Sachar DB, Koganei R, et al. Enterolithiasis, refractory anemia, and strictures of Crohn's diseases. J Clin Gastroenterol 1994;18:105–8.
9. Robert RJ, Sachar DB, Greenstein AJ. Severe gastrointestinal hemorrhage in Crohn's disease. Ann Surg 1991;213:207–11.
10. Warren R, Miller RH. Regional enteritis. N Engl J Med 1942;228:589–93.
11. Farmer RG, Hawk WA, Turnbull RB. Indication for surgery in Crohn's disease. Analysis of 500 cases. Gastroenterology 1976;71:245–50.
12. Van Patter WN, Bargen JA, Dockerty MB, et al. Regional enteritis. Gastroenterology 1954;25:347–450.
13. Daffner JE, Brown CH. Regional enteritis. I. Clinical aspects and diagnosis in 100 patients. Ann Int Med 1958;49:580–94.
14. Sparberg M. Kirsner JB. Recurrent hemorrhage in regional enteritis. Report of 3 cases. Am J Dig Dis 1966;2:652–7.
15. Robert HJ, Sachar DB, Aufses AH Jr, et al. Management of severe hemorrhage in ulcerative colitis. Am J Surg 1990;159:550–5.

16. Cicarelli O, Coley GM. Massive rectal bleeding in Crohn's colitis. Conn Med 1986;50:301–3.

17. Bruyns E, Lubbers EJC, van Tongeren JHM. Major hemorrhage in Crohn's disease. Neth J Med 1979; 22:67–71.

18. Jaffe BF, Youker JE, Margulis AR. Aortographic localization of controlled gastrointestinal hemorrhage in dogs. Surgery 1965;58:984–8.

19. Margulis AR, Heinbecker P, Bernard HR. Operative mesenteric arteriography in the search for the site of bleeding in unexplained gastrointestinal hemorrhage. Surgery 1960;48:534–9.

20. Nusbaum M, Baum S. Radiographic demonstration of unknown sites of gastrointestinal bleeding. Surg Forum 1963;14:374–5.

21. Browder W, Cerise EJ, Litwin MS. Impact of emergency angiography in massive lower gastrointestinal bleeding. Ann Surg 1986;204:530–6.

22. Orecchia PM, Hensley EK, McDonald PT, et al. Localization of lower gastrointestinal hemorrhage: experience with red blood cells labeled in vitro with technetium Tc 99m. Arch Surg 1985;120:521–624.

23. Szold A, Katz LB, Lewis BS. Surgical approach to occult gastro-intestinal bleeding. Am J Surg 1992; 163:90–3.

24. Lewis B, Waye J. Gastrointestinal bleeding of obscure origin: the role of small bowel enteroscopy. Gastroenterology 1988;94:1117–20.

25. Barkin J, Lewis B, Reiner D, et al. Diagnostic and therapeutic jejunoscopy with a new, longer enteroscope. Gastrointest Endos 1992;38:55–8.

30 Cancer

Adrian J. Greenstein

The surgical management of cancer occurring in Crohn's disease is complex. The myriad modes of presentation, the variety of anatomical sites, the presence or absence of fistulas or abscesses, and the possibility of multiple cancers make the operative care a challenge to the physician. Preoperative, operative, and postoperative care require expertise in Crohn's disease and a concomitant knowledge of oncologic surgery.

Historical Background

The occurrence of cancer in Crohn's disease was not appreciated until many years after the classic description of "regional enteritis" in 1932 (1). Warren and Sommers described the first case of carcinoma of the large bowel occurring in association with Crohn's disease (2). Including 21 new cases reported from the Mount Sinai Hospital (3) there are now over 149 patients in whom cancer of the large bowel has been reported in association with Crohn's colitis, ileocolitis, and even regional enteritis (4). The first report of cancer occurring in the jejunum in a patient with regional ileitis and jejunitis was that of Ginzburg et al. (5). Since that time, more than 100 cases of cancer of the small bowel have been reported in patients with Crohn's disease (6–8). Among these cases, 17 have occurred in excluded segments of bowel (6,9–11), of which 7 cases have been reported from our institution (12). Recently malignancies at various extraintestinal locations have been reported in association with Crohn's disease (13).

Cancer Risk

Early detection of cancer in Crohn's disease requires an appreciation of the risk of cancer in the various forms of Crohn's disease. Although precise calculation of the relative risk is difficult, estimates have varied from 6 to 320 times that of normal population, with most figures falling between 40 and 115 (14–17) for patients with small bowel Crohn's disease and between 6 and 20 for patients with large bowel Crohn's disease (12,18,19). Current estimates show an observed prevalence of 0.3% for small bowel adenocarcinoma and 1.8% for large intestinal adenocarcinoma in patients with Crohn's disease (20).

The incidence of cancer increases with longstanding duration of Crohn's disease. Hoffman et al. reported that 90% of their cases occurred more than five years, 70% more than 10 years, and 38% more than 20 years from the onset of disease, yielding a mean disease duration of 18 years (14). Beside duration, extension of disease appears to play a role in the development of cancer in Crohn's. In their study (21) Gillen et al. found that the relative risk of 4.9 for colorectal cancer increased to 13.3 for patients younger than 25 years at onset of Crohn's disease and to 18.2 if corrected for extensive colitis. If both factors were present the risk rose to 57.2. Thus in the presence of longstanding extensive colitis, especially with early onset of Crohn's disease, the risk seems clearly increased.

The risk appears increased in surgically bypassed bowel (12,22–24). Some authors have postulated that bypass with defunction and bacterial stasis has a carcinogenic effect (12). In addition, treatment with immunosuppressant for longer than six months has been associated with an increased risk of malignant transformation in Crohn's disease. Lashner (25), in a case-control study, recently demonstrated that prolonged (greater than 6 months) use of 6-mercaptopurine is significantly associated with the development of small bowel cancer in Crohn's disease. In the same study, he did not find any statistically significant association between development of small bowel carcinoma and prolonged use of prednisone, sulfasalazine, or metronidazole.

One question that remains unresolved, is the possible association of colorectal carcinoma with small bowel Crohn's disease (26). Seven (23%) of our patients had overt Crohn's disease confined to the small bowel, yet they developed five carcinomas in the colon and three in the rectum. It could be argued that colorectal cancer being a common disease, appeared only coincidentally in two patients, who were over 60 years of age, with short duration disease at the time of cancer diagnosis. However, three of the seven ileitis cases presented with colorectal cancers at ages 34, 38, and 42, suggesting a true increase in risk, and two developed cancer after 30, and 31 years of disease at ages 70 and 78 respectively. Moreover, there were no significant differences in age at onset of Crohn's disease, age at cancer, and duration of disease to cancer, between patients with ileitis and those with either ileocolitis or colitis. This finding once again raises the question of whether small bowel Crohn's disease may predispose to colorectal adenocarcinoma (26), a hypothesis consistent with the panenteric nature of this disease.

Although several studies prior to 1983 failed to demonstrate a statistically significant increase in incidence for extraintestinal cancers in patients with inflammatory bowel disease (8,27–29), a more recent study of 2000 patients has shown an increase in three specific tumor groups with Crohn's disease (4). The first group comprises squamocellular tumors arising from chronic inflammation such as squamous carcinoma of the anus and vulva (4,30) or peri-ileostomy carcinomas. The second group includes reticuloendothelial tumors such as lymphoma and leukemia (4,31). Finally, there may be an increased incidence of malignant melanoma (4,32).

Surveillance

Surveillance for cancer in patients with Crohn's disease remains controversial (33). In the 1980s Korelitz (34), and Shorter (35) suggested the need for surveillance, whereas Butt (36,37), Fielding (38), and Warren (2) did not advise prophylactic measures, although they recommended "vigilance." In 1985 Hamilton (39) suggested that cost-benefit studies of surveillance protocols were needed in well-defined Crohn's disease populations.

There are several factors which make it difficult to propose a rational surveillance program for Crohn's disease patients. These factors include the variety of cancers which occur in association with Crohn's disease: extraintestinal (4) and intestinal (8), and small (3,7,9,12) and large bowel (2,18,40,41) cancers. They also include several different modes of clinical presentation: cancers following long duration of disease (3), cancers coincident with onset of Crohn's disease (39,40,41), cancers remote from overt disease (7,8,39,42), and cancers in excluded segments (13). Finally, they include features that make the diagnosis difficult to establish even when a lesion is suspected and sought: the inaccessibility of small bowel to endoscopic examination, the difficulty of evaluating segments of bowel that are either bypassed (10–13,43) or proximal to strictures (4,44,45), the morphology of these tumors, often flat and difficult to differentiate from adjacent mucosa (24,41), and the confounding of cancer symptoms with those of the underlying bowel disease.

Despite these difficulties the following recommendations have been proposed. Regularly clinical check-ups should be instituted for patients with Crohn's disease, including examination of the abdomen and anovaginal area when perineal disease is present. An explanation should be sought for recurrence of old symptoms or for development of new symptoms, particularly stricture, fistula, intestinal bleeding, or weight loss, especially if these symptoms develop after a long period of quiescent disease. A high degree of suspicion should be maintained in patients with strictures and fistulas, especially in disease of long duration. Excluded segments should be removed whenever reoperation is being performed. Patients with perianal fistulae should be considered at some risk for malignant transformation of these areas of chronic inflammation.

A routine endoscopic surveillance program can be recommended for selected patients with longstanding (more than ten years), universal disease, especially with early onset. Biopsies must be taken from areas of raised mucosa, adenomatous polyps, and especially from areas of stricture and fistula formation. In view of the occurrence of carcinoma in overtly normal appearing bowel, biopsies of both normal and abnormal bowel should also be obtained and examined for dysplasia, carcinoma in situ, and infiltrating carcinoma. Colectomy should be advised if dysplasia develops. It remains to be seen whether small bowel enteroscopy will enable differentiation of benign from malignant strictures in the more proximal bowel.

The ratio of costs and risks to benefits has not been established for prophylactic colonoscopic surveillance, nor has an optimal surveillance regimen been determined. On an empirical basis, most surveillance programs commence after ten years of disease, often on an annual or biannual schedule. One could argue for earlier surveillance in view of the relative incidence of one third of cancers in Crohn's disease during the first decade (17). Newer and more sensitive indicators of premalignancy, such as DNA flow cytometry, cell turnover kinetics, mucin histochemistry, lectin binding, or monoclonal antibody identification of antigenic tumor markers, may ultimately supplant routine histologic examination for dysplasia as more effective screening techniques.

Intestinal Neoplasms

Small Bowel Adenocarcinoma

Most cancers of the small bowel in Crohn's disease are adenocarcinomas, usually in the terminal ileum or jejunum, and they are difficult if not impossible to diagnose at a curable stage. They differ from sporadic cancers of the small bowel in many respects (7,14). There is a male predominance of roughly 3:1 for small bowel carcinoma in Crohn's disease, in contrast with an equal distribution between sexes for patients with sporadic adenocarcinoma; there is a lower average age at diagnosis of cancer in Crohn's disease, 45 years versus 60 years; in concert with the anatomical distribution of the disease, the site of cancer in Crohn's disease is more distal, 76% vs. 20% (20,23,25,46–48); and the mean postoperative survival is shorter, eight months vs. approximately 32 months. There is also an increase in the proportion of multifocal (49) and mucinous cancers in association with Crohn's disease, and cancers with synchronous areas of dysplasia (23). Furthermore, sarcoma is an extremely rare form of small bowel cancer in Crohn's disease, whereas approximately one third of sporadic small bowel cancers are of this variety.

The most common clinical presentation of small bowel cancer is intestinal obstruction. Other important symptoms include diarrhea, weight loss, abdominal mass, and abdominal fistulas (9,20). These symptoms are also found in Crohn's disease without cancer. The possibility of the development of complicating cancer should be entertained if the development of these clinical features follows a long quiescent period (13). In addition, it is necessary to be especially suspicious of cases when the antiinflammatory therapy does not seem to achieve remission of obstructing symptoms, as this may be an indication that the stricture is not inflammatory, rather a fixed, neoplastic stricture.

Small bowel cancer is rarely suspected preoperatively, the diagnosis being made in less than 5% of reported patients. Intraoperative, postoperative, and autopsy diagnoses were made in 27%, 61%, and 7% respectively in the patients reviewed by Hoffman et al. for whom the timing of the diagnosis could be determined (14). Although these cancers may be difficult to appreciate on gross examination, all resected specimens with Crohn's disease should be opened and inspected by the operating surgeon prior to completion of the surgical procedure. The discovery of an unsuspected neoplasm may allow for completion of an otherwise incomplete surgical clearance.

Large Bowel Adenocarcinoma

The clinicopathological features of colorectal cancer occurring in Crohn's disease are difficult to differentiate from the clinical features of the underlying inflammatory bowel disease. Compared to sporadic cases, colorectal cancers in Crohn's disease have a bimodal age distribution, are located in the right colon in at least half of the cases, and are more frequently multiple (50,51).

It has been suggested that there are two separate populations among patients with colorectal cancer in Crohn's disease. First, there are those with onset of Crohn's disease over 60 years of age, in whom the vast majority have had a relatively short duration of disease and in whom the Crohn's disease and cancer symptoms occurred simultaneously. This group, for example, constitute approximately 20% of the patients in Hamilton's series (39). The second and much larger group consists of younger patients, usually with a long duration of disease. Examination of the literature prior to 1985 reveals that for all 29 patients under 60 years of age, for whom the duration of disease is recorded, the mean disease duration was 15 years, while for the 29 patients above 60 years of age, the mean disease duration was five years. This thesis has been supported by a recent publication by Kyle and Ewen who describe two such separate populations among patients who developed Crohn's colorectal carcinoma in their area (52). Since onset of Crohn's disease in the sixth decade of life is unusual, and the incidence of spontaneous colorectal cancer is higher in late decades, patients in this latter group could represent either coincidental spontaneous cancer, or colitis-associated cancers in a setting of longstanding undiagnosed Crohn's disease.

Cancers in Crohn's colitis usually develop without giving clinical evidence of their presence in their early stages. Advanced cases are characterized by obstructive symptoms, rapid weight loss, and abdominal masses. Colorectal cancers in Crohn's disease may occur in excluded distal bowel or in association with enterovesical or colovesical (13, 53), rectovaginal (53,54), colocutaneous (13,55), or perianal fistulas (13,30,54).

Extraintestinal Neoplasms

Squamous Carcinomas

Squamous cell cancers of the anus and perineal region usually develop in long-standing anoperianal disease. Cancers occurring at the site of an intestinal stoma are rare, but a number have been reported. Development of such cancers must be differentiated with biopsy from peristomal inflammatory complications as pyoderma gangrenosum, fistulas, and skin excoriation due to badly fitting appliances. Radical excision, including surrounding abdominal wall, with transposition of the stoma is required.

Reticuloendothelial Tumors

Lymphomas
Lymphomas, colonic or extraintestinal (31), occur uncommonly in both Crohn's disease and ulcerative colitis. It has been suggested that the incidence is above that expected (4). For intestinal lymphomas local excision is required, followed by radiotherapy when indicated, and chemotherapy (31).

Leukemias
Leukemias are more common in ulcerative colitis (4,56) than Crohn's disease and occasionally may exacerbate the hemorrhage due to gastrointestinal ulceration. In one such patient with leukemia in Crohn's disease total proctocolectomy was required for massive gastrointestinal hemorrhage. Appropriate chemotherapy is necessary to treat the underlying hematologic disorder (56).

Indications for Surgery

A. Absolute
1. Carcinoma proven by endoscopic biopsy.
2. Dysplasia, especially when associated with a mass or in the absence of acute inflammation.
3. A stricture that cannot be fully evaluated.
B. Relative
1. An excluded loop.
2. A poorly compliant patient on whom regular surveillance cannot be done.
3. High risk patients in whom accurate surveillance is impossible because of multiple large pseudopolyps.

Although most of the listed indications are self-explanatory, the presence of dysplasia and/or a tight stricture as indications to surgical intervention requires some elaboration.

Dysplasia is a preneoplastic epithelial change. Although the temporal development of an intestinal cancer from dysplastic epithelium has never been demonstrated, the presence of dysplasia has been reported in specimens of Crohn's disease complicated by cancer (23). In addition, accumulating evidence, obtained with modern molecular biology techniques, supports the concept of an orderly progression from normal epithelium, to dysplastic epithelium to an invasive cancer. In view of this modern evidence to well accepted concepts of tumorigenesis, and considering the expected long duration at risk for many young patients, the risk of failure by surveillance and the fact that unequivocal dysplasia is an already accepted indication to surgical treatment for ulcerative colitis, unequivocal dysplasia should also be considered an indication to surgical treatment in Crohn's disease.

Enteric strictures are one of the most common complications of Crohn's disease. The frequency of benign intestinal strictures in Crohn's disease, and the difficulty of differentiating them from malignant strictures makes this a topic of major importance in the attempt to diagnose cancers at an early and curable stage. Although there appears to be an association between stricture and cancer, it is not clear whether benign strictures degenerate into malignancy or whether cancers present as strictures.

Radiological examination is of value for detection of simple bowel stricture, but is not reliable for the differentiation of benign from malignant disease. When operating on small bowel stricture, especially when performing strictureplasty, small bowel cancer should be ruled out with frozen section biopsies (9).

Strictures in colorectal Crohn's disease are malignant in a high percentage of cases. Greenstein found nine malignant strictures in 132 patients with colonic Crohn's disease, for an incidence of 6.8% (45). Following radiological detection of a stricture, endoscopy with biopsies throughout the length of the stricture is essential. Multiple biopsies should be taken at the proximal and distal edges and from within the stricture in order to rule out dysplasia, carcinoma in situ, or frank adenocarcinoma. Surgery must be considered whenever the endoscopist cannot visualize and assess the entire stricture or the bowel proximal to it.

Operative Strategy

The objective of surgery for cancer in Crohn's disease is resection of the cancer for cure or, when indicated, palliation and removal of associated or discontinuous segments of inflammatory disease when necessary. Preoperative histologic diagnosis of a cancer still at a curable stage is rare and feasible only in colorectal cancer with colonoscopy; in these cases a preoperative carcinoembryonic antigen (CEA) level should be obtained and should be complemented by an abdominal and pelvic computed tomography (CT) scan if the tumor is located in the rectum to assess for local invasiveness and distant spread. The operative strategy should include a complete examination of the abdominal cavity and liver in order to detect possible metastatic disease. Histologic evidence of metastatic small or large bowel cancer can, at times, be obtained preoperatively by demonstrating liver metastasis on abdominal CT scan or malignant cells on paracentesis. Although surgical intervention is rarely indicated in the presence of malignant ascites, surgical resection of the primary tumor may afford palliation and a better quality of life even in the presence of liver metastasis.

In a number of patients the diagnosis is first appreciated or suspected at the time of the surgical procedure. Thus, in patients in whom the presence of cancer is possible, even if unproven, a formal cancer resection should be carried out. This applies to patients with extensive long-standing disease; those with internal enteroenteric or enterovesical fistulas with a concomitant mass, or with excluded loops; and patients with a non-negotiable stricture when an associated mass is present. Specimens should be opened and inspected as soon as resected in consultation with an experienced pathologist so that a complete oncologic clearance can be performed if necessary before closure of the celiotomy.

Operative Procedures

Segmental Resection

Segmental resection is the preferred surgical therapy for small bowel adenocarcinoma and for colonic cancer in segmental Crohn's disease. A small bowel resection or a hemicolectomy are all examples of segmental resections for limited Crohn's disease of the small bowel or colon with malignant degeneration. In patients with multiple small bowel strictures, concomitant strictureplasties should be performed in addition to the resection of the malignant stricture. Each stricture should be biopsied with frozen section evaluation to rule out the presence of synchronous cancers before a strictureplasty is carried out.

Squamous cell carcinoma of the anorectal and perineal region has historically been treated with abdominoperineal resection of the rectum including the affected perineum and a negative circumferential margin (30,57). This approach must be debated given the recent evidence that survival after chemoradiotherapy has yielded higher 5-year survival rates in non-Crohn's patients (58).

Subtotal Colectomy

Subtotal colectomy is the procedure of choice in the presence of Crohn's disease of the colon with malignant degeneration and sparing of the rectum. Following an abdominal colectomy with ileoproctostomy long-term surveillance with yearly endoscopy and biopsies of the remaining rectal segment is essential.

Total Proctocolectomy

This procedure is generally reserved for patients with pancolitis or with segmental colon and rectal disease or with colon and severe perianal disease.

Extensive En-Bloc Resections

At times nearby organs need to be resected along with the intestinal segment harboring the cancer because of malignant involvement, whether proven or suspected. This is often the case in the presence of a fistula. The association between cancer and fistulas has long been recognized (12,13,46,55). Unfortunately such cancers are often unresectable. However, it is possible on occasion to carry out a radical "en-bloc" resection including the fistula.

Palliative Procedures

When the cancer is very advanced or widely metastatic, surgical treatment may not offer any benefit to the patient. At times a palliative diverting stoma is all that may be performed or all that may be indicated.

Adjuvant Therapy and Long-Term Outcome

There is no data on the value and benefit of adjuvant therapy after curative resection of gastrointestinal cancers in Crohn's disease. Recommendation for adjuvant therapy after resection of sporadic colorectal cancer can be adopted for the occasional patient with cancer complicating Crohn's. These include a postoperative administration of 5-FU and levamisole in colon cancer, associated with radiation therapy to the pelvis in rectal cancer.

There is no experience with preoperative adjuvant therapy in rectal cancer complicating Crohn's disease. A potential disadvantage unique to the presence of Crohn's disease may be the worsening of Crohn's proctitis due to the effect of radiation therapy.

Long-term prognosis following surgical resection of a curable cancer is better in colorectal than small bowel tumors. Ribeiro and Greenstein has found a 56% five-year survival for colorectal cancer (3) and a 23% three-year survival for small bowel cancer (8). Mortality for cancers in excluded bowel was 100% for both small and large bowel by 18 months (3,8).

Following resection, long term surveillance for the possibility of recurrence of the primary cancer by routine CEA evaluation, as well as by CT scanning when necessary, are reasonable recommendations. Colonoscopy for detection of metachronous malignancy is also advisable on a yearly basis if limited segmental colonic resection has been carried out.

Conclusions

Cancer in inflammatory bowel disease is clearly increased in incidence in the intestinal tract, and probably in certain extraintestinal sites as well. The absolute number of patients developing such malignancies is small compared to the general population, but because of higher relative risks, younger ages of onset, distinctive clinicopathological features, and the difficulties of making a diagnosis, it is important that this complication of inflammatory bowel disease be widely appreciated.

There is increasing evidence that surveillance is indicated for patients with excluded bowel, long-standing (>10 years) and extensive disease, particularly in those with early onset of disease. Surgery for cancer in inflammatory bowel disease is based on a combination of principles for inflammatory bowel disease and oncologic surgery. The prognosis is no worse for colorectal cancers in Crohn's disease (except for those occurring in excluded bowel) than for sporadic cancers but it remains exceedingly poor for small bowel cancers.

References

1. Crohn BB, Ginzburg L, Oppenheimer GD. Regional ileitis. A pathologic and clinical entity. JAMA 1932; 99:1323–9.
2. Warren S, Sommers SC. Cicatrizing enteritis (regional enteritis) as a pathologic entity: analysis of one hundred and twenty cases. Am J Pathol 1948;24: 475–501.
3. Ribeiro MB, Greenstein AJ, Sachar DB, et al. Colorectal adenocarcinoma in Crohn's disease. Ann Surg 1996;223:186–93.
4. Nikias GW, Eisner T, Katz S, et al. Crohn's disease and colorectal carcinoma: rectal cancer complicating long-standing active perianal disease. Am J Gastroent 1995;90:216–9.
5. Ginzburg L, Schneider KM, Dreizin DH, et al. Carcinoma of the jejunum occurring in a case of regional enteritis. Surgery 1956;39:347–51.
6. Frank JD, Shorey BA. Adenocarcinoma of the small bowel as a complication of Crohn's disease. Gut 1973;14:120–4.
7. Greenstein AJ, Sachar DB, Smith H, et al. Patterns of neoplasia in Crohn's disease and ulcerative colitis. Cancer 1980;46:403–7.
8. Ribeiro MB, Greenstein AJ, Heimann TM, et al. Adenocarcinoma of the small intestine in Crohn's disease. Surg, Gynecol Obstet 1992;13:343–50.
9. Brown N, Weinstein VA, Janowitz HD. Carcinoma of the ileum 24 years after bypass for regional enteritis: a case report. Mt. Sinai J Med 1970;27:675–8.
10. Zisk J, Shore JM, Rosoff L, et al. Regional ileitis complicated by adenocarcinoma of the ileum: a report of two cases. Surgery 1960;47:970–4.
11. Senay E, Keohane M, Greenstein AJ. Small bowel carcinoma in Crohn's disease: distinguishing features and risk factors. Cancer 1989;63:360–3.
12. Greenstein AJ, Sachar D, Pucillo A, et al. Cancer in Crohn's disease after diversionary surgery: a report of seven carcinomas occurring in excluded bowel. Am J Surg 1985;135:86–90.
13. Greenstein AJ, Gennuso R, Sachar DB, et al. Extraintestinal cancers in inflammatory bowel disease. Cancer 1985;56;2914–21.

14. Hoffman JP, Taft DA, Weelis RF, et al. Adenocarcinoma in regional enteritis of the small intestine. Arch Surg 1977;112:606–11.

15. Greenstein AJ, Sachar DB, Smith H, et al. A comparison of cancer risk in Crohn's disease and ulcerative colitis. Cancer 1981;48:2742–5.

16. Korelitz B. Carcinoma of the intestinal tract in Crohn's disease: results of a survey conducted by the National Foundation for Ileitis and Colitis. (Editorial) Am J Gastroenterol 1983;78:44–6.

17. Fresco D, Lazarus SS, Dotan J, et al. Early presentation of carcinoma of the small bowel in Crohn's disease ("Crohn's carcinoma"): case reports and review of the literature. Gastroenterology 1982;82: 783–9.

18. Weedon DD, Shorter RG, Ilstrup DM, et al. Crohn's disease and cancer. New Engl J Med 1973;289:1099–102.

19. Gyde SN, Prior P, Macartney JC, et al. Malignancy in Crohn's disease. Gut 1980;21:1024–9.

20. Darke SG, Parks AG, Grogono JL, et al. Adenocarcinoma and Crohn's disease: a report of two cases and analysis of the literature. Br J Surg 1973;60:169–75.

21. Gillen CD, Andrews HA, Prior P, et al. Crohn's disease and colorectal cancer. Gut 1994;35:651–6.

22. Ribeiro MB, Greenstein AJ, Heimann TM, et al. Adenocarcinoma of the small intestine in Crohn's disease. Surg Gynecol Obstet 1991;173:343–9.

23. Hawker PC, Gyde SN, Thompson H, et al. Adenocarcinoma of the small intestine complicating Crohn's disease. Gut 1982;23:188–93.

24. Fleming KA, Pollock AC. A case of "Crohn's carcinoma." Gut 1975;16:533–7.

25. Lashner BA. Risk factors for small bowel cancer in Crohn's disease. Dig Dis Sci 1992;37:1179–84.

26. Kvist N, Jacobsen O, Norgaard P, et al. Malignancy in Crohn's disease. Scand J Gastroenterol 1986;21: 82–6.

27. Greenstein AJ, Sachar DB, Smith H, et al. A comparison of cancer risk in Crohn's disease and ulcerative colitis. Cancer 1981;48:2742–5.

28. Lennard-Jones JE, Stalder GA. Prognosis after resection of chronic regional ileitis. Gut 1967;8:332–6.

29. Prior P, Gyde SN, Macartney JC, et al. Cancer morbidity in ulcerative colitis. Gut 1982;23:490–7.

30. Slater G, Greenstein AJ, Aufses AH, Jr. Anal carcinoma in patients with Crohn's disease. Ann Surg 1984;199:348–50.

31. Greenstein AJ, Mullin GE, Strauchen JA, et al. Lymphoma in inflammatory bowel disease: a study of 9 cases. Cancer 1992;69:1119–23.

32. Greenstein AJ, Sachar DB, Shafir M, et al. Malignant melanoma in inflammatory bowel disease. Am J Gastroenterol 1987;82:964.

33. Cooper DJ, Weinstein MA, Korelitz BI. Complications of Crohn's disease predisposing to dysplasia and cancer of the intestinal tract: considerations of a surveillance program. J Clin Gastroenterol 1984;6: 217–24.

34. Korelitz BI. Carcinoma of the intestinal tract in Crohn's disease: results of a survey conducted by the National Foundation for Ileitis and Colitis. Am J Gastroenterol 1983;78:44–6.

35. Shorter RG. Risks of intestinal cancer in Crohn's disease. Dis Colon Rectum 1983;26:686–9.

36. Butt JH, Morson BC. Dysplasia and cancer in inflammatory bowel disease (editorial). Gastroenterol 1981;80:865–8.

37. Butt JH, Lennard-Jones JE, Ritchie JK. A practical approach to the risk of cancer in inflammatory bowel disease. Med Clin North Am 1980;64;1203–20.

38. Fielding JF, Prior P, Waterhouse JA, et al. Malignancy in Crohn's disease. Scand J Gastroenterol 1972;7: 3–7.

39. Hamilton SR. Colorectal carcinoma in patients with Crohn's disease. Gastroenterology 1985;89:398–407.

40. Perrett AD, Truelove SC, Massarella GR. Crohn's disease and carcinoma of the colon. Br Med J 1968;2:466–8.

41. Thompson EM, Clayden G, Price AB. Cancer in Crohn's disease—an "occult" malignancy. Histopathology 1983;7:365–76.

42. Radial RH, Goldman H, Ransohoff DF, et al. Dysplasia in inflammatory bowel disease: standardized classification with provisional clinical applications. Human Pathol 1983;14:931–68.

43. Kim U, Klein M, Baek S, et al. Carcinoma of the small intestine in Crohn's disease—occurrence in a bypassed loop. Mt. Sinai J Med 1976;43:461–6.

44. Yamazaki Y, Ribeiro MB, Sachar DB, et al. Malignant colorectal strictures in Crohn's disease. Am J. Gastroenterol 1991;86:882–5.

45. Greenstein AJ, Sachar DB, Kark AE. Stricture of the anorectum in Crohn's disease involving the colon. Ann Surg 1975;181:207–12.

46. Lightdale CJ, Sternberg SS, Posner G, et al. Carcinoma complicating Crohn's disease: report of seven cases and review of the literature. Am J Med 1975;59:262–8.

47. Sager GF. Primary malignant tumors of the small intestine: a 22 year experience with 30 patients. Am J Surg 1978;135:601–3.

48. McPeak CJ. Malignant tumors of the small intestine. Am J Surg 1967;114:402–11.

49. Richards ME, Rickert RR, Nance FC. Crohn's disease-associated carcinoma: a poorly recognized complication of Crohn's disease. Ann Surg 1989; 209:764–74.

50. Clemmensen T, Johansen A. A case of Crohn's disease of the colon associated with adenocarcinoma extending from cardia to the anus. Acta Pathol Microbiol Scand 1972;80:5–8.

51. Keighley MRB, Thompson H, Alexander-Williams J. Multifocal colonic carcinoma and Crohn's disease. Surgery 1975;78:534–7.

52. Kyle J, Ewen SWB. Two types of colorectal carcinoma in Crohn's disease. Ann R Coll Surg Engl 1992;74:387–90.

53. Buchmann P, Allan RN, Thompson H, et al. Carcinoma in a rectovaginal fistula in a patient with Crohn's disease. Am J Surg 1980;140:462–3.

54. Sher ME, Bauer JJ, Gelernt. Surgical repair of rectovaginal fistulas in patients with Crohn's disease: transvaginal approach. Dis Colon Rectum 1991;34:641–8.

55. Church JM, Weakley FI, Fazio VW, et al. The relationship between fistulas in Crohn's disease and associated carcinoma. Report of four cases and review of the literature. Dis Colon Rectum 1985;28:361–6.

56. Fabry TL, Sachar DB, Janowitz HD. Acute myelogenous leukemia in patients with ulcerative colitis. J Clin Gastroenterol 1980;2:225–7.

57. Connell WR, Sheffield MA, Kamm MA, et al. Lower gastrointestinal malignancy in Crohn's disease. Gut 1994;35:347–52.

Section III
Crohn's Disease

Part III
Strategy According to Specific Anatomical Sites

31 Gastroduodenal Crohn's Disease

David J. Schoetz

Crohn's disease occasionally involves the gastroduodenal region primarily. Until 1950 (1) primary gastroduodenal Crohn's disease was rarely reported. In 1954, van Patter and associates (2) reported a frequency of duodenal Crohn's disease of 0.5% in a series of 600 patients with gastrointestinal Crohn's disease. Since then, a number of authors (3–7) have added new cases to the existing literature. The reported frequency of gastroduodenal Crohn's disease varies between 0.5% and 4%. Nugent and Roy (8) have reported the largest single institutional experience of 89 cases from the Lahey Clinic between 1952 and 1986.

Enteric fistulas may secondarily involve the duodenum and stomach. In these instances, Crohn's disease primarily involves the transverse colon or a previous ileocolonic anastomosis; fistulization to a normal stomach or duodenum is a secondary phenomenon. The clinical presentation and treatment of entergastroduodenal fistulas are different from those of primary gastroduodenal Crohn's disease, and they are discussed separately in Chapter 26.

Clinical Features

Gastroduodenal Crohn's disease tends to affect young patients, with a median age at onset of symptoms of 26 years in the Lahey Clinic series (8). A male predominace of 1.7:1 was reported. In that series, 51.7% of patients had documented distal intestinal Crohn's disease that predated the duodenal involvement by a median of 4 years. An additional 30.3% had the diagnosis of duodenal and distal intestinal disease made simultaneously. Only seven patients (7.9%) did not have the develop-

ment of distal disease during a median follow-up time of 11.7 years (range, 6 to 14 years).

Although gastroduodenal involvement may be in any imaginable distribution, the most common pattern was contiguous antral and duodenal disease in 60%, with the remaining 40% having only duodenal involvement. Contiguous involvement of the proximal jejunum with distal duodenal disease is rare (8).

Regarding the distribution of distal Crohn's disease in these patients, the extent of extraduodenal disease is similar to that of patients without duodenal disease (8). Ileocolitis and terminal ileitis are seen with equal frequency, whereas proximal small bowel disease or colitis or both are seen less often.

Gastroduodenal Crohn's disease manifests itself with abdominal pain not unlike that of peptic ulcer disease. Nausea, vomiting, and weight loss are present in approximately two thirds of patients (Table 31.1). These latter symptoms, as well as persistent pyrosis, are indicators of significant gastric outlet obstruction. Although many patients will have occult blood in the stool, upper gastrointestinal hemorrhage resulting in hematemesis or melena is uncommon. Life-threatening hemorrhage is rare but has been reported (8,9). Unlike acid peptic disease of the duodenum in which free perforation of the ulcer is a well-recognized complication, free perforation from duodenal Crohn's disease is unusual (10). Similarly, acute pancreatitis resulting from duodenal Crohn's disease is unusual compared with the frequency of pancreatitis secondary to penetration of a posterior peptic ulcer into the pancreas (11).

In the absence of a preexisting diagnosis of

Table 31.1.   Symptoms of gastroduodenal Crohn's disease.*

Symptom	Number	Percent
Abdominal pain	70	79
Weight loss (>10 lb)	57	64
Nausea/vomiting	54	61
Hemorrhage	15	17

*From Nugent and Roy (8).

Crohn's disease, many patients with nonspecific symptoms consistent with peptic ulcer disease may have been treated with various acid reduction regimens before initiating the investigations that ultimately yield the correct diagnosis. Consequently, the initial presentation of gastric outlet obstruction may represent a delay in diagnosis, with the duodenal obstruction reflecting progression of the transmural inflammatory process. When the diagnosis of gastroduodenal obstruction is suspected or confirmed, appropriate testing is required to establish the correct nature of the underlying process. Barium contrast radiography of the upper gastrointestinal tract and flexible fiberoptic upper endoscopy are the two most useful diagnostic modalities available. These two tests are not mutually exclusive and should both be obtained in most instances. The former provides considerable information regarding the overall extent and severity of gastroduodenal involvement and a topographic roadmap for the endoscopist and surgeon, whereas the latter permits mucosal biopsies of directly visualized abnormalities while not necessarily accurately determining the total extent of the disease.

Radiology

Radiographic features of gastroduodenal Crohn's disease include a spectrum of abnormalities, beginning with thickened folds, modularity, and aphthous ulcers (Fig. 31.1). As the disease progresses, fissuring ulcers, cobblestoning, and stenosis become manifest (Fig. 31.2). Ultimately, gastric outlet obstruction develops, reflecting cicatrix formation with luminal compromise. These changes are more likely to involve the proximal rather than the distal duodenum (12).

The differential diagnosis, based on radiography alone, includes infiltrative carcinoma of the distal stomach (linitis plastica) and gastroduodenal lymphoma. Primary duodenal tumors, although rare, as well as pancreatic and biliary tumors that may extrinsically compress the duodenum, must also be considered but usually the clinical presentation is

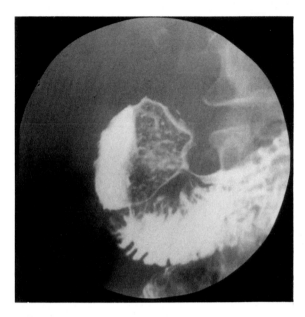

Fig. 31.1.   Early duodenal Crohn's disease with numerous aphthous ulcers and mucosal edema.

quite different. Acid peptic disease of the duodenum is the other primary consideration, although the length of duodenal involvement and concomitant gastric changes in Crohn's disease should make the distinction.

Endoscopy

With the advent of fiberoptic endoscopy, the ability to diagnose Crohn's disease of the duodenum accurately has been improved. In a series of 14 patients undergoing upper endoscopy, mucosal modularity was noted in 93%, aphthous ulcers in 64%, serpiginous ulcers in 55%, and luminal narrowing in 50% (13). In the Lahey Clinic series, abnormalities were found in 93% of patients (8).

At the time of endoscopy, multiple biopsy specimens should be obtained. Most often, pathologic changes will be nonspecific, with acute and chronic inflammation. Granulomas have been observed in between 15% and 68% of specimens (8,14).

It has been reported that patients with distal Crohn's disease are found to have abnormal upper endoscopic findings in 56% of patients in whom there was no clinical suspicion of gastroduodenal Crohn's disease (15). The described endoscopic changes are identical to those found in patients with known or suspected duodenal Crohn's disease, with granulomas in 19.5% of mucosal biopsies. As an inside, these authors suggest that upper endoscopy may assist in refining the diagnosis of indeterminate colitis.

Indications for Surgery

Operative intervention is indicated for at least one third of patients with intrinsic gastroduodenal Crohn's disease. Refractory gastric outlet obstruction was the primary reason for operation in 77% of a series of 22 patients undergoing surgery at the Lahey Clinic (16). Uncontrollable abdominal pain necessitated surgery in 18% of that series, and hemorrhage was the reason for urgent surgery in only one patient.

With the development of techniques to dilate intestinal strictures endoscopically, it is possible to consider applying these procedures before proceeding with major abdominal surgery (17). Since this treatment modality is relatively new, the long-term efficacy is unknown, and the complication rate is not described; however, for a fibrotic stricture of short length, without associated periduodenal inflammation, there may be a role for the endoscopic dilation.

Pitfall and Danger Point

Preoperative distinction between Crohn's disease and other causes of duodenal stricture is essential to guide the choice of operation. In the Lahey Clinic operative series, resective procedures were accompanied by appreciably higher morbidity than bypass procedures (16).

Operative Strategy and Technique

The preferred operation is gastrojejunostomy, operative details of which are explained below.

After thorough exploration of the abdomen, the lesser sac is entered by dividing the gastrocolic omentum from the stomach to expose the middle third of the greater curvature. To maximize dependent drainage, the gastrotomy is planned just posterior to the greater curvature. After the presence of proximal small bowel Crohn's disease is carefully excluded, the proximal jejunum is brought up in an ante- or retrocolic fashion and fixed to the stomach with interrupted sutures. Incisions are made into the gastric and small bowel lumens. Completion of the posterior inner layer by either a running or interrupted technique is followed by closure of the anterior layer in a similar fashion. Full-thickness sutures are essential for the inner layer. Finally, the outer anterior layer is completed with interrupted seromuscular sutures. After completion of the anastomosis, the stoma should be widely patent and on the most dependent portion of the gastric wall. The proximal jejunum should be without tension, and there should be no compression of the transverse colon.

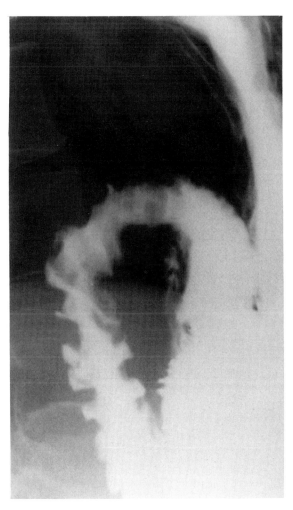

Fig. 31.2. Involvement of the proximal duodenum with deep ulcers and cobblestoning.

Treatment

Medical treatment of duodenal Crohn's disease is primarily with systemic corticosteroids. Most of the patients will obtain symptomatic relief with acid-reducing medications, such as H_2 blockers or omeprazole; certainly, these antacids should be continued during steroid treatment because of the reduction in capability of the mucosal barrier to protect itself from acid-induced damage. In patients without fixed outlet obstruction, corticosteroids are successful in treating more than 90% of affected individuals (8).

Attention must also be directed to the distal intestinal disease. Aminosalicylates, immunosuppressive agents, and metronidazole are prescribed as indicated for the intestinal disease. None of these agents have been studied as specific therapy for gastroduodenal disease, presumably because of the paucity of cases available for study by randomized prospective study.

Long-term follow-up data have been provided in a small series that has indicated that marginal ulceration was too large a risk to permit performance of gastrojejunostomy without vagotomy (18). On the other hand, the frequency of marginal ulceration at the Lahey Clinic was equivalent whether or not a truncal vagotomy was performed at the time of the bypass (16). Debate regarding the need for vagotomy continues because of the potential risk of the development of postvagotomy diarrhea after truncal vagotomy. This complication would be of particular consequence in an individual who may already have diarrhea as a result of previous bowel resections with or without the loss of the ileocecal valve.

It has been our recent policy to perform a highly selective vagotomy at the time of gastrojejunostomy for duodenal Crohn's disease. The anatomy of the left (anterior) vagus nerve indicates that a hepatic branch supplies the gallbladder and biliary tree. Of greater importance is the anatomy of the right (posterior) vagus nerve, with the celiac branch that supplies parasympathetic innervation to the bowel and other abdominal viscera. After identification of the anterior vagus nerve, division of branches of the nerve begins to the left of the crow's foot, which is approximately 7 cm from the pylorus. Care is taken to preserve the nerve of Laterjet and the hepatic branch. When dissection has been completed in a cephalad fashion so that the posterior leaf of the gastrohepatic ligament is exposed, the branches of the posterior vagus nerve are divided in a similar manner. Retraction of the gastrohepatic ligament to the right provides better exposure and countertraction. The dissection is continued across the gastroesophageal junction to the angle of His and the first short gastric vein. After all branches from the anterior esophagus have been cleared for a distance of 5 to 7 cm, the distal esophagus is retracted to the left, and all nerve branches to the posterior gastric fundus and distal esophagus are divided. A highly selective vagotomy preserves gallbladder and bowel function while effecting significant acid reduction.

With the description of the operation of strictureplasty to reestablish the intestinal lumen without resection, the technique has been applied to carefully selected patients with duodenal strictures (19). It has been suggested that strictureplasy is the procedure of choice for duodenal Crohn's disease (20), but the technical challenges associated with this operation for long strictures in the retroperitoneal portion of the duodenum will limit its application to those individuals with short fibrotic strictures in easily accessible portions of the

duodenum without significant phlegmonous reaction. In these cases, Heineke-Mikulicz strictureplasty is the strictureplasty of choice, although a Finney strictureplasty may have to be used for proximal duodenal lesions, extending into the gastric antrum (see Chapter 16). Alternatively, for strictures in the third or fourth portion of the duodenum, a side-to-side or Roux-en-Y duodenojejunostomy (Fig. 26.2) may obviate the need for a vagotomy. If strictureplasty is able to be accomplished, vagotomy should not be necessary and the dumping syndrome may be lessened.

In summary, gastroduodenal Crohn's disease is a fairly unusual site of primary intestinal involvement. It is usually associated with Crohn's disease elsewhere in the gastrointestinal tract. Diagnosis is by barium contrast radiography and upper endoscopy with biopsy. Medical management with acid reduction combined with systemic corticosteroids should be anticipated to relieve symptoms until gastric outlet obstruction supervenes. When this has occurred, gastrojejunostomy with highly selective vagotomy, strictureplasty, and side-to-side or Roux-en-Y duodenojejenostomy are the different surgical options. Endoscopic balloon dilation is a new technique that still needs to be evaluated in terms of efficacy and associated complications. The goal of therapy is relief of obstruction with ablation of abdominal pain. This can be accomplished with a high likelihood in nearly all instances.

References

1. Comfort MW, Weber HM, Baggenstoss AH, et al. Nonspecific granulomatous inflammation of the stomach and duodenum: its relation to regional enteritis. Am J Med Sci 1950; 220:616–32.
2. Van Patter WN, Bargen JA, Dockerty MB, et al. Regional enteritis. Gastroenterology 1954; 26:347–450.
3. McGarity WC. Regional enteritis of the duodenum. Surg Gynecol Obstet 1957; 105:203–9.
4. Edwards AM, Michalyshyn B, Sherbaniuk RW, et al. Regional enteritis of the duodenum: a review and report of five cases. Can Med Assoc J 1965; 93:1283–95.
5. Jones GW, Dooley MR, Schoenfield LJ. Regional enteritis with involvement of the duodenum. Gastroenterology 1966; 51:1018–22.
6. Wise L, Kyriakos M, McCown A, et al. Crohn's disease of the duodenum: a report and analysis of eleven new cases. Am J Surg 1971; 121:184–94.
7. Farmer RG, Hawk WA, Turnbull RB Jr. Crohn's disease of the duodenum (transmural duodenitis): clinical manifestations. Report of 11 cases. Am J Dig Dis 1972; 17:191–8.

8. Nugent FW, Roy MA. Duodenal Crohn's disease: an analysis of 89 cases. Am J Gastroenterol, 1989; 84:249–54.

9. Paget ET, Owens MP, Peniston WO, et al. Massive upper gastrointestinal tract hemorrhage: a manifestation of regional enteritis of the duodenum. Arch Surg 1972; 104:397–400.

10. Katz S, Talansky A, Kahn E. Recurrent free perforation in gastroduodenal Crohn's disease. Am J Gastroenterol 1983; 78:722–5.

11. Legge DA, Hoffman HN II, Carlson HC. Pancreatitis as a complication of regional enteritis of the duodenum. Gastroenterology 1971; 61:834–7.

12. Miller EM, Moss AM, Kressel HY. Duodenal involvement with Crohn's disease: a spectrum of radiographic abnormality. Am J Gastroenterol 1979; 71:107–16.

13. Danzi JT, Farmer RG, Sullivan BH Jr, et al. Endoscopic features of gastroduodenal Crohn's disease. Gastroenterology 1976; 70:9-13.

14. Rutgeerts P, Onette E, Vantrappen G, et al. Crohn's disease of the stomach and duodenum: a clinical study with emphasis on the value of endoscopy and endoscopic biopsies. Endoscopy 1980; 12:288–94.

15. Alántara M, Rodriguez R, Potenciano JL, et al. Endoscopic and bioptic findings in the upper gastrointestinal tract in patients with Crohn's disease. Endoscopy 1993; 25:282–6.

16. Murray JJ, Schoetz DJ Jr, Nugent FW, et al. Surgical management of Crohn's disease involving the duodenum. Am J Surg 1984; 147:58–65.

17. Williams AJ, Palmer KR. Endoscopic balloon dilatation as a therapeutic option in the management of intestinal strictures resulting from Crohn's disease. Br J Surg 1991; 78:453–4.

18. Ross TM, Fazio VW, Farmer RG. Long-term results of the surgical treatment for Crohn's disease of the duodenum. Ann Surg 1983; 197:399–406.

19. Alexander-Williams J, Haynes IG. Conservative operations for Crohn's disease of the small bowel. World J Surg 1985; 9:945–51.

20. Schoetz DJ Jr. Gastroduodenal Crohn's disease. Perspect Colon Rectal Surg 1992; 5:145–54.

32 Crohn's Anorectal Disease

David W. Dietz, Jeffrey W. Milsom, and Victor W. Fazio

Anorectal Manifestations of Crohn's Disease

Perianal Crohn's disease challenges even the most experienced of surgeons who treat inflammatory bowel disease. Malnutrition, poor wound healing, a propensity for recurrence, and the fear of serious anal sphincter impairment haunt both the patient and the surgeon and warrant a conservative approach. Fortunately, many patients with perianal Crohn's disease can be treated nonoperatively. When definitive surgical procedures are necessary, a number of recent reports have demonstrated that they can be performed with good results (1–5).

The frequency of anorectal manifestations in Crohn's disease varies widely in the literature, with a range between 8.5% to 93% (6). We reported an incidence of 56% in a group of 139 patients followed for more than 15 years at the Cleveland Clinic (7). The occurrence of anorectal pathology in Crohn's disease is related to several factors, including the pattern of involvement in the proximal bowel. Patients with Crohn's colitis are at the highest risk for developing perianal manifestations (47%) whereas the incidence is significantly less (25%) in those with isolated small bowel disease (8). Perianal disease usually arises after the diagnosis of Crohn's has been established in the proximal gastrointestinal tract, however anorectal problems are the first manifestation in 5% to 36% of cases (6,9,10).

A recent series of 129 patients with perianal Crohn's disease published by Platell et al. (1) illustrates the variety of anorectal lesions found in these patients and their relative frequency. The most common were perianal abscesses (29%), anal fis-sures (27%), low anal fistulas (26%), skin tags (5%), rectovaginal fistulas (5%), and high/complex anal fistulas (4%). Anal stenosis is also a common finding in patients with Crohn's disease, as are hemorrhoids. These anorectal manifestations can cause disabling symptoms, which are often exacerbated by the loose consistency of the patient's bowel movements related to more proximal disease. Thus, efforts to diagnose and treat this proximal disease are always of paramount importance in managing patients with anorectal Crohn's disease.

History and Physical Examination

Any prior diagnosis of inflammatory bowel disease or history of intestinal symptoms is obtained from the patient. Symptoms of the perianal disease are recorded, including presence and degree of pain, amount and character of discharge, fever, constitutional symptoms, and bowel habits. The patient is questioned for the presence of fecal soiling or incontinence, which can be secondary to sphincter injury caused by the disease itself, previous surgery, or the rigidity of a chronically inflamed rectum. A history of previous abdominal and perianal surgery is also gathered. Determining the current activity status of concurrent small and large bowel Crohn's, if present, is important in determining the overall strategy for the care of these patients.

A thorough examination of the anus and perineum is required in all patients suspected of having perianal Crohn's disease. If pain or anal stenosis precludes this in the office setting, an examination under anesthesia is performed.

Fig. 32.1. External examination of the perianal area in Crohn's disease may reveal edematous tags, macerations, external fistulous openings, and a "cyanotic" discoloration.

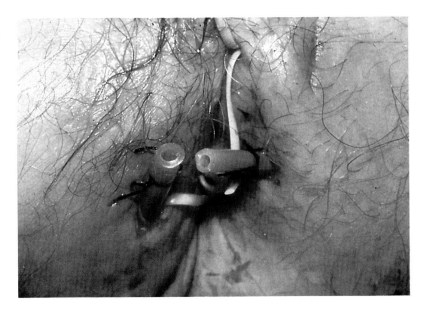

External examination may reveal perianal skin changes, including maceration, abrasions, and a "cyanotic" discoloration (Fig. 32.1). These lesions are nonspecific and reflect chronic infection or irritation secondary to diarrhea. External hemorrhoids may also be present. Edematous skin tags, 1 to 2 cm in size, may be seen protruding from the anal orifice and are one of the most common findings in patients with perianal Crohn's disease. A painful swelling with or without induration and overlying erythema is indicative of an anorectal abscess. If moderate to severe pain is present without swelling, an intersphincteric abscess should be suspected. Milder pain may be due to fissures. The external openings of fistulae may be visible on the perianal skin, and may extend to the perineum, genitalia, or thigh. These fistulae are often multiple and can be relatively innocuous. Predicting the course of the fistulous tract and its internal opening are difficult, as Goodsall's rule does not always apply to patients with Crohn's disease. Extensive probing in the office setting should not be attempted in friable tissues as there is a risk of creating false passages and little value accrues to the patient; it may also be quite uncomfortable for the patient. Probably greater than 90% of clinically important fistulae are detected by gentle probing or injection of the tracts with half-strength hydrogen peroxide in the operating room. Rarely, fistulograms (11), transanal ultrasound (12), and magnetic resonance imaging (MRI) (13) may be necessary to further define fistula tracts and search for occult abscesses.

Gentle separation of the buttocks may reveal an anal fissure. These lesions are typically deep with undermined edges but usually are not as painful as they appear. Fissures may be multiple and are not limited to the anterior or posterior midline as in patients without Crohn's disease. Digital rectal examination should be performed to assess the status of the sphincters. Anal stenosis may also be appreciated and is often high in the anal canal, at or above the dentate line.

Anoscopy and proctoscopy is performed to make a careful search for the internal opening of any fistulous tracts and to assess the rectum for inflammation and pliability. Every attempt is made to assess the amount of sphincter muscle involved. If Crohn's disease is suspected, biopsies are taken. Biopsy of the rectal mucosa has a higher yield than biopsy of the perianal lesions (14). In women, the rectovaginal septum should also be inspected from both the anorectal and vaginal sides for the presence of a rectovaginal fistula.

Any of the above findings in a patient with known Crohn's disease most likely represents anorectal manifestations of the same etiology but the differential should also include sexually-transmitted diseases, tuberculosis, hidradenitis suppurativa, leukemia, and anal cancer. Patients with Crohn's disease are at an increased risk for developing cancer and a number of different types of perianal carcinoma have been reported (15–17). These lesions may be related to chronic inflammation and irritation. The presence of mucinous discharge from a fistula tract or persistent induration in a nonsuppurative area raises the concern of cancer. Suspicious lesions should be biopsied.

In asymptomatic patients with no history of inflammatory bowel disease, certain findings should raise the suspicion of Crohn's. These include lack of pain, multiple lesions, fissures not located in the midline, deep ulcerations, skin discoloration, anal stricture, and complex fistulae. It is important to distinguish patients having perianal disease as their first manifestation of Crohn's from those with non-specific fissures, fistulae, and abscesses. The former group is approached in a conservative manner whereas the latter can undergo more aggressive or traditional surgical treatment. A history directed at bowel problems (notably diarrhea) and biopsy of the rectal mucosa and perianal lesions, along with sigmoidoscopy, offer the best chance at making this distinction (14,18,19).

Indices of Severity for Perianal Crohn's Disease

Several scoring systems have been devised to measure the severity of perianal Crohn's disease (20,21). The Perianal Crohn's Disease Activity Index proposed by the McMaster inflammatory bowel disease (IBD) Study Group is one example (Table 32.1). These schemes are meant to provide physicians with simple, objective assessments of disease activity that may aid in therapeutic decision-making and follow-up. They may also prove useful in determining and comparing outcomes during clinical trials and between institutions. These scoring systems await validation, however, and their value at this time remains questionable.

Indications for Surgery in Anorectal Crohn's Disease

The natural history of perianal Crohn's disease and the indications for operative therapy vary. Prompt surgical drainage is required in all patients with abscesses. These lesions will not resolve spontaneously and attempts at nonoperative management can lead to sphincter destruction or anal stenosis secondary to acute and chronic infection. Symptomatic fistulae also require surgical treatment with either setons, mushroom drains, or fistulotomy.

On the other hand, fissures and asymptomatic fistulae tend to be innocuous and may heal spontaneously or remain quiescent in response to medical management. Skin tags and hemorrhoids rarely cause symptoms and surgery is generally contraindicated for these lesions.

Table 32.1. Perianal Crohn's disease activity index.

Discharge
0	No discharge
1	Minimal mucous discharge
2	Moderate mucous or purulent discharge
3	Substantial discharge
4	Gross fecal soiling

Pain/restriction of activities
0	No activity restriction
1	Mild discomfort, no restriction
2	Moderate discomfort, some limitation of activities
3	Marked discomfort, marked limitation
4	Severe pain, severe limitation

Restriction of sexual activity
0	No restriction of sexual activity
1	Slight restriction of sexual activity
2	Moderate limitation of sexual activity
3	Marked limitation of sexual activity
4	Unable to engage in sexual activity

Type of perianal disease
0	No perianal disease/skin tags
1	Anal fissure or mucosal tear
2	<3 perianal fistulae
3	≥3 perianal fistulae
4	Anal sphincter ulceration of fistulae with significant undermining of skin

Degree of induration
0	No induration
1	Minimal induration
2	Moderate induration
3	Substantial induration
4	Gross fluctuance/abscess

Total score

Reprinted with permission from Irvine, et al.[20]

The philosophy towards the management of perianal Crohn's disease must be one of conservatism. The primary goal in treating these patients is to drain sepsis and relieve symptoms while preserving function of the sphincter mechanism. In the vast majority of cases, this goal can be met. Active Crohn's disease in the proximal bowel is usually treated first. This may allow healing of the perianal lesions in 47% to 80% of patients (22). We will present our approach to the management of these lesions below.

Manifestations of Anorectal Crohn's Disease Usually Treated Nonoperatively

Hemorrhoids and Skin Tags

External hemorrhoids and skin tags are common in patients with Crohn's disease, whereas internal hemorrhoids are unusual. These lesions rarely cause significant symptoms. Medical therapy consisting of sitz baths, topical agents, and control of diarrhea should be instituted. Hemorrhoidectomy in known Crohn's disease is contraindicated secondary to the risks of poor wound healing, anal stenosis, and sphincter injury. This concern is supported by a report from St. Mark's Hospital in which 11 of 20 patients with Crohn's disease suffered complications after hemorrhoidectomy. Six of these patients eventually required proctectomy as a direct result of the hemorrhoid surgery (23).

Fissures

Anal fissures in patients with Crohn's disease can be of two types. "Idiopathic" fissures are not related to the inflammatory bowel disease and are identical to those seen in normal patients. These fissures are typically shallow, located in the midline, and extend from just below the dentate line to the external margin of the anal canal. They usually respond to sitz baths, anesthetic and hydrocortisone ointments, bulk-forming agents, and control of diarrhea. Unfortunately, "idiopathic" fissures are rare in Crohn's disease.

The more common type of fissure seen in these patients is a distinct component of their Crohn's disease. "Crohn's" fissures are deep, wide, and sometimes multiple. They often occur laterally, away from the midline and are frequently accompanied by other components of perianal disease. Contrary to their angry appearance, however, these fissures are usually asymptomatic or cause only minor problems and should also be treated medically. If active Crohn's disease is present in the perianal region, oral metronidazole, 5-ASA enemas or suppositories, and immunosuppressive drugs may be indicated.

If pain is present, a thorough search for associated sepsis should be made. Any discovered abscesses must be drained surgically. Sexually-transmitted diseases and cancer are in the differential diagnosis and can be ruled out by serologic testing or appropriate biopsies.

Some patients with perianal Crohn's develop a unique type of anal canal ulcer which, in addition to being wide and penetrating, is very painful. These ulcers can involve extensive portions of the anal canal, and may even be circumferential. They usually do not respond to standard local therapy. Most will eventually require fecal diversion but we have used intralesional prednisolone (along with oral azathioprine) with significant relief of pain (24).

Rarely, a fissure will cause severe pain or bleeding and will be refractory to medical treatment. In these cases, anal dilatation or lateral internal sphincterotomy may be necessary. Sphincterotomy should only be undertaken when the patient's Crohn's disease is in remission, there is no diarrhea present, and hypertrophy of the lower one-third of the internal sphincter is causing high resting tone. Despite the most careful patient selection, sphincterotomy can still result in complications. Most surgeons will only perform this procedure on midline "idiopathic" strictures in patients with Crohn's disease. The recent report by Platell et. al. stated that 84% of their patients with anal fissures were treated nonoperatively. The remaining 16% required lateral internal sphincterotomy, which did heal the fissure in all cases (1). We prefer conservative two-finger dilatation to partial sphincterotomy in these cases. Topical nitroglycerine cream (0.2%) may also be helpful.

Anal Stenosis

Some degree of anal stenosis in patients with Crohn's disease is common, with a reported incidence of 26% (25). It usually occurs secondary to circumferential scarring precipitated by chronic perianal inflammation or previous surgical procedures. Anal stenosis can be relatively asymptomatic in some patients because of the soft nature of the stool. Symptoms are more likely to result from adjacent fissures, abscesses or fistulae than from the stenosis itself. Therefore, many Crohn's patients with anal stenoses require no specific treatment for this problem. Accompanying proctitis may be treated with sulphasalazine enemas or suppository preparations, oral metronidazole, or steroid enemas.

Patients who do have symptoms may be successfully treated with gentle finger dilatation under general anesthesia. This procedure can be repeated at intervals (determined by response to therapy) until symptoms resolve. We do not use mechanical dilators very often, in order to minimize the risk of sphincter injury. However, if symptoms persist or severe perianal sepsis develops, fecal diversion with a loop ileostomy may be indicated. Some patients may come to proctectomy or proctocolectomy.

A review of 44 patients with anorectal strictures secondary to Crohn's disease has been reported by Linares et al. (26). Ninety-eight percent of these patients had proctitis while 93% had additional perianal disease. Five of the patients underwent medical treatment only, which was successful in all cases. Dilatation was necessary in 33 patients; 15

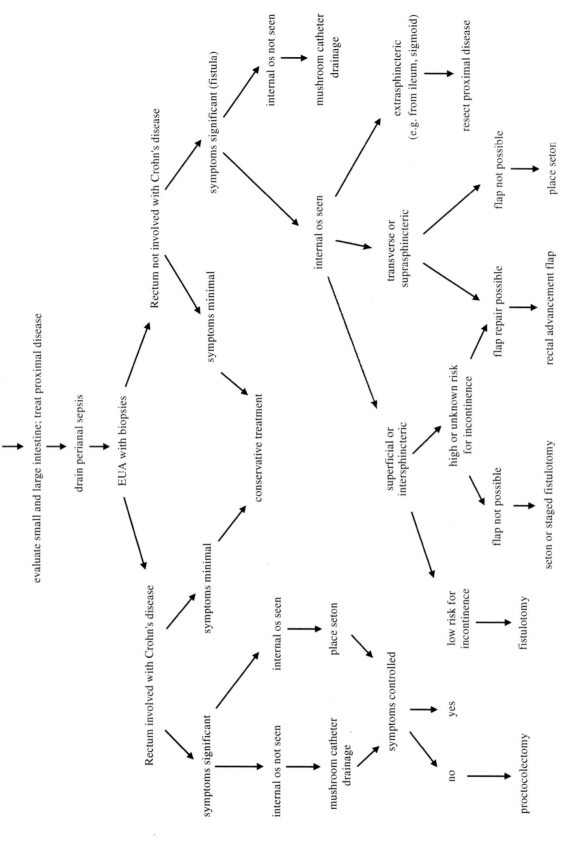

Fig. 32.2. Algorithm for surgical treatment of abscesses and fistulae in patients with anorectal Crohn's disease.

required only one treatment, eight required two, and 10 required three or more. The long-term success rate for dilatation was approximately 50%. Complications of dilatation were limited to exacerbation of perianal sepsis and occurred in 20%. Nineteen patients eventually required proctectomy, most often as a result of severe perianal sepsis.

Manifestations of Anorectal Crohn's Disease Usually Treated Operatively (Fig. 32.2)

Anorectal Abscesses and Fistulae—Treatment Strategy

Fistulae and their associated abscesses are the most common anorectal manifestations of Crohn's disease requiring surgical intervention. They are also the most difficult to treat. Fistulae in Crohn's disease can arise from the anal crypts or from full-thickness ulcerations of the low rectal mucosa. Fistulization proceeds through the perirectal tissues and may lead to the formation of an abscess that can be manifested clinically by pain, swelling, and fever. Often, however, the septic process will continue to spread without producing symptoms until it eventually erupts through the skin of the perianal area, perineum, genitalia, or thigh (22).

The first step in the treatment of a patient with suppurative perianal Crohn's disease presenting with an abscess is incision and drainage. For this step, we perform a limited incision close to the anal margin to evacuate the pus. Usually, a 10–16 French mushroom catheter is then inserted that can be left in the abscess cavity for several months if necessary (Fig. 32.3). If the fistula tract can be identified, a loose, noncutting seton may be placed to insure adequate drainage. Primary fistulotomy is not performed at this time. If there is cellulitis present, broad-spectrum antibiotics should be prescribed.

Once the acute process has resolved, attention can be turned toward treatment of the underlying fistula. Sound judgment is needed at this stage and is based on a number of factors including the anatomy of the fistula, extent and activity of the patient's Crohn's disease, status of the sphincter muscles, and, most importantly, the severity of symptoms. Using these criteria, several scenarios may be encountered.

Asymptomatic Low Fistulae

Low fistulae which are well tolerated by the patient do not require treatment. Keighley and Allan re-

ported on 40 patients with untreated low fistulae and found that 14 resolved spontaneously whereas 13 persisted but remained asymptomatic (22). If active Crohn's disease is present in the rectum, it should be treated with steroids or 5-ASA compounds (17).

Symptomatic Low Fistulae

Low intrasphincteric or transphincteric fistulae which cause troublesome symptoms should be treated by fistulotomy. Good results with this technique have been reported by a number of authors (27–33). In a recent series from McKee and Keenan, 21 of 34 low fistulae treated by fistulotomy healed permanently. Williams et al. found no adverse effects on sphincter function in 26 of 33 patients, and only minor incontinence in 3 (27). Any active Crohn's disease in the perianal area or rectum is addressed prior to surgery (33). Some groups have advocated lateral internal sphincterotomy to treat this group of patients (31), but this has not been our practice.

Complex Fistulae

"Complex" fistulae in Crohn's disease are those that are high and transphincteric, suprasphincteric, extrasphincteric, and rectovaginal. Anterior fistulae in females may also be considered complex, as the sphincters are relatively thin in this region. Fistula tracts with multiple external openings ("watering-can perineum") are also included in this category, as are recurrent fistulae.

The treatment of complex fistulae can be one of the most challenging facets of managing patients with Crohn's disease. The high internal opening increases the risk of incontinence with fistulotomy. Wound healing is also impaired. Anal stenosis, if present, may preclude good visualization of the anal canal, even in the operating room. The goal of therapy, therefore, often is not to eradicate the fistula but rather to alleviate symptoms. If a single fistula tract is present it can be treated by the insertion of a noncutting (loose) seton to insure adequate drainage and prevent recurrent abscess formation. A draining seton can be left in place indefinitely or until epithelialization of the tract allows its removal. This will convert the acute suppurative fistula into a chronic tract with well-controlled drainage.

The use of metronidazole or immunosuppressive agents have been advocated for the treatment of Crohn's fistulae. Several uncontrolled trials have reported symptomatic relief in greater than 90% and some degree of perianal healing in 50% to

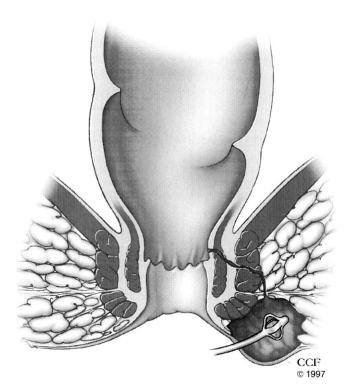

Fig. 32.3. A mushroom-shaped (dePezzar) latex catheter provides effective drainage of a perianal abscess related to Crohn's disease and may be left in place for several months if necessary.

CCF
© 1997

83% of patients treated with metronidazole. However, the drug must be given over many months, and the recurrence rate is high (up to 78%) after the drug is stopped (34,35). Unfortunately, chronic administration of metronidazole results in gastrointestinal symptoms, paresthesias, and other side effects. The mechanism whereby metronidazole promotes healing of perianal Crohn's disease is not known. Ciprofloxacin may be as effective as metronidazole but does not have the associated side effects (36). Imuran, 6-mercaptopurine, and cyclosporine have also been effective in initially closing some fistulae. Long-term results have not been as good, however, and side effects may be significant (18).

When adequate drainage of the tract has been achieved and rectal inflammation has quiesced, an endorectal advancement flap can be used in certain circumstances to close the internal opening of the fistulae. Counter drainage of the tract must be maintained until healing has occurred. Kodner, et al. (37) used advancement flaps to treat 24 patients with complex fistulae secondary to Crohn's disease. Primary healing occurred in 17 and eventual healing was obtained in 5 others for a final success rate of 92%.

In the case of multiple fistula tracts or those which continue to recur despite seton drainage and medical treatment, a more aggressive approach is required. Temporary fecal diversion may

need to be added in order to minimize ongoing contamination of the perianal region. Although this may not change the natural history of their disease, it may allow an improvement in the general condition of the patient. It may also provide a period of time for the patient to become psychologically adjusted to the idea of a permanent stoma, should it become necessary. In our practice, a laparoscopic loop ileostomy is the preferred method for diversion (see Chapter 25). A stoma may also permit advancement flap surgery to proceed "under the cover" of the stoma, giving it a greater chance to heal.

The success of any of these methods is largely dependent on the status of the patient's rectum. If the rectum is spared or the Crohn's disease is in remission, then chances for success are high. If these methods fail, however, or a watering-can perineum exists, then the patient is likely best served by proctectomy or proctocolectomy. In these cases, extensive destruction of the sphincters and perineum make further conservative therapy pointless. If active perineal sepsis is not present and the patient is reasonably fit, a one stage resection may be performed. If this is not the case, a subtotal colectomy and end-ileostomy can be done initially. This is followed by completion proctectomy when the perianal sepsis has quiesced and the general condition of the patient is improved.

Using a strategy of catheter drainage of abscesses, control of the fistula tract with setons, and intensive medical therapy, Fry et al. were able to avoid fecal diversion or proctectomy in 76% of their patients (5). Most of the 12% of patients requiring proctectomy did so for their rectal rather than perianal disease.

Recto- and Anovaginal Fistulae

Discharge of stool or gas from the vagina is the classic presentation of a recto- or anovaginal fistula. These fistulae usually arise from deep ulcerations in the rectal or anal mucosa that form tracts that eventually erode through the vaginal wall. They can rarely begin as cryptoglandular abscesses. As in all other types of Crohn's fistulae, severity of symptoms dictates the treatment. Asymptomatic lesions require no surgical treatment.

Symptomatic rectovaginal fistulae may cause dyspareunia, perineal pain, difficulty with hygiene, or repeated vaginal infections. Treatment during acute infection begins with catheter drainage of abscesses and insertion of noncutting setons. Medical therapy with 5-ASA compounds, metronidazole, or immunosuppressives is then undertaken. If this regimen fails to resolve the sepsis or discomfort associated with the fistula, temporary fecal diversion may be necessary.

Once infection is no longer present, a definitive repair can be attempted. If minimal to mild anorectal disease are present, we perform a transanal curvilinear rectal advancement flap. High and long fistula tracts are treated with a similar rectal advancement flap. A protecting stoma may or may not be created. In cases where there is severe ulceration of the anal mucosa, a sleeve advancement flap may be indicated with a temporary stoma. Using these techniques, we have achieved healing in 24 of 35 patients (68%) with Crohn's disease and anovaginal fistulae (38).

If all measures fail, or severe anorectal disease or poor sphincter tone with incontinence is present, total proctocolectomy is performed. The vaginal defect can be excised and closed primarily, or left open if sepsis is present in the surrounding tissues.

Hidradenitis Suppurativa in Crohn's Disease

Hidradenitis suppurativa is a chronic skin infection involving the apocrine sweat glands. This disease entity often involves the perineum and can be difficult to distinguish from perianal Crohn's. However, the fistulae associated with this disease should not extend more than two thirds of the way into the anal canal, as this is the limit of the apocrine glands. Fistulae in Crohn's disease typically extend to or above the level of the dentate line. In addition, the presence of granulomas on biopsy suggests Crohn's. It is important to make the distinction between these two diseases, if possible. Patients with hidradenitis who are mistakenly diagnosed with Crohn's disease may have surgery withheld unnecessarily, or be subjected to inappropriate medical therapy. Conversely, performing a radical resection for presumed hidradenitis in a patient who actually has Crohn's disease can be disastrous.

Hidradenitis suppurativa and Crohn's disease can also coexist. We have reported on a series of 61 patients with hidradenitis treated at the Cleveland Clinic (39), of which 24 (38%) also had a diagnosis of Crohn's. The Crohn's disease in these patients tended to be severe and usually predated the onset of hidradenitis. The coexistence of these diseases may lead to complications such as persistent perineal sepsis after proctectomy. An increased awareness of this possibility may allow more appropriate treatment.

Preoperative Preparation

Examination of the GI Tract

The entire gastrointestinal tract is studied in patients with symptoms of active inflammatory bowel disease prior to treatment of the perianal lesions. This evaluation consists of a colonoscopy along with enteroclysis or a small bowel follow-through to rule out diseased proximal bowel segments. Proctosigmoidoscopy is performed in patients presenting with perianal Crohn's to assess the status of the rectum and distal sigmoid colon.

Treat Active Small and Large Bowel Crohn's Disease

Active rectal inflammation will greatly reduce the chances of healing the perianal disease, especially after surgery. For this reason, preoperative treatment with steroids or 5-ASA compounds is imperative. Even the presence of active Crohn's disease in the more proximal large and small intestine may significantly decrease the chances for perianal healing. After resection of these diseased segments, however, spontaneous healing rates of 47% and 60% have been reported (40,41). In our practice, perianal Crohn's, in and of itself, is not sufficient indication for resection of proximal diseased bowel.

Maximize Nutritional Status

Malnutrition is common in patients with active Crohn's disease and may impair healing. The nutritional status is assessed preoperatively and malnutrition is corrected.

Skin Care

The condition of the perianal skin is optimized prior to operation. Sitz baths for patient comfort and frequent dressing changes to keep the area dry can be employed.

Mechanical Bowel Preparation

Magnesium citrate (12 oz.) or 90 cc of phosphosoda (Fleet's phosphosoda, Lynchburg, VA, USA) is used to prepare the bowel in all patients undergoing advancement flap repair, fecal diversion, or proctectomy. We avoid polyethylene glycol lavage in these patients, as it is usually not well-tolerated.

Antibiotics

Broad-spectrum intravenous antibiotics are given preoperatively and continued in the immediate postoperative period (at least 24 hours) for fistulotomies, advancement flaps, fecal diversions, and proctectomies. Ciprofloxacin (500 mg) and metronidazole (500 mg) is the preferred combination in our practice.

Pitfalls and Danger Points

1. Failure to identify and treat active rectal, colonic, or small bowel disease.
2. Failure to drain sepsis before any reconstructive procedure.
3. Overly aggressive surgery in inflamed tissue.
4. Damage to the sphincter mechanism.
5. Failure to identify a perineal neoplasm.

Useful Instruments and Techniques (Fig. 32.4)

1. Lighted Hill-Ferguson retractors (small, medium, and large).
2. Lacrimal duct probes.
3. Wing tip probes.
4. Currettes (short- and long- [uterine] handled).
5. Fine-tipped thin tonsil and right-angle clamps.
6. Blunt needle for peroxide injection.
7. Silastic setons.
8. Small mushroom catheter drains (10–16 F).
9. Perianal stay sutures for rectal advancement flaps.
10. Epinephrine (1:200.000) and saline to aid in elevating flap from underlying sphincter or rectovaginal septum when performing advancement flaps.
11. Pediatric anoscope for office visualization of low rectum/anal canal and to evaluate healing of rectovaginal fistula repairs.

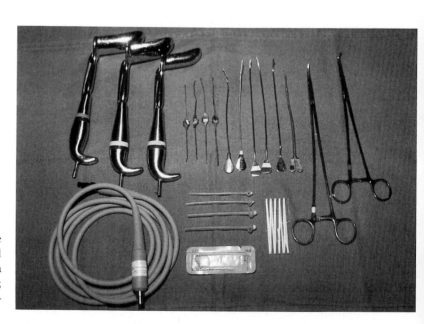

Fig. 32.4. A variety of surgical tools are necessary to effectively treat anorectal Crohn's disease: lighted retractors; fistula probes; mushroom-type latex catheters; long, thin, angled clamps; and setons (either silicone or silk).

Specific Operative Techniques— Abscesses, Anorectal Fistulae, and Rectovaginal Fistulae

Incision and Drainage of Abscesses (Fig. 32.5)

If the abscess is superficial, the procedure may be done in the office. However, in the case of a deeper abscess, the surgeon should not hesitate to schedule the patient for general anesthesia in order to effect thorough drainage. The patient is usually placed in the prone jackknife position. If possible, a thorough examination of the anal canal and distal rectum (described previously) is performed to identify associated fistulas, fissures, or inflammation. The skin is then prepared with 10% providone-iodine solution. A fluctuant point as close as possible to the anal verge is selected and the skin is anesthetized. A 1 cm radial stab incision is then made into the abscess cavity. After loculations are broken up by gentle finger exploration, a 10–16 F soft latex mushroom catheter (Bard Urological Catheter, C.R. Bard, Inc., Covington, GA, USA) is stretched over a probe and inserted into the cavity. The catheter is cut so that a length of 2 to 3 cm will protrude from the opening. The catheter is sutured in place with a 2–0 or 3–0 absorbable suture and a small absorbent dressing is placed over the wound. Disposable mesh underwear rather than adhesive tape is used to hold the dressing in place, since tape may not stick well and is painful to remove.

Fistulotomy for Low/Superficial Fistulae (Fig. 32.6)

General anesthesia is used. The patient is placed in the prone jackknife position and the skin is prepared with 10% providone-iodine solution. A fistula probe is carefully inserted into the external os and is passed through the tract until it emerges from the internal os. The probe should never be advanced forcefully or blindly. If the tract or its internal opening are difficult to ascertain, injecting hydrogen peroxide or methylene blue into the external os may be helpful. The fistulotomy is initiated at the external os by cutting down on the probe using a #15 blade scalpel or electrosurgery instrument. The tract is then unroofed, carrying the incision cephalad towards the internal os by following the probe. Meticulous hemostasis is essential so that any portion of the sphincter muscle encountered can be identified prior to being divided. If a significant portion of the external sphincter is encountered, the fistulotomy is stopped and a seton is inserted to drain the remainder of the tract. "Significant" sphincter is any

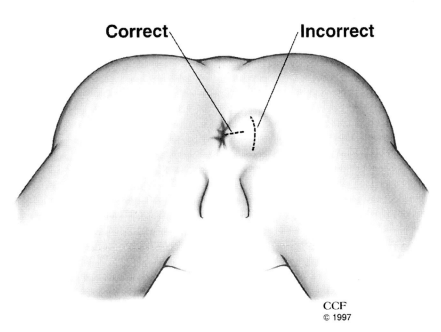

Correct   **Incorrect**

CCF
© 1997

Fig. 32.5. The perianal incision to drain an abscess in Crohn's disease should be placed as close as possible to the anal outlet and should be radial in orientation. This keeps the track as short as possible and minimizes risk of injuring branches of the pudendal nerve traveling to the anal sphincters.

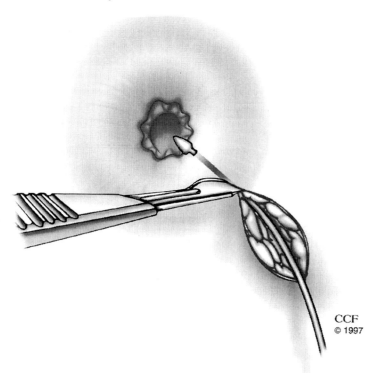

Fig. 32.6.   A fistulatomy over a probe is acceptable for a very low anorectal fistula. Only minimal sphincter muscle should ever be divided in a Crohn's patient, because recurrent fistula are common, and the risk of incontinence is higher than in the general populations.

CCF
© 1997

amount the surgeon believes may endanger reasonable continence postoperatively. Crohn's patients must have a "better" sphincter than most, owing to their generally loose stools. The unroofed fistula tract should be curetted. This careful approach will minimize the chances of rendering the patient incontinent.

Postoperative Care

If perianal sepsis is encountered during surgery, intravenous or oral antibiotics are continued postoperatively. Daily sitz baths are initiated. Loose bowel movements may be controlled with bulk-forming agents (e.g., psyllium) and loperamide or diphenoxylate hydrochloride with atropine sulfate, if necessary; if diarrhea is refractory, paregoric or tincture of opium can be used. The patient is seen in follow up every 2 to 3 weeks until healing is completed.

Complications

Infection is the most common postoperative complication of fistulotomy. Serious cases can be avoided by early follow-up and treatment when indicated. Postoperative incontinence should be a rare occurrence if the principles outlined above are followed. Careful questioning during preoperative visits can alert the surgeon to the patient who already has compromised sphincter function and no margin for error. Anal manometry may be of benefit.

Setons for Complex Fistulae (Fig. 32.7)

Draining setons and mushroom catheters should be used liberally in the treatment of patients with symptomatic fistulae secondary to Crohn's disease. A noncutting seton encircling the tract through the external and internal openings can ensure drainage to prevent recurrent abscess formation while the patient is being prepared for further surgery. Once the tract has epithelialized and sepsis has resolved, a definitive procedure can be contemplated. In patients with complex fistulae or severe active perianal disease that has not responded to medical therapy, treatment with a draining seton, possibly permanently, is indicated for symptomatic relief. We prefer to use silastic setons made of either fine tubing or thin, flat vessel loops (Surg-I-Loop, Scanlan International, St. Paul, MN, USA). Setons can be changed as needed. We believe there is no role for the use of cutting setons in patients with perianal Crohn's disease.

Postoperative Care

The patient is seen in follow-up every 2 to 3 weeks until the acute process has resolved and then every 3 to 6 months, thereafter. Maximal medical treatment is continued as previously outlined.

Complications

Complications as a result of seton drainage should be minimal. Incontinence or an exacerbation in

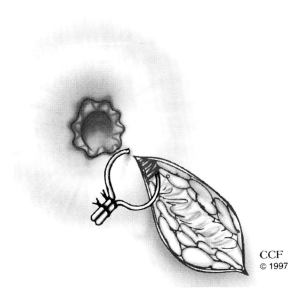

Fig. 32.7. A draining seton (a loosely applied one) is used whenever the surgeon is concerned about dividing the anal sphincter muscle. The seton should be lax and made of either silk (size #2) or silicone (vessel loop material used by vascular surgeons). The external portion of the track is opened to promote drainage.

the perianal disease may occur, but these will more likely be related to the natural course of the patient's Crohn's disease rather than to the surgical procedure.

Rectal Advancement Flaps for Complex and Rectovaginal Fistulae (Fig. 32.8)

A rectal advancement flap to cover the internal os of the fistula tract should only be attempted if there is minimal to no rectal disease present and anal symptoms are troublesome to the patient. At the Cleveland Clinic, we always use a transanal approach (rather than the transvaginal). The operation is performed with the patient in either the prone jackknife position (if the opening is anterior) or the lithotomy position using Lloyd-Davies stirrups (if the opening is posterior). In the area of the repair, the rectal wall, including muscularis propria, is infiltrated with 1:200,000 epinephrine to maintain hemostasis. Liberal amounts of saline can also be injected into the submucosa and rectal wall to increase flap thickness and facilitate dissection. A thick, broad-based, U-shaped flap is then elevated, beginning at the internal os of the fistula and continuing for 4 to 5 cm cephalad. The flap consists of mucosa, submucosa, muscle fibers of the internal sphincter, and the muscularis propria of the rectal wall (perirectal fat should be

encountered). Absolute hemostasis must be maintained by use of electrosurgery. The fistula tract is then curetted and closed in layers using 2-0 or 3-0 absorbable sutures and a mushroom catheter is inserted into the external opening to insure adequate counter drainage. In the case of a rectovaginal fistula, the tract is also cored out, closed in layers, and the vaginal mucosa is left open for drainage. The distal end of the flap is then trimmed (angled thoracic surgery scissors may be quite helpful), elevated, and pulled down over the repaired defect and secured with 2-0 chromic sutures.

In the case of complex fistulae or extensive anal canal ulceration, modifications of this technique are necessary. One of the authors (VF) has described a procedure in which the diseased anal mucosa is completely excised and a circumferential sleeve of rectum is advanced downward and sutured to the neodentate line (38) (Fig. 32.8). Fecal diversion should be considered after any of these advancement flap repairs if the operation has not been technically perfect.

Postoperative Care
The patient is kept on clear liquids only for the first 48 hours postoperatively. Medical constipation can be considered for the initial 48 hours using an agent such as loperamide or codeine. The urinary catheter is removed as soon as the patient is able to ambulate. Intravenous antibiotics are given until discharge from the hospital, typically on postoperative day 3; oral antibiotics are usually not prescribed. Patients are sent home on a program consisting of sitz baths, bulk-forming agents, and stool softeners with drainage catheters left in place. The patient should be seen back in the office in 10 to 14 days at which time the repair can be inspected (a pediatric anoscope is helpful to assess the flap). If adequate healing has taken place, drainage catheters can be removed. Any medical treatment of the patients Crohn's disease initiated prior to surgery should be continued for at least 3 to 4 months postoperatively.

Complications
Again, infection is the most common complication. If not recognized promptly and treated, dehiscence of the flap can result. Flap necrosis can also occur if the flap becomes elevated by hematoma. The incidence of this can be minimized by maintaining strict hemostasis during the dissection and returning the patient to the operating room early on to drain any suspected infection.

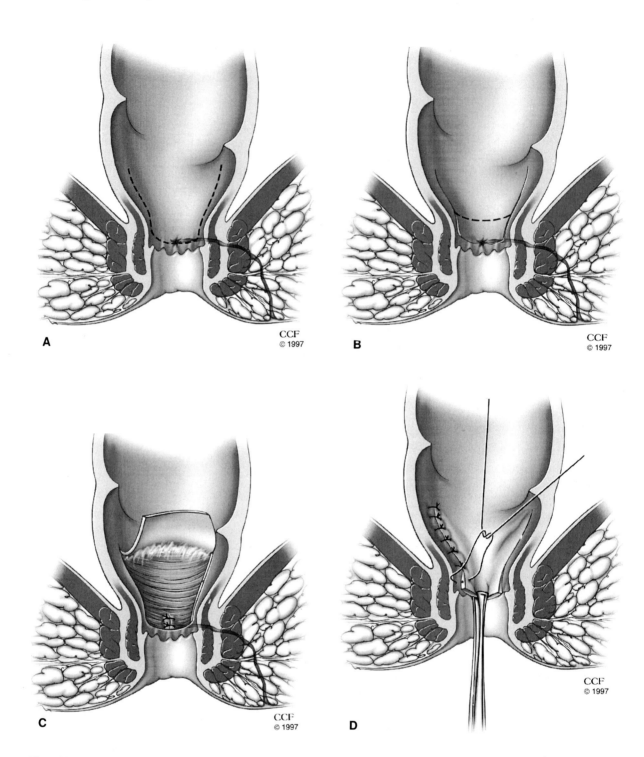

Fig. 32.8. Rectal Advancement Flap Procedure in Crohn's anorectal fistula: consideration for the procedure is only undertaken when the anorectal disease is quiescent. (A) Initially, a thick broad-based U-shaped flap is chosen, with the apex of the flap at the internal fistulous opening. (B) Scarring on inflammation of the flap adjacent to the internal opening is trimmed off.

(C) The flap is raised for a distance cephalad of about 4–6 cm and the internal opening is closed with size 2-0 absorbable sutures. (D) The flap is gently advanced over the internal opening and closed with a series of interrupted size 3-0 sutures (running sutures are also acceptable). This type of flap generally will easily slide over the internal opening and cover it without tension.

Fecal Diversion

If the terminal ileum is not involved with Crohn's disease, we prefer a laparoscopic loop ileostomy for temporary fecal diversion (Chapter 25). A loop ileostomy is easier for the patient to manage and it does not require an intraabdominal procedure for reversal. The creation of a stoma is not intended to heal the fistula. We use temporary diverting stomas in two settings; to protect a definitive repair and to decrease major perianal sepsis prior to planned proctocolectomy. In the latter instance, this may provide the patient with a period of adjustment prior to creation of a permanent stoma.

Advantages of the laparoscopic approach include a minimal incision remote from the stoma site, rapid return of bowel function, less adhesion formation, and a quick return to normal activity. We have recently reported our initial experience in 13 patients undergoing laparoscopic fecal diversion for the treatment of perianal Crohn's disease (42).

Proctectomy

We perform an intersphincteric proctectomy at the Cleveland Clinic, as described by Turnbull and Fazio (43). The internal sphincter is excised along with the rectum while the external sphincter, levator muscles, and puborectalis are retained. This minimizes the chance of postoperative sexual dysfunction in these patients. A pelvic drain is placed and exited through an abdominal stab wound. The levators are closed from both the abdominal side and perineal aspect. All fistula tracts are widely drained and the skin edges are left open.

Conclusions

The management of patients with anorectal manifestations of Crohn's disease is complex and fraught with dangers. After a thorough history and physical examination, the surgeon, gastroenterologist, and patient together should formulate a carefully thought-out plan of action. This plan should take into account the patient's symptoms, severity of disease, and the likelihood of a definitive surgical procedure to cause further harm. The goals of treatment should be realistic and clear. Once the acute suppuration has been treated with drainage, medical therapy can be undertaken to treat the underlying Crohn's disease. Great patience is required during this period of time. A definitive operation is contemplated only if the tissues can be returned to a healthy state. If these general principles are followed, complications will be minimized and good results can be achieved.

References

1. Platell C, Mackay J, Collopy B, et al. Anal pathology in patients with Crohn's disease. Aust NZ J Surg 1996;66:5–9.
2. Williamson PR, Hellinger MD, Larach SW, et al. Twenty-year review of the surgical management of perianal Crohn's disease. Dis Colon Rectum 1995;38:389–92.
3. Pescatori M, Interisano A, Basso L, et al. Management of perianal Crohn's disease. Dis Colon Rectum 1995;38:121–4.
4. McKee RF, Keenan RA. Perianal Crohn's disease—is it all bad news? Dis Colon Rectum 1996;39:136–42.
5. Fry RD, Shemesh EI, Kodner IJ, et al. Techniques and results in the management of anal and perianal Crohn's disease. Surg Gynecol Obstet 1989;168:42–8.
6. Williams DR, Coller JA, Corman ML, et al. Anal complications in Crohn's disease. Dis Colon Rectum 1981;24:22–4.
7. Harper PH, Fazio VW, Lavery IC, et al. The long-term outcome in Crohn's disease. Dis Colon Rectum 1987;30:174–9.
8. Rankin GB, Watts D, Melnyk CS, et al. National cooperative Crohn's disease study: extraintestinal manifestations and perianal complications. Gastroenterology 1979;77:914–20.
9. Kodner IJ. Perianal Crohn's disease. In: Inflammatory Bowel Diseases, 1996.
10. Homan WP, Tang CK, Thorbjarnarson B. Anal lesions complicating Crohn's disease. Arch Surg 1976;111:1333–5.
11. Weisman RI, Orsay CP, Pearl PK, et al. The role of fistulography in fistula-in-ano. Dis Colon Rectum 1991;24:181–4.
12. Solomon MJ, McLeod RS, Cohen EK, et al. Reliability and validity studies of endoluminal ultrasonography for anorectal disorders. Dis Colon Rectum 1994;37:546–51.
13. Jenss H, Starlinger M, Skaleij M. Magnetic resonance imaging in perianal Crohn's disease [letter]. Lancet 1992;340:1286.
14. Abcarian H. Perianal Crohn's disease. Sem Colon Rectal Surg 1994;5(3):210–5.
15. Ball CS, Wujanto R, Haboubi NY, et al. Carcinoma in anal Crohn's disease: discussion paper. J R Soc Med 1981;81:217–9.
16. Preston DM, Fowler EG, Lennard-Jones JE, et al. Carcinoma of the anus in Crohn's disease. Br J Surg 1983;70:346–7.
17. Slater G, Greenstein A, Aufses AJ Jr. Anal carcinoma in patients with Crohn's disease. Ann Surg 1984;199:348–50.
18. Nivatvongs S. Crohn's disease. In: Gordon PH, Nivatvong S, eds. Principles and practice of surgery for the colon, rectum, and anus. St. Louis, Q.M.P., 1992.

408   D.W. Dietz, J.W. Milsom, and V.W. Fazio

19. Alexander-Williams J, Buchmann P. Perianal Crohn's disease. World J Surg 1980;4:203–8.

20. Jan Irvine E, et al. for the McMaster IBD study group. Usual therapy improves perianal Crohn's disease as measured by a new disease activity index. J Clin Gastroenterol 1995;20(1):27–32.

21. Allan A, Linares L, Spooner HA, et al. Clinical index to quantitate symptoms of perianal Crohn's disease. Dis Colon Rectum 1992;35:656–61.

22. Allan A, Keighley MRB. Management of perianal Crohn's disease. World J Surg 1988;12:198–202.

23. Jeffrey PJ, Ritchie JL, Parks AG. Treatment of hemorrhoids in patients with inflammatory bowel disease. Lancet 1977;1:1084–5.

24. Hughes LE, Donaldson DR, Williams JG, Taylor BA, et al. Local depot methylprednisilone injection for painful anal Crohn's disease. Gastroenterology 1988;94:709–11.

25. Wolff BG, Culp CE, Beart RW, et al. Anorectal Crohn's disease: a long-term perspective. Dis. Colon Rectum 1985;28:709–11.

26. Linares L, Moreira LF, Andrews H, et al. Natural history and treatment of anorectal strictures complicating Crohn's disease. Br J Surg 1988;75:653–5.

27. Williams JG, Rothenberger DA, Nemer FD, et al. Fistula-in-ano in Crohn's disease: results of aggressive surgical treatment. Dis Colon Rectum 1991;34:378–84.

28. Marks CG, Ritchie JK, Lockhart-Mummery HE. Anal fistulas in Crohn's disease. Br J Surg 1981;68:525–7.

29. Bernard D, Morgan S, Tasse D. Selective surgical management of Crohn's disease of the anus. Canadian J Surg 1986;29:318–22.

30. Hobbiss JH, Schofield PF. Management of perianal Crohn's disease. J R Soc Med (London) 1982;75:414–7.

31. Sohn N, Korelitz BI, Weinstein MA. Anorectal Crohn's disease: definitive surgery for fistulas and recurrent abscesses. Am J Surg 1980;139:394–7.

32. Levien DH, Surrell J, Mazier WP. Surgical treatment of anorectal fistula in patients with Crohn's disease. Surg Gynecol Obstet 1989;169:133–6.

33. Morrison JG, Gathright JB, Ray JE, et. al. Surgical management of anorectal fistulas in Crohn's disease. Dis Colon Rectum 1989;32:492–6.

34. Bernstein LH, Frank MS, Brandt LJ, et al. Healing of perineal Crohn's disease with metronidazole. Gastroenterology 1980;79:357–65.

35. Brandt LJ, Bernstein LH, Boley SJ, et al. Metronidazole therapy for perineal Crohn's disease. A follow up study. Gastroenterology 1982;83:383–7.

36. Turunen U, Farkkila M, Seppala K. Long-term treatment of perianal or fistulous Crohn's disease with ciprofloxacin. Scand J Gastroenterol Suppl 1989;24:144.

37. Kodner IJ, Mazor A, Shemesh EI, et al. Endorectal advancement flap repair of rectovaginal and other complicated anorectal fistulas. Surgery 1993;114:682–90.

38. Hull TL, Fazio VW. Surgical approaches to low anovaginal fistula in Crohn's disease. Am J Surg 1997;173:95–8.

39. Church JM, Fazio VW, Lavery IC, et al. The differential diagnosis and comorbidity of hidradenitis suppurativa and perianal Crohn's disease. Int J Colorect Dis 1993;8:117–9.

40. Hellers G, Bergstrand O, Ewerth S, et al. Occurrence and outcome after primary treatment of anal fistulae in Crohn's disease. Gut 1980;21:525–7.

41. Heuman R, Bolin T, Sjodahl R, et al. The incidence and course of perianal complications and arhthralgia after intestinal resection with restoration of continuity for Crohn's disease. Br J Surg 1981;68:528–30.

42. Ludwig KA, Milsom JW, Church JM, et al. Preliminary experience with laparoscopic intestinal surgery for Crohn's disease. Am J Surg 1996;171:52–6.

43. Turnbull RB, Fazio VW. Advances in the surgical techique of ulcerative colitis surgery-endoanal proctectomy and two-directional myotomy ileostomy. Surg Ann Nygus LM, ed., NY: Appleton-Century-Crofts-Pub., Division of Prentice-Hall, 1975;315–29.

33 Ileoanal Pouches

M.R.B. Keighley, S. Korsgen, and H.T. Tan

Background

Few surgeons and no self-respecting gastroenterologist would advise an ileal pouch for patients known to have Crohn's disease (1). This dogma was first challenged in reservoir ileostomy on the grounds that the quality of life was so much better in patients with a Kock pouch compared with conventional ileostomy and that individuals should be given the right to choose, particularly if the risks of recurrent Crohn's disease or Crohn's complications are likely to be low (2). Thus it was suggested that reservoir ileostomy might be considered in patients who had no evidence of ileal Crohn's disease despite histological evidence of Crohn's colitis and who had had no complications for ten years with a conventional ileostomy (3). Despite this, the literature is full of disasters amoungst patients having a Kock pouch who eventually turned out to have Crohn's disease. In these patients there was a high incidence of abdominal sepsis, fistulas, obstruction, and metabolic sequelae (4,5,6).

There are now a variety of reports of unsuspected Crohn's disease occurring in the ileal pouch or in the ileum above the pouch following restorative proctocolectomy and ileoanal anastomosis where the original histology in the colectomy specimen or in the proctectomy specimen suggested ulcerative colitis (7–12). One of the most common forms of presentation has been late pouch vaginal fistula (13,14) or chronic pelvic or perineal fistulas in both sexes. A few patients have developed obstructive pouchitis with ulceration and bowel thickening, some of whom have been improved by antimicrobial agents or steroid medication. There are also a few patients who have developed obstruction in the ileum, in or more commonly above the pouch, that may be a source of sepsis or fistulas. Another group comprises patients with megaloblastic anemia or other metabolic sequelae of Crohn's disease (15).

We should recognize that many patients develop pouch vaginal, pouch perineal, and pouch vesical fistulas without there being any evidence of Crohn's disease (16). Likewise, patients may develop pouch anal stenosis, chronic pouchitis, pelvic sepsis, and chronic ileoanal dehiscence without there being any evidence of Crohn's disease at all (17). It is also important that cases labeled as Crohn's disease should conform to the known pattern of the disease's natural history. Hence, a single granuloma from a pouch biopsy in a patient with poor pouch function should not be assigned as Crohn's disease unless there is progressive deterioration of function, fistulas, obstruction, or where pouch excision clearly indicates macroscopic as well as histolopathologic evidence of Crohn's disease.

Crohn's Disease

A diagnosis of Crohn's disease is one based on macroscopic appearances and thus radiology of the gut, histopathology, and natural history. It is inappropriate to use histology alone as the final arbiter since in as many as 10% to 15% of proctocolectomy resection specimens ulcerative colitis and Crohn's disease cannot be distinguished and pathologists will not agree. The importance of macroscopic appearances cannot be overstated, if there is discontinuous disease skip lesions, transmural inflammation, linear ulceration, cobblestoning of the mucosa, ileal or appendiceal involvement, most patients have a natural history that is compatible with Crohn's disease. Even if the appearance of the colon and the histology are unequivocal ulcerative colitis, 5% to 10% of patients followed up for more than 20 years after proctocolectomy will develop ileal disease, usually just proximal to the abdominal wall and are reclassified as Crohn's disease.

The histological features which favor Crohn's disease are deep fissured ulcers, panmural inflammation and submucosal fibrosis, noncaseating epitheloid granulomas, crypt abscesses, and focal lymphocytic infiltration forming microgranulomata.

Indeterminate Colitis: How Does It Relate to Crohn's Colitis?

Indeterminate colitis is poorly defined and interpreted differently by separate histopathologists (see Chapter 4 for an extensive discussion on this) (18). Some merely use the term to describe slightly atypical colitis, whereas others confine indeterminate colitis to pathology that is more likely to be Crohn's disease but where all the diagnostic features are not present and thus a confident diagnosis of Crohn's disease on the material available cannot be made (19,20). It is hardly surprising therefore to find that in some institutes reporting indeterminate colitis, the natural history for patients having restorative proctocolectomy closely follows the colitic population (21), whereas in others the natural history is much closer to patients who eventually turn out to have Crohn's disease (11,22). In view of the discrepancy in reporting indeterminate colitis amongst pathologists, we believe that the term should either be used to describe a form of bowel disease that cannot be labeled as ulcerative colitis or Crohn's disease until sufficient time has elapsed to clarify the diagnosis, otherwise the term should not be used at all. In our own review (23), we found that many cases of indeterminate colitis behaved like Crohn's disease and

in most of these cases the final diagnosis has now been changed to Crohn's disease. However, in others, the label of indeterminate colitis remains but continued surveillance now suggests that the patient probably does not have Crohn's disease. Thus in our more recent update we acknowledge a category of patients where the final diagnosis must be classified as "unknown."

Current Data from the Birmingham Gastrointestinal Unit

We have reviewed our own experience of Crohn's disease in 32 patients beings considered for or having had a restorative proctocolectomy (Table 33.1). In this review we have deliberately excluded patients with indeterminate colitis based on the fact that our pathologists were unable to definitely label these patients as having Crohn's disease.

Crohn's Disease at Initial Laparotomy

There were 166 patients operated on between 1983 and 1993 who have all been followed up for a minimum of two years having surgery for presumed ulcerative colitis. Eleven patients had features of Crohn's disease at the time of colectomy; five of these individuals had obvious ileal disease proven on subsequent histology and six of the patients had features of colonic Crohn's disease with involvement of the appendix, linear ulcers, rectal sparing, or segmental distribution where Crohn's disease was proven on resection histology. *None* of these patients went on to restorative proctocolectomy and have been treated by subtotal colectomy or by proctocolectomy.

No Evidence of Crohn's Disease at Initial Laparotomy

The remaining 155 patients all had macroscopic features of ulcerative colitis and had an ileal pouch

Table 33.1. Diagnosis of Crohn's disease: planned restorative proctocolectomy (*n* = 166). Birmingham GI Unit 1983–1993.

Preoperative Crohn's disease	11 At first laparotomy - 5 ileal disease.
	- 6 colonic disease with features of Crohn's disease (no restorative proctocolectomy done).
Known Crohn's disease	2 from restorative proctocolectomy specimen.
	2 from colectomy specimen.
	4 from rectal excision specimen.
	13 from complications. All previous resection specimens labeled ulcerative colitis.
Possible Crohn's disease	3 possible cases of Crohn's disease. Suspected but unproven.

Fig. 33.1. A pouch-vaginal fistula occurring late after restorative proctocolectomy can be the initial manifestation of Crohn's disease. Crohn's may also manifest itself in the small bowel proximal to the bowel.

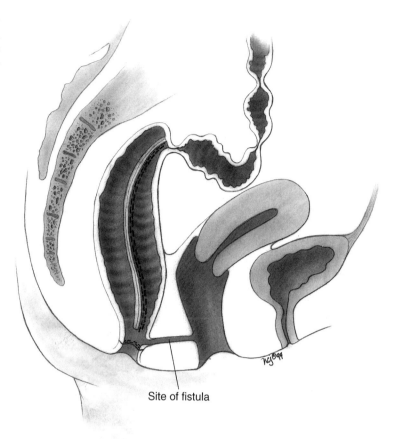

Site of fistula

and ileoanal anastomosis. Twenty-one of these patients (13.5%) are now known to have Crohn's disease. Eleven of these were women, four of whom presented with pouch vaginal fistulas as their first manifestation of Crohn's disease (see Fig. 33.1). In only one of them was local treatment successful in curing the pouch vaginal fistula.

One-Stage Restorative Proctocolectomy

Eight of the 21 patients had a one stage restorative proctocolectomy in whom three had features of Crohn's disease in the initial proctectomy specimen. The remaining five were only discovered as having Crohn's disease as a result of further surgery for complications necessitating resection or biopsy (Table 33.2). Of those discovered as having Crohn's disease in the proctocolectomy specimen, one still has a loop ileostomy above an insitu pelvic pouch, the remaining two have a functioning pouch but suffer from intermittent diarrhea. The five other cases in this group have developed complications. One had a pouch cutaneous fistula with features of Crohn's disease on pouch biopsies and from the fistula but the fistula has been successfully excised and the patient now has good pouch func-

tion. One patient developed a pouch vaginal fistula, biopsy from which suggested Crohn's disease. She subsequently underwent pouch excision when Crohn's disease was confirmed. Two patients suffered incapacitating diarrhea after restorative proctocolectomy and eventually requested pouch excision when Crohn's disease was discovered in the pouch. The last patient in this group developed a stricture above the ileal pouch with radiographic features typical of small bowel Crohn's disease (X-ray (Fig. 33.1)). She became symptomatic and underwent a strictureplasty in the involved ileal segment above the pouch in which

Table 33.2. Subtotal colectomy or restorative proctocolectomy.

8 one stage restorative proctocolectomy	Crohn's disease identified in 3 cases who might have been prevented by subtotal colectomy.
13 previous colectomy	Crohn's disease only identified in 2 cases. (4 cases identified at rectal excision and pouch construction.)

Crohn's disease was confirmed on biopsy. Currently she remains well with good pouch function.

Previous Colectomy

There are 13 patients now classified as having Crohn's disease who had a preliminary colectomy before rectal excision and pouch construction. Two of these patients had Crohn's disease in the colectomy specimen. Despite counseling, both patients elected to have a pouch even though there was a high suspicion of Crohn's disease. However, because the small bowel radiology was normal, there was no evidence of macroscopic small bowel disease at the second laparotomy, and the patient had a profound desire to avoid a permanent stoma, the rectum was removed and a pouch constructed. Both of these patients have satisfactory pouch function at three- and seven-year follow-ups respectively.

In the remaining 11 cases there was no evidence of Crohn's disease in the colectomy specimen, but in four of these cases Crohn's disease was identified in the rectal excision specimen at the time of pouch construction. The outcome in these four additional cases was uncomplicated in all cases though some of these do suffer from intermittent diarrhea. None have so far developed complications and all are satisfied with the functional outcome.

The remaining seven patients had no evidence of Crohn's disease in the colectomy specimen or in the proctectomy specimen. One of these patients had a long efferent limb which caused impaired evacuation. When it was excised and a new ileoanal anastomosis fashioned, Crohn's disease was reported in the excision specimen from the efferent limb. This individual has satisfactory pouch function and so far has not developed complications. There were three patients in this group who developed a pouch vaginal fistula. Two of them had florid Crohn's disease in the pouch complicated by stenosis requiring pouch excision. One patient has a healed pouch vaginal fistula but there is obvious small bowel Crohn's disease above the pouch which is currently defunctioned with a loop ileostomy. In view of the likely deleterious outcome if the loop ileostomy is closed, this patient has accepted an almost certain permanent loop ileostomy but an intact pouch and a healed pouch vaginal fistula. One patient had severe pelvic sepsis eventually requiring disconnection of the pouch anal anastomosis, and delivery of the pouch to the abdominal wall as an end-ileostomy. She continued to have pelvic sepsis despite this and subsequent reoperation revealed obvious Crohn's disease in

the ileum above the pouch with a fistula into the bladder. Another patient has developed a stricture with typical radiological features of Crohn's disease in the ileum just proximal to the pouch. He has a megaloblastic anaemia from B12 and folate deficiency but has not yet required further surgical resection. Finally, there is another patient who developed a leak from the ileoanal anastomosis. The pouch-anal anastomosis was disconnected and the end of the pouch was brought up as an end-ileostomy. Subsequently the pouch was reconnected to the anal canal. Following this he developed enterocutaneous and an enterovesical fistula from a long efferent limb appendage of a J-pouch which was excised. There was evidence of Crohn's disease, in this specimen, and the patient currently suffers from diarrhea, though he is not prepared to contemplate pouch excision or a proximal stoma.

Possible Crohn's Disease

There are three patients who are thought might have Crohn's disease of the distal pouch. All have a

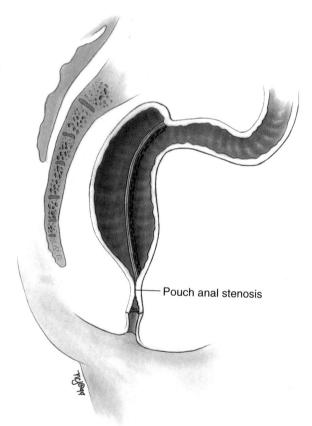

Fig. 33.2. A distal pouch-anal stenosis may also be an early feature of Crohn's disease after restorative proctocolectomy.

Table 33.3. Current outcome of Crohn's patients who have undergone restorative proctocolectomy (*n* = 21).

3 functioning pouch. Bowel frequency <7 day.
5 functioning pouch. Bowel frequency >7 day <10 day.
4 functioning pouch. >10 day.
2 permanent loop ileostomy.
5 pouch excision for complications—4 pouch vaginal fistulas. 1 sepsis and ileal disease.
2 pouch excision for poor function.

mild stricture in the distal part of the pouch (Fig. 33.2) and marked inflammatory change on endoscopy. The features are highly suggestive of Crohn's disease but an absolute diagnosis has not yet been established. All of these patients suffer from diarrhea, urgency and episodes of incontinence.

Current Outcome

The current outcome of our patients known to have Crohn's disease (*n* = 21) are shown on Table 33.3. Three have a functioning pouch with a bowel frequency less than seven times a day. Five have a functioning pouch with a bowel frequency greater than seven times a day but less than ten times a day. Four have a functioning pouch with a bowel frequency greater than ten times a day. Two patients have a permanent loop ileostomy. Five have had pouch excisions for complications, four for pouch vaginal fistula and one for chronic sepsis. Two patients have had pouch excision for poor function.

The time interval between pouch construction and features of Crohn's disease in the thirteen individuals who had no evidence of Crohn's disease either in the colectomy or proctectomy specimen was three years (range 6 months to 7 years).

Data from Other Centers

The Cleveland Clinic reported that 54 of 1005 patients (5%) having restorative proctocolectomy were classified as having indeterminate colitis and 67 of 1005 patients (7%) are now known to have Crohn's disease. Pouch excision was recorded in 34 patients, largely for pouch vaginal fistulas, persistent perianal or pelvic sepsis, recurrent pouchitis or incontinence. Pouch excision was reported in 1.8% of patients with ulcerative colitis, in 1.9% of those with indeterminate colitis, compared with 25.4% in those with known Crohn's disease. Thus, over a quarter of patients having pouch surgery finally classified as having Crohn's disease failed. Complications, particularly from sepsis, was more common in Crohn's disease but function and quality of life in the functioning pouches with Crohn's disease were comparable to patients with known ulcerative colitis or indeterminate colitis (24).

At St Marks Hospital the long term results of 110 patients are recorded. Only three of these cases were classified as having indeterminate colitis at the time of the resection and none had evidence of Crohn's disease in the resection histology. Subsequently six cases of possible Crohn's disease had been identified in the 16 patients whose pouch failed. Failure in this series was usually due to chronic sepsis often accompanied by some features of Crohn's disease (25).

Diagnostic Dilemmas

There is often some difficulty in establishing a final diagnosis from a resection performed for fulminating colitis. In these circumstances it can be more difficult to distinguish between Crohn's disease and ulcerative colitis especially as the colon may be dilated, there may be extensive mucosal loss and because in many patients there are features of colonic ischaemia (26).

There may be diagnostic difficulty in patients with radiological features and histopathology compatible with ulcerative colitis who have perianal disease (24). We believe these individuals present a high risk group. Certainly, all perianal sepsis should be thoroughly eliminated for at least a year before contemplating restorative proctocolectomy. However, not all such patients eventually turn out to have Crohn's disease. Despite this, they may still lose their pouch from recurrent sepsis. Of our 155 patients followed up for at least two years, five had active perianal disease before pouch construction. Only one of these still has a functioning pouch, the remainder developed recurrent sepsis around the pouch anal anastomosis necessitating pouch excision, yet in none of them was there evidence of Crohn's disease.

Radiologic features of the colon may sometimes be more helpful than repeated biopsies in discovering Crohn's disease. After all, good double contrast radiology correlates very closely with the macroscopic features of the colon at resection. Admittedly, good endoscopy can be just as informative, but it is subject to the experience of the endoscopist, knowledge of the particular location in the colon, the quality of bowel preparation, and the ability of the examiner to reach the cecum. Biopsies are limited to the mucosa of the bowel and therefore cannot exclude panmural disease. The ability to positively diagnose Crohn's disease also depends on the number and quality of the biopsies.

Frozen sections are used in some institutions as a means of attempting to differentiate Crohn's disease from ulcerative colitis (7). A positive diagnosis of Crohn's disease is very helpful but a negative frozen section report cannot reliably eliminate the risk of Crohn's disease. In this author's view it is absolutely essential that the ileum should be carefully inspected during laparotomy and if necessary an on table endoscopy of the ileum performed. It is also our own view that the colon should be opened and visually and manually inspected by the surgeon after the colectomy since the macroscopic appearance of the colon may be just as informative of the risk of Crohn's disease as frozen section biopsies. If there is any doubt about the underlying diagnosis, for instance, with linear ulcers in the colon, inflammation of the appendix, a segmental distribution of disease, gross panmural thickening, or if there is a cobblestone appearance of the mucosa, we would strongly advise a subtotal colectomy and ileostomy rather than a single stage restorative proctocolectomy (27). Incidentally, we have routinely biopsied the small bowel in all 155 cases here reported to exclude microscopic Crohn's disease, but in none of them was there evidence of Crohn's disease despite the subsequent outcome of Crohn's disease in 21 cases.

Should Preliminary Colectomy Be Routine?

In our series of 155 patients having restorative proctocolectomy for presumed ulcerative colitis, 68 had a single stage restorative proctocolectomy whereas 87 had a staged procedure with a preliminary colectomy. Eight cases of Crohn's disease appeared in the 68 having a single stage restorative proctocolectomy (11.7%) compared with 13 of 87 having a staged procedure (14.9%). This actually would seem to give a higher risk of Crohn's disease for the staged procedure than for single stage restorative proctocolectomy. However, of the eight cases of Crohn's disease in those having a one stage restorative proctocolectomy, only three were in fact reported from the resection whereas the rest were

diagnosed either at pouch excision or as a consequence of complications such as stricture, fistula, chronic sepsis, or malabsorption. Similarly, of the 13 cases of Crohn's disease occurring in the staged procedure group only two were actually discovered in the colectomy specimen. Four were eventually evident from the proctectomy specimen whereas the remaining seven only were diagnosed as a result of complications. Thus we do not think that a preliminary elective colectomy necessarily protects against misdiagnosis (28).

Accuracy of diagnosis is less certain in acute colitis. One stage restorative proctocolectomy in acute colitis is still very rarely advised in the United Kingdom, though its protagonists are increasing in number in the United States of America (26). Twenty-four patients with acute ulcerative colitis having restorative proctocolectomy subsequently were reviewed and four of them (17%) finally showed features of Crohn's disease. Thus, many still believe that synchronous restorative proctocolectomy is rarely advised for fulminating colitis especially as up to 20% of these patients may eventually turn out to have Crohn's disease (27).

Counseling

It is important to tell patients being considered for pouch surgery for presumed ulcerative colitis that between 7% and 13% will eventually be found to have Crohn's disease and if this should occur 25% to 40% will eventually fail from sepsis, fistulas, chronic pouchitis, or poor pouch function. If there is histological evidence of Crohn's disease in a colectomy specimen in those having a staged procedure, most will be advised not to have a pouch. However, some patients will not accept this and will want to know what will happen if a pouch is made. Our data indicates that seven of eight patients having pouch surgery when the diagnosis of Crohn's disease had been established beforehand, so far, have excellent function without complications. Thus at the moment, in our series, the outlook is better (87% success) for patients having restorative proctocolectomy when a diagnosis of Crohn's disease was known beforehand than in those patients who were eventually found to have Crohn's disease from additional histologic material or complications (42% success rate only).

Patients with known Crohn's disease are more likely to develop pelvic or perineal sepsis, fistulas, stenosis, small bowel strictures, chronic pouchitis, and sometimes features of malabsorption. Furthermore these patients are more likely to have an inferior functional result particularly diarrhea, urgency, and soiling (23).

Complications

If a patient develops a pouch vaginal fistula always suspect Crohn's disease. Multiple biopsies should be taken. It is usually wise to defunction the pouch by loop ileostomy. If the sepsis can be controlled by drainage and defunction then it might be worth attempting to close the defect by advancement flap or repair (13,29) but it would be sensible to keep the pouch defunctioned and to warn the patient that the success rate is often less than 50% (14).

If a patient develops severe pelvic or perianal sepsis in suspected Crohn's disease after restorative proctocolectomy it would be worthwhile defunctioning the pouch and eradicating the sepsis where possible by repeated drainage provided there is evidence of improvement. If despite these measures the sepsis is progressive the patient should be considered for pouch excision because if not, sepsis tends to relentlessly recur causing malnutrition and chronic ill health.

Occasionally pouch strictures may be managed by pouch strictureplasty. Certainly ileal strictures just above the pouch may be amenable to strictureplasty in the short term but resection is probably not advised because of the risks of severe diarrhea afterwards.

Conclusion

Rarely should restorative proctocolectomy be advised if a diagnosis of Crohn's disease is known prior to surgery. On the other hand, this is just the group where in our experience the functional results have in fact been better than in those individuals discovered to have Crohn's disease later as a result of complications.

One stage restorative proctocolectomy in an emergency situation should be resisted in nearly all cases. Under these circumstances the diagnosis is not known for certain and there is a greater chance that the underlying diagnosis might be Crohn's disease than in patients having elective resection after full radiological and histopathologic workup. In the elective situation there is no evidence from our data that synchronous colectomy and rectal excision with pouch construction is associated with a greater risk of Crohn's disease than in a staged procedure with a preliminary colectomy. If a one stage proctocolectomy is being undertaken and if the operative findings in any way suggest a diagnosis of Crohn's disease (possible small bowel in-

volvement, appendiceal involvement, segmental disease, linear ulceration, relative rectal sparing) then it would be wiser to perform a preliminary subtotal colectomy and ileostomy rather than a single staged procedure. At all times it is the duty of the surgeon to inspect the resection specimen before pouch construction. If any questions about the diagnosis exists intraoperatively, either frozen section should be used to confirm the diagnosis of Crohn's or pouch construction should be aborted.

There are many patients who develop pelvic and perineal sepsis following restorative proctocolectomy who have no evidence of Crohn's disease. However, these complications should alert the clinician as to the possibility of underlying Crohn's disease. Indeed, in patients developing pouch vaginal fistulas after restorative proctocolectomy over half are likely to have underlying undisclosed Crohn's disease responsible for the fistula and under these circumstances the chances of successful reconstructions or repair are small.

Finally, there are a group of patients who develop clear evidence of Crohn's disease after pouch construction who have either acceptable function or whose Crohn's complications may be amenable to further surgical treatment without necessarily jeopardizing the chances of retained pouch function. However, each case must be evaluated on its merits. If further reconstructive surgery is to be contemplated, full gut endoscopy or radiology would be strongly advised and a cautious outcome should be expressed to the patient since the prognosis in this group is poor and many eventually require pouch excision.

References

1. Wexner SD, Wong WD, Rothenberger DA, et al. The ileoanal reservoir. Am J Surg 1990;159:178–83.
2. Kock NG. Continent ileostomy. Prog Surg 1973;12:180–201.
3. Gerber A, Apt MK, Craig PH. The Kock continent ileostomy. Surg Gynecol Obstet 1983;156:345–50.
4. Gelernt IM, Bauer JJ, Kreel I. The reservoir ileostomy: early experience with 54 patients. Ann Surg 1977;185:179–84.
5. Goldman SL, Rombeau JL. The continent ileostomy: a collective review. Dis Colon Rectum 1978;21:594–9.
6. Failes DG. The continent ileostomy—an 11 year experience. Aust NZ J Surg 1984;54:345–52.
7. Dozois RR. Ileal 'J' pouch-anal anastomosis. Br J Surg 1985;72(suppl.):S80–S82.
8. Nicholls RJ, Pescatori M, Motson RW, et al. Restorative proctocolectomy with a three loop ileal reservoir for ulcerative colitis and familial adenomatous polyposis. Ann Surg 1984;199:383–8.

9. Rothenberger DA, Long WD, Buls JG, et al. Restorative proctocolectomy with ileal reservoir and ileoanal anastomosis for ulcerative colitis and familial polyposis. Dig Surg 1984;1:19–26.

10. Pemberton JH, Kelly KA, Beart RW Jr, et al. Ileal pouch-anal anastomosis for chronic ulcerative colitis. Long term results. Ann Surg 1987;206:504–13.

11. Koltun WA, Schoetz DJ Jr, Roberts PL, et al. Indeterminate colitis predisposes to perineal complications after ileal pouch-anal anastomosis. Dis Colon Rectum 1991;34:857–60.

12. Deutsch AA, McLeod RS, Cullen J, et al. Results of the pelvic-pouch procedure in patients with Crohn's disease. Dis Colon Rectum 1991;34:475–7.

13. Keighley MRB, Grobler SP. Fistula complicating restorative proctocolectomy. Br J Surg 1993;80(8):1065–7.

14. O'Kelly TJ, Merrett M, Mortensen NJ, et al. Pouch-vaginal fistula after restorative proctocolectomy: aetiology and management. Br J Surg 1994;81:1374–5.

15. Hyman NH, Fazio VW, Tuckson WB, et al. Consequences of ileal pouch-anal anastomosis for Crohn's colitis. Dis Colon Rectum 1991;34:653–7.

16. Groom JS, Nicholls RJ, Hawley PR, et al. Pouch-vaginal fistula. Br J Surg 1993;80(7):936–40.

17. Kohler L, Troidl H. The ileoanal pouch: a risk-benefit analysis. Br J Surg 1995;82:443–7.

18. Price AB. Overlap in the spectrum of nonspecific inflammatory bowel disease—"colitis indeterminate." J Clin Pathol 1978;31:567–77.

19. Lewin K, Swales JD. Granulomatous colitis and atypical ulcerative colitis. Gastroenterology 1966;50:211–23.

20. Lee KS, Medline A, Shockey S. Indeterminate colitis in the spectrum of inflammatory bowel disease. Arch Pathol Lab Med 1979;103:173–6.

21. McIntyre PB, Pemberton JH, Wolff BG, et al. Indeterminate colitis: long-term outcome in patients after ileal pouch-anal anastomosis. Dis Colon Rectum 1995;38:51–4.

22. Wells AD, McMillan I, Price AB, et al. Natural history of indeterminate colitis. Br J Surg 1991;78:179–81.

23. Grobler SP, Hosier KB, Affie E, et al. Outcome of restorative proctocolectomy when the diagnosis is suggestive of Crohn's disease. Gut 1993;34:1384–8.

24. Fazio VW, Ziv Y, Church JM, et al. Ileal pouch-anal anastomosis complications and function in 1005 patients. Ann Surg 1995;222(2):120–7.

25. Setti-Carraro P, Ritchie JK, Wilkinson KH, et al. The first 10 years' experience of restorative proctocolectomy for ulcerative colitis. Gut 1994;35:1070–5.

26. Ziv Y, Fazio VW, Church JM, et al. Safety of urgent restorative proctocolectomy with ileal pouch-anal anastomosis for fulminant colitis. Dis Colon Rectum 1995;38:345–9.

27. Lucarotti ME, Freeman BJC, Warren BF, et al. Synchronous proctocolectomy and ileoanal pouch formation and the risk of Crohn's disease. Br J Surg 1995;82:755–6.

28. Keighley MRB, Grobler S, Bain I. An audit of restorative proctocolectomy. Gut 1993;34:680–4.

29. Makowiec F, Jehle EC, Becker HD, et al. Clinical course after transanal advancement flap repair of perianal fistula in patients with Crohn's disease. Br J Surg 1995;82:603–6.

Section III
Crohn's Disease

Part IV
Recurrent Disease

34 Operative Strategy in Recurrent Crohn's Disease

Ridzuan Farouk and Roger R. Dozois

Crohn's disease is a panenteric chronic inflammatory disease with an inherent tendency to recur after previous medical or surgical therapy. Indeed, two patients described by Crohn and his associates in their original publication had recurrent disease (1). Most of these recurrences are within the 8- to 10-year period after surgery (2–4). The chronicity of the condition, its ability to recur, and its tendency to affect more than one site in the gastrointestinal system suggest that a conservative approach may be preferable whenever surgery is contemplated. Thus, the patient should be fully informed of potential sequelae from surgery, including recurrence, and the decision to operate should include a risk assessment in which the potential disadvantages of surgery outweigh the status quo.

It is perhaps a misnomer to talk of "recurrent Crohn's disease" as opposed to "recurrent symptomatic Crohn's disease." Indeed, in 92% of patients with active disease, corticosteroids may induce remission, but 71% of patients still have active lesions at endoscopic examination (5). After ileocolic resection, most patients have endoscopically detectable recurrence in the neoterminal ileum within 1 year, although only a minority have symptoms (6).

The common indications for surgery in patients with recurrent Crohn's disease are similar to those for patients presenting with the disease for the first time. These indications primarily are for complications of the disease, such as perforation, abscess, fistula, obstruction, and hemorrhage. Relative indications for consideration of surgery result from failure of medical therapy to adequately palliate symptoms, for example, weight loss and malnutrition, diarrhea and fecal incontinence, refractory

anemia, chronic pain, and growth retardation or "failure to thrive." Except for patients in extremis, the decision to operate and its timing may vary considerably among individual physicians and surgeons. In addition to these indications, the specter of postoperative complications arising as a result of inadequately resected disease as well as technical complications adds another dimension to further surgery in Crohn's disease. The primary purpose of this review is to address the issue of surgical strategies for recurrent disease rather than surgery for technical complications or inadequately resected disease.

Patterns and Incidence of Recurrent Disease

Patterns of recurrence reflect previously recognized distributions of disease. Disease in patients presenting for the first time is confined to the small intestine in approximately 30%, affects the colon, rectum, and anus in 30%, and affects the small and large bowels in 40% (3,7). Patients with ileocolic disease appear to have the highest recurrence rates after surgery: 53%, compared with 45% for colonic and 44% for small intestinal patterns (8). Second recurrences tend to be more evenly distributed, with rates of 35% for the ileocolic pattern, 34% for the large bowel, and 38% for the intestine (8).

Agrez et al. (9) identified 103 residents of Olmsted County, Minnesota, which is served by the Mayo Clinic in Rochester, with the diagnosis of Crohn's disease since 1935. Forty-two of these patients had undergone one or more surgical procedures. Thirty-six had at least one definitive resec-

420 R. Farouk and R.R. Dozois

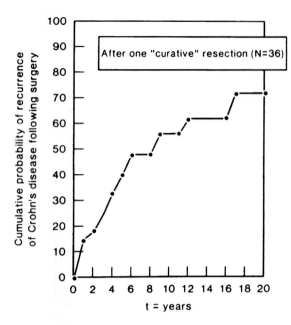

Fig. 34.1. Cumulative risk of recurrent Crohn's disease in 103 patients in Olmsted County, Minnesota, after one "curative" operation. (From Agrez MV, Valente RM, Pierce W et al. Mayo Clin Proc 1982;57:747–52. By permission of Mayo Foundation.)

tion (Fig. 34.1). Eight of these patients subsequently underwent a second definitive procedure. The likelihood of an operation was greatest within the first year of diagnosis. The proportions of patients in whom recurrent disease developed after the first and second operations were 50% and 37%, respectively (Fig. 34.2). Approximately half the patients who experienced a recurrence underwent further surgery. Patients aged 40 years or older appeared to fare best with respect to recurrent disease.

Any discussion about rates of recurrence cannot be totally separated from the issue of extent of previous resections. Controversy still exists about whether microscopic disease at the resection margin affects the risk of recurrent disease (2,10,11). A retrospective review at the Mayo Clinic of 710 patients undergoing surgery for Crohn's disease identified 42 patients with residual anastomotic disease. The recurrence rate at 8 years with only microscopic involvement of the resection margin was 89.4%, which was substantially higher than the previously reported institutional rate of 55% at 10 years (2) (Fig. 34.3). The issue has not been fully settled, but at present a 2-cm margin free of macroscopic disease appears to be a sensible compromise when resection is considered (12). Finally,

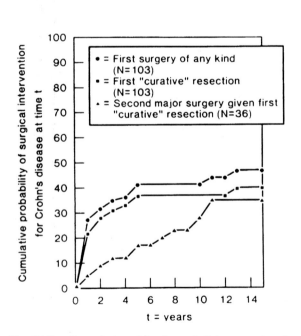
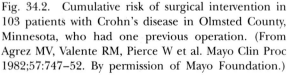

Fig. 34.2. Cumulative risk of surgical intervention in 103 patients with Crohn's disease in Olmsted County, Minnesota, who had one previous operation. (From Agrez MV, Valente RM, Pierce W et al. Mayo Clin Proc 1982;57:747–52. By permission of Mayo Foundation.)

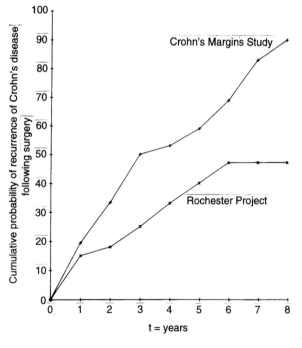

Fig. 34.3. Cumulative probability of recurrence of Crohn's disease after surgery. (From Wolff BG, Beart RW Jr, Frydenberg HB et al. Dis Colon Rectum 1983;26:239–43. By permission of American Society of Colon and Rectal Surgeons.)

the true risk of recurrence has been found to be greater than expected when disease is searched for prospectively by invasive means regardless of symptoms (5).

Indications for Surgery

Recurrent disease alone does not justify further surgery. Between 1988 and 1995, 682 patients with recurrent Crohn's disease were assessed at the Mayo Clinic (unpublished data). Of these, 326 underwent surgery for recurrent disease. The operations are summarized in Table 34.1. Up to 30% of patients with distal ileal disease required more than one resection at 10-year follow-up, and 5% required more than three resections (13). The risk of short-gut syndrome is high, with up to 1.5% of all patients eventually acquiring this problem (14). Complications such as perforation, major hemorrhage, or progressive toxic megacolon despite adequate medical therapy are the only absolute indications for further surgery. Obstruction due to stricture formation or septic complications, such as abscess formations may respond to more conservative therapy, such as parenteral nutrition and medical therapy for stricture and radiologically guided percutaneous drainage and antimicrobial therapy for control of sepsis. These patients may nevertheless require surgery, although the intervening period can allow for improvement in nutritional status, control of sepsis, and stabilization of any coexisting medical conditions. The time used for the stabilization of the patient may also permit sufficient delay until the abdomen can be safely reentered and a stoma can possibly be avoided.

Fistula formation due to recurrent disease, either enterocutaneous or internal (enteroenteric, enterovesical, and others), may require further surgery. Internal fistulas occur in up to one third of patients with Crohn's disease, and enterocutaneous fistulas may affect up to 15% of all patients (7). The commonest form of enteroenteric fistula is the ileosigmoid fistula; fistulas between loops of small bowel are also common. Gastric and duodenal fistulas are less common, occurring in 0.6% and 0.5% of all patients, respectively. Colovesical fistulas are not uncommon, accounting for 5.8% of all cases in the Mount Sinai series (7). Most of these patients are operated on because of symptoms or recurrent sepsis (15), although surgery may be deferred for up to 5 years (7).

Attempts have been made to separate the initial presentations of Crohn's disease into a sepsis-fistula group and a more indolent obstructing group as a means of predicting which patients are most likely to have recurrent disease (16). Such observations, not confirmed by McDonald et al. (17), have been supported by a long-term study from Switzerland (18).

Surgical Strategies

Indications for surgery may be divided classically into emergent and elective indications or be based on the anatomical site of the disease. When celiotomy is necessary, a midline incision should be used to ensure adequate access throughout the peritoneal cavity and to preserve the flanks for stoma sites. This chapter deals with surgical management of recurrent disease on the basis of anatomical site.

Gastroduodenal Crohn's Disease

Surgery for gastroduodenal Crohn's disease is often a "first time" procedure, and recurrent surgery is not a major issue. This situation is unlike that in the rest of the enteric tract, because the disease is bypassed rather than resected. The presenting features are similar to those of peptic ulceration, namely, pain, stricture, and bleeding. The incidence of this disease affecting the gastroduodenal region is between 0.5% and 4% of all cases (19). Concurrent disease, which predominantly affects the small bowel, is common in these patients. One-third of patients are operated on, most for gastric outlet obstruction (20).

The primary aim at surgery is to distinguish between peptic ulcer disease and Crohn's disease. The former usually requires a form of vagotomy with resection, whereas the latter most often requires bypass surgery. The morbidity for resectional surgery in patients with Crohn's disease is four times higher than that with bypass alone (20). If the patient has Crohn's disease and has had a

Table 34.1. Summary of operations for recurrent Crohn's disease performed in 326 patients at Mayo Medical Center between 1988 and 1995.

Type of operation	No. of patients
Vagotomy and gastroenterostomy	3
Proximal small bowel resection	16
Strictureplasty	17
Distal small bowel resection	108
Segmental colectomy	132
Protocolectomy and Brooke ileostomy	27
Perianal fistula surgery	23

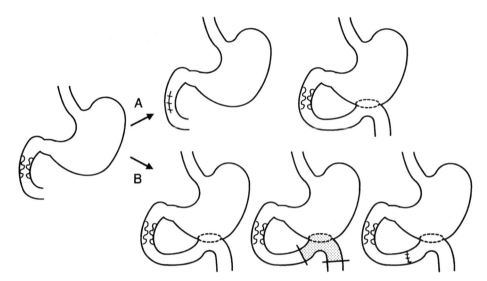

Fig. 34.4. Surgical options for recurrent gastroduodenal Crohn's disease. (A) Recurrence at a duodenal strictureplasty site is treated by gastroenterostomy and, preferably, proximal gastric vagotomy. (B) Recurrence at a previous gastroenterostomy site is treated by takedown and resection of the previous anastomosis and formation of a new gastroenterostomy.

previous duodenal strictureplasty and now has gastric outlet obstruction, bypass gastrojejunostomy should be performed (Fig. 34.4). Whether a vagotomy should be added is debatable, but if one is contemplated, a highly selective vagotomy is preferred. Denervation of only the proximal portion of the stomach may avoid the potential for small bowel motility disorders; avoidance may be crucial because of disease elsewhere in the small intestine (20). If a patient has had a previous gastroenterostomy and disease recurs at the anastomosis, resection may be necessary, followed by creation of a new anastomosis between uninvolved stomach and small intestine.

Fistula formation does not immediately indicate the need for surgery (21). Preliminary treatment with corticosteroids, sulfa compounds, and total parenteral nutrition may resolve the problem. Gastroenteric fistulas tend to develop from the transverse colon (16). Duodenoenteric fistulas usually involve the second and third parts of the duodenum because of its proximity to the colon and small bowel. At the Mayo Clinic, only 16 of 6313 patients treated for Crohn's disease between 1975 and 1994 were found to have a duodenal fistula. Four of these patients had undergone previous ileocolic resection. At the time of presentation, the extent of active Crohn's disease included ileocolic (15 patients), duodenal (3 patients), gastroduodenal (1 patient), and perianal (1 patient)

disease (22). When surgical treatment is required, the existence of Crohn's disease should be established within the stomach or duodenum or both. Most often, the stomach and duodenum are uninvolved and can be simply disconnected from the primary source of the disease, which is resected. The defect can be closed primarily after freshening of the edges, with care taken to avoid pancreatic injury, and omentum interposed to avoid direct contact with the site of any other anastomosis.

Small Bowel Crohn's Disease

The risk of short-bowel syndrome should be considered and discussed with any patient who has recurrent Crohn's disease of the small bowel and is being considered for surgery. Relative indications against operative treatment include rapid recurrence after previous surgery, lack of evidence of obstruction on the basis of endoscopic or radiologic evaluation, and lack of an adequate trial of medical therapy. The timing of surgery is also crucial, because the morbidity incurred after the first 10 days of previous surgery up to 6 months after the last laparotomy can be substantial. Nonobstructing, nonhemorrhaging segments usually respond to medical therapy.

Short, fibrous strictures, whether single or multiple, may be adequately addressed by endoscopic balloon dilatation (23) or operatively by strictureplasty (24,25). If resection is performed, a 2-cm margin of bowel free from macroscopic disease is usually sufficient. It is important during surgery to closely examine the remaining bowel, by a balloon pull-through technique, for submucosal strictures not apparent by either radiologic examination or direct palpation of the external surface of the bowel. If a stricture is detected, a longitudinal enterotomy is made, extending 1 cm on either side, and closed transversely. With this technique, the incidence of recurrent stricture is low (24), although about half the patients require reoperation for recurrent disease at other sites. At the Mayo Clinic, 35 patients underwent 71 strictureplasties between 1985 and 1991. Bowel with active disease was concomitantly resected in 67% of these procedures. The perioperative complication rate was 14%, and the rate of recurrence of symptoms at 3 years was 20%. Six patients required reoperation (25). Enterocutaneous fistula and intraabdominal sepsis are the primary complications of this technique. The incidence of suture line leakage has been reported to be between 0% and 8% (12,24,25). Strictureplasty is an important method of conserving small bowel length, particularly in patients who have undergone one or more previous resectional operations.

Enteroenteric fistulas confined to the small bowel are frequently asymptomatic and found coincidentally by radiologic examination. Alone, they are not an indication for surgery, although they usually indicate the severity of the patient's penetrating intestinal disease. As a reflection of this, most patients ultimately require surgery (7,21).

Fistulas involving the small bowel usually originate from the terminal ileum, and the affected distal site of the fistula usually requires only disconnection and simple repair. The exception to this rule is the ileosigmoid fistula, with which contiguous resection of the sigmoid colon may also be required (15). Ninety patients with this complication were treated at the Mayo Clinic between 1975 and 1995. The condition was diagnosed preoperatively in 77% of the patients studied. Sigmoid repair was performed in 43 patients (47.8%), sigmoid resection in 32 (35.6%), colectomy in 12 (13.3%), and no operation in 3 (3.3%) (26). Reasons for resection rather than simple repair included significant purulence or inflammation, a large fistulous defect, a defect on the mesenteric border of the colon, and active sigmoid Crohn's disease. The repair and resection groups were otherwise similar in age, duration of disease, and preoperative symptoms.

The primary choices that the surgeon faces in dealing with recurrent disease are whether a septic focus needs to be drained and whether diseased segments can be dealt with by strictureplasty or by resection (Fig. 34.5). If reobstruction occurs at the site of a previous strictureplasty, resection may be the only option (Fig. 34.6). Also, the surgeon should be concerned about the admittedly remote, but definite, possibility of cancer complicating areas of long-standing disease. Intestinal bypass is rarely practiced because of a perceived higher risk of morbidity and reoperation as well as a high risk of subsequent development of malignant disease in the bypassed segment. Such malignant lesions are difficult to diagnose and are associated with a poor prognosis (27).

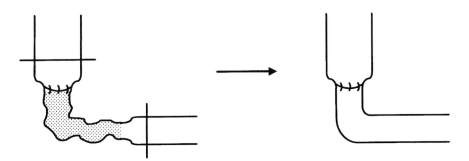

Fig. 34.5.   Recurrence of small bowel Crohn's disease, usually at a site proximal to the previous anastomosis, is treated by segmental resection and primary anastomosis with a 2-cm macroscopic clearance of disease.

Small Bowel

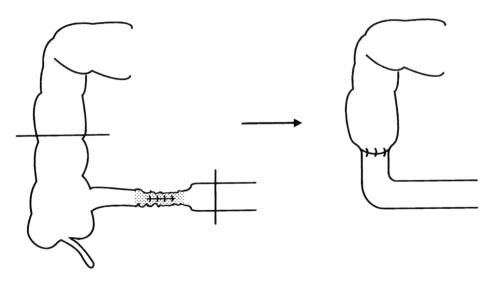

Fig. 34.6.   Recurrence of symptoms from small bowel Crohn's disease at the site of a previous strictureplasty is treated by segmental resection and primary anastomosis.

Colonic Crohn's Disease

The indications for surgery in patients with recurrent colonic Crohn's disease are not different from those for small bowel disease, namely, perforation, fistula, abscess formation, major hemorrhage, obstruction, and failure of medical therapy. Failure of medical therapy includes the specific complication of toxic colitis with megacolon.

In one series of patients with a previous segmented colectomy, 81% had preservation of intestinal continuity at 5-year follow-up (28). At the Mayo Clinic, 22 of 49 evaluable patients who underwent segmental colonic resection between 1976 and 1985 and were reassessed after a mean of 14 years (range, 9 to 19 years) had no evidence of recurrent disease and required no further therapy (29). Of the remaining 27 patients, 11 were successfully treated for recurrence by medical means alone. Only 7 of the 16 patients who underwent further surgical treatment eventually required a stoma. Mean time to recurrence of disease was 44 months, and time to recurrence of disease requiring surgery was 51 months.

Stricture formation may require surgery because of obstructive symptoms or the risk of coexisting cancer. Colonic stricture formation may be primary or associated with the site of a previous anastomosis. In very selected patients, such strictures may be managed nonoperatively if there are few obstructive symptoms and the colon can be kept under continuing colonoscopic surveillance. Pa-

tients with ileocolitis and Crohn's colitis have an increased relative risk of 3.2 and 5.6 times, respectively, for the subsequent development of colonic carcinoma, compared with a relative risk of one for ileitis alone (30). The strong suspicion of coexisting cancer should be kept at the forefront, because cancer has been shown to be present in 6.8% of all primary strictures (31). After ileocolonic resection, symptomatic stricture can occur in up to 69% of patients after 20-year follow-up (32).

The surgical options in patients with recurrent disease have to be weighed against the psychologic and surgical morbidity associated with a stoma. Colonic strictures or strictures at an ileorectal eusrasmoni may be dealt with by endoscopic balloon dilatation, which satisfactorily relieves symptoms in about two thirds of patients. The primary early complications of this method are perforation and hemorrhage; restricture is a longer term risk (33). Strictureplasty is not a real option for colonic strictures because of the risk of coexisting cancer, the higher risk of sepsis, and the lesser need to conserve bowel length. The only exception is an ileocolic anastomotic stricture, which tends to occur just proximal to the previous anastomotic site. Strictureplasty has been described as providing better outcome than endoscopic balloon dilatation for this circumstance (34). Patients who have a localized stricture due to recurrent disease with sparing of the colon elsewhere may be suitable for segmental resection, particularly if the ileocolic valve and the right colon with its absorptive function can

Colon and Rectum

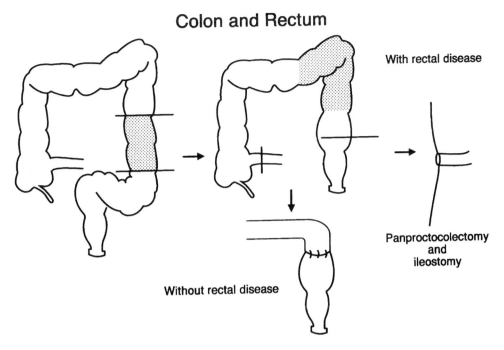

Fig. 34.7. Recurrent colonic Crohn's disease initially treated by segmental resection. The surgical options are dictated by the state of the rectum. With no or minimal rectal disease, treatment may be by completion colec-tomy and ileorectostomy. With severe rectal or anal disease, treatment is best done by completion proctocolectomy with a Brooke ileostomy.

be spared. The recent finding that maintenance therapy with higher doses of mesalamine reduces the incidence of short-term relapse of Crohn's may make rejuvenated resection a more attractive option (39). For more diffuse disease, ileorectostomy and panproctocolectomy are the only surgical options. Recurrent disease at the anastomotic site in patients with an ileorectostomy may be managed by segmental resection and reanastomosis if the disease is localized and the rectum spared or by proctocolectomy and ileostomy if the rectum is diseased (Fig. 34.7).

Perianal Crohn's Disease

The true incidence of perianal disease is unknown, but it is estimated to be a complication in 23% to 38% of patients with Crohn's disease (3,35). In 64% of patients from one series, perianal disease was preceded by enterocolic disease (35). The time from initial diagnosis to the appearance of perianal disease was at least 5 years in half the patients studied and between 1 and 5 years in one third (35). Almost all patients with the diagnosis of Crohn's disease based on perianal disease have enterocolic disease by 5 years. Between 1988 and 1995, 25 patients with recurrent perianal disease were treated at the Mayo Clinic. Three patients required proctocolectomy (Table 34.1).

Rectal Crohn's disease influences the outcome of perianal disease as well as the options for treatment. Proctitis causes diarrhea, tenesmus, incessant mucus discharge, and perhaps, incontinence, all of which exacerbate the patient's symptoms. Endorectal advancement flaps for fistula are not a real option with proctitis, although cutaneous anal advancement flaps may still be considered for fissures. Similarly, proctitis may delay fistulotomy; a seton may be used instead and the proctitis treated first (36). In severe anorectal inflammation with sepsis, diversion of the fecal stream combined with drainage and prolonged antibiotic therapy may be contemplated. Relapses are common, however, after stoma closure. In such patients or in patients with recurrent symptomatic perianal disease associated with proctitis, proctectomy may ultimately be the only solution (37).

The strategy for treatment of anorectal Crohn's will be fully discussed in Chapter 32.

Crohn's Disease after Ileal-Pouch Anal Anastomosis

Crohn's disease remains a contraindication for ileal-pouch/anal anastomosis. The distinction between ulcerative colitis and Crohn's disease can be difficult, however, and some patients with Crohn's disease inadvertently undergo ileal-pouch/anal anastomosis. At the Mayo Clinic, 37 patients with colitis that later proved to be Crohn's disease had this procedure (38). Histologic reexamination of the resected colon showed features of ulcerative colitis in 22 patients, indeterminate colitis in nine, and Crohn's disease in six. A J-pouch was constructed in 35 patients, an S-pouch in one patient, and a W-pouch in the remaining patient. In the postoperative period, complex fistulae developed in 11 of the 37 patients: pouch-cutaneous in six, pouch-vaginal in four, and pouch-vesical in one. Crohn's disease recurred in the pouch in 20 patients, in the anal canal in four, in the pouch and anal canal in 10, and in the small bowel in three. After an average follow-up of 10 years (range, 3 to 14 years), 20 patients continued to have a functioning pouch (54%), with a bowel frequency of seven stools per day (range, 3 to 10 stools). Seven patients had a defunctioning procedure and 10 had excision of the pouch, for a failure rate of 46%.

Conclusions

Surgery for recurrent Crohn's disease is limited to specific symptomatic complications of the disease. For small bowel disease, the option of strictureplasty is a genuine attempt at conserving bowel length. The recent use of high-dose mesalamine prophylaxis to reduce the recurrence rate of the disease is an exciting development, although the period of follow-up is short and subgroup analysis is limited because of small numbers of patients (39). This approach nevertheless may improve the option for segmental rather than total colectomy and proctectomy, avoiding or at least delaying a stoma whenever possible. This option may further increase the likelihood of a conservative approach and reduce the inherently mandatory role for surgery in Crohn's disease, at least in recurrent disease.

References

1. Crohn BB, Ginzburg L, Oppenheimer GD: Regional ileitis: a pathologic and clinical entity. JAMA 1932;99:1323–9.
2. Wolff BG, Beart RW Jr, Frydenberg HB, et al. The importance of disease-free margins in resections for Crohn's disease. Dis Colon Rectum 1983;26:239–43.
3. Farmer RG, Whelan G, Fazio VW. Long-term follow-up of patients with Crohn's disease. Relationship between the clinical pattern and prognosis. Gastroenterology 1985;88:1818–25.
4. Goligher JC. The long-term results of excisional surgery for primary and recurrent Crohn's disease of the large intestine. Dis Colon Rectum 1985;28:51–5.
5. Modigliani R, Mary JY, Simon JF, et al. Clinical, biological, and endoscopic picture of attacks of Crohn's disease. Evolution on prednisolone. Gastroenterology 1990;98:811–8.
6. Rutgeerts P, Geboes K, Vantrappen G, et al. Predictability of the postoperative course of Crohn's disease. Gastroenterology 1990;99:956–63.
7. Greenstein AJ. The surgery of Crohn's disease. Surg Clin North Am 1987;67:573–96.
8. Whelan G, Farmer RG, Fazio VW, et al. Recurrence after surgery in Crohn's disease. Relationship to location of disease (clinical pattern) and surgical indication. Gastroenterology 1985;88:1826–33.
9. Agrez MV, Valente RM, Pierce W, et al. Surgical history of Crohn's disease in a well-defined population. Mayo Clin Proc 1982;57:747–52.
10. McLeod RS. Resection margins and recurrent Crohn's disease. Hepatogastroenterology 1990;37:63–6.
11. Kotanagi H, Kramer K, Fazio VW, et al. Do microscopic abnormalities at resection margins correlate with increased anastomotic recurrence in Crohn's disease? Retrospective analysis of 100 cases. Dis Colon Rectum 1991;34:909–16.
12. Fazio VW, Tjandra JJ, Lavery IC, et al. Long-term follow-up of strictureplasty in Crohn's disease. Dis Colon Rectum 1993;36:355–61.
13. Andrews HA, Keighley MR, Alexander-Williams J, et al. Strategy for management of distal ileal Crohn's disease. Br J Surg 1991;78:679–82.
14. Hellers G. Crohn's disease in Stockholm county 1955–1974. A study of epidemiology, results of surgical treatment and long-term prognosis. Acta Chir Scand Suppl 1979;490:1–84.
15. McNamara MJ, Fazio VW, Lavery IC, et al. Surgical treatment of enterovesical fistulas in Crohn's disease. Dis Colon Rectum 1990;33:271–6.
16. Greenstein AJ, Lachman P, Sachar DB, et al. Perforating and nonperforating indications for repeated operations in Crohn's disease: evidence for two clinical forms. Gut 1988;29:588–92.
17. McDonald PJ, Fazio VW, Farmer RG, et al. Perforating and nonperforating Crohn's disease. An unpredictable guide to recurrence after surgery. Dis Colon Rectum 1989;32:117–20.
18. Aeberhard P, Berchtold W, Riedtmann HJ, et al. Surgical recurrence of perforating and nonperforating Crohn's disease. A study of 101 surgically treated patients. Dis Colon Rectum 1996;39:80–7.
19. Schoetz DJ Jr. Gastroduodenal Crohn's disease. Perspect Colon Rectal Surg 1992;2:145–54.
20. Murray JJ, Schoetz DJ Jr, Nugent FW, et al. Surgical management of Crohn's disease involving the duodenum. Am J Surg 1984;147:58–65.
21. Broe PJ, Bayless TM, Cameron JL. Crohn's disease: Are enteroenteric fistulas an indication for surgery? Surgery 1982;91:249–53.

22. Dominguez JM, Frizelle FA, Wolff BG. Duodenal fistulas in Crohn's disease (abstract). Dis Colon Rectum 1996;39:A36.

23. Williams AJ, Palmer KR. Endoscopic balloon dilatation as a therapeutic option in the management of intestinal strictures resulting from Crohn's disease. Br J Surg 1991;78:453–4.

24. Alexander-Williams J, Haynes IG. Conservative operations for Crohn's disease of the small bowel. World J Surg 1985;9:945–51.

25. Spencer MP, Nelson H, Wolff BG, et al. Strictureplasty for obstructive Crohn's disease: the Mayo experience. Mayo Clin Proc 1994;69:33–6.

26. Young-Fadok TM, Wolff BG, Meagher A, et al. Surgical management of ileosigmoid fistula in Crohn's disease (abstract). Dis Colon Rectum 1996;39:A38.

27. Hawker PC, Gyde SN, Thompson H, et al. Adenocarcinoma of the small intestine complicating Crohn's disease. Gut 1982;23:188–93.

28. Longo WE, Ballantyne GH, Cahow CE. Treatment of Crohn's colitis. Segmental or total colectomy? Arch Surg 1988;123:588–90.

29. Prabhakar LP, Laramee C, Nelson H, et al. Avoiding a stoma: the role for segmental colectomy in Crohn's colitis (abstract). Dis Colon Rectum 1996;39:A23.

30. Ekbom A, Helmick C, Zack M, et al. Increased risk of large-bowel cancer in Crohn's disease with colonic involvement. Lancet 1990;336:357–9.

31. Yamazaki Y, Ribeiro MB, Sachar DB, et al. Malignant colorectal strictures in Crohn's disease. Am J Gastroenterol 1991;86:882–5.

32. Trnka YM, Glotzer DJ, Kasdon EJ, et al. The long-term outcome of restorative operation in Crohn's disease: influence of location, prognostic factors and surgical guidelines. Ann Surg 1982;196:345–55.

33. Breysem Y, Janssens JF, Coremans G, et al. Endoscopic balloon dilation of colonic and ileocolonic Crohn's strictures: long-term results. Gastrointest Endosc 1992;38:142–7.

34. Sharif H, Alexander-Williams J. Strictureplasty for ileocolic anastomotic strictures in Crohn's disease. Int J Colorectal Dis 1991;6:214–6.

35. Williams DR, Coller JA, Corman ML, et al. Anal complications in Crohn's disease. Dis Colon Rectum 1981;24:22–4.

36. White RA, Eisenstat TE, Rubin RJ, et al. Seton management of complex anorectal fistulas in patients with Crohn's disease. Dis Colon Rectum 1990;33:587–9.

37. Bayer I, Gordon PH. Selected operative management of fistula-in-ano in Crohn's disease. Dis Colon Rectum 1994;37:760–5.

38. Sagar PM, Dozois RR, Wolff BG. Long-term results of ileal pouch-anal anastomosis in patients with Crohn's disease. Dis Colon Rectum 1996;39:893–8.

39. McLeod RS, Wolff BG, Steinhart AH, et al. Prophylactic mesalamine treatment decreases postoperative recurrence of Crohn's disease. Gastroenterology 1995;109:404–13.

Section IV
Inflammatory Bowel Disease: Surgical Treatment

Part I
General Complications

35 Septic Complications

David A. Rothenberger and Kemal I. Deen

The frequency of septic complications following surgical operations for inflammatory bowel disease is not significantly higher than the frequency of septic complications following small bowel and colonic surgery for other benign or malignant disorders in similar risk patients. However, the consequences of sepsis in patients with inflammatory bowel disease can be dire because of preexisting malnutrition, long-standing corticosteroid and immunosuppressive therapy, and alterations in host defense mechanisms [1].

Infection after operation may arise from either the patient's own microflora or the hospital environment, including hospital personnel. Microbial colonization of the human gut occurs during and immediately after birth. When established, the normal flora of the gut is composed of bacteria and some yeasts. Humans are not thought to have a normal viral flora. The oral cavity flora consists of aerobes and anaerobes. However, the lumen of the normal stomach is relatively free of microbial colonization due to its acid pH. The lumen of the proximal small intestine contains an average of 10^2 organisms per milliliter, composed chiefly of aerobes and gram-positive organisms. There is a transient increase in the bacterial content of the proximal small bowel following a meal thought to result from swallowing saliva and oral microflora. Intestinal obstruction increases the bacterial content of the proximal small bowel. The bacterial content of the distal small bowel is greater and approaches that of the colon in the region of the ileocecal valve. An incompetent valve or surgical removal of the ileocecal valve increases small bowel colonization by bacteria. In the colon there is a remarkable increase in the number of bacteria,

and anaerobic organisms dominate: *Bacteroides spp.*, *Peptostreptococcus spp.*, *Clostridium spp.*, and *Fusobacterium spp.* Predominant colonic aerobes are *Escherichia coli*, *Streptococci*, *Staphylococci*, *Proteus* and *Pseudomonas spp.* [2]. There is no difference in the fecal flora of patients with ulcerative colitis, Crohn's colitis, or a normal colon [3].

Emergency operations and prolonged procedures increase the risk of bacterial contamination of previously sterile areas. Whereas spillage of enteric content into the peritoneal cavity and wound results in direct bacterial contamination, more recent evidence suggests that bacterial translocation to adjacent lymphatics and the bloodstream may also contribute to sepsis following surgery [4].

A swift diagnosis and control of the origin of infection complemented by appropriate antibiotic therapy usually leads to resolution of a postoperative infection with minimal metabolic consequences to the patient. However, delay in diagnosis is not uncommon and is often due to occult foci of sepsis that cannot be easily identified or lack of clinical suspicion that a postoperative infection is developing. In these patients there may be a subtle but progressive deterioration in their general status that may predispose to worsening of the infectious complication. Eventually, entry of bacteria into the bloodstream and multiplication of organisms within the blood that release large amounts of endotoxin may cause cardiac muscle toxicity, renal hypoperfusion, and, ultimately, death from multisystem failure.

This chapter discusses surgical site infections, including superficial and deep wound infections, organ or space abscess formation, anastomotic dehiscence, and enterocutaneous fistula complications following surgery for inflammatory bowel disease. The etiology, diagnosis, and management of these conditions are described.

Surgical Site Infections

Definitions

The Centers for Disease Control and Prevention recently revised the definition of surgical wound infection by introducing the term surgical site infection (SSI) to encompass superficial incisional, deep incisional, and organ/space infections arising within 30 days after the operative procedure (5). Superficial incisional SSIs involve only the skin and subcutaneous tissue of the wound, whereas deep incisional SSIs involve the fascial and muscle layers of the incision. Organ/space SSIs involve any organ or space other than the incision that is opened or manipulated during the operative procedure.

A superficial incisional SSI requires at least one of the following (6):

1. Purulent drainage from the superficial incision.
2. Organisms isolated from an aseptically obtained culture of fluid or tissue from the superficial incision.
3. At least one of the following signs or symptoms of infection: pain or tenderness, localized swelling, redness, or heat and superficial incision is deliberately opened by surgeon, *unless* culture of the incision is negative.
4. Diagnosis of superficial incisional SSI by the surgeon or attending physician.

A deep incisional SSI requires at least one of the following (6):

1. Purulent drainage from the deep incision but not from the organ/space component of the surgical site.
2. A deep incision spontaneously dehisces or is deliberately opened by a surgeon when the patient has at least one of the following signs or symptoms: fever (over 38°C), localized pain, or tenderness, unless culture of the incision is negative.
3. An abscess or other evidence of infection involving the deep incision is found on direct examination, during reoperation, or by histopathologic or radiologic examination.
4. Diagnosis of a deep incisional SSI by a surgeon or attending physician.

An organ/space SSI requires at least one of the following (6):

1. Purulent drainage from a drain placed through a stab wound into an organ/space.
2. Organisms isolated from an aseptically obtained culture of fluid or tissue in the organ/space.
3. An abscess or other evidence of infection involving the organ/space on direct examination, during reoperation, or by histopathologic or radiologic examination.
4. Diagnosis of an organ/space SSI by a surgeon or attending physician.

Risk Factors

The likelihood that a given patient will develop a postoperative SSI is dependent on bacteria-related, patient-related, and operation-related risk factors (6). The greater the number of organisms and the more virulent the bacteria, the greater the risk of an SSI. Anaerobes cannot grow in the oxygen concentrations found in most wounds and thus most wound infections are due to aerobic organisms. Highly encapsulated strains of bacteria are more resistant to host defense mechanisms.

Bacteria that produce exotoxins are potentially more virulent than those without that ability. Tables 35.1 and 35.2 summarize the available information regarding patient-related and operation-related risk factors. The classification of the surgical wound as clean, clean-contaminated, contaminated, and

Table 35.1.   Host-related risk factors for surgical wound infection.*

Risk factor	Relation to wound infection
Morbid obesity	Definite
Old age	
Prolonged preoperative stay	
Infection at other sites	
ASA class	
Disease severity index	
Low albumen	Likely
Malnutrition	
Cancer	Possible
Diabetes mellitus	
Patient age	Other possible
Having three or more discharge diagnoses	
Immunosuppressive therapy	
Number of organs injured (blunt trauma)	
Shock (gunshot wound)	

*Data from Table 22.4 in Howard and Lee (6).

Table 35.2. Operation-related risk factors for surgical wound infection.*

Risk factor	Relation to wound infection
Prolonged duration of surgery	Definite
Razor shaves	
Intraoperative microbial contamination	
Surgical wound class	
Low abdominal operative site	
Specific type of surgical procedure	
Tissue trauma	Likely
Prolonged hospital admission	
Multiple procedures	
Low procedure volume	Possible
Unskilled surgeon	
Foreign material	
Poor hemostasis	
Failure to obliterate dead space	
Number of people in operating room	
Emergency surgery	
No preoperative shower or scrub	
Drains	
Glove punctures	

*Data from Table 22.3 in Howard and Lee (6).

dirty/infected is a definite risk factor. By definition, operations on the alimentary tract are at best clean-contaminated. Table 35.3 provides useful benchmark wound infection rates by wound class.

Efforts have been made to develop a risk index accounting for patient and operation-related risk factors. No single system has proven superior, but Haley et al. (7) identified four risk factors of approximately equal weight that increased the risk of an SSI: 1) an abdominal operation, 2) operative time over two hours, 3) a contaminated or dirty/infected wound class, and 4) the presence of more

than three diagnoses on the discharge face sheet (i.e., comorbidity) (8).

Wound Infections

Etiology: Wound infections account for up to 20% of all infections after surgery for inflammatory bowel disease (9). The spectrum of organisms cultured from such infections is wide (see Table 35.4). The origin of a wound infection may be the bowel flora, in which case gram-negative aerobic and anaerobic bacteria are most commonly

Table 35.3. Wound infection rates.*

Wound class	NAS-NRC[a] 1964 (n = 15,613)	Cruse and Foord[b] 1980 (n = 62,937)	SENIC[c] 1983 (n = 59,352)	Olson and Lee[d] 1990 (n = 36,439)	Culver et al.[e] 1991 (n = 84,691)
Clean	5.1	1.5	2.9	1.3	2.1
Clean-contaminated	10.8	7.7	3.9	2.4	3.3
Contaminated	16.3	15.2	8.5	7.9	6.4
Dirty	28.0	40.0	12.6	—	7.1

[a]Report of an ad hoc committee of Committee on Trauma, Division of Medical Sciences, National Academy of Sciences—National Research Council. Postoperative wound infections: the influence of ultraviolet irradiation of the operating room and of various other factors. Ann Surg 1964;160:1.

[b]Cruse PJ, Foord R. The epidemiology of wound infection: a 10-year prospective study of 62,939 wounds. Surg Clin North Am 1980;60:27.

[c]Haley RW, Culver DG, White JW, et al. The efficacy of infection surveillance and control programs in preventing nosocomial infections in US hospitals. Am J Epidemiol 1985;121:182.

[d]Olson MM, Lee JT. Continuous, 10-year wound infection surveillance. Results, advantages, and unanswered questions. Arch Surg 1990;125:794.

[e]Culver DH, Horan TC, Gaynes RD, et al. Surgical wound infection rates by wound class, operative procedure, and patient risk index. Am J Surg 1991;91:152S.

*Data taken from Table 22.2 in Howard and Lee (6).

Table 35.4. Morphologic, metabolic, and staining properties in bacteria found in surgical infection.

	Bacilli (rods)	Cocci (spheres)
Gram positive	Clostridium perfringens** Clostridium tetani** Actinomyces israelii**	Staphylococcus aureus *epidermidis Streptococcus pyogenes pneumoniae faecalis *viridans Peptostreptococcus supp.**
Gram negative	Escherichia coli Proteus mirabilis Klebsiella aerogenes Enterobacter spp. Pseudomonas aeruginosa Hemophilus influenzae Acinetobacter spp. Bacteroides spp.** Fusobacterium spp.**	Veilonella spp.

*Organisms that are commensals in skin that can cause infection in immunosuppressed patients and those with indwelling lines.
**Organisms that obtain nutrition chiefly by anaerobic metabolism.

cultured. Infection may originate from the patient's skin flora or from a member of the operating team, in which case gram-positive organisms are more likely to be cultured. *Staphylococcus aureus* is most notable and present in the anterior nares, axilla, and umbilicus, whereas *Clostridia spp.* are generally found below the level of the umbilicus. Bacterial phage typing can confirm the suspicion that a wound infection originated from a member of the surgical team. Infection of a surgical wound may also occur after surgery. Such infections are nosocomial in origin and involve strains of bacteria that are often resistant to conventional antibiotic therapy. Transmission of hospital infection may be by fomites and cross contamination by members of staff. Occasionally, clinically significant wound infections may be caused by skin contaminants such as *Staphylococcus epidermidis*, which produce slime to facilitate adherence of bacterial cells to the wound.

Clinical manifestations: Most wound infections present within four to six days after operation, although some may not present for several weeks. They typically present with edema, erythema, pain, and drainage. Cellulitis is variable but may be the only manifestation. Fever and leukocytosis may be present. Infection of the deep wound may present with wound dehiscence or pus draining between fascial sutures.

Some wound infections present early and run a fulminant, life-threatening course (10). Streptococcal infections may produce rapidly progressing cellulitis, lymphangitis, and blood-filled blebs around the wound within a day of an operation. Abscess formation is uncommon but there may be a thin, watery, purulent exudate heralding underlying tissue gangrene and necrotizing fasciitis.

Clostridial infections are rare but usually occur after colon surgery or trauma. Skin changes may be minimal, thus hiding the underlying necrotizing process that can be extreme and quickly fatal if not recognized and treated. Palpation of subcutaneous air or the presence of thickened, edematous skin in a septic patient should suggest the diagnosis. Necrotizing wound infections can also be caused by mixed aerobic and anaerobic bacteria.

Management of superficial wound infections: A superficial incisional SSI can usually be treated at the bedside or in the outpatient clinic. Minor erythema and minimal edema at the wound edges should alert the clinician to the possibility of a developing superficial wound infection. If there is no wound drainage, close observation of the wound is advised. If minor cellulitis is present, an antibiotic effective against staphylococci and streptococci is instituted. Minor cellulitis will usually respond quickly to antibiotic therapy. If the erythema, edema, or cellulitis progress, if drainage develops, or if the patient develops wound pain, fever or leukocytosis, the diagnosis of a more serious wound infection is likely.

The wound is opened initially only at sites of drainage, fluctuance, tenderness, or induration. After removal of one or two sutures or staples, a Q-tip swab is easily inserted into the wound to open it and allow drainage of infected material. The swab is used to obtain a culture if it appears antibiotics are necessary. In many cases of superficial wound infections, opening of the wound allows the patient to recover uneventfully without the need for antibiotics or expensive cultures. Immunosuppressed or septic patients should be hospitalized for treatment with intravenous antibiotics instituted after obtaining wound cultures. The opened wound is examined to determine whether all purulent material has been drained, the fascia is intact, further debridement of necrotic or devitalized tissue is necessary, and there is evidence of an underlying deeper source of infection, such as an abscess or enteric fistula. If necessary, the entire length of the wound is opened superficially. It is irrigated with sterile saline and dressed (not packed tightly) with sterile gauze. Wound edges should not be allowed to desiccate. When the infection is controlled, the wound will heal by secondary intention. Alternatively, the wound may be re-closed when granulation tissue appears healthy and there is no sign of infection.

Management of deep wound infections: A deep incisional SSI involves all layers of the anterior abdominal wall. It is best treated in the hospital setting. Deep wound infections may result in necrosis of the fascia or weakening of the fascial sutures. Dehiscence or pus draining between fascial sutures may best be treated by removal of fascial sutures to assure adequate drainage. If the defect is small, the fascia may be left open to promote drainage. Major wound dehiscence or bowel herniation or evisceration requires reoperation and reclosure. Necrotic tissue, including fascia, must be debrided. Primary closure is accomplished by first placing and then serially tying interrupted fascial sutures and retention fascial sutures. If tension is present, lateral fascial relaxing incisions or synthetic mesh are used to achieve closure. Rarely, the dehisced wound is treated by open packing, allowing for secondary closure. A ventral hernia will result but can be repaired electively if the patient survives the infectious complication.

Failure to obtain cultures in cases of deep wound infection may lead to difficulties in identifying the original source of infection because antibacterial therapy may alter the microbial flora. Identification of organisms causing infection is also important to assess patterns of bacterial resistance to antibiotic agents in the hospital and in the evaluation of cross infections. In the presence of minimal discharge a wound swab may be obtained. This should be transported to the laboratory immediately. In case of delay, specimens should be stored in a transport medium at 4°C, although this may lead to an overgrowth of the patient's own flora. It is preferable to send whole pus or slough from the wound in a sterile container rather than a swab. Pus will preserve the reducing environment that pathogens require to survive and will also help prevent desiccation. In the presence of fever, blood should be obtained for aerobic and anaerobic culture. In case of transportation delay, blood culture specimens should be stored at room temperature and not in the refrigerator. Antibiotic therapy that is deemed appropriate may then be commenced. In the case of bowel-related infection, this is usually a combination of a second or third generation cephalosporin combined with metronidazole.

Prevention: Polk and Lopez-Mayer demonstrated that preoperative prophylactic antibiotics greatly reduced wound infections after elective colectomy (11). Some studies have shown the benefit of using a single agent effective against aerobes and anaerobes (12). Earlier data on prophylaxis suggested the need for two postoperative doses of intravenous antibiotics, but more recent studies have shown that a single preoperative dose is as effective (13). There are no studies in which the risk of wound infection has been assessed if an operative procedure is prolonged. Many surgeons give a second dose of antibiotic if an operation lasts more than two or three hours.

Preoperative mechanical bowel preparation is designed to empty the colon of all bulk fecal matter and to make the remaining contents less infective by reducing the absolute numbers of gut bacteria. This is thought to reduce the incidence of wound infection, anastomotic leak, and intraabdominal sepsis. It has been noted that bowel preparation does not decrease bacterial concentration, which is a key factor determining the incidence of septic complications (14). It was for this reason that oral antibiotic agents were added to the bowel preparation regimen as they can reduce the residual bacterial concentration. Most randomized trials of preoperative oral antibiotics have shown a reduction in infection rate.

Antibiotics and bowel preparation are useful in preventing septic complications, but surgical technique is probably much more important. Gentle handling of tissues, securing hemostasis, and irrigating to dilute inoculation of bacteria and remove blood and devitalized tissue are effective means of preventing postoperative infections.

The greatest risk of wound infection arises from spillage of bowel content from an enterotomy or colotomy. This is most likely to occur during emergency operations, operations on obstructed bowel, and reoperations in patients particularly with Crohn's disease or in those with extensive adhesions. During emergency operation for obstructed bowel, care should be taken in entering the peritoneal cavity to prevent accidental enterotomy. Obstructed bowel full of feces should not be delivered through the anterior abdominal wall during creation of a stoma due to the risk of accidental perforation or slippage from a bowel clamp. It is wise to decompress obstructed bowel of gas with a large bore needle and to perform on-table lavage in some instances to reduce the fecal content of proximal bowel; this enables easier handling of obstructed colon and reduces the risk of spillage (15). Fecal spillage may also occur during bowel resection if intestinal clamps are applied too close to bowel edges, allowing them to slip off. During resection and anastomosis, some routinely cleanse the bowel with either chlorhexidene and cetrimide solution or povidone iodine.

Organ/Space Infections

Etiology: Following surgery for inflammatory bowel disease, intraperitoneal, retroperitoneal, or visceral abscesses may develop with or without concomitant wound infection (see Table 35.5). Intraabdominal abscesses represent the successful result of normal host defense mechanisms in the peritoneal cavity to wall off infections from the rest of the peritoneal cavity by inflammatory adhesions, loops of intestine and their mesentery, the omentum, and other viscera. The contents of the abscess cavity locally prevent complete resolution of the infection so therapeutic intervention is necessary.

Abscesses typically arise as a sequela to diffuse peritonitis or to a bacterial innoculum deposited within the peritoneal cavity as a result of a bowel perforation, fecal spillage during surgery, or from a leaked anastomosis. Postoperative abscesses account for 46% to 74% of all intraabdominal abscesses and over 30% of such abscesses result from a leaked anastomosis, usually after colorectal resections (16–18). Visceral abscesses, most commonly due to hematogenous or lymphatic spread of bacteria to an organ, occur most often in the liver but sometimes develop in retroperitoneal viscera, such as the pancreas. Crohn's disease may produce tubo-ovarian infections or uterine, bladder, retroperitoneal, or other fistulas. If not recognized at laparotomy or if incompletely treated, postoperative abscesses can develop in these sites.

The bacteria that cause postoperative abscesses represent a mix of anaerobic and aerobic gut flora.

Table 35.5.   Organ/space infections following surgery for inflammatory bowel disease.

I. Intraperitoneal
  A. Subphrenic
    1. Left:
      Subdiaphragmatic
      Lesser sac
    2. Right:
      Subdiaphragmatic
      Subhepatic
  B. Pelvic
    1. Pouch of Douglas in women
    2. Rectovesical pouch in men
  C. Paracolic gutter
  D. Mesenteric
    1. Intermesenteric
    2. Intramesenteric
II. Retroperitoneal
  A. Paracolic
  B. Psoas
  C. Ileocecal
III. Visceral
  A. Hepatic
    1. Single
    2. Multiple
  B. Ovarian
  C. Other

In the postoperative patient, antibiotic-resistant organisms may be present, especially if a patient received broad-spectrum antibiotics preoperatively, or if antibiotics were instituted postoperatively to "treat the fever" rather than draining and culturing an abscess.

Clinical manifestations and diagnosis: The presence of a high intermittent temperature after surgery should arouse suspicion of an abscess. The patient may complain of abdominal pain and tenderness, anorexia, and a sense of being ill. In the postoperative state, a physical examination is especially unreliable, but a mass may be palpable on abdominal or pelvic/rectal examination. The diagnosis is further supported by a neutrophilic leukocytosis, often in excess of 15,000 cells/mm^3. A blood smear may show the presence of toxic granules in neutrophils which also show a left shift, indicating immature forms in the peripheral blood. In contrast, in older people there may be no fever and the total leukocyte count may be less than normal, indicating a poor immunologic response in the presence of severe infection.

Usually, a plain film of the abdomen is not diagnostic of an abscess, but a mottled appearance within extralumenal gas collections is highly suggestive of an abscess. Dilated loops of small bowel may be evident adjacent to the abscess cavity in which an air fluid interphase may be observed.

Intraperitoneal abscesses are often found at a site remote from the original source of the infection because the intraperitoneal circulation brings fluid to dependent sites in the pelvis and lateral gutters. The peritoneal circulation favors unilateral spread of exudate. The site of an abscess may evoke a specific clinical response. For instance, pain from a subdiaphragmatic abscess may be referred to the shoulder. Diaphragmatic irritation may cause frequent hiccups, cough, or tachypnea. Auscultation of the ipsilateral lung base may reveal reduced basilar breath sounds, and a chest film may show elevation of the ipsilateral hemidiaphragm and a pleural effusion. Pelvic abscesses may cause a deep, visceral pelvic pain. Irritation of the adjacent rectum may lead to tenesmus, whereas irritation of the bladder causes increased frequency with micturition. Congestion of the vagina may result in vaginal bleeding.

Delay in diagnosis of a postoperative abscess is common and often results in significant additional morbidity and even multiorgan failure, septic shock, and death (19). Delay in diagnosis is due to many factors—symptoms may be masked by analgesics; signs of infection are difficult to evaluate in a postoperative patient, especially if antibiotics are being administered; and abscesses are sometimes occult. The single most important factor in the delay is probably the surgeon's reluctance to admit the possibility of a complication. Olson and Allen reported that the median time from initial operation to clinical recognition of an abscess was eight days, compared to a median time of four days from initial operation to symptoms of an abscess (18, 20). Clinical suspicion of an abscess should prompt immediate radiologic testing to confirm the diagnosis.

Radiologic investigations: Scanning of the abdomen and pelvis by ultrasonography (US), computed tomography (CT), or magnetic resonance imaging (MRI) will usually reveal the location of a clinically significant abscess. Furthermore, scanning may provide information such as dimensions of the abscess, presence of loculations and feasibility to safely perform percutaneous aspiration and drainage of the abscess. Ultrasonography is rapid, noninvasive, relatively inexpensive, and it does not expose the patient to irradiation, but it has several disadvantages. It is difficult to assess patients with drains, open wounds, or stomas because of the lack of acoustic windows. It is extremely operator-dependent. Ultrasonography is poor in identifying retroperitoneal and peripancreatic abscesses, chiefly because of poor resolution of these areas and overlying bowel gas, which is common in critically ill patients with an ileus. CT with enhancement of images using intravenous and bowel contrast is the most accurate technique available to diagnose intraabdominal abscesses (21). Gas filled structures and abdominal wall defects do not interfere with CT. CT provides better resolution of retroperitoneal structures compared with US. CT has been employed most commonly as a guide to percutaneous drainage of abscesses. MRI is costlier but has no danger of irradiation. It also provides superior soft tissue definition compared with CT.

Role of scintigraphy: Despite the availability of several radiologic investigations, it may not be possible to identify localized collections of pus in all cases. Interloop abscesses, which represent four percent of all abscesses, are poorly visualized by CT (22). Radionuclide scans have been used to identify occult intraabdominal abscesses (23). Labeled leukocytes would be expected to concentrate in the abscess and then manifest as an area of increased radioactivity compared with surrounding tissue. However, increased concentrations of leukocytes may also be visualized in the spleen and liver, which makes it difficult to diagnose an abscess in these regions. Gallium 67 citrate, technetium 99 and indium 111 have been employed as nuclear markers. Technetium 99 has the advantage of a shorter half life (24). Lantto reported that technetium 99 labeled leukocyte scans were superior to indium 111 leukocyte scans in acute abdominal sepsis and inflammatory bowel disease (24). The method is sensitive but not specific, implying that a normal scan result does not exclude an abscess.

Management: Appropriate treatment of a patient with an intraabdominal abscess includes general supportive care, intravenous antibiotic administration and drainage by either percutaneous or operative means. The overall status of the patient determines the type of supportive care needed. This may vary from merely providing maintenance fluids to providing emergency fluid resuscitation, invasive monitoring, ventilator support, and other aggressive supportive measures. Nutritional support is critical since most patients with an abscess have not had adequate caloric intake for five to ten days and sepsis will further aggravate this deficit. Total parenteral nutrition is usually necessary in this setting because the associated ileus or anastomotic leak prevents use of enteral feedings. Antibiotic therapy is directed initially against a combination of anaerobic and aerobic bacteria. As soon as culture results are available, adjustments in the regimen can be made.

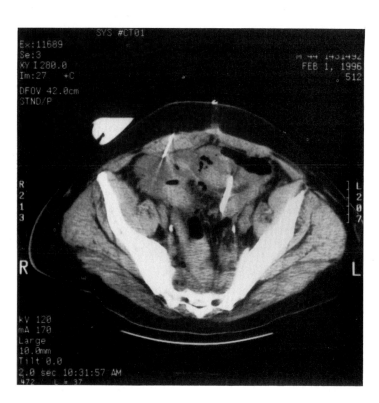

Fig. 35.1. This CT scan shows two drainage catheters placed into separate intraabdominal abscess collections.

Drainage of the abscess cavity remains the key to successful treatment. Previously, the majority of intraabdominal abscesses were drained by an open operation. Minimally invasive drainage by repeated needle aspiration or insertion of a drainage catheter into the abscess cavity under radiologic guidance has added a new dimension to therapy (see Fig. 35.1). Pus is aspirated and sent for microbiologic analysis. The distal tip of the catheter curves into a "pig tail" when the stillete from within it is withdrawn, thus preventing dislodgement. The catheter is left in until there is clinical resolution of sepsis and drainage is minimal and nonpurulent, which may be from a few days to a few weeks. It is also possible to assess healing of the abscess by instilling radiologic contrast into the cavity. Added advantages of percutaneous drainage are avoidance of anesthesia in patients who are often ill, avoidance of laparotomy, and virtually a zero risk of wound infection. In a proportion of patients, residual collections may require repeated percutaneous drainage, whereas some others may require open drainage by laparotomy.

We recently reported our experience at the University of Minnesota with percutaneous drainage of 111 abdominal abscesses in 82 patients, some following surgery for inflammatory bowel disease. The presence of fecal material, fistula connections with the abscess, multiloculated abscess cavities, multiple abscesses and an abscess diameter of greater than 10 cm were found to be associated with a high failure rate (25).

If percutaneous drainage is not possible or if it fails to eradicate sepsis, laparotomy is undertaken to drain all abscesses and control the source of infection. Peritoneal lavage with copious volumes of warm saline, sometimes mixed with an antibacterial agent, e.g., povidone iodine solution or a cephalosporin, will help to dilute the bacterial content within the peritoneal cavity. Fecal diversion is usually necessary if a bowel fistula or a leaking anastomosis is in continuity with the abscess cavity. A pelvic abscess, if large enough, may be drained through the suprapubic route, although usually drainage is achieved by the transperineal or transrectal route.

The clinical response to drainage of pus is usually dramatic and is noted by defervescence, normalization of leukocyte counts and the return of the patient's sense of well-being in 24 to 48 hours. Appropriate antibiotic therapy for up to two weeks is usually employed as an adjunct to drainage of pus. It is particularly indicated in the immunocompromised, steroid-dependent, or diabetic patient. However, in established abscesses, antibiotic therapy is no substitute for drainage. Furthermore, injudicious use of broad-spectrum antibiotics often leads to unnecessary delays in diagnosis and may promote growth of antibiotic-resistant organisms.

Anastomotic Dehiscence

Dehiscence of an anastomosis is a dreaded complication of bowel resection and anastomosis for Crohn's disease or ulcerative colitis. Its etiology is multifactorial. Meticulous anastomotic technique to achieve a watertight seal with a well preserved blood supply to the bowel edges, the absence of tension, and the absence of distal obstruction remain the cornerstones to success of any anastomosis. A conservative approach is advised during emergency operations and in the presence of generalized abdominal sepsis, suboptimal physiologic conditions, or poor bowel preparation. It may be appropriate to postpone an anastomosis in such situations and instead construct a stoma. Alternatively, one may consider a primary anastomosis but with proximal diversion, especially after high-risk anastomoses such as an ileoanal procedure. Although proximal diversion does not prevent a leak, it can protect the patient from major morbidity and even death associated with a dehiscence.

Small Bowel Anastomotic Dehiscence

Leaks following a small bowel anastomosis are usually due to a technical error or nondiagnosed concomitant pathology. Most leaks occur after non-elective operations. For Crohn's disease, emergency small bowel resection is usually undertaken for perforation of a segment of bowel, sepsis, or obstruction that is not responding to steroid therapy. In the elective situation, leakage is rare unless there has been an occult injury to the bowel or distal obstruction is left untreated. Distal obstruction must be excluded during operation by careful examination of the entire small intestine. Absence of strictures in the distal duodenum and in the recto sigmoid may at times be difficult to assess by examination or palpation only. Passage of a catheter with an inflatable balloon via the oral route or passage of a scope through the anus may reveal strictures not detected otherwise. Some have reported leakage following closure of a loop ileostomy that may be due to improper technique, fibrosis, and diminished vascularity of bowel edges or obstruction in the defunctioned efferent limb (21).

A variety of methods have been employed to perform small bowel anastomoses, but there are no data to show that one is superior to the other. However, when anastomosis of edematous bowel is undertaken and there is concern that staples may not hold, it may be wise to employ a two-layered technique provided that sufficient lumen through the anastomosis is preserved. Suture ligation of the thickened, edematous mesentery provides secure hemostasis and may prevent mesenteric hematoma formation that can produce ischemia at the anastomosis. An anastomotic leak may thus be avoided.

Large Bowel Anastomotic Dehiscence

Large bowel anastomoses are more risky than those of small bowel with clinically significant leaks noted in 3% to 23% of patients after colectomy (26–29). One third to one half of patients with a leaked colonic anastomosis die, and thus anastomotic leak accounts for up to 50% of all operative mortality after colectomy (30). Sepsis causes an increase in collagen lysis and a decrease in collagen synthesis, and thus it is not surprising that the prime factor contributing to anastomotic leakage at operation is peritonitis. Extraperitoneal anastomoses leak more often than intraperitoneal anastomoses presumably because they are more difficult to perform, are surrounded by dead space that is not exposed to the intraperitoneal defense mechanisms, and are missing the serosa that may help anchor anastomotic sutures or staples (30,31). Hypoxia impairs anastomotic healing and because colonic blood flow is particularly sensitive to hypovolemia, hypoxia undoubtedly contributes to many colonic anastomotic leaks. Preoperative hematocrit of less than 35%, intraoperative blood loss of over 10% of blood volume, intraoperative transfusion of more than two units, or intraoperative hypotension all are associated with an increased risk of leak (30). Starvation and hypoalbuminemia have also been associated with an increased leak rate (28,32). Some studies have suggested an increased anastomotic leak rate in patients dependent on steroids, but others have not confirmed such a relationship (27,28). While single-layer, double-layer, hand-sutured, and stapled colonic anastomoses may be equally secure, there is evidence that inverting anastomoses are superior to everting anastomoses (31).

Segmental resection of large bowel may have to be undertaken for Crohn's disease, but anastomosis does not carry a greater risk of dehiscence compared with resection and anastomosis for other benign and malignant diseases of the large bowel in patients with similar degrees of illness. Subtotal colectomy with Hartmann pouch is an option in emergency surgery for inflammatory bowel disease. Karch et al. reviewed their experience of 114 patients having this operation (33). There was a 2.6% incidence of pelvic sepsis consequent to suture line leakage from the rectal stump. Leakage from the rectal stump was found to occur in 3 of 73 patients in whom the rectum was not decompressed by transanal catheter drainage compared with none of 41 patients in whom catheter drainage of the rectum appeared to be protective against rectal stump leakage. An alternative operation is subtotal colectomy with mucus fistula, but it has the potential disadvantage of leaving a longer segment of diseased colon within the abdomen. Ileorectal anastomosis following subtotal colectomy for inflammatory bowel disease is usually a safe anastomosis, providing the rectum is reasonably healthy.

Ileal-Anal Pouch Anastomotic Dehiscence

Anastomotic leakage following an ileal pouch-anal anastomosis procedure may occur in as many as 12% of patients (34). Leakage leads to major morbidity including abscess formation, local or generalized peritonitis, chronic sepsis, fistulas, and anastomotic stricture. Ultimately pouch excision may be necessary. The ileal-pouch/anal anastomosis is extraperitoneal, and some believe that all extraperitoneal anastomoses should be protected by a proximal stoma. In contrast, others believe that a selective policy to create a proximal stoma only in high-risk situations is the appropriate choice. Although there is no consensus, a review of the literature suggests several indications for proximal diversion of the fecal stream, including prolonged pelvic dissection, undue hemorrhage and pelvic hematoma, intraoperative hypotension and vital sign instability, elderly patients and patients on high-dose steroids and immunosuppression (35–37). Furthermore, technical factors such as anastomotic tension or questionable anastomotic integrity as evidenced by incomplete stapler "donuts" or leakage of air on testing the anastomosis under water are indications for proximal fecal diversion, especially if primary repair is not feasible. Despite this, the role of loop ileostomy in reducing sepsis and anastomotic dehiscence complications remains uncertain. In a randomized controlled trial of loop ileostomy for ileal-pouch/anal anastomosis, Grobler et al. showed no difference in septic complications and dehiscence in patients with and without loop ileostomy, albeit in a small sample. Instead, these authors showed that loop ileostomy was related to a greater incidence of complications following closure (34).

Role of Omentum

The omentum has been thought to provide greater security to bowel anastomoses chiefly by reducing dead space adjacent to it, thus minimizing hematoma formation (38). In a randomized trial of omentectomy during restorative proctocolectomy with ileal anal anastomosis, Ambroze et al. found a greater incidence of septic complications in patients having omentectomy (38).

Role of Drains

Drains are placed adjacent to an anastomosis in the hope of reducing perianastomotic fluid collection that may become infected and secondarily rupture through the suture line. This is thought to be especially useful if the anastomosis is extraperitoneal. Some surgeons advocate perianastomotic drains so that if a leak occurs, a controlled fecal fistula is produced as opposed to development of peritonitis or an abscess, had no drain been present. However, there is evidence that drains stimulate collagenase activity that may lead to disruption of the anastomosis (39). Furthermore, there is no clear evidence that pelvic drainage prevents leaks or abscesses. Sagar et al. in a randomized trial of pelvic drainage following anterior resection have shown that residual fluid volume in the pelvis measured by ultrasound was similar in patients, irrespective of pelvic drainage (40). Most surgeons agree that if a perianastomotic drain is used, it should be the closed suction type and not the open drainage systems that are more apt to promote entry of bacteria into the peritoneal cavity.

Diagnosis and Management

The presentation of a leaked anastomosis is highly variable, depending on the degree of the leak and the location of the anastomosis. Debas and Thomson classified clinically apparent anastomotic leaks as a minor separation, major separation, or gross necrosis of the bowel (29).

Minor separation occurred in one-third of patients with anastomotic leak and often presented approximately one week after surgery as a fecal fistula through a previous drain site or through the incision. Most such patients are not ill although they may have a low-grade fever, minimal leukocytosis, and mild abdominal discomfort. Such fistulas usually heal spontaneously with nonoperative management. Occasionally, proximal small bowel fistulas produce a high output and require eventual surgery to achieve closure.

Major anastomotic separations occurred in over half of all leaks and usually presented within a few days of surgery with fever, leukocytosis, and toxicity. About one third of such leaks result in peritonitis that necessitates immediate laparotomy. In the remainder the clinical picture may be confusing. Aggressive use of diagnostic studies, including a gentle digital rectal examination, a water-soluble contrast enema, and CT scan, will usually confirm the clinical suspicion of a disrupted anastomosis. Considerable judgment and frequent evaluations of the patient are required to properly manage such situations. In many cases, the leakage is walled off by omentum and adjacent bowel, producing a localized abscess adjacent to the anastomosis. There may be localized abdominal or pelvic tenderness, but there is no diffuse peritonitis. Laparotomy may be ill advised in such patients. If the infection can be controlled by antibiotics and if abscesses can be drained percutaneously or transanally, many leaked anastomoses can be salvaged without further surgery.

Gross necrosis of at least one segment of a colon anastomosis occurred in 10% of cases of leaked anastomoses studied (29) and produced early diffuse peritonitis resulting ultimately in death in all such cases. Intraabdominal leakage from an anastomosis producing peritonitis or sepsis that is not easily controlled medically demands correction by immediate reoperation. Exploration within a few days or weeks of surgery can be hazardous due to postoperative bowel adhesions, separation of which causes excessive bleeding and carries the risk of accidental enterotomy. Localized collections of stool or pus must be drained. With a major leak, proximal diversion is performed. If there is a complete anastomotic disruption or bowel necrosis, the anastomosis should be taken down and the ends exteriorized, or a Hartmann pouch should be constructed. Supportive care, including broad-spectrum antibiotics and total parenteral nutrition, is critical to achieve recovery.

Enterocutaneous Fistula

Etiology

Enterocutaneous fistula is an abnormal connection between bowel and the skin surface. It usually results from an anastomotic dehiscence. Crohn's disease may lead to fistula formation irrespective of a surgical procedure. In some cases, if underlying Crohn's disease is not recognized, an enterocutaneous fistula may result from an uncomplicated procedure. An often quoted example is an enterocutaneous fistula developing after an appendectomy undertaken for acute appendicitis in which underlying ileocecal Crohn's disease was not recognized.

In ulcerative colitis an enterocutaneous fistula occurs most often following ileal-pouch/anal anastomosis. Keighley et al. reviewed their experience of fistulas after J-pouch anal anastomosis (41). Fistulas originated from several sites: ileal-anal ana-

stomosis, staple line of a J-pouch, and pouch appendage. Iatrogenic small bowel injury was another cause of fistula. Suture or staple line leakage was identified as the cause of fistula formation in the majority, but in a proportion of patients, cryptoglandular infection at the dentate line was thought to complicate the postoperative course.

Once a fistula is established, several factors may be responsible for its persistence. Chronic sepsis either within the fistula track or adjacent to the fistula must be identified. Often a collection of pus may be present adjacent to the track that feeds the fistula, or the presence of a foreign body, including suture material, may continue the active infection. There may be bowel obstruction distal to the site of fistula that prevents it from healing because the fistula functions as a vent for bowel effluent. Long-standing fistula tracks may have epithelialized, thus preventing healing. Furthermore, the fistula track may have become the site of active disease, such as Crohn's or malignancy.

Diagnosis and Management

Adoption of a methodical approach to the diagnosis and management of enterocutaneous fistula complicating surgery will usually provide the surgeon with control over the problem. The main issues to resolve are to identify the source of fistula, delineate the anatomy of the fistula track, assess bowel to exclude active underlying disease and bowel obstruction distal to the fistula track, identify occult sepsis either within the fistula track or adjacent to it, and assess the patient for comorbid conditions that influence wound healing, e.g., malnutrition, immunosuppression, and diabetes mellitus.

The history will most likely indicate the source of fistula. Its anatomy may be outlined by employing contrast radiography, including sonograms, contrast enhanced CT or MRI. This will outline the complexity of the fistula together with areas of cavitation that represent an abscess. If soft tissue structures need to be visualized in relation to the fistula track, MRI is probably the investigation of choice. In the anorectum, it is essential to visualize a fistula in relation to the anal sphincters so that surgical treatment of the fistula may avoid concomitant sphincter injury. This may be achieved with endorectal ultrasound. The fistula track may be conveniently delineated by image enhancement using hydrogen peroxide injected into the fistula opening. Endorectal ultrasound has also been employed in the assessment of sepsis following ileal anal pouch surgery. Solomon et al. were able to differentiate peripouch inflammation from abscess in relation to a pouch (42). More recently, MRI using image enhancement with an endorectal copper coil has been beneficial in imaging the pelvis. This may be useful in cases where resolution from ultrasound is poor or unreliable, such as above the level of the pelvic floor. In complex fistulas drainage and surgical debridement should always be accompanied by microbiologic analysis of organisms. In the presence of a cyclical fever, blood cultures should be taken for aerobic and anaerobic organisms. This will help direct appropriate antibiotic therapy. Tissue from the fistula should also be sent for histology in the case of complex and long-standing fistulas to exclude Crohn's disease or malignancy. The patient's nutritional, fluid, and electrolyte status should be assessed.

Management of an enterocutaneous fistula is based on the likelihood of spontaneous closure of the fistula and on an understanding of the problems it poses for patients. If workup reveals a complete or near complete distal obstruction, active disease or malignancy, or anastomotic necrosis and wide dehiscence, spontaneous closure will not occur. Early operative intervention is performed as soon as the patient is properly resuscitated. In the absence of such findings, conservative therapy is directed to keep up with fluid and electrolyte losses; to support nutrition via enteral or parenteral nutrition; to control skin excoriation at the site of fistula drainage with appropriate skin barriers and ostomy appliances; to reduce the volume of fistula output by use of H2 blockers or proton pump inhibitors to inhibit gastrointestinal, biliary and pancreatic secretions; and to control infection by drainage and curettage of the fistula track and any associated abscesses (43–45).

Conservative management is highly successful and over 90 percent of fistulas will close within four to six weeks of presentation (45). Small bowel fistulas close spontaneously less often than do esophageal, gastric, or colonic fistulas. If a fistula fails to close in four to six weeks, or if sepsis persists or recurs, laparotomy is usually needed to resolve the problem. Proximal fecal diversion and drainage may be necessary. Ideally, the source of the fistula can be resected and bowel continuity restored with a primary anastomosis. Judgment is necessary to decide whether this can be accomplished with one operation.

In fistulas of the anal canal, the choice lies between fistula track incision or excision for low fistulas involving minimal sphincter muscle and seton fistulotomy or advancement flap for tracks that encompass the bulk of sphincter muscle. Purulent collections that are high in the anal canal

may be drained percutaneously under ultrasound guidance using a wide bore needle. Complex Crohn's disease fistulas may have to be managed by abdominoperineal excision.

Conclusion

Surgical operations for Crohn's disease and ulcerative colitis incur the risk of septic complications. Infection may originate from the patient's own skin microflora, members of the surgical team, and the hospital environment. Hence, antibiotic prophylaxis plays a key role in preventing wound infection. If a surgical site infection develops, management will vary considerably, depending on whether it is a superficial or deep wound infection or an organ/space infection. If antibiotics are necessary, they should be as specific as possible. The majority of intraabdominal abscesses may now be managed by percutaneous drainage.

Anastomotic dehiscence following surgery for inflammatory bowel disease is usually due to a technical error or poor judgment when a surgeon performs an anastomosis in less than ideal circumstances. Steroid and immunosuppressant therapy may occasionally contribute to anastomotic disruption.

Enterocutaneous fistula most commonly results from suture line disruption after surgery. The aim of management should be to identify its source, map fistula track anatomy, manage sepsis and exclude obstruction at a site distal to the origin of the fistula. Appropriate management without the need for relaparotomy is often highly successful.

References

1. Hodgson HJF. Immunological aspects of inflammatory bowel disease. In: Bouchier IA, Allan RN, Hodgson HJF, Keighley MRB, eds. Textbook of Gastroenterology. London: Bailliere Tindall, 1984: 902–5.
2. Gorback SL. Intestinal microflora. Gastroenterology 1971;66:1110–29.
3. Walker AP, Condon RE. Infections of the colon. In: Howard RJ, Simmons RL, eds. Surgical Infectious Diseases. 3rd ed. Norwalk, CT: Appleton & Lange, 1995:1122.
4. Sedman PC, Macfie J, Sagar P, et al. The prevalence of gut translocation in humans. Gastroenterology 1994;107:643–9.
5. Horan TC, Gaynes RP, Martone WJ, et al. CDC definitions of nosocomial surgical site infections, 1992: a modification of the CDC definitions of surgical wound infections. Infect Control Hosp Epidemiol 1992;13:606.

6. Howard RJ, Lee JT. Surgical wound infection: epidemiology surveillance, and clinical management. In: Howard RJ, Simmons RL, eds. Surgical Infectious Diseases. 3rd ed. Norwalk, CT: Appleton & Lange, 1995:402–5.

7. Haley RW, Culver DH, Morgan WM, et al. Identifying patients at high risk of surgical wound infection. A simple multivariate index of patient susceptibility and wound contamination. Am J Epidemiol 1985;121:206.

8. Haley RW, Culver DG, White JW, et al. The efficacy of infection surveillance and control programs in preventing nosocomial infections in US hospitals. Am J Epidemiol 1985;121:182.

9. Wettergren A, Gyrtrup HJ, Grossman E, et al. Complications after J-pouch ileoanal anastomosis: stapled compared with handsewn anastomosis. Eur J Surg 1993;159:121–4.

10. Bubrick MP, Hitchcock CR. Necrotising anorectal and perineal infections. Surgery 1979;86:655.

11. Polk HC, Lopez-Mayer JF. Postoperative wound infection: a prospective study of determinant factors and prevention. 1969;66:97.

12. Gortz G, Boese-Landgraf J, Hopfenmuller W, et al. Ciprofloxacin as single dose antibiotic prophylaxis in colorectal surgery: results of a randomized, double blind trial. Diagn Microbiol Infect Dis 1990;13:181–5.

13. Lumley JW, Siu SK, Pillay SP, et al. Single dose ceftriaxone as prophylaxis for sepsis in colorectal surgery. Aust NZ J Surg 1992;62:292–6.

14. Dickman MD, Chappelka AR, Schaedler RW. Evaluation of gut microflora during administration of an elemental diet in a patient with an ileoproctostomy. Am J Dig Dis 1975;20:377.

15. Rothenberger DA, Mayoral J, Deen KI. Obstruction and perforation. In: Williams NS, ed. Colorectal Cancer. London: Churchill Livingstone, 1995:123–33.

16. Deveney CW, Lurie K, Deveney KE. Improved treatment of intraabdominal abscess. Arch Surg 1988;123:1126.

17. Olak J, Christou NV, Stein LA, et al. Operative vs. percutaneous drainage of intraabdominal abscesses. Comparison of morbidity and mortality. Arch Surg 1986;121:141.

18. Olson MM, Allen MO. Nosocomial abscess. Results of an eight-year prospective study of 32,284 operations. Arch Surg 1989;124:356.

19. Polk HC, Shields CL. Remote organ failure: a valid sign of occult intraabdominal infection. Surgery 1977;81:310.

20. Nathens AB, Ahrenholz DH, Simmons DL, et al. Peritonitis and other intraabdominal infections. In: Howard RJ, Simmons RL, eds. Surgical Infectious Diseases. 3rd ed. Norwalk, CT: Appleton & Lange, 1995:959–1009.

21. Knochel JO, Koehler PR, Lee TG. Diagnosis of abdominal abscesses with computed tomography, ultrasound, and In-111 leukocyte scans. Radiology 1980;137:427.

22. Baker ME, Blinder RA, Rice RP. Diagnostic imaging of abdominal fluid collections and abscesses. CRC Crit Rev Diagn Imaging 1986;25:233.

23. Peters AM. The utility of [99 Tc] HMPAO—leukocytes for imaging infection. Seminars in Nucl Med 1994;24:110–27.

24. Lantto E. Investigation of suspected intraabdominal sepsis: the contribution of nuclear medicine. Scan J Gastroenterol (suppl) 1994;203:11–14.

25. Bernini A, Spencer MP, Wong WD, et al. CT guided percutaneous abscess drainage in colorectal disease: factors associated with outcome. Dis Colon Rectum 1997;40:1009–13.

26. Jonsell G, Edelmann G. Single-layer anastomosis of the colon: a review of 165 cases. Am J Surg 1978; 135:630.

27. Schrock TR, Deveney CW, Dunphy JE. Factors contributing to leakage of colonic anastomoses. Ann Surg 1973:123:513.

28. Morgenstern L, Yamakawa T, Ben-Shoshan M, et al. Anastomotic leakage after low colonic anastomosis: clinical and experimental aspects. Am J Surg 1972;123:104.

29. Debas HT, Thomson FB. A critical review of colectomy with anastomosis. Surg Gynecol Obstet 1972;135:747.

30. Walker AP, Condon RE. Infections of the colon. In: Howard RJ, Simmons RL, eds. Surgical Infectious Diseases. 3rd ed. Norwalk, CT: Appleton & Lange, 1995:1105–65.

31. Goligher JC, Lee PWG, Simpkins KC, et al. A controlled comparison of one- and two-layer techniques of suture for high and low colorectal anastomoses. Br J Surg 1977;64:609.

32. Irvin TT, Goligher JC. Aetiology of disruption of intestinal anastomoses. Br J Surg 1973;60:461.

33. Karch LA, Bauer JJ, Gorfine SR, et al. Subtotal colectomy with Hartmann's pouch for inflammatory bowel disease. Dis Colon Rectum 1995;38:635–9.

34. Grobler SP, Hosie KB, Keighley MR. Randomized trial of loop ileostomy in restorative proctocolectomy. Br J Surg 1992;79:903–6.

35. Wexner SD, James K, Jagelman DG. The double stapled ileal reservoir and ileoanal anastomosis: a prospective review of sphincter function and clinical outcome. Dis Colon Rectum 1991;34:487–94.

36. Deen KI, Williams JG, Grant EA, et al. Randomized trial to determine the optimum level of pouch-anal anastomosis in stapled restorative proctocolectomy. Dis Colon Rectum 1995;38:133–8.

37. Sagar PM, Lewis W, Holdsworth PJ, et al. One-stage restorative proctocolectomy without temporary defunctioning ileostomy. Dis Colon Rectum 1992;35:582–8.

38. Ambroze WL, Wolff BG, Kelly KA, et al. Let sleeping dogs lie: the role of the omentum in the ileal pouch-anal anastomosis procedure. Dis Colon Rectum 1991;34:563–5.

39. Hawley PR, Faulk WP, Hunt TK, et al. Collagenase activity in the gastrointestinal tract. Br J Surg 1970;57:896–900.

40. Sagar PM, Couse N, Kerin M, et al. Randomized trial of drainage of colorectal anastomosis. Br J Surg 1993;80:769–71.

41. Keighley MR, Grobler NSP. Fistula complicating restorative proctocolectomy. Br J Surg 1993;80:1065–7.

42. Solomon MJ, McLeod RS, O'Connor BI, et al. Assessment of peripouch inflammation after ileoanal anastomosis using endoluminal ultrasonography. Dis Colon Rectum 1995; 38:182–7.

43. Sitges-Serra A, Guirao X, Pereira JA, et al. Treatment of gastrointestinal fistulas with Sandostatin. Digestion 1993;54(Suppl 1):38–40.

44. Kocak S, Burin C, Karayalcin K, et al. Treatment of external biliary, pancreatic and intestinal fistulas with a somatostatin analog. Dig Dis 1994;12(1):62–8.

45. Barnes SN, Kontny BG, Prinz RA. Somatostatin analog treatment of pancreatic fistulas. Int-J-Pancreatol 1993;14(2):181–8.

36 Management of the Persistent Perineal Wound

Lawrence J. Gottlieb and Sandeep S. Jejurikar

Since the introduction of abdominoperineal resection for rectal carcinoma by Ernest Miles in 1908 (1), many patients and their surgeons have been frustrated and challenged by persistent perineal wounds. Initially, primary closure of the perineal wound following proctectomy was advocated. However, due to an unacceptably high incidence of severe wound complications and mortality, this practice was replaced by open packing of the perineal wound and subsequent secondary healing. This open technique remained the surgical standard of care until the early 1960s, when primary closure of the perineal wound with closed suction drainage was reintroduced by Burge and Tompkin (2). Their success has made primary closure following proctectomy the procedure of choice over the past three decades. Successful primary closure of the perineum results in less postoperative perineal pain, shorter inpatient hospital stays, and shorter convalescence when compared to open packing. Unfortunately, this closure is not always successful and a significant number of these patients subsequently develop persistent perineal wounds.

The persistent perineal wound following rectal extirpation for inflammatory bowel disease remains a major cause of postoperative disability for many patients and a difficult surgical challenge. These patients typically suffer from chronic pelvic pain, persistent foul-smelling drainage requiring frequent dressing changes, daily hydrotherapy and Sitz baths, long-term antimicrobial therapy, and an inability to have an acceptable quality of life. In addition, these patients may be at increased risk for local infection and systemic sepsis.

The open perineal wound typically closes by descent of the small intestines and the peritoneal floor, posterior migration of the urogenital structures, and superior movement of the soft tissues of the buttock. Watts initially defined a wound that is unhealed at six months following proctocolectomy as a persistent perineal sinus (3). This is typically a wound of the dorsal perineum with the anterior wall consisting of the vagina, cervix, and uterus in the female, and the bladder, seminal vesicles, and prostate in the male. The wound is bordered laterally and posteriorly by the bony ischium, coccyx, and sacrum. A perineal sinus may be adjacent to the small intestines which settle in the inferior pelvis following proctocolectomy. A fibrotic, unyielding wall subsequently forms, which prevents collapse and closure of the wound.

Risk Factors

Magnitude of perineal resection, underlying condition and management of the perineal wound influence the rate of perineal wound healing. Perineal wound breakdown after primary closure following proctectomy is invariably related to a failure to obliterate dead space and the subsequent development of a fluid collection in this space. These wounds frequently become secondarily infected. The consequent inflammation leads to increased fibrosis and scar formation. The chronically infected, fibrosed cavity bound by the rigid bony pelvis leads to a persistent draining wound.

Intersphincteric, perimuscular excision vs. wide excision of the rectum, has resulted in a decreased frequency of persistent perineal wounds (4). With intersphincteric proctectomy, the rectum and anal canal are separated from the pelvic musculature along the embryonic plane of fusion so that accurate and safe rectal mobilization is accomplished without damage to the pelvic floor. The remaining levator muscle mass and perirectal adipose tissue may be approximated in several layers. Better obliteration of dead space in the perineum is most likely the reason for the lower incidence of perineal wound problems using this operative approach.

The persistent perineal wound has proven to be more common in patients with inflammatory bowel disease than in patients with malignancy, polyposis coli, or other diagnoses.

Broader et al. reported that chronic treatment with corticosteroids after proctocolectomy delayed wound healing (5). Watts et al. also demonstrated a strong correlation with the use of preoperative steroids in inflammatory bowel disease and the development of a persistent perineal wound (3). However, other investigators have found no such correlation (6,7).

Persistent wounds are more likely to occur in patients with Crohn's disease than in those with ulcerative colitis. Primary healing of the perineal wound within six months has been reported in 44% to 82% of patients with ulcerative colitis and 21% to 85% in patients with Crohn's disease (Table 36.1). This may be due to the propensity for anorectal transmural involvement, fistulae formation, the presence of chronic perineal sinuses, abscess formation, and the need for a wider perineal resection in Crohn's disease.

Oshitani et al. recently demonstrated that patients with Crohn's disease who developed perineal fistulae had a significantly lower activity of blood coagulation Factor XIIIa (8). This factor also functions in wound healing as a glue to connect collagen, fibronectin, and fibrin to form a stable fibrin network during the blood coagulation that follows

tissue destruction. It may be that a relative deficiency of this factor may result in perineal healing problems.

Patients that have had open packed wounds instead of primarily closed wounds demonstrate a significant delay in perineal wound healing. Jalen et al. demonstrated that only 40% of patients that underwent primary closure of the perineum following proctocolectomy for ulcerative colitis were unhealed at 6 months whereas 63% of patients that underwent open packing of the perineal wound were unhealed during the same interval (9). Other studies have reported similar results (3,5).

Treatment Options

Nonoperative therapy may be appropriate in selected patients. Dressing changes with topical antimicrobials will frequently treat the troublesome symptomatology of perineal wounds. This treatment regimen usually takes from 6 to 18 months until healing is achieved. Unfortunately, many of these patients continue to have chronic sinus tracts and require surgery for closure anyway. Although some patients would prefer daily local wound care for more than one year rather than surgery, one can not predict with confidence how long it will take for local therapy to completely affect healing. Nonsurgical treatment is further complicated in patients who, in addition to their persistent perineal wounds, suffer from multiple abscesses and sinus tracts of the buttock and perineal skin. This skin condition is not unlike that seen in hidradenitis suppurativa.

Surgical options previously advocated for the persistent perineal wound included debridement and curettage, excision and primary closure, and serial debridement with skin grafting. Corman et al. in the late 1970s advocated performing curettage at regular six-month intervals until healing was achieved (7). Unfortunately, this therapy was usually prolonged for years.

Excision and closure of the persistent perineal sinus was advanced by Ferrari and DenBesten in 1980 (10). Using this technique, they were able to achieve healing within two weeks in a series of seven patients. Unfortunately, many reports by other authors have demonstrated this technique to be uniformly unsuccessful (2,11).

Serial debridement with skin grafting in conjunction with the systemic administration of adrenocorticotropic hormone has been reported by Anderson and Turnbull to decrease the morbidity of the persistent perineal wound (12). However, only seven of 48 patients experienced complete healing.

Table 36.1. Healing of the perineal wound following proctocolectomy for inflammatory bowel disease.

Author	% healed within 6 months	
	Ulcerative colitis	Crohn's disease
Hughes 1965	81.7	
Watts et al. 1966	75.3	
Jalen et al. 1969	45.3	
Roy et al. 1970	81.6	76.3
de Dombal et al. 1971		57.4
Ritchie 1971	54.5	21.1
Broader et al. 1974	80.5	84.6
Irvin and Goligher 1975	69.7	69.7
Corman et al. 1978	44.4	27.9
Lubbers 1981	73.9	60.0

McLeod et al. reported the same technique in nine patients, but almost half of them required multiple procedures (13).

Marsupialization of the perineal sinus with coccygectomy was shown to be effective by Silen and Glotzer, but the healing period was exceptionally prolonged (14). In some patients this process took up to two years.

All of the aforementioned surgical therapies usually required multiple operations, had a protracted healing period, and ultimately had a high failure rate.

Principles of Wound Management

Reliable wound closure requires adherence to basic principles of wound management, which include optimizing both systemic and local factors. Prior to surgical intervention, adverse systemic factors should be addressed. Cardiac, pulmonary, renal, hepatic, and hematopoietic function should be maximized. Patients should be metabolically stable and nutritionally replete. Tobacco use should be eliminated. Patients on systemic corticosteroids should be supplemented with vitamin A.

Once systemic factors are optimized, the perineal wound may then be surgically addressed. Principles of wound management must include obtaining and maintaining bacteriologic balance in the wound, adequate debridement, and obliteration of dead space with well-vascularized tissue.

Bacteriologic control of the wound is essential for successful wound healing to occur. Bacterial levels in the wound may be assessed by obtaining quantitative tissue culture. Wound infection is defined as greater than 10^5 organisms per gram of tissue. Whether or not a particular organism will penetrate tissue depends upon the balance between host defenses and the biologic behavior of any particular microorganism. Bacteriologic balance is defined as less than or equal to 10^5 organisms per gram of tissue on quantitative tissue culture. Systemic antibiotics do not achieve adequate tissue levels in this clinical situation. Infected perineal wounds are best treated with topical antimicrobial agents that penetrate into granulating and fibrosed wounds such as silver sulfadiazine (Silvadene) or mafenide acetate (Sulfamylon).

Adequate debridement of these wounds includes surgical removal of all devitalized and infected tissue. Ideally, all scar tissue should also be removed. Unfortunately, this is sometimes limited by the involvement of unresectable adjacent structures.

Since the fibrotic and bony constraints of the perineal wound preclude soft tissue collapse and adherence, the dead space must be filled with imported, well-vascularized, pliable soft tissue. The advent of muscle, musculocutaneous, and fasciocutaneous flaps has revolutionized the management of the persistent perineal wound.

Wound debridement with immediate or delayed muscle flap closure has been used successfully in other chronically infected wounds including osteomyelitis of the lower extremities, pressure sores of the trunk, and postoperative sternal infections. Pliable, well-vascularized flaps not only serve to eliminate the dead space that exists in the chronic wound, but also provide improved blood supply to the wound, thereby increasing oxygen tension and improving leukocyte delivery and function (15). As with other wound problems the key to success is adequate debridement and obliteration of dead space. Placing a well-vascularized flap in an inadequately debrided wound is doomed to fail.

Flap Options

A variety of flaps may be employed to provide stable and long-lasting wound coverage following perineal debridement. These flaps may be utilized to treat persistent perineal wounds at any time in their course, as long as the aforementioned tenets of wound management are followed. It is possible to achieve reliable one-stage closure in these patients with these principles and techniques. Furthermore, cooperation between the general surgeon and the reconstructive surgeon may make flap closure at the time of proctocolectomy possible for carefully selected high risk patients.

Gracilis Muscle Flap

Bartholdson and Hulten initially described the gracilis muscle flap for perineal reconstruction in 1975 (16). This long, strap-like fusiform muscle lies along the medial side of the thigh and knee and serves to adduct the thigh, flex the leg, and medially rotate the leg. It attaches proximally at the body and inferior ramus of the pubis and distally to the superior part of the medial surface of the tibia. A line from the pubic tubercle to the insertion of the semitendinosus tendon marks the superior edge of the gracilis. The dominant vascular pedicle of the gracilis muscle flap is the medial femoral circumflex artery and vein, which are branches off the profunda femoris artery and vein. The pedicle usually arises between the adductor longus and adductor brevis muscles. (Fig. 36.1).

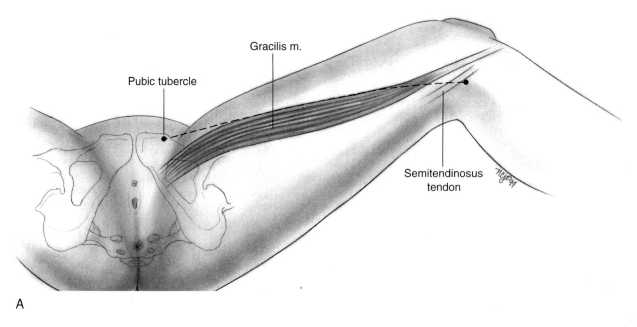

A

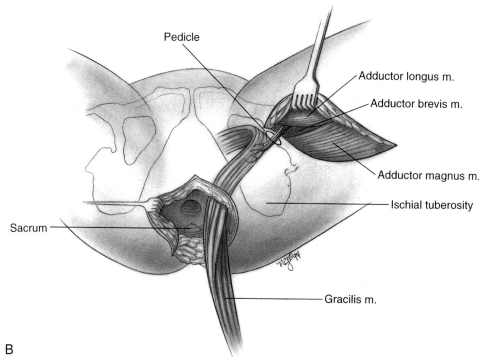

B

Fig. 36.1.   Use of the Gracilis muscle flap for closure of a persistent perineal sinus. (From Ryan, JA, Am J Surg 1984;64–70.)

The gracilis flap may be transferred as muscle only or as a myocutaneous unit. The muscle is typically exposed through a longitudinal thigh incision and is divided near the knee. The inclusion of a skin island tends to limit the degree to which the muscle can be transposed into the perineal wound. Furthermore, the cutaneous vascular supply is frequently precarious and unreliable. In general, males are preferred gracilis donors due to the greater muscle bulk present. Bilateral gracilis muscles may be used for larger defects.

Some authors consider the gracilis muscle the flap of choice for many chronic perineal wounds. Ryan accumulated a series of 15 patients that underwent gracilis flap reconstruction following chronic perineal wound problems and reported that 93% of patients benefited from this method of reconstruction (17).

The principle drawback to the gracilis muscle flap is that it frequently may not provide sufficient bulk to fill the dead space in large, complex perineal wounds. In addition, the proximal two thirds of the gracilis muscle, which represents the main bulk of the flap, may not reach the deepest point of the perineal wound due to its low axis of rotation. Finally, the vascularity of the distal third of the flap may be unreliable. The inability of this flap to adequately obliterate the dead space of deep, complex perineal wounds has led many reconstructive surgeons to be cautious in utilizing this flap.

Gluteal Thigh Flap

This deepithelialized fasciocutaneous flap, based on the descending branch of the inferior gluteal artery, includes the skin and subcutaneous tissue of the proximal posterior thigh. In patients with a poorly developed descending branch of the inferior gluteal artery, the inferior portion of the gluteus maximus muscle should be incorporated in the pedicle. The posterior cutaneous nerve of the thigh is intimately associated with the vascular pedicle (Fig. 36.2). This sensory nerve provides the opportunity of transferring a sensate flap.

The point of rotation of the flap is five centimeters above the ischial tuberosity, which overlies the emergence of the inferior gluteal artery from underneath the piriformis muscle. The central axis of the flap is midway between the greater trochanter and the ischial tuberosity and is perpendicular to the gluteal crease. The flap is centered over the thigh as the knee is approached.

The donor site can usually be closed primarily. In general, the donor sites of obese females are closed more easily than those of muscular males. To facilitate direct donor site closure, the flap should be designed to be less than 12 cm in width. The flap may be extended to within 8 cm of the popliteal fossa, and in theory the entire posterior thigh skin can be elevated and sustained on the vascular pedicle.

The gluteal thigh flap has excellent soft tissue bulk, and usually no functional deficit is noted postoperatively. In 1980, Hurwitz et al. demonstrated the reliability, versatility, and low morbidity of the gluteal thigh flap in a series of 19 patients with 21 buttock and perineal wounds closed in a single stage (18).

This flap is considered by many to be the gold standard for the chronic, deep midline perineal defect. Others feel that deepithelialized fasciocutaneous flaps have a limited ability to contour to the walls of complex defects thereby decreasing their efficacy in totally obliterating dead space.

The skin paddle of the gluteal thigh flap is an excellent option when extra skin is needed for closure of perineal wounds. In addition, the fascia of the gluteal thigh flap may be used to repair perineal floor defects (Fig. 36.3).

Gluteus Maximus Muscle and Musculocutaneous Flap

The gluteus maximus muscle is one of the largest muscles in the body. It attaches proximally at the iliac crest, dorsal surface of the sacrum and coccyx, and the sacrotuberous ligament. Most of its fibers insert in the iliotibial tract which inserts into the lateral condyle of the tibia. The principle actions of the gluteus maximus muscle are to extend the thigh and assist in its lateral rotation, steady the thigh, and assist in raising the trunk from the flexed position. The gluteus maximus muscle has a dual blood supply from the superior and inferior gluteal vessels. Either the inferior or superior portions of the gluteus maximus muscle may be utilized without functional compromise, even in the ambulatory patient.

In 1978, Shaw and Futrell suggested use of the inferior one third of the gluteus maximus muscle for closure after marsupialization of the perineal sinus tract (19). Sproles and Gough reported the use of the gluteus maximus turnover flap for closure of the persistent perineal wound in 1980 (20). They utilized a semicircular incision from the proximal end of the perineal wound, over the buttock, and down to the greater trochanter. A large flap of skin and subcutaneous fat is raised to expose the gluteus maximus muscle. The lower third of the muscle is detached distally along the iliotibial tract and mobilized, taking care to preserve its blood supply from the inferior gluteal vascular pedicle. The mobilized muscle is then folded into the perineal wound and held in place without tension using suture. The subcutaneous fat is then closed over the perineal wound after closed suction drains are applied and the buttock flap is rotated medially to achieve primary closure of the skin. They were able to achieve primary healing at three weeks in all patients.

Baird et al. reported a series of 16 patients in which the inferior gluteal myocutaneous flap was utilized to close large perineal wounds (21). A split-muscle technique is employed. The deep portion of the gluteus maximus is preserved in the donor site to provide protection to underlying structures

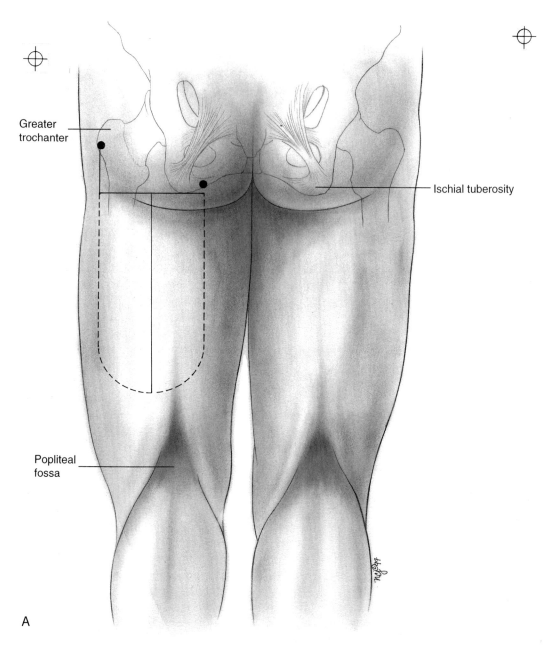

A

Fig. 36.2A.   Gluteal thigh flap—The greater trochanter and ischial tuberosity are identified. A vertical line between these two points marks the central axis of the flap. The distal extent of the flap can be within 8 cm of the popliteal fossa. (From Hurwitz DJ, Swartz WM, and Mathes SJ. Plas Reconstr Surg 1982;68:521–30.)

while the superficial muscle provides adequate vascular supply to the overlying skin paddle. This myocutaneous flap can then be transposed into the perineal defect. In this series, all but one patient achieved complete healing of the perineal wound.

The authors' preference is to utilize the inferior gluteus maximus muscle. The muscle is mobilized through the midline perineal wound. To facilitate exposure, dissection, and elevation of the lateral, distal aspect of the inferior gluteus maximus muscle from the iliotibial tract, a counter-incision is made in the upper lateral posterior thigh. By detaching the origin and insertion of the inferior portion of the gluteus maximus muscle, leaving it attached only by its vascular pedicle, the flap will be able to fill the dead space of very large and deep perineal or pelvic wounds (Fig. 36.4).

With these techniques, the attachment of the superior portion of the gluteus maximus muscle to the iliotibial tract is preserved and hip stability is maintained. Patients have no functional deficits

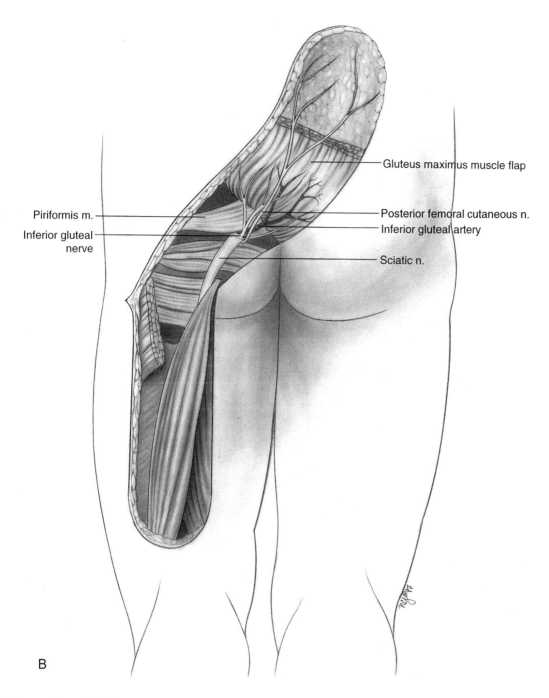

Piriformis m.

Inferior gluteal nerve

Gluteus maximus muscle flap

Posterior femoral cutaneous n.

Inferior gluteal artery

Sciatic n.

B

Fig. 36.2B. Gluteal thigh flap—The vascular pedicle and posterior cutaneous nerve are identified on the under surface of flap. Although, as shown, the original description of this flap includes elevation of the distal portion of the inferior gluteal muscle, this flap may be elevated as an island based only on the descending branch of the inferior gluteal artery and vein.

and a return to normal unrestricted physical activity can be expected.

Gluteus Maximus V-Y Advancement Flaps

Shallow perineal defects may be closed utilizing single or bilateral gluteus maximus V-Y advancement flaps (Fig. 36.5A,B). The origins of the gluteal muscles are detached from their attachment to the sacrum, advanced medially and secured to each other in the midline. V incisions are made in the posterior/lateral buttock skin down to the gluteal muscle. The musculocutaneous unit is advanced

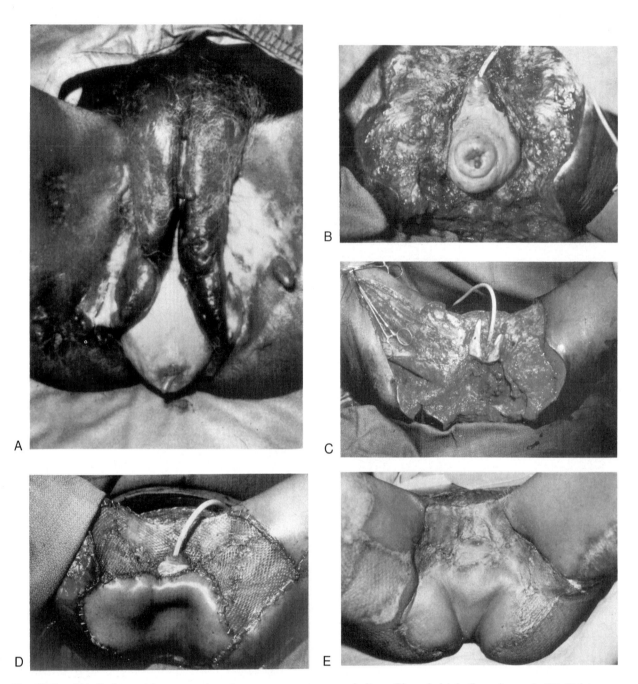

Fig. 36.3.   (A) Patient with severe chronic, recurrent perineal Crohn's disease. Status post proctectomy with perineal hernia and prolapsed uterus. (B) Wound following total vulvectomy and debridement of perineal and buttock skin. (C) Wound following vaginal hysterectomy. Tenuous closure of pelvic floor with remnants of pubo-coccygeal sling. Gluteal thigh flap elevated. (D) Pelvic floor reconstructed with gluteal thigh fascial-cutaneous flap. Fascia of the flap secured circumferentially to remnants of pelvic supporting structures. (E) 10-months follow-up demonstrating good support of pelvic floor.

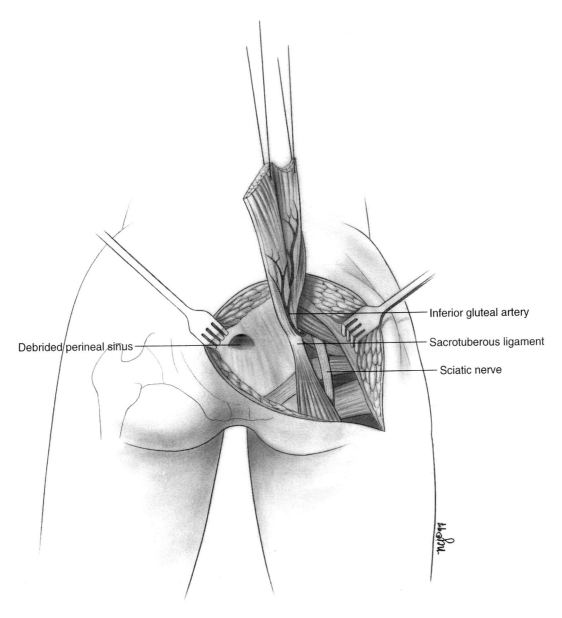

Fig. 36.4. The gluteus maximus musculocutaneous flap. (From Baird WL, Hester TR, Nahai F et al. Arch Surg 1990;125:1486–9.)

medially and a midline skin closure is performed without tension. The donor site is closed as a Y. In deeper wounds with a skin replacement requirement, the V-Y advancement flap may used in combination with a contralateral flap to fill dead space (Fig. 36.5C).

Gluteal-Posterior Thigh Chimera Flap

If additional skin is required to accomplish perineal wound closure without tension, the gluteal thigh flap may be elevated in combination with a gluteal muscle flap based on the same pedicle (Fig. 36.6). The pedicle of the gluteal thigh flap, the descending branch of the inferior gluteal artery, can be separated from beneath the gluteal muscle (Fig. 36.7). This branch may be dissected to its take-off from the inferior gluteal artery as it emerges from underneath the piriformis muscle. This single pedicle chimera flap allows independent placement of the muscle in the cavity and the skin paddle on the surface.

A combination of the aforementioned techniques can be employed to close difficult perineal wounds in a creative and individualized manner.

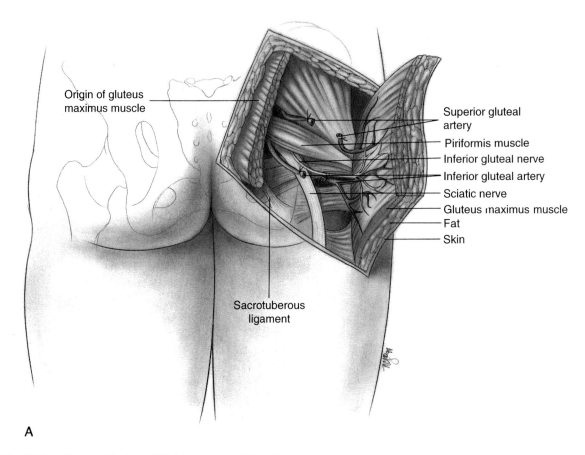

Origin of gluteus
maximus muscle

Superior gluteal
artery
Piriformis muscle
Inferior gluteal nerve
Inferior gluteal artery
Sciatic nerve
Gluteus maximus muscle
Fat
Skin

Sacrotuberous
ligament

A

Fig. 36.5.   Gluteus Maximus V-Y Advancement Flap (A) Diagram of anatomy (Reprinted with permission from Ramirez, OM, Orlando JC, and Hurwitz DJ. Plas Reconst Surg 1984;74:68.) (B) Schematic of bilateral gluteus maximus V-Y advancement myocutaneous flaps. (C) V-Y advancement flap to minimize midline skin closure tension while a contralateral flap was used to fill pelvic dead space.

Rectus Abdominis Muscle Flap

The rectus abdominis muscle is a wonderful option with much versatility for treating pelvic and perineal problems. Based on the inferior epigastric artery and vein it may be passed into the pelvis to close the pelvic floor, fill dead space or provide a well vascularized barrier for gastrointestinal/genitourinary (GI/GU) fistulae. This muscle flap is best employed prophylactically in high risk patients at the time of proctectomy, when dead space and potential perineal wound problems are anticipated. As a delayed or secondary procedure, the advantages of this flap must be weighed against the potential difficulties and morbidity of having to re-enter the lower abdomen and mobilize the bowel to provide space to pass this flap into the pelvis. In addition, adjustments may need to be made regarding placement of the anterior abdominal wall stoma. Occasionally, in very large pelvic wounds, the bulk of a single rectus abdominis muscle is inadequate to totally obliterate the dead space.

Omentum

The use of the omentum in perineal reconstruction is limited for a variety of reasons. Similar to the rectus flap, it is best used prophylactically when dead space and potential perineal wound problems are anticipated. In delayed reconstructions, harvesting of the omentum requires repeat laparotomy. In addition, it frequently is of poor quality following a previous laparotomy, was previously resected, or was transposed to the inferior pelvis during proctocolectomy.

Conclusion

The persistent perineal wound results in a significant amount of morbidity and anxiety in the af-

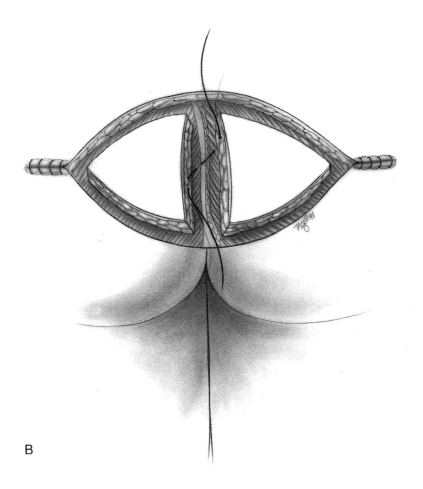

B

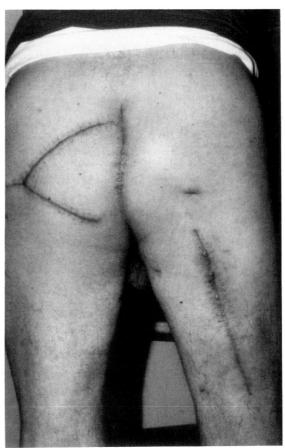

C

Fig. 36.5. (*Continued*)

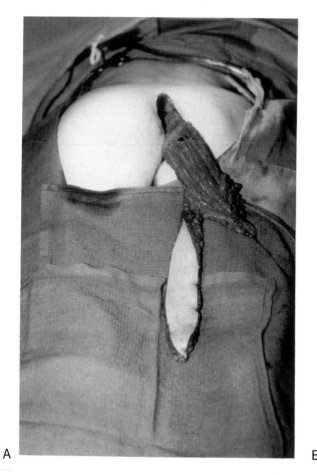

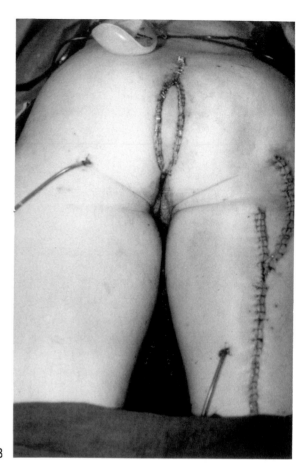

Fig. 36.6.   (A) Gluteal-posterior thigh chimera flap elevated in a 45-year-old female with 10 year history of a painful persistent perineal wound following proctocolectomy. The patient had previously undergone numerous surgical procedures in the past. (B) Following extensive debridement of the complex deep presacral sinus tract with coccygectomy, the left inferior gluteal muscle was transposed to the pelvis obliterating dead space and the skin, based on the descending branch of the inferior gluteal vascular bundle was used to close the skin without tension. At one-year follow-up patient is pain free with a healed wound.

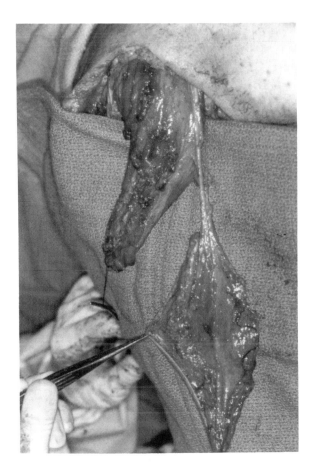

Fig. 36.7. Descending branch of inferior gluteal vascular bundle dissected off of gluteal muscle to facilitate independent use of muscle and skin of left inferior gluteal-posterior thigh chimera flap.

flicted patient following proctocolectomy for inflammatory bowel disease. Fortunately, treatment has progressed in the last few decades from repeated unreliable procedures to successful one-stage closure utilizing modern principles of wound management.

References

1. Miles WE. A method of performing abdominoperineal excision for carcinoma of the rectum and of the terminal portion of the pelvic colon. Lancet 1908;2:1812–3.

2. Saha SK, Robinson AF. A study of wound healing after abdominoperineal resection. Br J Surg 1976;63:555.

3. Watts JM, DeDombal FT, Goligher JC. Long term complications and prognosis following major surgery for ulcerative colitis. Br J Surg 1966;53:1014.

4. Zeitels JR, Fiddian-Green RG, Dent TL. Intersphincteric proctectomy. Surgery 1984;96:617–23.

5. Broader JH, Masselink BEA, Oates GD, et al. Management of the pelvic space after proctectomy. Br J Surg 1974;61:94–7.

6. Manjoney DL, Koplewitz MJ, Abrams JS. Factors influencing perineal wound healing after proctectomy. Am J Surg 1983;145:183–9.

7. Corman ML, Veidenheimer MC, Coller JA, et al. Perineal wound healing after proctectomy for inflammatory bowel disease. Dis Colon Rectum 1978;21:155–9.

8. Oshitani N, Kitano A, Hara J, et al. Deficiency of blood coagulation factor XIII in Crohn's disease. Am J Gastroenterology 1995;90:1116–8.

9. Jalen AN, Smith CV, Ruckley CW, et al. Perineal wound healing in ulcerative colitis. Br J Surg 1969;56:749.

10. Ferrari BT, DenBesten L. The prevention and treatment of the persistent perineal sinus. World J Surg 1980;4:167–72.

11. Irvin TT, Goligher JC. A controlled clinical trial of three different methods of perineal wound management following excision of the rectum. Br J Surg 1975;62:287.

12. Anderson R, Turnbull RB. Grafting the unhealed perineal wound after coloproctectomy for Crohn disease. Arch Surg 1976;111:335–8.

13. McLeod RS, Palmer JA, Cohen Z. Management of chronic perineal sinuses by wide excision and split-thickness skin grafting. Can J Surg 1985;28:315–7.

14. Silen W, Glotzer DJ. The prevention and treatment of the persistent perineal sinus. Surgery 1974;75:535–42.

15. Feng LJ, Price D, Mathes SJ. Relationship of blood flow and leukocyte mobilization in infection. Surg Forum 1983;33:603.

16. Bartholdson L, Hulten L. Repair of persistent perineal sinuses by means of a pedicle flap of musculus gracilis. Scand J Plast Reconstr Surg 1975;9:74–6.

17. Ryan JA. Gracilis muscle flap for the persistent perineal sinus of inflammatory bowel disease. Am J Surg 1984;148:64–70.

18. Hurwitz DJ, Swartz WM, Mathes SJ. The gluteal thigh flap: a reliable, sensate flap for the closure of buttock and perineal wounds. Plas Reconstr Surg 1981;68:521–30.

19. Shaw A, Futrell JW. Cure of chronic perineal sinus with gluteus maximus flap. Surg Gynecol Obstet 1978;147:417–20.

20. Sproles GJ, Gough IR. The gluteus maximus muscle in the management of persistent perineal sinus. Aust NZ J Surg 1980;50:197–9.

21. Baird WL, Hester TR, Nahai F, et al. Management of perineal wounds following abdominoperineal resection with inferior gluteal flaps. Arch Surg 1990;125:1486–9.

37 Ileostomy

Tracy L. Hull

The first ileostomies were described in the late 1800s. They initially were used to relieve an obstruction from cancer (1,2). As the use of ileostomies evolved, the ileum was simply brought through a defect made in the abdominal wall. Without any type of maturation, such stomas at approximately one week postoperatively developed a type of pseudo-obstruction at the level of the stoma with a high loss of watery fluid, abdominal cramping, and stoma swelling. "Ileostomy dysfunction" (3) was the term coined to describe this phenomena and the etiology was from serositis. In 1941, Dragstedt applied a skin graft to the exposed serosa to prevent this problem (4). In the 1950s, Crile and Turnbull further refined the maturation process by describing an eversion technique where the seromuscular coat was removed from the distal ileum and the mucosa was everted as a sliding graft (5). The current practice of everting the bowel and suturing it to the dermis was described by Brooke in 1952 (6). Even though this procedure is over 40 years old it is still the most common method employed to construct an ileostomy. Four or five centimeters of terminal ileum are exteriorized beyond the skin such that with eversion and suturing of the bowel edge to the dermis a two or three centimeter ileostomy protrudes.

Besides the end ileostomy described by Brooke, other types of ileostomies include a loop ileostomy and a loop end ileostomy. The loop ileostomy is usually constructed proximal to a complex perianal reconstruction, to divert the fecal stream for patients with Crohn's perianal sepsis, and in the first stage of the pelvic pouch procedure. A loop of terminal ileum is identified and sutures are placed to delineate the proximal and distal ends. The bowel is brought out through an abdominal wall opening and a rod placed beneath the bowel. A transverse opening is made over the efferent end and the proximal bowel is everted. The dominant end is the afferent end which protrudes. The nonfunctioning end is the recessive efferent end.

The loop end ileostomy is used if the distal end of ileum becomes ischemic with resection of the mesentery when preparing the bowel for eversion or there is excessive tension when bringing the bowel to the abdominal surface. These circumstances usually occur in obese patients or patients with a thick, short, or fatty mesentery. To construct a loop end ileostomy, a loop of ileum is identified which will reach the surface of the skin with sufficient length so that the stapled efferent limb will be in the abdominal cavity. Orientation sutures are placed and the loop of bowel is brought onto the skin's surface and a rod placed beneath it. The stoma is matured as with the loop ileostomy described above.

Classic "ileostomy dysfunction" is now rare with eversion techniques which prevent serositis. Other complications can occur with some reporting 20% to 30% of patients experiencing a stoma related problem (1). Another study using life table analysis predicts that at 20 years after ileostomy construction 76% of patients with ulcerative colitis will have had a stoma related complication and of these 28% will require revisional surgery. When considering Crohn's disease, 59% will have a stoma related complication and 16% will require stoma revision (7). These stoma related complications can be the result of technical error at the time of stoma construction; recurrent disease; or the result of poor stoma care which can range from inadequate patient education to neglect by the patient.

Table 37.1. Guidelines for stoma siting.*

1) Visibility to patient.
2) Siting in the supine sitting and standing positions.
3) Optimal site at the mound of the infraumbilical fat fold, away from scars, creases, bony prominences, and damaged skin.
4) Stoma site within boundary of rectus muscle.
5) Allow for possible future weight gain.

*Data from Fazio and Tjandra (8).

Table 37.2. Early complications.

Ischemia
Bleeding
Mucocutaneous separation
Parastomal suppuration
Fistula

Complications can be divided into early and late complication but prevention is really the first line of treatment. Prevention begins with the anticipation of the need to construct a stoma and allows a site to be chosen preoperatively. The site ideally is over the mound of the infraumbilical fat fold and centered over the rectus muscle. In obese patients the site may need to be supraumbilical if the abdominal contour and panniculus changes when the patient changes positions. The patient should be able to clearly see the site and it should be away from scars, creases, bony prominence, and damaged skin. Fazio believes when considering positioning of a stoma, the least important consideration is the transrectus location, whereas the most important concern should be patient visibility of the stoma site (8). Another consideration is that many patients will gain weight after surgery to treat inflammatory bowel disease. Therefore, when constructing the stoma allowance should be made for future weight gain (8). (Table 37.1)

Early Complications

Early complications are listed in Table 37.2. Each will be discussed separately.

Ischemia: Insufficient blood supply is the obvious underlying cause of ischemia. It can range from superficial slough to general necrosis. The incidence of ischemia is unknown probably because many episodes of minor slough of mucosa do not require more than expectant management. Necrosis was reported to be 1% in one study (7). It is important to examine any stoma for ischemic changes. At the time of construction if doubt exists, using a needle to prick the mucosa looking for prompt bleeding is reassuring. In the postoperative period, the secretions should be cleaned off the mucosa to assess the color. Again if doubt exists using a needle to prick the mucosa can help determine blood flow. If there is true necrosis, it is important to delineate the depth. If it is superficial or above the fascia expectant management may be enough keeping in mind this may result in a strict-

ured stoma or a flush ileostomy. Any stoma that is necrotic at or below the fascia needs prompt revision to prevent perforation that can lead to peritonitis. Sometimes it is difficult to determine how deep below the skin surface the necrosis extends. In these circumstances, placing two cotton swabs on opposite sides of the mucosa and prying the mucosa back will help. Sometimes a small empty test tube (the type used on the hospital floor to collect a patient's blood sample) can gently be inserted into the stoma orifice and a light shined down the lumen to look at the color of the mucosa beneath the skin surface.

During the construction of an end stoma if ischemia is a concern, this usually can be circumvented by constructing a loop stoma. This is especially true if trimming the mesentery from the distal bowel end seems to exacerbate the problem. This type of ischemic effect is further compounded by bringing the stoma through a narrow fascial opening and further compressing the bowel and mesentery against the abdominal wall aperture. Therefore, the blood supply also needs to be assessed after the bowel is brought through the abdominal wall. On rare instances even a loop stoma will become dusky when attempting to place a rod beneath the bowel. This usually occurs in the morbidly obese patient with a large panniculus and a thick fatty mesentery. In this type of patient placing the stoma in the upper quadrant or the upper midline wound will help decrease the problem. If it does not alleviate the ischemia, the stoma should be brought out through the upper aspect of the midline incision and a long trocar is used to stabilize the stoma. The long trocar is placed through the skin lateral to the incision and through the deeper mesentery of the loop stoma to eliminate the tension on the surface blood vessels. The other end is brought out through the other side of the incision. (The patient looks like there is an arrow through the upper abdomen.) The loop stoma can be matured in the usual fashion and the rod is removed according to the normal postoperative timetable.

Bleeding is usually from the cut edge of the bowel. It usually stops spontaneously or with gentle compression. At times suture ligature is needed. If the bleeding is from the subcutaneous fat, gentle packing after removing a mucocutaneous suture may control the problem. Rarely return to the operating room is needed to find and control the bleeding point.

Mucocutaneous separation involves separation of the mucosa from the skin. It is the result of excessive tension on the sutures or infection. It usually involves a limited dimension of the circumference of the stoma and can be managed in conjunction with the enterostomal therapy nurse. The area is cleaned and if there is a large enough defect, it is filled with paste material such as stomahesive or karaya gum powder. The stomaplate is placed over the defect. Some areas of separation are small but have a large cavity beneath the surface which can be filled with purulent material when discovered. These usually respond to initial flushing with saline then drainage with a small mushroom tipped catheter. The catheter is included in the pouching apparatus. If the separation is large, serositis may develop or after healed there may be a stricture.

Parastomal suppuration and fistula: Approximately 1% to 7% of patients with an ileostomy will have parastomal suppuration and/or a fistula (7,8). Considering each process separately, an early abscess around the stoma may be from a fistula or an infected hematoma. If possible the abscess should be drained with an incision placed outside the stomaplate. Usually a mushroom tipped catheter can be placed in the cavity for sufficient drainage. If there is a small cavity and mucocutaneous separation, placing the mushroom tipped catheter in the mucocutaneous defect and including it in the pouching mechanism is sufficient. Treatment of an infected parastomal hematoma should bring prevention to mind. Meticulous hemostasis is important. Irrigation of the subcutaneous fat after the bowel has been brought through but before eversion may help. When constructing the stoma, preservation of the subcutaneous fat eliminates dead space formation where fluid can collect.

An early fistula on the other hand is usually from a technical error. It can result from a missed serosal tear/enterotomy or a suture which has pulled out of the bowel. (A remote fistula is usually secondary to recurrent Crohn's disease or rarely traumatic instrumentation of the stoma.) If the fistula can be easily pouched with the stoma no further treatment may be needed. Usually segmental resection is required. If the need for a resection is determined before the seventh postoperative day, the operation can usually be done as a local procedure mobilizing around the stoma site only. If the need for revision is determined after the seventh postoperative day, it is usually best to wait at least 6 to 8 weeks prior to revision to allow for the normal postoperative inflammation around the stoma to subside before an attempt at revision is carried out.

Late Complications

Late complications are listed in Table 37.3.

Bleeding is usually the result of irritation at the edge of the stoma. This may be from a mucosal laceration from the appliance or from trauma from a poorly fitting appliance. This can usually be treated by an adjustment in the appliance. At times hypertrophied tissue on the stoma can bleed from minor trauma. This tissue can usually be sharply excised with the scissors and the base treated with silver nitrate to eliminate bleeding.

It may be difficult to detect when bleeding is from within the stoma. Ileoscopy is helpful to detect recurrent Crohn's disease which can lead to bleeding. If more proximal Crohn's disease is suspected, then a small bowel series is needed. It is important to remember that peptic ulcer disease may also present with stomal bleeding so a thorough work-up for any source of upper gastrointestinal bleeding may be needed. This may include upper gastrointestinal endoscopy.

A rare form of stomal bleeding occurs in patients with portal hypertension. This may be seen in alcohol abusers, ulcerative colitic patients with primary sclerosing cholangitis and cirrhosis, or patients with inherent liver disease which leads to cirrhosis. These conditions can lead to parastomal varices which can repeatedly bleed. Nonoperative management, such as sclerotherapy injection of varices, has variable results (9). Portasystemic disconnection is another temporizing measure. In this approach the mucosa is disconnected from the skin and the subcutaneous veins oversewn. The dissection may need to be continued down to the

Table 37.3.   Late complications.

Bleeding
Stricture
Small bowel obstruction/bolus obstruction
Parastomal abscess/ulcer
High ileostomy output
Ileostomy prolapse/parastomal hernia
Retraction
Skin irritation
Cancer

fascia until the stoma is completely mobilized. Then the stoma is again matured as before (10). Liver transplantation or shunting is a more permanent approach to control of this type of bleeding. For patients who can not be treated by other measures, percutaneous transhepatic embolization of varices has been successful (11).

Stricture of the ileostomy results from ischemia, parastomal suppuration, recurrent Crohn's disease, or rarely a tight opening of the fascia or skin. It is reported in 5% to 24% of patients with an ileostomy (8). When obstructive symptoms cannot be managed with a low residue diet and gentle dilatation, stomal revision is necessary. Attempts at local revision by mobilizing the stoma circumferentially from the skin to the fascia, resecting the stricture, and rematuration may be successful. If unsuccessful, a formal laparotomy may be needed.

Small bowel obstruction/bolus obstruction: A mechanical small bowel obstruction may result from adhesions, recurrent Crohn's disease, or from a volvulus. It occurs in 10% to 21% of patients (7,8). It is felt that obliteration of the mesenteric defect by fixation of the ileal mesentery to the peritoneum during end ileostomy formation prevents the small bowel from volvulizing through the lateral space but in a study by Leong closure of the lateral space did not reduce the probability of developing an intestinal obstruction (7). This mesenteric fixation is not needed if a loop stoma is performed. As with any bowel obstruction treatment initially is with nasogastric decompression, intravenous fluids, and surgery if ischemia is suspected or the patient does not respond to conservative treatment. For patients suspected of having recurrent Crohn's disease treatment with steroids, may offer relief. At times if there is a question between recurrent Crohn's disease versus adhesions causing the obstruction, a nuclear medicine scan may demonstrate inflammation which would be seen with recurrent Crohn's disease and not with an adhesive obstruction (12).

A bolus obstruction from undigested food such as raw carrots or nuts can cause an intrinsic bowel obstruction. This usually causes an abrupt cessation of stoma output accompanied by cramping abdominal pain. Therefore a careful dietary history is important in assessing a patient with an ileostomy and small bowel obstruction. The obstruction usually occurs at a point of angulation or narrowing such as the fascial level. A digital exam is first done to assess the stoma and the fascial opening. Stomal irrigation is the first step of therapy. A 24 French foley is inserted in the stoma and irrigated with tap water (100 to 200 cc). If particulate material is re-

turned (especially if it resembles the suspected food culprit) the irrigation is continued until the return is clear and the blockage is eliminated. If the obstruction is suspected to be more proximal, a gastrograffin small bowel study may be both diagnostic and therapeutic (8).

Parastomal abscess/ulcer outside of the immediate postoperative period usually implies recurrent Crohn's disease. As expected it occurs more significantly in patients with an ileostomy for Crohn's disease than ulcerative colitis. Leong found a cumulative probability of 12% of patients developing this problem if followed for 20 years (7). Local trauma or sepsis can also lead to this problem. Management consists of debridement of the overlying or nonviable tissue. Adjustments in the pouching system in conjunction with the enterostomal therapy nurse is essential. If the defect is small, a patch of Telfa (Kendall Healthcare Products Co., Mansfield, MA) over the defect allows placement of a Stomahesive wafer (ConvaTec Inc., Princeton, NJ) (13). For larger defects (over 2 cm) the Perry model 51 system (Perry products, Minneapolis, MN) maintains a seal with a latex sleeve which is attached to the mucosa rather than the peristomal skin. The device is also stabilized with a double belt fixation and allows medicated pads to be placed on the skin without interfering with the seal of the appliance (8). Most ulcers will heal within three months. Even many from recurrent Crohn's disease will heal sufficiently to allow pouching of the stoma. If a fistula is noted, as long as it does not interfere with pouching, nothing further needs to be done after the skin has healed. For ulcers and fistula which prohibit adequate pouching of the stoma, a work-up for recurrent Crohn's disease is undertaken with endoscopy and contrast studies. Surgical revision usually entails moving the stoma to another location and resecting the recurrent disease.

Ulceration from peristomal pyoderma gangrenosum may occur in patients with inflammatory bowel disease. It occurs more commonly in women and can occur when the inflammatory bowel is in remission. These ulcers start as small pustules and rapidly enlarge with undermining of the skin and large irregular erythematous ulcers. The rapid development of these ulcers is considered a hallmark (14). Histologic findings are nonspecific and include lymphocytic vasculitis, neutrophilic abscess, or a polymorphous infiltrate (15). Treatment involves aggressive local care and initial local injection of intralesional steroids (triamcinolone acetonide solution 10 to 30 mg/ml) (14,16). If this fails high dose systemic steroids (prednisone 20 to

100 mg/day) is initiated. Up to one third of cases require multiple medications for treatment. In addition to the prednisone, these include minocycline HCl, dapsone, clofazimine, sulfasalazine, and cytotoxic agents (17,18). Recurrence of the problem after surgical revision is commonly seen.

Ulceration from a poorly fitting stoma appliance may be seen on the undersurface of the stoma and simply require an adjustment in the appliance size. This must be distinguished from apthus ulceration from recurrent Crohn's disease or hypertrophied polyps. A thorough history can also uncover an unsuspected source of trauma leading to skin ulceration (i.e., in patients who lift weights and inadvertently traumatize their peristomal skin).

High ileostomy output can be a major source of morbidity for patients with an ileostomy. Normal output ranges from 500 to 800 cc daily for an established stoma. High output is greater than 1000 cc daily (19). Loss of sodium and water from an ileostomy is high and about 120mM/liter is lost. Renal compensation prevents sodium depletion. High ileostomy output usually results from short bowel syndrome, stenosis of the stoma, gastroenteritis, recurrent Crohn's disease, partial small bowel obstruction, resolution of an ileus, or idiopathic etiology. The first line of treatment includes antidiarrheal medications and electrolyte replacement. Antidiarrheal medications include loperamide hydrochloride (imodium) or diphenoxylate hydrochloride with atropine sulfate (lomotil) up to eight pills daily. The next line of antidiarrheal medication would include codeine sulfate or phosphate 15 to 60 mg every four to eight hours (20). This can be given in addition to the loperamide hydrochloride and/or diphenoxylate hydrochloride with atropine sulfate. Tincture of opium can also be used in a dose of 0.3 to 1 mL four times daily. This small dose of opiate is effective for diarrhea but does not produce euphoria or dependence (20). The above medications may be needed longterm especially if it allows the patient to sustain their nutrition and hydration without intravenous supplementation. Some patients however must have supplementation with hyperalimentation or intravenous fluids on a long term basis.

Use of octreotide to decrease ileostomy output has been described but the long term value is not clear (21,22). We have used octreotide in doses of 50 micrograms one to four times daily subcutaneously for short term treatment (less than three months) of high ileostomy output. All patients had undergone proctocolectomy and formation of a pelvic pouch with pouch anal anastomosis and loop ileostomy. Because of the body habitus or a short mesentery the ileostomy was placed more proximal than the ideal location just above the ileal pouch. No adverse problems were encountered but liver function tests were monitored weekly during treatment.

Ileostomy prolapse and/or parastomal hernia is generally felt to result from a stoma aperture which is too large, obesity, or an aperture which is placed outside of the rectus muscle. However Leong found the incidence of parastomal herniation or prolapse was not reduced by siting the stoma through the rectus muscle versus the oblique muscle (7).

The incidence of prolapse ranges from 1% to 12% (8), but overall it appears to be less frequent than retraction (2). A prolapse can be fixed or sliding. A fixed prolapse need only be repaired if it is bothersome to the patient. Repair is usually accomplished locally by eversion of the stoma after taking down the mucocutaneous junction. The excessive ileum is resected and a new stoma constructed (2). With a sliding prolapse, large amounts of bowel can be involved and ischemia can result. It usually is seen after previous revisions and inadequate abdominal fixation may contribute to this problem (23). Since large amounts of bowel may be involved and recurrence may happen, simply resecting the prolapse is not always optimal. If the abdominal wall opening is too wide repair may be sufficient treatment. Fixation to the abdominal wall through a laparotomy may be needed to manage a sliding prolapse (23). Refixation with strips of polyglactin may also be used (2). Linear fixation with a knifeless GIA stapling device with three rows of staples applied the length of the stoma has also been described (23).

Parastomal herniation should be managed nonoperatively with an abdominal wall binder if it does not interfere with pouching and does not cause symptoms. The incidence of herniation is 1% to 11% (7,8). There are several repair options. The simplest involves making an incision locally and extending it as needed for adequate visualization. The hernia can be repaired primarily with nonabsorbable sutures or prosthetic mesh. Several methods of applying the mesh include bringing the bowel out through a defect created in the center of the mesh while the edges of the mesh are sutured to the fascial defect; bringing the bowel out next to the edge of the mesh while the remainder of the edge is sutured to the fascial defect; or creating two strips of mesh 3 cm wide and placing them on either side of the bowel suturing each strip to the fascial defect and then together around the bowel (24). Repair of the hernia either primarily or with mesh may need to be done through a laparotomy if local repair is not feasible. The other alternative method of repair is laparotomy and stoma relocation. Rubin found that fascial repair had a 76% recurrence vs. a 33% recurrence rate if stoma relocation was used. He concluded that stoma relocation should be used for first time hernia repairs. For recurrent parastomal hernias failure rates were 100% for direct fascial repair, 71% for stoma relocation, and 33% for repair with prosthetic material. Therefore, if a recurrent parastomal hernia occurred he recommended repair with a prosthetic material (25).

Retraction occurs in 5% to 19% of patients with an ileostomy (8). This complication makes pouching difficult because the effluent of an ileostomy is watery and if the ileostomy does not protrude leakage under the stomaplate with destruction of skin will occur. The retraction can be intermittent or fixed. Weight gain, poor stoma siting, parastomal hernia, recurrent Crohn's disease and inadequate initial stoma length all can predispose to retraction. Attempts at management of this problem include a convex stomaplate or convex inserts which help protrude the stoma. A belt may also be helpful. If the leakage and soilage which results in skin excoriation cannot be managed by skilled enterostomal nursing—revision is necessary. Local revision using a circumferential incision around the stoma and mobilizing it to allow for sufficient protrusion with maturation is the easiest type of revision. Intraabdominal tethering, associated Crohn's disease, or the need to repair an associated parastomal hernia may mandate a laparotomy and ileal exteriorization. Repair of the hernia can be accomplished by the methods described previously. To prevent recurrence of the retraction the use of polyglactin 910 mesh has been described (26). Three strips of mesh are sewn longitudinally to the serosal surface of the ileum. The bowel is then attached to the fascia by sutures placed through the bowel, mesh, and fascia. At the Cleveland Clinic to prevent recurrence, we prefer to use a two-directional myotomy incision made with the electrocautery and placed on the serosal surface of the ileum which is external to the abdominal wall (8).

Skin irritation usually results from leakage of ileostomy effluent under the stomaplate. Ileostomy effluent contains active pancreatic enzymes which can digest skin so even minor irritation should be treated promptly. Other sources of skin irritation include fungal and bacterial rashes, allergic reaction to pouching equipment, and heat excoriation from the pouch collection bag. Leong found this to

be the most common complication in ileostomy patients occurring in 34% of his studied (7). As previously stated hernia, stoma prolapse, and retraction can lead to skin irritation. Most skin problems can be managed with relevant stoma education and modification of stoma equipment. Assistance from enterostomal therapy nurses is invaluable when managing this problem. Skin which is constantly macerated will develop pseudoepitheliomatous hyperplasia or a painful thickening of the skin (8). This is usually treated by applying a proper appliance and if the skin is severely destroyed a Perry model 51 (as described previously) (8).

When constructing the stoma, a technical error which can cause difficulty pouching in the future involves the maturation process. When placing the suture to the abdominal skin, the surgeon should never take full thickness bites of the skin but rather a subcuticular bite (of the dermis). Full thickness bites can lead to implantation of the ileal mucosa on the surface of the skin. This mucosa then secretes mucous and makes sealing and fitting of the stomaplate difficult if not impossible. The only treatment for this problem is excision. If large defects are made with excision, a rotational flap may be necessary. Even with excision ileal mucosa may be buried deep and grow again to the surface to cause problems. Severe cases may require stoma relocation (8).

Cancer of an ileostomy is not common after a stoma constructed for inflammatory bowel disease. However adenocarcinoma in a stoma which has been in place for greater than 20 years has been reported in at least 14 patients. Patients develop an exophytic mass which makes pouching difficult. This leads them to seek medical attention. The first case was reported in 1969 and with the completion of this "biologic latency" period which began in the 1950s when the Brooke ileostomy was introduced (27), there may be a dramatic increase in this problems over the next ten years. Therefore, adenocarcinoma must be considered in any unusual stoma mass (28).

In conclusion, there have been many changes in the construction of an ileostomy since the late 1800s. However, there have been few changes in stoma construction since the 1950s when the Brooke ileostomy was popularized. One study has estimated that by 20 years after stoma construction, 59% of patients with an ileostomy for Crohn's disease and 76% of patients with an ileostomy for ulcerative colitis will experience a stoma related complication (7). Of these 16% to 28% will require revisional surgery (7). Many complications may be avoided with thoughtful planning of the stoma site and careful technical construction. The enterostomal therapy nurse is an essential member of the surgical team to provide preoperative and postoperative support and education. In attempting to manage some complications nonoperatively, the enterostomal therapy nurse is invaluable to assist in appropriate pouching devices. Some patients however, will ultimately need surgery for ileostomy revision.

References

1. Nadler LH. General considerations and complications of the ileostomy. Ostomy/Wound Management 1992;38:18–22.

2. Bubrick MP, Rolstad BS. Intestinal stomas, In: Gordon PH, Nivatvongs S, eds. *Principles and practice of surgery for the colon, rectum, and anus.* St. Louis: Quality Medical Publishing, 1992;856–74.

3. Warren R, McKittrick LS. Ileostomy for ulcerative colitis. Technique, complications and management. Surg Gynecol Obstet 1951;93:555–67.

4. Dragstedt LR, Dack GM, Kirsner JB. Chronic ulcerative colitis: a summary of evidence implicating *Bacterium necrophorum* as an etiologic agent. Ann Surg 1941;114:653.

5. Crile G Jr, Turnbull RB Jr. The mechanism and prevention of ileostomy dysfunction. Ann Surg 1954; 140:459–65.

6. Brooke BN. The management of an ileostomy including its complications. Lancet 1952;2:102–4.

7. Leong APK, Londono-Schimmer EE, Phillips RKS. Life-table analysis of stomal complications following ileostomy. Br J Surg 1994;81:727–9.

8. Fazio VW, Tjandra JJ. Prevention and management of ileostomy complications. J ET Nurs 1992;19:48–53.

9. Morgan TR, Feldshon SD, Tripp MR. Recurrent stomal bleeding: successful treatment using injection sclerotherapy. Dis Colon Rectum 1986;29:269–70.

10. Beck DE, Fazio VW, Grundfest-Bromatowski S. Surgical management of bleeding stomal varices. Dis Colon Rectum 1988;31:343–6.

11. Samaraweera RN, Feldman L, Widrich WC, et al. Stomal varices: percutaneous transhepatic embolization. Radiology 1989;170:779–82.

12. Nelson RL, Subramanian K, Gasparaitis A, et al. The Indium-111 labeled granulocyte scan in patients with

13. Fazio VW. Complications of intestinal stomas. In: Ferrari BT, Ray JE, Gathright JB, eds. *Complications of colon and rectal surgery: prevention and management.* Philadelphia: WB Saunders, 1985;227–50.

14. Cairns BA, Herbst CA, Sartor BR, et al. Peristomal pyoderma gangrenosum and inflammatory bowel disease. Arch Surg 1994;129:769–72.

15. Lever WF, Schaumburg-Lever G. Histopathology of the skin. Philadelphia: JB Lippincott, 1990;214–5.

16. Keltz M, Lebwohl M, Bishop S. Peristomal pyoderma gangrenosum. J Am Acad Dermatol 1992;27:360–417.

17. Schwaegerte SM, Bergfeld WF, Senitzer D, et al. Pyoderma gangrenosum: a review. J Am Acad Dermatol 1988;18:559–68.

18. Callen JP. Pyoderma gangrenosum and related disorders. Adv Dermatol 1989;4:51–70.

19. Kodner IJ. Stoma complications. In: Fazio VW, ed. *Current therapy in colon and rectal surgery.* Philadelphia: MC Decker, 1990;424.

20. AMA Drug Evaluations, 5th ed. American Medical Association, Chicago, 1983;1287–9.

21. Mulvihill SJ. Perioperative use of octreotide in gastrointestinal surgery. Digestion 1993;54(suppl 1): 33–7.

22. Kusuhara K, Kusunoki M, Okamoto T, et al. Reduction of the effluent volume in high-output ileostomy patients by a somatostatin analogue, SMS 201–995. Int J Colorect Dis 1992;7:202–5.

23. Corman M. Intestinal stomas. In: *Colon and rectal surgery,* 3rd ed. Philadelphia: JB Lippincott, 1993; 1118–21.

24. Byers JM, Steinberg JB, Postier RG. Repair of parastomal hernias using polypropylene mesh. Arch Surg 1992;127:1246–7.

25. Rubin MS, Schoetz DJ, Matthews JB. Parastomal hernia: is stoma relocation superior to fascial repair? Arch Surg 1994;129:413–9.

26. Truedson H, Press V. A new method of stomal reconstruction in patients with retraction of conventional ileostomy. Surg Gynecol Obstet 1986;162:60–1.

27. Carey PD, Suvarna SK, Baloch KG, et al. Primary adenocarcinoma in an ileostomy: a late complication of surgery for ulcerative colitis. Surgery 1993;113: 712–5.

28. Starke J, Rodriguez-Bigas M, Marshall W, et al. Primary adenocarcinoma arising in an ileostomy. Surgery 1993;114:125–8.

38 Urinary and Sexual Complications

Anthony J. Thomas Jr. and Dominick J. Carbone Jr.

Genitourinary complications have long been recognized as some of the most serious extraintestinal manifestations of inflammatory bowel disease (IBD). In 1936, just four years after Crohn, Ginzburg and Oppenheimer's original description of regional enteritis, Ten Kate recorded the first documented case of an enterovesical fistula secondary to IBD (1). This was followed in 1943 by Hyams' original report of ureteral obstruction resulting from chronic ileitis and in 1962 by Deren's paper on nephrolithiasis as a complication of ulcerative colitis and regional enteritis (2,3). Other authors throughout this century have continued to emphasize significant genitourinary complications associated with or resulting from surgery for IBD (4,5).

This chapter is intended to be a guide that will enable the surgeon to anticipate, avoid, and deal with some of the most significant urologic problems associated with IBD, including those related to sexual and reproductive function. These latter complications often cause the greatest distress in this young, sexually active patient population.

Urinary Complications

Urinary retention: Voiding problems are not uncommon after surgery for IBD, especially following total proctocolectomy. Up to 16% of patients may have difficulty voiding in the postoperative period. Although both men and women are at risk for this complication, older men may be at greatest risk due to benign prostatic enlargement (6,7).

Although prevention of urinary retention is not always possible, knowledge of the neuroanatomy and attempts to avoid the responsible nerves may minimize the problem. During surgery, dissection should be carried out as close to the rectum as possible and anterior to the endopelvic fascia in order to avoid damage to the pelvic autonomic nerves at the level of the sacral promontory or lateral and anterior to the rectum in the retrovesical and retrouterine spaces (8).

Even with the most skilled dissection, however, retention may still occur in the absence of apparent injury to the pelvic plexus. Contributing factors can include bladder overdistention, diminished awareness of bladder sensation, poor preoperative bladder contractility due to processes such as diabetes, inhibition of the micturition reflex secondary to pain, or preexisting outlet obstruction caused by benign enlargement of the prostate (9). Some of these problems may be anticipated and avoided by the preoperative placement of an indwelling catheter. Though no studies have been carried out on IBD patients specifically, the urologic literature demonstrates significantly reduced rates of postoperative retention in orthopedic patients who are treated with 24 to 48 hours of postoperative bladder decompression by continuous catheter drainage as opposed to intermittent catheterization. Of note is the fact that there appears to be no increase in the incidence of urinary tract infection related to this (10,11).

Alpha adrenergic blockade has been shown to be effective prophylaxis against urinary retention in some patients. In a retrospective review of colorectal patients treated with and without perioperative phenoxybenzamine therapy, Goldman found a 19.2% incidence of retention in patients receiving phenoxybenzamine versus a 54.7% incidence in those who did not (12). A recent meta-analysis demonstrated a 29.1% reduction in the postoperative retention rate in patients receiving this medication (13). Petersen reported similar success in a randomized trial using prazosin in patients undergoing joint replacement surgery (14). Newer alpha blockers such as terazosin and doxazosin have not yet been studied in this regard, but they should work as well or better than the older drugs with fewer side effects. The precise mechanism of action of the alpha blockers is still a matter of some debate but they have been clearly shown to decrease bladder outlet resistance.

Bethanechol and other parasympathomimetic agents have historically been recommended for the treatment of postoperative urinary retention for the patient who is awake and alert and without evidence of urinary obstruction (9). Review of the urologic literature, however, demonstrates little to no evidence supporting the use of bethanechol or any other parasympathomimetic (15). Barrett was unable to demonstrate any significant efficacy in terms of improving flow or reducing residual volume in a randomized, double-blind trial in female patients (16). Nevertheless, anecdotal reports of success with bethanachol and its analogues in the treatment of urinary retention persist and these medications certainly have their advocates in the general surgical community. The potential side effects of these parasympathomimetic agents are not insignificant and include flushing, nausea, vomiting, diarrhea, GI cramps, bronchospasm, headache, salivation, sweating, and visual disturbances. Intramuscular and intravenous use are contraindicated and may cause catastrophic side effects, including circulatory failure and cardiac arrest (17).

Urinary retention that persists beyond 48 to 72 hours should precipitate urologic consultation. In general, it is not necessary for many of these patients to undergo a complete urologic investigation unless there was a significant preoperative voiding problem, such as neurogenic voiding dysfunction or an obstructive voiding pattern. In these cases, upper tract evaluation and appropriately timed urodynamic studies are in order. The majority of voiding difficulties are often transient, and despite the desire of all involved to "do something," most of these patients are best served with expectant, conservative management such as intermittent self catheterization (9). There are, however, certain cases that may appear to require surgery to alleviate obstruction. It is imperative in these cases that urodynamic testing be done first to determine if the bladder has normal detrusor tone. If little or no detrusor activity is demonstrated by cystometry, per-

forming a prostatectomy is unlikely to be of any benefit, as the problem is more likely one of detrusor dysfunction.

Nephrolithiasis: The incidence of urinary tract calculi is higher in patients with IBD than in the general population, rising still higher in those who have undergone intestinal resection or ileostomy. Bambach reported the following stone formation rates in postoperative IBD patients: 6.7% in patients who had small bowel resections, 8.9% of those who underwent ileostomies, and 14.8% of patients with both small bowel resections and ileostomies (18).

The stones formed in postoperative IBD patients are primarily uric acid and calcium oxalate. In general, patients with ileostomies are at increased risk for uric acid stones whereas those with multiple ileal resections but without ileostomies tend to form calcium oxalate stones.

Uric acid stones tend to form in states of low urine volume, low urine pH, and high uric acid concentration (19,20). Large volume alkaline fluid loss from an ileostomy produces precisely this state of low-volume acidic urine, thus favoring uric acid stone formation. Clarke reported patients with ileostomies produce an average of 1082 mL urine/day, compared with 1340 mL/day in the control population. The mean urine pH of patients with ileostomies was 5.05, well below the 5.7 pKa of uric acid (21). In addition, uric acid crystals may promote nephrolithiasis by serving as a nidus for the deposition of calcium oxalate via the phenomenon of epitaxy (22). To date, there has been no evidence that patients with continent (Kock) ileostomies are at any lower risk for uric acid stone formation. Stern reported no significant difference in either mean uric acid concentration or mean daily volume of urine excretion between the two populations (23).

Management of uric acid stones in IBD patients should be primarily aimed at prevention. Patients need to be advised to ingest large amounts of fluid in order to increase urine volume (22,23). In addition, potassium citrate in divided doses ranging from 30 mEq to 60mEq/day may be administered to alkalinize the urine (24). Potassium citrate may have an added therapeutic benefit of inhibiting calcium oxlate stone formation (25).

The mechanism of calcium oxalate stone formation in IBD is less clear. Three major theories exist; the most accepted is known as the solubility concept. Normally, calcium and oxalate combine in the lumen of the intestine to form the relatively insoluble calcium oxalate, which is then eliminated in the feces. In patients with IBD, especially those who have undergone resection of the terminal ileum, nonabsorbed fatty acids are available to bind calcium, leaving oxalate unbound. Unbound oxalate is then freely absorbed in the colon, ultimately producing hyperoxaluria that leads to stone formation (26,27). Allison and Clayman suggested that a deficiency of *Oxalobacter formigenes,* an anaerobic bacteria that metabolizes oxalic acid in the colon, may contribute to oxalate hyperabsorption in IBD patients (28). Finally, it has also been postulated that the excess bile salts and fatty acids may have a direct irritative effect on the colonic mucosa, enhancing its permeability (29). In all likelihood, the solubility concept, the bacterial deficiency, and the direct effect of bile salts and fatty acids act in concert to cause the intestinal hyperabsorption of oxalate, with the solubility concept being most important (30).

Management of the IBD patient with calcium oxalate nephrolithiasis may be a difficult clinical problem. Dietary restriction of oxalate should be beneficial, but in practice, this is generally not the case. Low oxalate diets are notoriously unpalatable and compliance is low. Studies have demonstrated that the therapeutic effect of the low oxalate diet is not maintained after discharge from a metabolic unit (31). A more successful form of dietary therapy has been to reduce fat malabsorption by either substituting medium chain triglycerides or simply reducing dietary fat (32).

Another strategy has been to bind the excess oxalate and thus diminish oxalate absorption. This may be accomplished by supplementing the diet with cations to bind the oxalate, specifically calcium or magnesium. Both Earnest and Stauffer have demonstrated reductions in urinary oxalate excretion with increased oral calcium in patients with ileal resections (33,34). Barilla and Hylander, however, have shown that the beneficial effect of this therapy may be at least partly obviated by the concomitant rise in urinary calcium (35,36). Magnesium has also been suggested as an oxalate binder, but there are concerns that its tendency to exacerbate diarrhea may minimize its potential benefit.

Cholestyramine has been investigated as a potential oxalate binder, and studies have demonstrated a reduction in the mean 24-hour urinary oxalate excretion with this drug (37,38). Cholestyramine also increases bile salt loss and may therefore increase the pool of fatty acids capable of binding calcium, thus diminishing its therapeutic effect. To date, there is no single accepted management strategy for eneteric hyperoxaluria.

Rectourethral fistulas: The overall incidence of genitourinary fistulas associated with Crohn's disease ranges from 1.6% to 10% (30,40). Although rectourethral fistulas secondary to Crohn's disease are uncommon occurrences, they can be a complicated management problem for both the colorectal surgeon and the urologist. Rectourethral fistulas may present with pneumaturia, fecaluria, or leakage of urine from the rectum during micturition. They have also been associated with urinary tract infections and epididymitis (41,42). Diagnosis may be difficult, as the patient is often assumed to have the more common enterovesical fistula. Thorough examination of the rectum, careful proctoscopy and methodical cystourethroscopy will generally demonstrate the lesion (43).

Various methods of treatment, ranging from medical therapy to radical surgery, have been described. As is so often the case in IBD, therapy must be individualized. Rampton has reported the successful treatment of a postoperative rectourethral fistula in Crohn's disease with metronidazole therapy alone (44). Santoro has documented significant improvement at a follow-up of 15 months (45). Indeed, a number of authors have recommended systematic medical therapy prior to any surgical intervention in all forms of perirectal Crohn's disease (46,47). Side effects from the medication, primarily paresthesias, can occur in up to 50% of patients (48,49). Recent reports have also indicated that cyclosporine may play a role in the treatment of fistula of Crohn's disease; however, none of the patients reportedly treated with this medication had rectourethral fistulas (50,51). There is also considerable concern over the well documented nephrotoxic effects of cyclosporine, which may not be reversed by dose reduction (52).

Surgery has been considered the cornerstone of therapy for rectourethral fistulas in Crohn's disease, but precisely which procedure to perform has been a matter of some debate. Historically, radical operations with fecal diversion have been favored, particularly when flagrant proctitis is present (53,54). Alperstein successfully used a staged approach involving diverting ileostomy and total proctocolectomy followed by primary repair (55). Talamani also reported on a patient managed with a staged approach; the patient suffered a recurrence after three years requiring management with a permanent sigmoid colostomy (56).

The current trend has been toward local management without fecal diversion in the absence of active rectal disease. At the Mayo Clinic, four patients were treated successfully with simple division and repair via a perineal approach (57). Fazio and colleagues reported on the successful management of 3 patients with rectourethral fistulas via anterior rectal advancement flaps similar to those performed for rectovaginal fistulas (58,59,60).

Sexual and Reproductive Dysfunction

Male Sexual and Reproductive Dysfunction

A thorough understanding of the anatomy and physiology of erection and ejaculation will minimize the occurrence of sexual dysfunction after surgery for IBD. The parasympathetic nerves responsible for erection arise from the second, third, and fourth sacral spinal cord segments. These preganglionic nerves then enter the pelvic plexus. The pelvic plexus is located between the rectum and posterior-lateral position of the bladder. The nerves then exit the pelvic plexus and descend towards the penis in the plane between the prostatic capsule and the endopelvic fascia. These nerves are known as the nervi eregentes. They then run along the posterolateral aspect of the prostate, and once beyond the apex of the prostate, the nerves penetrate the tunica albuginea of the corpus spongiosum as the cavernous nerves (61,62). The sympathetic nerves are responsible for the deposition of semen in the posterior urethra as well as closure of the bladder neck to produce antegrade ejaculation. They originate from the eleventh thoracic to the second lumbar spinal segments. These preganglionic fibers synapse with postganglionic fibers in the preaortic plexus. The postganglionic fibers descend into the pelvis and lie just beneath the peritoneum anterior to and on either side of the aorta, coalescing in the superior hypogastric plexus at the bifurcation of the aorta en route to the end organs. Within the thin adventitial tissue of the end organs, there is another synaptic junction, the short adrenergic fibers, branches of which innervate the individual smooth muscle cells (63,64) (Fig. 38.1).

During surgery for IBD, particularly extirpation of the colon and rectum, injury to either or both the sympathetic or parasympathetic fibers may occur (Fig. 38.2). Most frequently, the parasympathetic nerves are damaged just inferior to the peritoneal reflection on either side of the rectum, although the sympathetic fibers may be injured near the promontory of the sacrum or just anterolateral to the rectum. Therefore, dissection of the mesentery and peritoneal attachments should always be performed as close to the rectum as possible in order

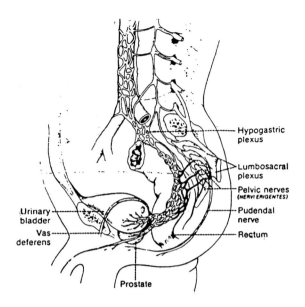

Fig. 38.1. The hypogastric (sympathetic) and pelvic nerves (parasympathetic) lie close to the rectum before traveling to the bladder and sexual organs.

order to minimize damage to the nerves below. Ligation of the superior hemorrhoidal vessels should likewise be performed close to the bowel wall so that the layer of tissue overlying the sacral promontory is not violated. Finally, when dissecting the rectum free from the prostate, the surgical plane should be kept immediately adjacent to the rectal wall, staying posterior to the fascia of Denonvilliers' thereby sparing the nerves in this area (65,66).

Although colorectal surgeons and their patients reluctantly accept the frequent occurrence of sex-

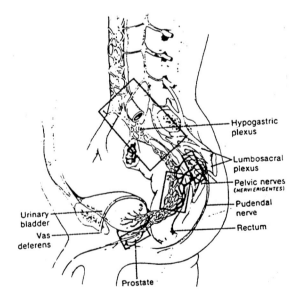

Fig. 38.2. The sacral promontory region (large box) and the lateral stalk region (small box) are areas that are particularly prone to injury at the time of proctectomy.

ual dysfunction as a consequence of their cancer surgery, it is particularly distressing when erectile or ejaculatory complications after surgery for IBD, given the young, active nature of the patient population. Fortunately, the rate of impotence following proctocolectomy for IBD is relatively low. In Watts' series, 11 of 41 men experienced some impairment of sexual function after proctocolectomy. This appeared to be age related, with only 5 of 33 men younger than 50 reporting any dysfunction. Of these five, two were anejaculatory, two suffered transient impotence, and one man under the age of 50 was rendered permanently impotent (67). More recent series demonstrate an even lower incidence of postproctocolectomy sexual dysfunction. Corman reported an extremely low incidence of impotence following proctocolectomy for IBD, with only 1 out of 76 men experiencing transient impairment of erectile function (68). Bauer's series of 135 males treated with proctectomy included four patients (3%) who suffered a permanent deficit in either erectile or ejaculatory function. Two men, ages 32 and 30, were able to sustain an erection but had retrograde ejaculation; two others, ages 19 and 44, were impotent (65). Fazio and Montague reported the incidence of sexual dysfunction after proctocolectomy for IBD was 11%. It was, in all cases, partial and transient. Conversely, the rate of sexual dysfunction following abdominoperineal resection of the rectum for carcinoma was 50% and it was generally permanent (66).

If impotence should occur in the young male patient, a period of observation is always warranted, as the dysfunction is often transient. Should the dysfunction persist beyond 3 to 6 months, urologic consultation is advised. After careful screening to rule out other causes of impotence, a variety of therapeutic options are available. Injection of the corpora with a vasodilatory drug such as prostaglandin or papaverine may be the first option. These substances act by doing what the nerves are supposed to do, i.e., increase blood flow to the penis. Young patients with good penile blood supply and pure neurogenic impotence represent excellent candidates for self-injection therapy. Alternatively, the patient may prefer the surgical placement of either a malleable or an inflatable penile prosthesis (Figs. 38.3 and 38.4). Patient-partner satisfaction rates are particularly good for the multi-component inflatable penile prosthesis, with over 90% of couples reporting satisfaction with the device after surgery (69).

Although damage to the parasympathetic nerves may result in impotence, injury to the sympathetic nerves can produce ejaculatory dysfunctions. Retrograde ejaculation results from a failure of the bladder neck to close synchronous with the rhythmic contractions of the ischiocavernosus and bulbocavernosus muscles that expel the semen from the urethra. Sympathomimetic medications, such as phenylpropanolamine, pseudoephedrine, ephedrine, and imipramine, may be of some benefit in restoring antegrade ejaculation (70,71,72). If medical therapy fails, several techniques may be used to retrieve and process the sperm from the bladder for use with artificial insemination (73,74,75). More extensive damage to the sympathetic nerves may result in a complete lack of seminal emission into the posterior urethra. Sympathomimetic medications can be tried, but in these cases they are much less successful than with retrograde ejaculation. Proctocolectomy does not allow rectal probe electrostimulation of ejaculation and patients desirous of trying to establish a pregnancy can choose to undergo sperm aspiration from the vas deferens or epididymis with either intrauterine insemination or in vitro fertilization (76). It is not unreasonable to consider offering the young male patient an opportunity to cryopreserve sperm before the surgery if he or his surgeon feel more comfortable based on prior experience and level of anxiety.

It should also be noted that some of the medications used in the treatment of IBD may adversely affect fertility. Patients taking sulfasalazine can exhibit a wide variety of abnormalities in their semen, including decreases in sperm concentration, motility and percent of normal forms, each of which can impact on fertility (77,78). Most studies show resolution of these changes following discontinuation of the drug.

Female Sexual and Reproductive Dysfunction

Several studies have demonstrated a relatively high degree of baseline sexual dysfunction and dyspareunia in female patients with IBD. Moody has shown that 24% of female patients with Crohn's disease had either infrequent or no intercourse compared with 4% of controls (79). Weber and Fazio demonstrated that 55% of women with IBD report pain on penetration and 50% complain of abdominal pain during sexual intercourse (80). Gruner and colleagues have ascribed this high rate of dyspareunia to inflammation in the rectal segment (81).

Most reports demonstrate marked improvement in female sexual function following almost all

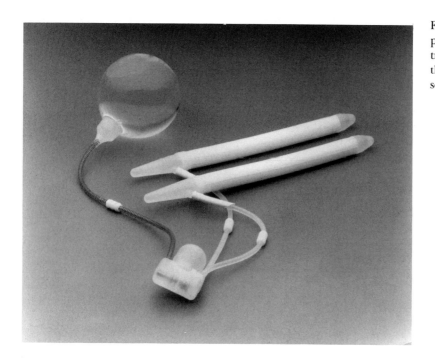

Fig. 38.3. An inflatable penile prosthesis permits erection to be triggered by an inflated balloon that is surgically placed in the scrotum.

forms of surgery for IBD, presumably due to resection of the involved rectal segment. These studies also demonstrate no impairment of fertility. Sjogren interviewed 30 women following pelvic pouch surgery for IBD and found that following closure of the temporary ileostomy, 23 (77%) reported an increase in sexual desire and 28 (93%) could experience orgasm (82). Metcalf and colleagues reported similar success in patients undergoing proctocolectomy with a continence-preserving procedure (50 Kock pouches, 50 ileoanal anastomoses) for IBD. Frequency of inter-

course increased while the incidence of dyspareunia decreased in both groups. They also noted no impairment in postoperative fertility (83). Keighley also noted no deleterious effects on postoperative fertility following restorative proctocolectomy. In a series of 168 patients who underwent this procedure over a nine-year period, ten females who attempted pregnancy were able to have children after the operation, eight with an uncomplicated vaginal delivery (84).

Surgery for IBD has been reported to produce some deleterious effects on the sexual function of

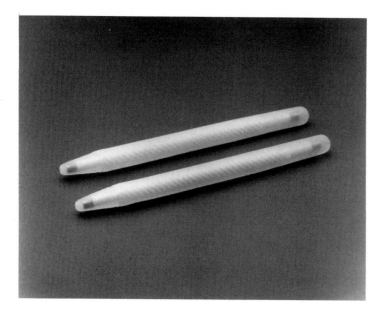

Fig. 38.4. A malleable penile prosthesis is much simpler than the inflatable type, although patient-partner satisfaction may be lower.

certain women. Some instances of retained menstrual blood, colpitis, chronic vaginal discharge and persistent dyspareunia have been reported after proctectomy. In some cases, these symptoms may result from dorsocaudal dislocation of the vagina which produces an almost horizontal position of the vagina. Postoperative scarring may also cause the posterior fornix to become adherent to the coccyx, causing the vagina to become angulated and leading to the formation of a pouch containing air, retained secretions, and menstrual blood (85,86).

Kylberg has devised a perineal colpoplasty designed to reverse the complications of proctectomy. It involves resection of the coccyx and placement of a muscle flap from the gluteus maximus between the posterior fornix of the vagina and the lower part of the sacrum. This causes the vagina to lie in a more vertical position and avoids direct contact with the coccyx and the perineal skin preventing angulation and dyspaerunia (86).

Sjodahl reported on a series of 9 patients treated with the Kylberg perineal colpoplasty from 1972 through 1983. Eight of the nine women were free of symptoms. Two had developed wound infections, one had a perineal sinus tract, and another required reoperation at six months for relapsing symptoms but was ultimately rendered pain free (86).

Conclusion

Surgery for IBD carries with it significant risks of genitourinary side effects including urinary retention, stone disease, fistula formation, and sexual dysfunction. These potential complications should be discussed with the patient when considering whether or not to perform surgery for IBD. Although some problems, such as urinary retention, are transient and often have little impact on the patient's ultimate outcome, others, such as erectile impotence, may significantly affect the patient's quality of life. The likelihood of the complication, the extent of the corrective measures needed to reverse it, and most importantly, the patient's ability to deal with an adverse outcome all need to be weighed when planning surgery in the IBD patient.

References

1. Ten Kate J. Twee Gevallen van Ileitis Terminalis. Nederl Tijdschr Geneesk 1936;80:51.
2. Hyams JA, Weinberg SR, Alley JL. Chronic ileitis with concomitant ureteritis: case report. Am J Surg 1943;61:117.
3. Deren JJ, Porusch JG, Levitt MF, et al. Nephrolithiasis as a complication of ulcerative colitis and regional enteritis. Ann Int Med 1962;56:843.
4. Ginzburg L, Oppenheimer GD. Urological complications of regional ileitis. J Urol 1948;59:948.
5. Shield DE, Lytton B, Weiss RM, et al. Urologic complications of inflammatory bowel disease. J Urol 1976;115:701.
6. Baumrucker GO, Shaw JW. Urological complications following abdominoperineal resection of the rectum. Arch Surg 1972;67:502.
7. Tank ES. Urinary tract complications of anorectal surgery. Am J Surg 1972;123:118.
8. Block GE, Hurst GE. Complications of the Surgical Treatment of Ulcerative Colitis and Crohn's Disease. In: Inflammatory Bowel Disease, 4th ed., Kirsner JB, Shorter RG. 1995;898. Wms & Wilkins, Baltimore MD.
9. Wein AJ. Neuromuscular dysfunction of the lower urinary tract and its treatment. In: Cambell's Urology, 7th ed. (in press).
10. Carpiniello VL, Cendron M, Altman HG, et al. Treatment of urinary complications after total joint replacement in elderly females. Urology 1988;32:186.
11. Michelson JD, Lotke PA, Steinberg ME. Urinary bladder management after total joint replacement surgery. N Engl J Med 1988;319:321.
12. Goldman G, Kahn PJ, Kashton H, et al. Prevention and treatment of urinary retention and infection after surgical treatment of the colon and rectum with alpha adrenergic blockers. SGO 1988;166:647.
13. Velanovich V. Pharmacologic prevention and treatment of postoperative urinary retention. Infect in Urol 1992;3:87.
14. Petersen MS, Collins DN, Selakovich WG, et al. Postoperative urinary retention associated with total hip and knee arthroplasties. Clin Ortho Rel Res 1991;269:102.
15. Finkbeiner AE. Is bethanechol chloride clinically effective in promoting bladder emptying? A literature review. J Urol 1985;134:443.
16. Barrett DM. The effects of oral bethanechol chloride on voiding in female patients with excessive residual urine: a randomized double-blind study. J Urol 1981;126:640.
17. Taylor P. Cholinergic agonists. In: Gilman AG, Rall TW, Nies AS, Taylor P, eds. Goodman and Gilman's The pharmacological basis of therapeutics, 8th ed. New York: Pergamon Press, 1990;122.
18. Bambach CP, Robertson WG, Peacock M, et al. Effect of intestinal surgery on the risk of urinary stone formation. Gut 1981;22:257.
19. Broadus AE, Thier SO. Metabolic basis of renal stone disease. N Engl J Med 1979;300:839.
20. Clarke AM, Chirnside A, Hill GL, et al. Chronic dehydration and sodium depletion in patients with established ileostomies. Lancet 1967;2:740.

21. Clarke AM, McKenzie RG. Ileostomy and the risk of urinary uric acid stones. Lancet 1969;2:395.

22. Ryall RL, Grover PK, Marshall VR. Urate and calcium stones—picking up a drop of mercury with one's fingers? Am J Kid Dis 1991;17:426.

23. Stern H, Cohen Z, Wilson DR, et al. Urolithiasis risk factors in continent reservoir ileostomy patients. Dis Colon Rectum 1990;23:556.

24. Sakhaee K, Nicar M, Hill K. Contrasting effects of potassium citrate and sodium citrate therapies on urinary chemistries and crystallization of stone-forming salts. Kidney Int 1983;24:348.

25. Pak, CY, Peterson R. Successful treatment of hyper-uricosuric calcium oxalate nephrolithiasis with potassium citrate. Arch Int Med 1986;146:863.

26. Banner, MP. Genitourinary complications of inflammatory bowel disease. Rad Clin NA 1987;25:199.

27. Fukushima T, Ishiguro N, Matsuda Y, et al. Clinical and urinary characteristics of urolithiasis in ulcerative colitis. Am J Gastroenterol 1982;77:238.

28. Allison MJ, Cook HM, Milne DB, et al. Oxalate degradation by gastrointestinal bacteria from humans. J Nutr 1986;116:455.

29. Dobbins JW, Binder HJ. Effect of bile salts and fatty acids on the colonic absorption of oxalate. Gastroenterology 1976;70:1096.

30. Preminger GM. Medical management of urinary calculus disease Part II: Classification of metabolic disorders and selective medical management. AUA Update Series 1995;14:46.

31. Ernest DL. Perspectives on incidence, etiology, and treatment of enteric hyperoxaluria. Am J Clin Nutr 1977;30:72.

32. McLeod RS, Churchill DN. Urolithiasis complicating inflammatory bowel disease. J Urol 1992;148:974.

33. Earnest DL, Williams HE, Admirand WM. Treatment of enteric hyperoxaluria with calcium and medium chain triglycerides. Clin Res 1975;23:130A, abstract.

34. Stauffer JQ. Hyperoxaluria and intestinal disease. The role of steatorrhea and dietary calcium in regulating intestinal oxalate absorption. Am J Dig Dis 1977;22:921.

35. Barilla DE, Notz C, Kennedy D, et al. Renal oxalate excretion following oral oxalate loads in patients with ileal disease and with renal and absorptive hypercalciurias: effect of calcium and magnesium. Am J Med 1978;64:579.

36. Hylander E, Jarnum S, Frandsen I. Urolithiasis and hyperoxaluria in chronic inflammatory bowel disease. Scand J Gastroenterol 1979;14:475.

37. Smith LH, Fromm H, Hoffmann AF. Acquired hyperoxaluria, nephrolithiasis, and intestinal disease: description of a syndrome. N Engl J Med 1972;286:1371.

38. Stauffer JQ, Humphreys MH, Weir GJ. Acquired hyperoxaluria with regional enteritis after ileal resection. Role of dietary oxalate. Ann Int Med 1973;79:383.

39. Gjone E, Orning OM, Myren J. Crohn's disease in Norway 1956–63. Gut 1966;7:372.

40. Karamohandani MC, West CF. Vesicoenteric fistulas. Am J Surg 1984;147:681.

41. Culp OS, Calhoun HW. A variety of rectourethral fistulas: experiences with 20 cases. J Urol 1964;91:560.

42. Tiptaft RC, et al. Fistulas involving rectum and urethra: the place of Parks operation. Br J Urol 1983;55:711.

43. McVary KT, Marshall FF. Urinary Fistulas. In: Adult and Pediatric Urology, 3rd ed. Gillenwater J, Grayhack JT, Howards S, Duckett J, eds. 1996;1355–77.

44. Rampton DS, Denyer ME, Clark CG et al. Rectourethral fistula in Crohn's disease. Br J Surg 1982;69:233.

45. Santoro GA, Bucci L, Frizelle PA. Management of rectourethral fistulas in Crohn's disease. Int J Colorectal Dis 1995;10:183.

46. Goebell J. Perianal complications in Crohn's disease. Neth J Med 1990;37:S47.

47. Ursing B, Kamme C. Metronidazole for Crohn's disease. Lancet 1975;1:775.

48. Bernstein LH, Frank MS, Brandt LJ, et al. Healing of perineal Crohn's disease with metronidazole. Gastroenterology 1980;83:357.

49. Brandt LJ, Bernstein LH, Boley SJ, et al. Metronidazole therapy for perineal Crohn's disease: a follow-up study. Gastroenterology 1982;83:383.

50. Brynskov J. Cyclosporin for inflammatory bowel disease: mechanisms and possible actions. Scand J Gastroenterol 1993;28(10):849.

51. Present D, Simon L. Efficacy of cyclosporine in treatment of fistula of Crohn's disease. Dig Dis Sci 1994;39:374.

52. Lobo AJ, Juby LD, Smith AH, et al. Effect of oral cyclosporin on renal function in Crohn's disease. Dig Dis Sci 1993;38:1624.

53. Smith JBP, Williams RE, DeDombal AT. Genitourinary fistulae complicating Crohn's disease. Br J Urol 1972;44:657.

54. Kyle J. Urinary complications of Crohn's disease. World J Surg 1980;4:153.

55. Alperstein G, Daum F, Aiges H, et al. Urethroperineal-rectal fistula in Crohn's disease. J Pediatr Surg 1983;18:311.

56. Talamini MA, Broe PJ, Cameron JL. Urinary fistulas in Crohn's disease. SGO 1982;154:553.

57. Thompson JS, Beart RW. The management of acquired rectourinary fistula. Dis Colon Rectum 1982;25:689.

58. Jones IT, Fazio VW, Jagelman DG. The use of transanal rectal advancement flaps in the management of fistulas involving the anorectum. Dis Colon Rectum 1987;30:919.

59. Ozuner G, Hull TL, Cartmill J, et al. Long-term analysis of the use of transanal rectal advancement flaps

for complicated anorectal/vaginal fistulas. Dis Colon Rectum 1995;39:10.

60. Fazio VW, Jones IT, Jagelman DG, et al. Recto-urethral fistulas in Crohn's disease. SGO 1987;164: 148.

61. Lue TF. Physiology of Erection and Pathophysiology of Impotence. In: Campbell's Urology, 6th ed. Walsh P, Retik J, Stamey T, Vaughan D, eds. WB Saunders Co, Philadelphia, 1992;707.

62. Walsh PC, Donker PJ. Impotence following radical prostatectomy: insight into etiology and prevention. J Urol 1982;128:492.

63. Hinman F. Autonomic nervous system. In Atlas of Urosurgical Anatomy. WB Saunders Co, Philadelphia, 1993;44.

64. Tanagho E. Anatomy of the lower urinary tract. In: Campbell's urology. Walsh P, Retik J, Stamey T, Vaughn D, eds. WB Saunders Co, Philadelphia, 1992;1(6):40–59.

65. Bauer JJ, Gelernt IM, Salky B, et al. Sexual dysfunction following proctocolectomy for benign disease of the colon and rectum. Ann Surg 1983;197:363.

66. Fazio VW, Fletcher J, Montague D. Prospective study of the effect of resection of the rectum on male sexual function. World J Surg 1980;4:149.

67. Watts JM, de Dombel PT, Goligher JC. Early results of surgery for ulcerative colitis. Br J Surg 1966;53:1005.

68. Corman ML, Veidenheimer MC, Coller, JA. Impotence after proctectomy for inflammatory disease of the bowel. Dis Colon Rectum 1978;21:4118.

69. Malloy TR, Wein AJ, Carpiniello VL. Reliability of AMS 700 inflatable penile prosthesis. Urology 1986;27:385.

70. Brooks ME, Sidi A. Treatment of retrograde ejaculation using imipramine (letter). Urology 1981;18:633.

71. Proctor KG, Howards SS. The effect of sympathomimetic drugs on post-lymphadenectomy aspermia. J Urol 1983;129:837.

72. Thiagarajah S, Vaughan ED, Kitchin JD. Retrograde ejaculation: successful pregnancy following combined sympathomimetic medication and insemination. Fert Steril 1978;30:96.

73. Cameron MC, Gillett WR. The recovery of sperm, insemination and pregnancy in the treatment of in-fertility because of retrograde ejaculation. Fert Steril 1985;44:844.

74. Mahadeven M, Leston JF, Trounsen AO. Noninvasive method of semen collection for successful artificial insemination in a case of retrograde ejaculation. Fert Steril 1981;36:243.

75. Ingerslev HJ. Retrograde ejaculation: successful artificial homologous insemination. Lancet 1985;1: 519.

76. Belker AM, Sharins RJ, Bustillo M, et al. Pregnancy with microsurgical vas aspiration from a patient with neurologic ejaculatory dysfunction. J Androl 1994; 15:6S.

77. Riley SA, Lecarpentier J, Mani V. Sulfasalazine induced seminal abnormalities: results of mesalazine substitution. Gut 1987;28:1008.

78. Ragni G, Bianchi Porro G, Ruspa M. Abnormal semen quality and lower serum testosterone in men with inflammatory bowel disease treated for a long time with sulfasalazine. Andro 1984;16:162.

79. Moody GA, Mayberry JF. Perceived sexual dysfunction amongst patients with inflammatory bowel disease. Digestion 1993;54:256.

80. Weber AM, Ziegler C, Belinson JL, et al. Gynecologic history of women with inflammatory bowel disease. Ob & Gyn 1995;86:843.

81. Gruner CPN, Naas R, Fretheim B, et al. Marital status and sexual adjustment after colectomy: results in 178 patients operated on for ulcerative colitis. Scand J Gastroenterol 1977;12:193.

82. Sjogren B, Foppan B. Sexual life in women after colectomy—proctomucosectomy with S-pouch. Acta Obstet Gyn Scand 1995;74:51.

83. Metcalf AM, Dozois RR, Kelly KA. Sexual function in women after proctocolectomy. Ann Surg 1986;204: 624.

84. Keighley MR, Grobler S, Bain I. An adult of restorative proctocolectomy. Gut 1993;34:680.

85. Nilsson LO, Kock NG, Kylberg F, et al. Sexual adjustment in ileostomy patients before and after conversion to continent ileostomy. Dis Colon Rectum 1981;24:287.

86. Sjodahl R, Per-olof N, Olaison G. Surgical treatment of dorsocaudal dislocation of the vagina after excision of the rectum. Dis Colon Rectum 1990;33:672.

Section IV
Inflammatory Bowel Disease: Surgical Treatment

Part II
Septic Complications Following Restorative Proctocolectomy

39 Dehiscence of Ileoanal Anastomosis

David C.C. Bartolo

The ileoanal anastomosis is technically demanding, and the outcome is highly dependent on the expertise of the operating surgeon. Refinements of technical aspects have in recent years reduced the incidence of anastomotic failure.

When restorative proctocolectomy was first introduced by Parks and Utsunomiya in the late seventies, the operation involved a long complex mucosectomy where ten or more centimeters of rectum were retained. The mucosectomy left a raw muscular tube that was often highly vascular. The ileal-pouch that was placed within this cavity was greatly at risk from so called cuff abscesses that inevitably drained through the anastomosis leading to chronic septic sequelae. The use of shorter cuffs has been associated with fewer septic complications without adversely affecting function. It was initially considered that a long cuff of retained rectum was essential for adequate continence and satisfactory anorectal function.

Pelvic Sepsis

Sepsis in the pelvis after pouch-anal anastomosis may result because of infection of a pelvic hematoma, or because of anastomotic dehiscence. This may in turn arise from the pouch itself, or more commonly from the ileoanal anastomosis. The perimuscular dissection, in which the operation of rectal excision proceeds between the mesorectum and the rectal muscle tube has the advantage that it carries a lower risk of injury to the pelvic nerves. On the other hand, careful dissection in the anatomic plane allows accurate nerve identification and preservation, and in expert hands does not increase the incidence of sexual dysfunction. The advantage is easier hemostasis with consequent lower risks of hematomas and pelvic sepsis.

Leakage from the pouch itself should be exceptionally rare with attention to detail during construction of the pouch. Care must be taken to ensure a complete suture line. At completion of the anastomosis, it is our normal practice to measure the capacity of the pouch. The volumes are normally between 250 to 300 mL. A dilute solution of povidone iodine is injected into the pouch until it is fully distended. This allows any leak which may have occurred for technical reasons to be identified and oversown. The pouch must not have been traumatized during dissection, and it should have a good blood supply, since ischemia will predispose to late leakage from the pouch. The blind end of a J-pouch is an area for problems to develop. It may be stapled or closed with interrupted inverting seromuscular sutures. An example of a transient leak is shown in Fig. 39.1. This patient had a one stage restorative proctocolectomy carried out with a covering loop ileostomy for severe acute chronic colitis that failed to respond to high dose steroid therapy. She made an apparently excellent postoperative recovery. Six weeks postoperatively when the contrast study was done, a small leak was demonstrated from the blind end of the J-pouch, shown below the sacrum on the top radiograph. This was managed by delaying closure for one month by which time complete resolution occurred as demonstrated on the lower radiograph. The author has also seen two patients who presented with sinuses extending to the abdominal wall that presented late after ileostomy closure. These were thought initially to be suture sinuses, but exploration showed they were connected to the

477

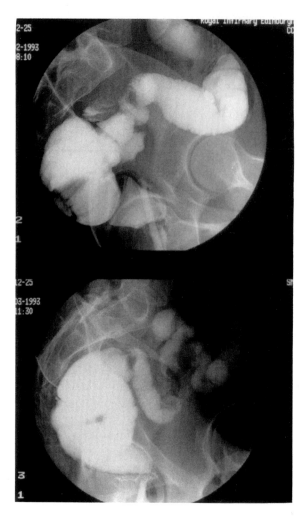

Fig. 39.1. Transient leak from the blind end of a J-pouch.

blind limb of the J-pouch. Oversewing of the affected area through healthy freshened gut tissues resolved the problem in both patients.

Ileoanal Anastomotic Dehiscence

There is increasing evidence that septic complications are more common when the pouch is constructed in indeterminate colitis (1) and Crohn's disease. Thus avoidance of anastomotic dehiscence is related to case selection. Careful technique is essential. If a mucosectomy is carried out, meticulous hemostasis should be secured. Access to the mucosa for dissection is facilitated by use of the Lone Star retractor (Lone Star Medical Products Inc, Houston, TX, USA). Small hooks attached to elastic tubes are placed at the dentate line, and a series of eight of these are held in place by a ring retractor placed around the anal canal. The anastomosis then proceeds with good exposure. Prob-

lems will occur if there is tension because of inadequate length of small bowel in bringing the pouch down to the anus. The main disadvantage of this retractor is that by everting the anus, the distance the pouch has to be brought down is increased so the problem will be exacerbated. One option under such circumstances is to place all the sutures in and tie them after removal of the retractor and hooks. Under no circumstances should an anastomosis be accepted if it is under tension, since postoperative complications are almost certain to ensue. If there is obvious tension, then further mesenteric lengthening maneuvers should be attempted. The author finds that release of the origin of the superior mesenteric artery will provide elongation. This maneuver together with extensive mobilization behind the pancreas and duodenum helps considerably. Selective vascular division may be necessary. Before doing this it must be ascertained that there is an adequate collateral flow. Illumination of the mesentery, together with removal of mesenteric fat will help to identify the blood supply and confirm the collateral anatomy. In principle, the higher the vessel ligation, the more length is gained. On the other hand, higher vessel ligation, especially on the main course of the superior mesenteric artery may jeopardize the blood supply to the pouch. Temporary occlusion with vascular clamps is advisable prior to selective vascular division. Ideally, the ileocolic artery and its arcade should be preserved during colectomy. If the main artery is kept intact, and the cecum is excised by ligating the vessels close to the bowel wall, then an excellent input to the terminal ileum will be preserved that may allow division of the superior mesenteric artery distal to the ileocolic artery. This has been used on rare occasions in thick set males with short mesenteries with excellent results. Clearly it is a procedure to be adopted when simpler measures will not suffice. Planning vascular divisions is essential, since there is no room for error. If for example a rather cautious division has produced inadequate length, further ligations may make part of the pouch critically ischemic and ruin the operation.

If access is difficult, and the anastomosis cannot be carried out easily, a helpful maneuver is to use Gelpie retractors, and the assistant is asked to push the retractor inwards, thus reducing length and pushing the anus towards the pouch. This allows the pouch to be sutured endoanally with less difficulty. If at completion, the pouch is bow-stringed across the pelvis, problems are almost inevitably going to follow, and it would be preferable to revise the anastomosis after obtaining adequate length or abandoning the anastomosis. It should be born in mind that aborting the ileoanal operation and establishing an end ileostomy for a period of 1 to 2 years will almost certainly result in significant mesenteric lengthening. This may permit a relatively easy anastomosis to be made without tension some time in the future. A well constructed anastomosis should leave the pouch lying in contact with the sacrum without tension. Tension is the principle reason for dehiscence. It is not the only explanation, since the problem occurs for other reasons. Ischemia of the pouch at the apex where the anastomosis is constructed will result if excessive numbers of sutures are inserted and or tied too tightly. These will lead to areas of necrosis that will cause dehiscence and septic sequelae. Poor nutritional status in poorly selected patients will mean the individual does not have the physical resources to heal satisfactorily in areas where minor imperfections would otherwise be overcome in a healthier individual.

Pelvic sepsis and anastomotic dehiscence are clearly closely intertwined. The data on the former are more accurately reported in the literature. The incidence varies between 3% to 33% (2). There is substantial evidence that its incidence falls with increasing surgical experience. Thus Keighley reported pelvic sepsis in 12%, 6%, and 2% respectively in his first, second, and third consecutive cohorts of 50 patients (3).

Anal and distal rectal mucosectomy is conventionally followed by a sometimes difficult sutured anastomosis at the dentate line. Access in fat or muscular patients is potentially very difficult, particularly if problems have been experienced in obtaining adequate length when constructing the pouch. The management of low rectal cancer with anastomoses stapled to the anus suggested that this approach could be employed in restorative proctectomy. Heald and Allen (4) described how the rectum could be excised and an ileoanal anastomosis constructed using a circular stapling gun, thus avoiding the need for a perineal phase to the operation. The essential differences between this and traditional mucosectomy are first, no muscular rectal cuff is left behind and second, a variable amount of anal transitional zone mucosa is preserved.

It is claimed that the stapling technique possesses several advantages. The technique is quicker than mucosectomy and hand-sewn anastomosis. Construction is reliable and reproducible, and provides the option of omitting a temporary loop ileostomy. The anal transitional zone contains sensory receptors that contribute to the defecation sam-

pling reflex (5). Avoiding a perineal phase reduces the degree and duration of sphincter stretching.

The major disadvantage is the preservation of potentially diseased transitional or colonic mucosa. In familial adenomatous polyposis, polyps may either be left or perhaps subsequently arise with obvious malignant potential. In ulcerative colitis, diseased mucosa is inevitably retained but whether or not this matters for either symptomatic control or malignant risk is controversial.

Following Heald's description of this technique, there has been a continuing debate surrounding the risks of retaining variable amounts of colitic mucosa below the anastomosis. This leads to two potential problems. The first is persistent active colitis in the retained rectal cuff which may be problematic if more than a few millimeters have been left. The second and potentially more serious is the risk of malignancy in the retained cuff. There is an obvious difference in constructing the anastomosis at the top of the anal columns, with a true ileoanal anastomosis, and an ileodistal-rectal anastomosis where rectum is left behind.

The stapled ileoanal technique was popularized by the Leeds group (6) who, in common with other authors (7,8) have used a double-stapling technique. Although the level above the dentate line at which the transverse staple gun is placed is routinely checked per annum, the eventual level of the ileoanal anastomosis is variable. A randomized study of patients from St Mark's undergoing stapled ($n = 17$) or manual ($n = 15$) anastomoses showed wide scatter for the stapled group: median 2 cm, range 0.2 to 4 cm above the dentate line.

We have routinely employed a single-stapling technique, with the aid of a reusable purse-string device (Davis and Geck, UK) applied across the anorectal junction. This is just as easy to use in the depths of the pelvis as the 30 mm transverse staplers, and simpler than a hand-applied whip stitch recommended by some authors (4,9). The position of the purse-string device is checked per annum to be approximately 2 cm above the dentate line so as to leave a safe margin to be removed by the 31 or 33 mm circular staplegun. This results in an anastomosis lying 1 to 2 cm above the dentate line. One of the problems highlighted by Nicholls is the difficulty in placing the staple line at the precise intended point. When the intention was to construct this 1 cm above the dentate line, there was considerable variation. If the anastomosis is too low, then a significant amount of internal sphincter will have been excised and this has been shown by Keighley to result in poor control in patients in whom the anastomosis is stapled at the dentate line, compared to those where it was placed at the top of the anal canal.

Despite theoretical reasons why function might be better if the anal transitional zone is preserved and an endoanal procedure avoided, evidence of improved clinical function is hard to come by. Our own experience includes two series in which all operations were undertaken or directly supervised by the author. In the first series, 60 patients had stapled (n = 14) or hand-sewn (n = 46) anastomoses. In the second series, a further 102 patients underwent stapled (n = 91) or hand-sewn (n = 11) anastomoses. Median emptying frequency was 5/24 hours and there was no difference in the proportion of patients suffering anal seepage, nor in the ability to discriminate and pass flatus successfully. Urgency to evacuate and the awareness of the need to evacuate were similar in both groups.

Malignant Risk

It is very difficult to quantify the risk of malignancy in residual colonic epithelium above the dentate line (see also Chapter 10). Restorative proctocolectomy is still a fairly new procedure and cancers may arise in colitic mucosa many years after diagnosis. One cancer has arisen in a rectal cuff 4 years after mucosal proctectomy and ileoanal pouch for severe dysplasia (10). The patient had an occult Dukes C cancer of the ascending colon discovered at subtotal colectomy 7 years before the pouch procedure and it is possible that the second cancer antedated the pouch procedure. Certainly islands of mucosa can be left after mucosectomy and it is uncertain whether the malignant risk is any higher after preserving a 1 cm cuff of transitional mucosa. King et al. (11) examined the anal mucosa in 16 consecutive proctocolectomy specimens and found moderate dysplasia in four and in one of these an unsuspected adenocarcinoma of the anal canal extending down to the dentate line. If colonic dysplasia is recognized preoperatively, our policy is to perform mucosectomy down to the dentate line. In our second series, moderate or severe dysplasia was found on colonoscopic biopsies in 4/91 patients. All four patients plus one other had moderate or severe dysplasia in the colectomy specimen (5%). Tsunoda et al. (12) studied 118 patients with colitis, only three (3%) of whom had dysplasia within the anal strippings. Two of these patients had cancers elsewhere in the colon but so did six others with no dysplasia within the anal canal.

The long-term cancer risks from leaving up to 2 cm of rectum are not known. Clearly, those patients who have either cancer or dysplasia should have mucosectomies to ablate all of the colitic mucosa. Overall, the number with dysplasia is low, but this may change over 20 to 30 years after surgery when diseased rectum is left in situ.

This debate will undoubtedly continue for some time to come, and it is obviously important for the surgical community to document the outcome of large numbers of patients over prolonged periods.

Complications

Technical differences between stapling and endoanal anastomosis might be expected to influence the incidence of certain complications, particularly anastomotic leak, pelvic sepsis, pouch-vaginal fistula, and anastomotic stricture. Major complications are relatively uncommon after restorative proctocolectomy and small studies are unlikely to reveal differences. In the St. Mark's randomized study (8), pelvic sepsis occurred with 3/17 stapled and 3/15 manual anastomoses. Keighley et al. (13) reported pelvic sepsis in 16/65 hand-sewn procedures. In our second series, pelvic sepsis occurred after 5/91 stapled procedures (three anastomotic leaks) and 0/11 endoanal procedures (no leaks). Seow-Choen et al. reported one pouch-vaginal fistula after double stapling. The overall incidence of this complication at St. Mark's was 9.7% (15 among 155 females). In contrast, Keighley et al. (13) reported three pouch-vaginal fistulae after 65 manual anastomoses. In our two series, there were four pouch-vaginal fistulae. One occurred after stapling and three after hand-sewn procedures.

There is concern that anastomotic stricture may be more common after stapling. This complication has been reported in about 7% to 15% of patients after restorative proctocolectomy (14–16) although many require repeat dilatations only. With the single-stapling technique in the author's hands, 2/91 patients developed significant strictures requiring surgical revision with good eventual outcome in our second series. Thus, the overall incidence of complications with both single and double stapling appears similar to that experienced with hand-sewn endoanal anastomosis.

The stapled ileoanal anastomosis carries the advantages that it is easier to construct, is associated with fewer problems related to tension, there is no mucosectomy, nor is there a rectal cuff to encourage sepsis. Thus this approach has been associated with a much lower incidence of anastomotic dehiscence in some series. The reduction in the prevalence of this complication has encouraged surgeons to expand the place of this operation to the semi-urgent patient who would formerly have undergone a staged procedure with preliminary colectomy and ileostomy. The avoidance of a loop ileostomy has also been popularized by some, but clearly requires considerable experience on the part of the surgeon to determine which patients should be thus managed.

Avoidance of an Ileostomy (see also Chapter 10)

There has been considerable debate surrounding the need for a protective loop ileostomy. The arguments for avoiding a temporary stoma have centered around the high morbidity reported by some following loop ileostomy closure. We reported a series of ileostomy closures with low morbidity, and found most patients were able to leave hospital soon after the procedure, so adopted a conservative approach (17). Over the last five years, we have increasingly avoided a stoma if the operation proceeded satisfactorily. Our policy is as follows: patients who are severely ill with toxic megacolon undergo a colectomy and ileostomy with a view to reconstructive surgery electively; the remainder have a restorative proctocolectomy or rectal excision and reconstruction if the colectomy has been carried out elsewhere.

Between June 1990 and March 1995, 102 patients (57 male, 45 female) underwent restorative proctocolectomy. Age ranged between 12 to 76 (median 36) years. Indications were ulcerative colitis ($n = 83$); indeterminate colitis ($n = 4$); familial adenomatous polyposis (FAP), ($n = 5$); ideopathic megacolon and/or slow transit constipation ($n = 6$); Hirschsprungs' disease ($n = 1$); diffuse angiodysplasia ($n = 1$); cancer and multiple polyps ($n = 2$). Seventy-two did not have a temporary loop ileostomy. Two patients with FAP had mucosectomies, and did not have loop ileostomies, whereas the remainder had a covering loop stoma. Of the 72 without an initial stoma, six (8%) required reoperation and formation of a loop ileostomy for the following reasons: two patients developed partial dehiscences at the anastomosis; one patient had pelvic sepsis; one stoma was raised following a small bowel perforation; one patient developed a pouch vaginal fistula, and one required defunctioning because of a painful anastomotic ulcer. All these stomas have now been closed following successful resolution of the problems.

Two patients in the defunctioned group had anastomotic sinuses which were managed by delayed stoma closure. Similarly, a radiological leak from the blind end of the J-limb was managed by deferring closure with good results.

Management of Anastomotic Dehiscence

This will depend on whether the patient has a defunctioning ileostomy or not. There is little doubt that the intensity of patient management is considerably greater when no stoma is raised. The author has adopted a selective policy with regard to stomas. In brief, patients with toxic colons undergo only a colectomy and ileostomy. Those who are urgent but not desperately ill will have a restorative proctocolectomy and loop ileostomy, so long as conditions are optimal, and the patient's nutritional indicators such as serum albumin are reasonable. The majority of elective cases in recent years have not had a routine stoma. When the operation is done in a single stage, or electively following earlier colectomy, a No. 30 soft Foley catheter is inserted in the pouch. The self-retaining balloon is not inflated, so the catheter is sutured to the perianal skin with No. 1 silk, and the catheter is held in place with waterproof adhesive tape. The catheter is left in situ for approximately 5 days. The decision to remove it is somewhat arbitrary. Bypass of pouch contents and discomfort will prompt removal. If the catheter was draining freely and the patient fails to evacuate spontaneously, it should be reinserted by 12 to 18 hours to avoid the risk of excessive pressure build up.

The indicators of sepsis are a fever, tachycardia, and a leucocytosis. Incontinence or impairment of control are possible indicators of a leak or sepsis. Similarly, excessive frequency and inadequate emptying indicate that an anastomotic problem may have developed. Digital examination may be unclear. If any doubt exists, then a contrast study will identify complications in most instances. Figure 39.2 demonstrates a leak behind the pouch. This took a large amount of contrast to demonstrate, but usually a large volume of contrast inserted is not recommended. It can be seen that the pouch is well applied to the sacrum, and the cavity is very small. This patient did not have an ileostomy, and was managed with a large pouch catheter for 4 days to divert the fecal stream, with complete resolution of the problem. When digital examination detects a significant defect in the staple or suture line, in a patient in whom an ileostomy has not been raised, then it is wise to reoperate on the patient with some urgency to construct a defunctioning stoma. This is particularly important in females with anterior defects where delay may result in the development of a pouch vaginal fistula.

Early action will largely avert later difficulties, and will also facilitate the abdominal procedure.

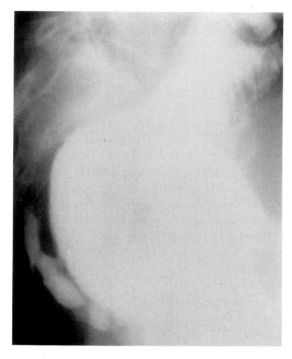

Fig. 39.2.   Small leak managed conservatively.

Bringing out a loop ileostomy in a septic patient with edematous small bowel can be extremely difficult to achieve satisfactorily and is one of many penalties paid for procrastination. The patient should be examined under anaesthesia, and an assessment is made of the extent of the defect and pelvic sepsis. The author takes the view that if an apparently satisfactorily constructed anastomosis has failed, then there is no merit in attempting to resuture it. Moreover, the tissues will be in a poor state, and attempts to resuture it may well exacerbate the problem. The pouch should be emptied, since retained contents will lead to continuing pelvic sepsis. The pelvis should be lavaged and drainage may be appropriate. Small defects dealt with in this manner will not normally pose long term problems. Late presentations are considerably more complex to manage.

The scenario here is that there will have been a leak which causes sepsis in relation to it. The resulting cavity will produce induration outside the pouch, and ultimate function will be poor unless it can be resolved satisfactorily. A small cavity can be curetted until resolution. More complex cavities need more aggressive management. An indwelling drain such as a mushroom catheter can be used, and allows daily irrigation. With such a cavity, the probability is relatively high that induration and stenosis will develop. Once the acute sepsis has re-

solved, then something must be done to deal with the fibrosis that will affect pouch motility and efficacy of evacuation. This will present a problem that may not be easy to solve without the risk of loosing the pouch. It may be possible to mobilize the pouch from below and advance part over the fibrotic segment. Alternatively, a trans-abdominal approach may be required. This may necessitate exteriorizing the pouch as an end stoma. The pelvic sepsis can be dealt with, and at a later stage, a new ileoanal anastomosis is constructed. This represents quite a high price for the patient to pay, and it may be that they will opt either to accept inferior function or have a permanent ileostomy. An alternative would be to convert the pouch to a continent ileostomy.

Case Illustration

Figure 39.3 depicts a pouch with considerable forward displacement and a small cavity which is arrowed, and outlines contrast leaking from the anastomosis. This patient did not have an ileostomy, and presented late with symptoms of frequency and urgency that would not normally be expected in a patient who did not have pouchitis. The size of the leak appears to be quite small, but the most obvious feature is the distance between the pouch

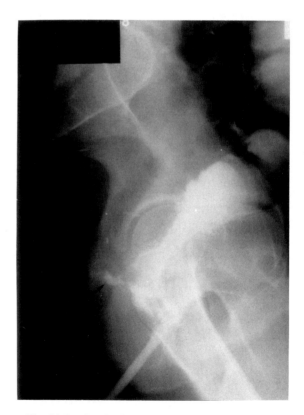

Fig. 39.3.   Leak with extensive peripouch sepsis.

and the sacrum. Examination under anesthesia revealed a considerable amount of induration behind the pouch. Exploration of the cavity with curettage removed septic granulation tissue. The cavity was drained with a small indwelling Foley catheter to provide adequate drainage. Several examinations under anaesthesia were carried out with curettage of the cavity until it was small enough to heal spontaneously with complete resolution of sepsis and restoration of satisfactory function.

Anastomotic Stenoses

Most stenoses will respond to simple dilatation in the office setting, and do not recur. Significant stenoses will need more aggressive measures to optimise pouch function. If recurrence occurs following dilatation, then division of the stricture is indicated. Incision of the stricture in three quadrants will normally suffice in short web like strictures. If the stenosis is more complex or has followed sepsis, then some sort of strictureplasty will be required. The management will depend on whether the stenosis is anal or pouch anal.

Anal Stenosis

It is likely that in such a case, that there has been ulceration of the anal canal with fibrous scarring and stenosis. Crohn's disease will have to be excluded, but some patients with ulcerative colitis develop a florid anal inflammatory disorder which may cause considerable management problems. Manual dilation is mentioned only to condemn it. Patients with ileal pouches are dependent on good internal sphincter function, and destroying the internal sphincter by forceful dilation is likely to render them incontinent. The approach used by the author is to excise the scar tissue, taking care to preserve the underlying internal sphincter. Island flaps are raised from the buttocks on either side, and advanced into the anal canal. The mobilized skin on a healthy pedicle is anastomosed to the pouch at the proximal end of the anal canal. The flaps should be constructed with a broad base just beyond the lower end of the external sphincter from which they must be released to allow adequate length. A triangular flap allows the donor defect to be closed as a V-Y plasty. Adequate illumination and exposure is essential for satisfactory endoanal surgery. The prone-jackknife position is advisable for ease of access and mobilizing the flaps. In addition, Gelpie retractors, and a lighted suction irrigator (Davis & Geck, Portsmouth, UK), helps to provide a clear field.

Pouch Anal Stenosis

An example of a pouch anal stenosis is demonstrated in Fig. 39.4. It can be seen that there is a small posterior sinus at the level of the anastomosis, but there is also a significant stenosis approximately 2 cm in length. This patient also presented late with impaired function. He had undergone an urgent stapled restorative proctocolectomy and pouch for severe acute colitis without an ileostomy. His initial progress had been uneventful. He presented several weeks after surgery and the findings were as shown on the X-ray. Examination under anaesthesia revealed a cavity which was managed along the lines outlined above. In this case the cavity was much smaller and easier to resolve. This left the management of the stenosis to be resolved. The approach used was to incise the fibrous scar tissue between the pouch and the anal canal deeply to allow entry into a healthy plane of tissue between the pouch and the sacrum, to allow the pouch to be mobilized and advanced distally. Suture was then possible to the dentate line following mucosectomy. The method of carrying out strictureplasty will vary according to the individual case. In this

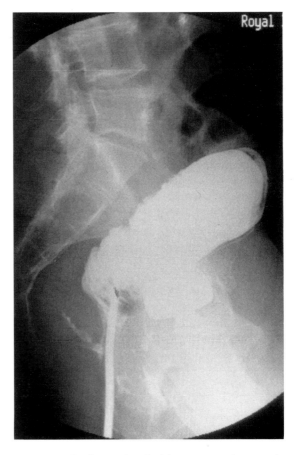

Fig. 39.4. Leak associated with anastomotic stenosis.

instance, longitudinal incisions were made in the three and nine o'clock positions. This allowed release of the pouch that was then advanced as described above. If adequate mobilization cannot be achieved from below, then a combined abdominal and transanal approach may be required.

Conclusions

Anastomotic complications may be very difficult to manage, and moreover may jeopardize pouch function. The worst scenario results in pouch excision. A temporary loop ileostomy does not prevent anastomotic complications, but does reduce the morbidity arising because of them. The authors view is that the wisest course of action in the majority is to raise an ileostomy that can often be closed in 8 weeks. This gives the patient the opportunity to experience life with a stoma that may help put less than ideal-pouch function in perspective if ultimately a decision has to be made between continuing with a pouch or opting to have a permanent stoma. In selected patients who have already had a colectomy, consideration may be given to performing the operation without a loop stoma. The surgeon adopting such a policy should be prepared to reoperate to raise a stoma at the first sign of morbidity related to the anastomosis.

References

1. Pezim ME, Pemberton JH, Beart RW Jr. Outcome of "indeterminate colitis" following ileal pouch anal anastomosis. Dis Colon Rectum 1989;32:653–8.
2. Lindqvist K, Nilsell K, Liljeqvist L. Cuff abscess and ileoanal anastomotic separations in pelvic pouch surgery. An analysis of possible etiological factors. Dis Colon Rectum 1987;30:355–9.
4. Heald RJ, Allen DR. Stapled ileoanal anastomosis: a technique to avoid mucosal proctectomy in the ileal pouch operation. Br J Surg 1986;73:571–2.
5. Miller R, Bartolo DCC, Cervero F, et al. Anorectal sampling: a comparison of normal and incontinent patients. Br J Surg 1988;75:44–7.
6. Johnston D, Holdsworth PJ, Nasmyth DG, et al. Preservation of the entire anal canal in conservative proctocolectomy for ulcerative colitis: a pilot study comparing end-to-end ileoanal anastomosis without mucosal resection with mucosal proctectomy and endoanal anastomosis. Br J Surg 1987;74:940–4.
7. Kmiot WA, Keighley MRB. Totally stapled abdominal restorative proctocolectomy. Br J Surg 1989;76:961–4.
8. Seow-Chen A, Tsunoda A, Nicholls RJ. Prospective randomized trial comparing anal function after hand-sewn ileoanal anastomosis with mucosectomy versus stapled ileoanal anastomosis without mucosectomy in restorative proctocolectomy. Br J Surg 1991;78:430–4.
9. Fazio VW, Tjandra JJ, Lavery IC. Techniques of pouch construction. In: Restorative Proctocolectomy. Nicholls R, Bartolo D, Mortensen N, eds. London: Blackwell, 1983;18–44.
10. Stern H, Walfisch, Mullen B, et al. Cancer in an ileoanal reservoir: a new late compilation? Gut 1990;31:473–5.
11. King DW, Lubowski DZ, Cook TA. Anal canal mucosa in restorative proctocolectomy for ulcerative colitis. Br J Surg 1989;76:970–2.
12. Tsunoda A, Talbot IC, Nicholls RJ. Incidence of dysplasia in the anorectal mucosa in patients having restorative proctocolectomy. Br J Surg 1990;77:506–9.
13. Keighley MRB, Winslet MC, Flinn R, et al. Multivariate analysis of factors influencing the results of restorative proctocolectomy. Br J Surg 1989;76:740–4.
14. Galandiuk S, Scott NA, Dozois RR, et al. Ileal pouch-anal anastomosis. Ann Surg 1990;212:446–54.
15. Keighley MRB, Grobler S, Bain I. An audit of restorative proctocolectomy. Gut 1993;34:680–4.
16. Setti-Carraro P, Ritchie JK, Wilkinson KH, et al. The first 10 years' experience of restorative proctocolectomy for ulcerative colitis. Gut 1994;35:1070–5.
17. Lewis P, Bartolo DCC. Closure of loop ileostomy after restorative proctocolectomy. Ann R Coll Surg Engl 1990;72:263–5.

40 Perineal Complications after Ileal Pouch-Anal Anastomosis

Jeffrey W. Milsom

Despite the fact that the restorative proctocolectomy (RP) has become the therapy of choice in the surgical management of ulcerative colitis, there remains an appreciable complication rate following the operation of up to 50% (1–5). The development of a fistula or abscess in the perineal or vaginal areas following RP heralds a potentially serious problem in the patient, since such an event not only may lead to a significant amount of pain and discharge, but nearly always requires further corrective surgery, and implies some degree of failure of the ileal pouch-anal anastomosis. It also looms as one of the most common reasons for pouch "failure," meaning that the pouch must be removed because of an inability to surgically correct this problem by other means (1,4).

The incidence of fistula or abscess to the perineum or vagina varies in the literature, but ranges from about 2% to as high as 16% (1–6). Generally speaking, this type of problem presents itself within several months of the ileostomy closure (after a two stage procedure), or early on (within days to weeks of ileal pouch surgery) after a one stage procedure. Despite this concern, there remains a considerable amount of expertise in the management of these problems to suggest that the vast majority of fistulas arising after RP can be successfully treated without the need for permanent functional loss or loss of the pouch itself. The purpose of this chapter, therefore, is to outline the underlying causes of these fistulas, then to suggest appropriate management of them.

Etiology of Perineal Complications after Restorative Proctocolectomy

The underlying cause of an abscess or fistula in the perineum or vagina after RP bears directly on the timing of its appearance after surgery and any associated abnormalities seen in this area. Fistulas and abscesses seen early after RP or after subsequent ileostomy closure (within one month after the operation) are almost certainly due to an infectious complication related to the anastomosis. Perineal complications seen after this time may be related to one of the following: (1) occult dehiscence of the anastomosis with or without associated stricturing; (2) cryptoglandular disease as in the non-IBD population; and (3) complex etiology such as Crohn's disease; or rarely (4) trauma related to childbirth. Treatment is naturally related to the etiology and will be discussed below.

Clinical Presentations

Patients developing perianal abscesses or fistulas after RP do not usually have symptoms that differ markedly from symptoms of non-RP patients who have similar problems. There may be some confusion as to perianal symptomatology in RP patients, since they often have a mild to moderate amount of irritation or discomfort in the perianal skin after surgery resulting from loose bowel movements. Complaints about pain, fever, or purulent drainage from the perineum or vagina must alert the surgeon to the possibility that an infectious problem may be developing, and thus the patient should be seen as soon as this is practical.

A careful examination should be carried out where the surgeon has the proper instruments to examine the patient comfortably and thoroughly. If the patient is so uncomfortable that a thorough exam is not possible, then he/she is scheduled for an examination in the operating room under general anesthesia.

The vaginal septum should be carefully evaluated in all female RP patients with the possibility of a perineal complication. Some thickening may be noted even after uneventful surgery, but usually this is not marked. Tenderness is distinctly abnormal, even early after RP surgery. Any amount of cloudy drainage from the vagina is highly suspicious for a fistula, especially if the patient has a history of any passage of air from the vagina.

If an examination fails to disclose any signs of infection or fistula, but clinical suspicion is high, then a water soluble contrast enema should be ordered. The procedure should be done by a radiologist familiar with the ileoanal procedure, and a soft latex catheter with an inflatable balloon at its tip (10–16 French size) should be used. This may demonstrate a sinus tract or fistula that was not clinically apparent, although the yield is probably low if the examination was done under anesthesia.

Treatment Strategies

General Principles

If the patient is febrile and has an obvious infection, then antibiotics are begun either orally or systemically as per the clinical decision of the treating surgeon. If a serious infection is present with a major soft tissue component, then we would prefer to use systemic antibiotics and treat the patient as an inpatient in the hospital setting. Generally we use a broad spectrum antibiotic active against gram positive and gram negative organisms, plus metronidazole. If no definite abscess, fistula, or soft tissue infection is found, but we are still considering an infectious component, then we would probably still consider an empiric trial of oral antibiotics for 7 to 10 days, using a combination of ciprofloxacin 500 mg bid and metronidazole 500 mg tid, requesting the patient to be seen in the office within one or two weeks of initiating therapy.

When an abscess is encountered, then we advocate simple drainage of the area over the point of maximal fluctuance, trying to drain any perianal abscess as near to the anal margin as possible, so as to not create a long fistulous tract. Once a small opening is made, then a mushroom catheter is inserted into the depths of the cavity and sutured in place using a 2-0 or 3-0 braided absorbable suture. The drain is cut off about 2 cm above the skin. This is a simple technique that avoids the need for packing the wound, which may be very uncomfortable. If the procedure is possible in the outpatient setting and the patient is not systemically ill, then he/she is sent home on oral antibiotics and instructed to soak in a warm Sitz bath or tub of water at least three times a day, with visits to the outpatient area weekly or every two weeks.

If a definite fistula is noted (either perianal or pouch-vaginal) in the presence of active infection, then an alternative might be to place a seton drain, completely traversing the fistula and draining it at the same time. This may be more uncomfortable to position in the outpatient setting, and often requires a general anesthetic. The procedure is described in detail in Chapter 35. As in all infectious or fistulous complications of inflammatory bowel disease (IBD), a biopsy should be obtained in order to attempt to make a diagnosis of Crohn's disease, even though the absence of granulomas does not exclude it as a diagnostic consideration. Postoperative care is similar to that after mushroom drain placement.

It is very important to emphasize that the acute infectious complication occurring after RP must be dealt with in an expeditious fashion, so that any infectious process is limited and quickly placed under control. The potential for infection to cause scarring of the perianal area, including the anal canal, anal sphincters, and the low pouch area must be minimized since these patients already have a continence mechanism that has been somewhat altered by the ileal pouch surgery. Thus it is reasonable to hospitalize most of these patients if there is any significant soft tissue component to their infection, and place them on systemic antibiotics. Additionally, if the infection is extensive, or if drainage is significant from a vaginal fistula, then it is wise to consider (re)establishing the loop ileostomy coincident with treating the infection.

In summary, the principles of acute management of perineal complications include: (1) careful examination; (2) immediate drainage of any purulent collection with drain placement; (3) antibiotics; and (4) diversion with loop ileostomy as indicated, especially in vaginal fistula. The patient's perineal tissues are then given the opportunity to resolve the acute inflammatory process before definitive therapy is undertaken. This healing period should usually last for a minimum of two to three months, depending on the extent of inflammation present.

If Crohn's disease is a possibility, then the patient should be advised as such and medical therapy specific for this disease should be considered. This could include prolonged oral metronidazole therapy, topical antiinflammatory medication to the anal canal or pouch, or consideration for use of an immunosuppresive such as 6-mercaptopurine.

Definitive Therapies

Once the acute infectious process has resolved, it is reasonable to consider definitive repair of the fistulous problem, since success rates in pouch-vaginal fistulas (meaning healing of the fistula with reestablishment of intestinal continuity) range from at least 50% (7) to as high as 85% (5), with similar success rates for pouch or ano-perineal (1,4,6). The type of repair contemplated will depend on the location of the fistula, the degree of anal stenosis present and whether or not Crohn's disease is a possibility. There are three main surgical options: (1) simple fistulotomy; (2) transanal advancement flap procedures (there are several types); and (3) Abdominal-anal revision with advancement of the pouch to cover the internal opening of the fistula. There are other surgical repairs (transvaginal approach (8), fibrin glue, gracilis muscle interposition (9) but these are rarely used).

The preoperative evaluation should include a thorough examination including endoscopy of the pouch and a water soluble contrast enema of the pouch to search for occult branching of the fistula and for any presacral component to the fistula. "Pouchography" by contrast enema can frequently be falsely negative (9), so it is only an ancillary test, and may help with assessment of pouch configuration (size and distensibility). Signs of Crohn's disease are searched for, since the latter might sway the surgeon away from surgical therapy. If the anal canal is scarred, or the infection was remarkable during the acute event, then it may be reasonable to consider an examination under anesthesia solely to assess the anal canal, ileal pouch, and the vagina so as to plan thoroughly for a later operation and to discuss matters fully with the patient prior to definitive therapy. If a proximal stoma was not used at the onset of the problem, then it may also be wise to consider this concomitant with the definitive repair if a high fistula or extensive scarring is present.

For nearly all patients, we perform a thorough mechanical preparation of the intestinal tract prior to operation (if not diverted), then perform an irrigation of the pouch on the operating table once the patient is under general anesthesia, generally in the lithotomy position. If the fistula is located anteriorly, then the patient is positioned in the prone-jackknife position. A urinary catheter is placed, then the perianal area is infiltrated using a local anesthetic with epinephrine (we use bupivicaine with epinephrine 1:100,000 solution). Anal effacement sutures are helpful in exposing the anal margin area and lighted anoscopes (Hill-Ferguson retractors; see Chapter 35) are very useful in viewing the canal. If some degree of anal stenosis is present, dilation with lubricated gloved fingers is preferable to blind insertion of dilators since this is likely to be a more controllable dilating maneuver. Once the index finger can be inserted, a small anoscope can then be used to directly view the canal, and probes inserted from the external opening, can search for the fistula. We may use a variety of maneuvers to find the internal opening (see Chapter 35), but forceful blind probing should not be attempted because of the possibility of creating a false passage. We generally use perioperative prophylactic antibiotics, beginning at least one hour before the surgery, and giving two doses postoperatively. We continue the antibiotics for 3 to 5 days for more extensive procedures, especially if there has been any contamination during the operation.

Repair of the Simple Anal Fistula

If a patient truly has developed a simple fistula-in-ano, then it is reasonable to consider fistulotomy as a treatment option, especially if the fistula is posterior and involves only a minimal amount of sphincter muscle. This situation does occur in RP patients, and has been used as a reparative technique in reported series ranging from 0% to 57% of cases (1,4). The policy at the Cleveland Clinic has been to use this sparingly if at all since these patients must maintain all sphincter reserve possible. Principles involved are similar to conventional fistula surgery, keeping the above principles in mind. If there is any question about whether to divide the sphincter, then an error on the side of conservatism is advised, meaning use of a flap procedure with primary repair of the fistula and no division of any muscle.

Transanal Advancement Flap Procedures

These procedures are the most common operations used when a vaginal or perineal fistula occurs

488 J.W. Milsom

after RP and the tissues have recovered from any
acute infection (4,5,7,10). Using the above general
principles, we locate the fistula and infiltrate local
anesthetic into the region of the internal opening
of the fistula and 4 to 5 cm above it, into the wall of
the pouch and the soft tissues beneath it. There are
three distinct types of advancement flaps that may
be used in the repair of the pouch-anal or pouch-
vaginal fistula: (1) advancement flap of the lowest
portion of the pouch to lie over the internal opening; (2) advancement of the anal skin from below
the anastomosis to above the internal opening; (3)
complete circumferential transanal pouch advancement. We will discuss the indications for
each, and proceed with the steps needed to safely
accomplish each of them.

Advancement of a Pouch-Based Flap

This is a flap that may be used for closure of an
internal opening of a fistula leading to either the
perineum or the vagina. It is indicated for such a
purpose if the condition of the pouch is healthy
and neither scarred nor inflamed. Likewise, if
there is significant scarring or stenosis of the anal
canal (usually related to previous sepsis) then it will
be difficult to safely visualize the pouch and thereafter mobilize a flap from it. This flap is used when
the fistula is the simplest type that requires an advancement flap procedure.

The procedure should be set up as in the general principles outlined above, using anal effacement sutures, appropriate positioning of the patient, and infiltration of the anal canal and flap
area with local anesthesia. The shape we have used
in our department has been a wide U-shaped or
"smile"-shaped flap that encompasses the full-
thickness of the pouch wall. The procedure begins
with a careful examination of the anal and perianal
skin, and of the vagina in females. Lighted anal
retractors are used, and gentle probing of the
fistula is carried out with a small probe. Occasionally, a thin-tipped curved clamp may also be useful
in delineating a tract. Once located, the tract is
curetted of granulation tissue, which is sent along
with any other inflamed tissue for biopsy.

Next, using electrosurgery, the scar tissue surrounding the internal opening is dissected away
from the underlying sphincter muscle out to normal tissue in both the pouch region as well as the
anal canal (Fig. 40.1). The electrosurgery is also
used to make the initial incisions laterally from this
area to define the pouch. Dissection is then carried
both cephalad and caudally to free the normal
tissues from adherent structures, using fine dissecting scissors to mobilize the pouch away from the
underlying sphincters, then out into the perirectal
fat (laterally or posteriorly) or into rectovaginal
septum (anteriorly). Control of the depth of dissection may be accurately maintained anteriorly by
placing a finger into the vagina (experienced assistant) while the surgeon dissects up the plane of the
septum. The flap is freed for a distance for about

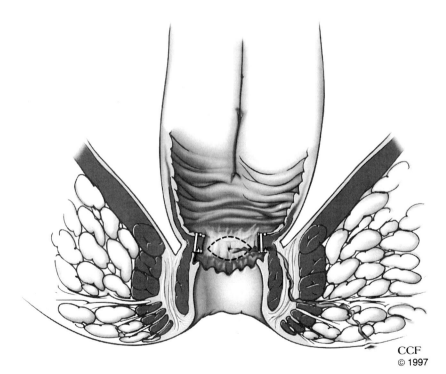

CCF
© 1997

Fig. 40.1. Advancement flap scar is
dissected away from internal opening.

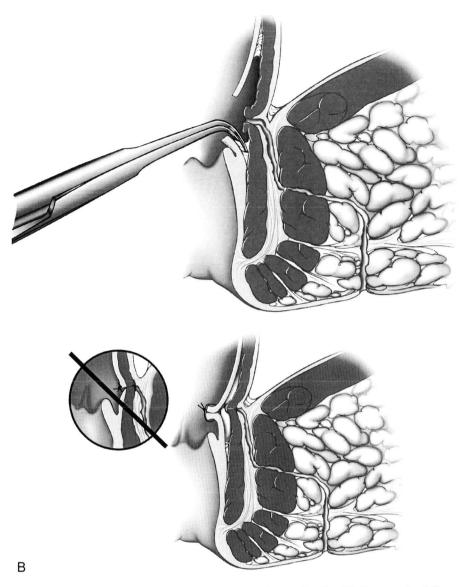

B

Fig. 40.2.   (A) Using thorek curved scissors to dissect distally. (B) Prevents buckling.

5 or 6 cm so it may easily reach into the anal canal without tension. This is gauged by pulling caudally on the pouch with an atraumatic instrument such as a Babcock or Allis-type clamp. The anoderm is next mobilized caudally using sharp dissection with a small scalpel blade or a scissor with an acutely-angled tip, e.g., thorek scissors (Fig. 40.2). This is a key step in helping the flap lie down over the internal opening without tension, and in allowing for closure of the internal opening without buckling the edge of the anoderm into it.

Advancement of the flap begins with two or three size 2-0 braided absorbable sutures being placed into the posterior of the flap at about its midportion, then placing the second bite of these sutures below the closed internal opening (Fig. 40.3). All sutures are first placed, then tied.

Then the flap is sewn into position using 3-0 absorbable sutures in a running fashion, placing sutures first at the corners and the midpoint of the "smile," then running them together from the ends to the middle (Fig. 40.4). Interrupted sutures are placed as necessary to ensure good apposition of the edges of the flap. For pouch-perineal fistulas, the external track is drained with a small mushroom catheter, placing the tip just outside the sphincter muscles, and sewing it in place with a 3-0 braided absorbable suture.

If the complication leading to the fistula has been a major problem for the patient, or if the procedure has been difficult, serious consideration should be given to diversion with a loop ileostomy coincident with the procedure.

Postoperative care is conducted as described

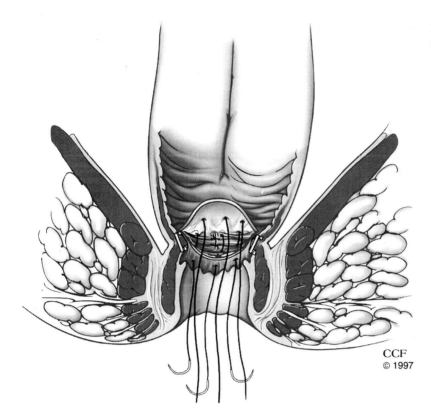

Fig. 40.3.   Placing sutures on serosal side of flap.

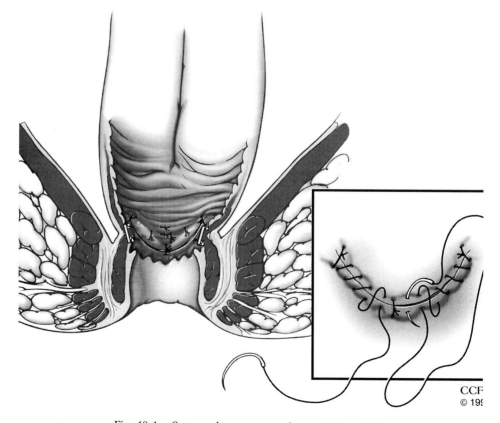

Fig. 40.4.   Suture placement at edges and in middle.

above. Antibiotics are given longer than one day only if there has been serious contamination. The patient is kept in the hospital for 1 to 3 days, depending on the extent of dissection and if a stoma has been created. Clear liquids are begun immediately after surgery, and the diet is advanced on the second postoperative day if no fever is present and the patient is doing well otherwise.

Anal Advancement Flap

This procedure is used in cases where there is significant scarring of the anal canal, with or without anal stenosis present, or where there is significant inflammation of the distal portion of the pouch such that it could be extremely difficult to mobilize and advance distally.

The procedure is set up in the same fashion as the pouch advancement, and in fact the surgeon may be initially prepared to perform the latter, only to find that there is too much stenosis or inflammation. Thus the anal advancement procedure should be in the surgeon's "armamentarium" when confronting pouch-related fistulas.

Once the decision is made to perform this flap, a more narrow U-shaped flap is traced out in the anal canal, still keeping the base rather wide (Fig. 40.5). This caudally-based flap is only taken down to the internal sphincter, then allowed to thicken once the lower edge of the flap dissection proceeds below the muscle. All scar around the internal opening is excised, and the lower edge of the pouch is

certainly freed from the sphincters so the internal opening may be closed without drawing the pouch into the closure. The internal opening is closed as described above and the flap is well mobilized so as to reach the pouch without tension. Suturing it in place proceeds in a mirror fashion to the technique described above. Consideration for diversion should follow criteria as mentioned above.

Postoperative care is as in the pouch advancement procedure as described above.

Transanal Pouch Advancement

This is the most complex of transanal repairs and constitutes a major anal operative procedure. It is used when there is a complex anal fistula to either the vagina or the perineum, and concomitant scar or inflammation that is circumferential or nearly so. This type of procedure should only be contemplated if a concomitant stoma is performed (or already exists) and the patient is prepared for a laparotomy if the procedure is not possible by the transanal route alone. The degree of severity of the anal canal and distal pouch scarring when this type of pouch is used also means that the patient should be mentally prepared for a permanent stoma if the procedure is not possible. The general risks of pelvic surgery should also be discussed with the patient, including potential for sexual and bladder dysfunction, pelvic hemorrhage, ureteric or urethral injury, and the potential for worsening of incontinence for stools.

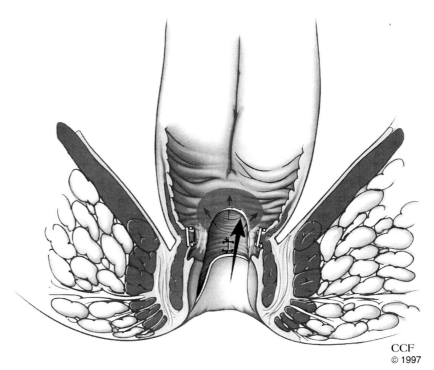

Fig. 40.5.   The anal advancement flap: U-shaped.

CCF
© 1997

Preoperative preparations are as for the previously described anal procedures. The anus is carefully effaced with circumferential sutures (usually six to eight), then the anal canal is carefully evaluated and dilated with digital exam, then a small lighted retractor is used to inspect the canal and distal pouch. After infiltration of local anesthetic, the scar in the canal is carefully excised using scalpel dissection starting distally, taking care not to excise any sphincter muscle (Fig. 40.6). The dissection is carried cephalad to the top of the scarred area (which may be 2 to 4 or 5 cm) then several centimeters beyond, so that the entire pouch is freed from both the sphincters and pelvic floor (Fig. 40.7). Pelvic fat should be visible around the pouch. A careful method of dissection entails continuing to work from normal tissues to abnormal, so that planes may be recognized and buttonholing of the pouch can be avoided. A finger in the vagina can help define the proper plane in this area, as described in the previous section.

As the pouch is dissected from surrounding tissues, the edges of each quadrant are grasped with long Allis-type clamps, which permits gentle traction to be placed on the tissues as well as to allow proper orientation. The distal aspect of the repair, the anal canal, should also be mobilized so that good apposition of the tissues are possible when the pouch edges are sewn in place. The internal opening of the fistula is closed as described above, in two layers.

Once the pouch is mobilized and will freely reach distally to cover the internal opening and the defect left by the scar excision, 2-0 braided absorbable sutures are placed into each of the four quadrants of the pouch (full thickness) and as many as four more are placed between the initial sutures if it seems there will be any difficulty in seeing the distal edge of the pouch once the sutures are tied. The next key point to tying the sutures down with the minimum tension on the tissue is to place the second bite of all of the sutures into the anoderm (catching a little internal sphincter with each of them). **Before** tying down on any of the stitches, the perianal stay sutures are then released so as relieve as much tension on the tissue as possible, and the sutures are tied circumferentially about the anal canal (Fig. 40.8). Additional sutures are

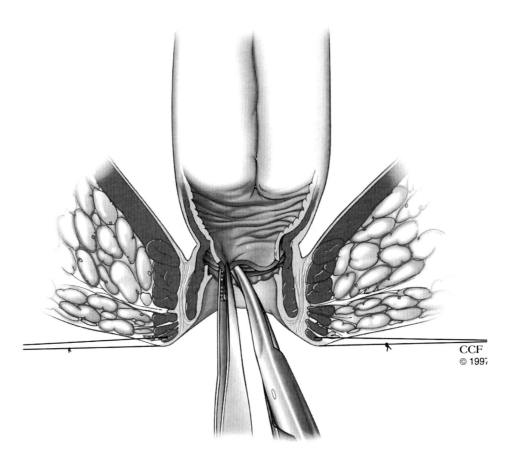

Fig. 40.6.   Scar in anal canal is excised first distally in initiating the pouch advancement.

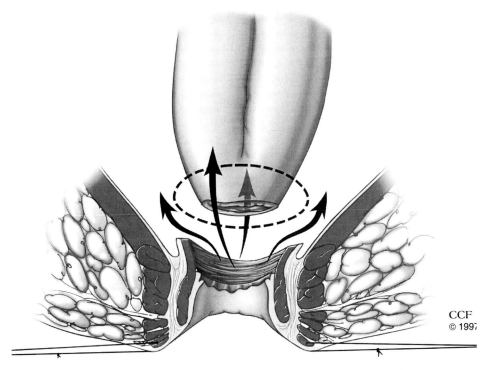

Fig. 40.7.   Pouch advancement: entire pouch is freed from the sphincters.

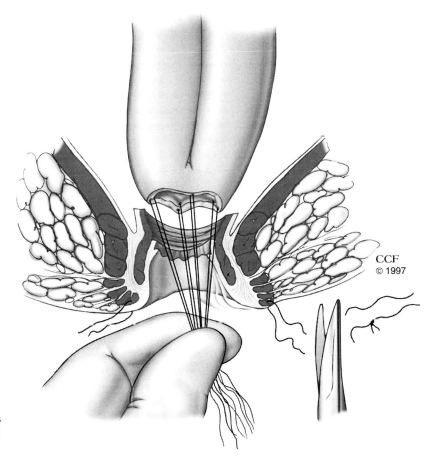

Fig. 40.8.   Before tying down the sutures of the pouch advancement, the perianal stay sutures are released.

placed between these initial sutures in order to achieve good apposition of the edges of the repair. If it is obvious that adequate pouch mobilization will not be possible, i.e., that the transanal approach will not suffice to free the pouch sufficiently to draw it down over the repaired internal opening and the excised scar area in the anal canal without tension, or if there has been accidental tearing, shredding, or buttonholing of the pouch while mobilizing it, then serious consideration must be given to proceeding on to a laparotomy with an abdominal approach to mobilizing the pouch. This procedure will be described in the next section below.

Because of the extensive nature of this operation, we prefer to leave these patients in the hospital for at least 2 or 3 days, giving them the same basic care as patients described earlier. Since all of these patients will have diversion by a loop ileostomy, if they are comfortable, showing no signs of infection, and can care for their stoma reliably, they can be safely discharged home with plans for a routine follow-up in two to three weeks' time.

Abdominal-Anal Revision of the Restorative Proctocolectomy

If the situation arises that the pouch simply cannot feasibly be mobilized from the perineal aspect in order to repair the defect in the anal canal as well as the internal opening of the fistula, then a laparotomy with complete mobilization of the pouch transabdominally must be considered. This repair permits optimal freeing up of the pouch from the pelvic tissues, and furthermore will allow mobilization of the superior mesenteric artery pedicle as well. It has been described for use in treating chronic pelvic abscesses related to the pouch as well as fistulas and strictures related to it (9,11–13).

The procedure involves initial mobilization of the pouch from the anal aspect, then performance of the laparotomy with the patient being maintained in the modified lithotomy position so as to permit simultaneous operating from both aspects as needed once the abdominal mobilization is begun. Ureteric stents are placed at the outset of the operation if extensive adhesions are anticipated. Adhesions are lysed and the superior mesenteric artery is identified proximally and traced into the pelvis. Generally, the pouch is freed from the pelvic tissues rather easily, except where there has been pelvic infection. Thus the mobilization should proceed from normal to abnormal, and generally from posterior to anterior until the pelvic floor is reached circumferentially. The level of dissection is checked with one hand of the surgeon in the pelvis, and one passed transanally after a second glove is placed over it (Fig. 40.9). The pouch is discon-

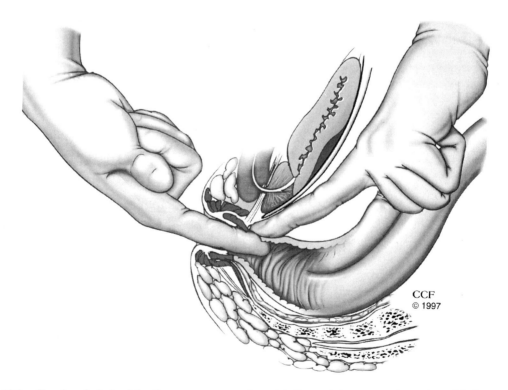

Fig. 40.9.   Two-handed check by the surgeon—one in pelvis from abdomen, and one in pelvis from anus.

nected from the pelvic floor and brought up into the operative field. Any pelvic abscess cavity is curretted or debrided.

The pouch is then trimmed of any scar on its distal aspect, and enterotomies are closed. Insufflation of the pouch should be performed using saline via a bulb syringe to ensure that no enterotomies have been missed. The base of its mesentery is then fully mobilized up to the pancreas, and a trial of making the pouch reach to the pelvic floor is performed by passing a long Allis or Babcock type clamp transanally and pulling down on the pouch.

If a difficult anastomosis is anticipated, then quadrant sutures can be placed into the pouch from the abdominal aspect prior to passing the pouch to the perineal surgeon. The anastomosis is then performed as described in the previous section, using every maneuver to relieve tension on the anastomosis when the sutures are tied down.

Finally, if it is possible, an omental pedicle is placed into the pelvis so as to lie over the area of previous scar or sepsis. It can be sutured into place with several sutures of absorbable material. A closed suction drain is also placed and brought out through a separate stab wound in the lower abdomen.

Results of the Various Operations for Perineal Complications after Restorative Proctocolectomy

The outcome of the various operations used in the treatment of perineal/vaginal fistulas may be broadly divided into perineal approach results and abdominal-anal operation results, since few authors have selected out results for each individual operation (partially based on the fact that these operations are not performed frequently by anyone). In a very general sense, salvage operations performed transanally have been associated with a range of outcomes, with Paye et al. reporting zero of five successful repairs (9), and in our series of vaginal fistulas at the Cleveland Clinic a success rate of 85% (10 of 12 patients) if the diagnosis was not Crohn's, and a success rate of 25% (3 of 12 patients) if Crohn's was present (14). O'Kelly et al. of Oxford reported healing of all 5 of five vaginal fistulas presenting within several weeks after RP, using an endovaginal flap procedure (not described in this chapter, but obviously an option). Two cases in their series presented six or more months after RP and were found to be Crohn's patients, ultimately requiring pouch excision. These results contrast with those reported by Wexner et al. in 1989 from a multiinstitutional study of

21 patients with pouch-vaginal fistulas, where a 50% success rate was seen, with transvaginal repair the least successful procedure (7). Much of the variability relates to whether or not Crohn's is present.

Results after the more extensive abdominal-anal procedure are somewhat less successful, with rates ranging from 50% to 80% (9,11,15). This is not surprising, given the serious nature of the fistulous disease in these patients.

One question that remains largely unanswered is what the ultimate functional outcome is after the repair of a fistula is undertaken. Although it seems that results are probably reasonably good, this is not an issue that has been carefully evaluated in the literature up to this point.

In summary, it appears that the majority of patients developing perineal complications after RP do have options that will allow them to be cured of their problem. Fistulas presenting many months after the procedure are likely to be associated with Crohn's disease, and a cautious approach is advised in this circumstance. Pouch excision may become necessary, but the excision rate in most of the large series is less than 40% (1,3,4). Thus a pouch-related fistula is not synonymous with ultimate failure of the pouch.

Although perineal complications thankfully appear only rarely after restorative proctocolectomy, if a stepwise and methodical approach is used, most of these patients can be expected to gain good function of their pouch and avoid a permanent stoma.

References

1. Galandiuk S, Scott NA, Dozois RR, et al. Ileal pouch-anal anastomosis: reoperation for pouch-related complications. Ann Surg 1990;212:446–52.
2. Keighley MRB, Grobler S, Bain I. An audit of restorative proctocolectomy. Gut 1993;34:680–4.
3. Mikkola K, Luukkonen P, Jarvinen HJ. Long-term results of restorative proctocolectomy for ulcerative colitis. Int J Colorect Dis 1995;10:10–14.
4. Foley EF, Schoetz DJ, Roberts PL, et al. Rediversion after ileal pouch-anal anastomosis. Dis Colon Rectum 1995;38:793–8.
5. Ozuner G, Hull T, Lee P, et al. What happens to a pelvic pouch when a fistula develops? Dis Colon Rectum 1997;40:543–7.
6. Rothenberger DA, Gemlo BT, Deen KI. Complications after ileal pouch-anal anastomosis. In Fazio VW, Allen CD, Keighley MRB, Hanauer S, eds. Inflammatory bowel disease. London: Churchill Livingstone International, 1996;793–801.

7. Wexner AD, Jensen L, Rothenberger DA, et al. Long-term functional analysis of the ileoanal reservoir. Dis Colon Rectum 1989;32:275–81.

8. O'Kelly TJ, Merrett M, Mortensen NJ, et al. Pouch vaginal fistula following restorative proctocolectomy. Br J Surg 1994;81:1374–5.

9. Paye F, Penna C, Chiche L, et al. Pouch-related fistula following restorative proctocolectomy. Br J Surg 1996;83:1574–7.

10. Fleshman JW, McLeod RS, Stern H. Improved results following use of an advancement technique in the treatment of ileoanal anastomotic complications. Int J Colorectal Dis 1988;3:161–5.

11. Sagar PM. Long-term results of ileal pouch anal anastomosis in patients with Crohn's disease. Dis Colon Rectum 1996;39:893–8.

12. Fazio VW, Tjandra JJ, Lavery IC, et al. Long-term follow-up for strictureplasty in Crohn's disease. Dis Colon Rectum 1993;36:353.

13. Fazio VW, Tjandra JJ. Pouch advancement and neo-ileoanal anastomotic suture for anovaginal fistula complicating restorative proctocolectomy. Br J Surg 1992;79:694–6.

14. Lee PY, Fazio VW. Pouch-vaginal fistula following restorative proctocolectomy: characteristics and outcome. Dis Colon Rectum 1995;38:P13.

15. Wu J. Strictureplasty in Crohn's disease. In Cameron JL, ed. Current surgery therapy. Philadelphia, BC Decker, 1997; in press

41 Pouchitis

Jacques Heppell and Keith A. Kelly

The surgical treatment of ulcerative colitis has evolved considerably over the past few decades. Although proctocolectomy with Brooke ileostomy was the standard operation of the past, surgeons now often employ proctocolectomy with ileal-pouch/anal canal anastomosis. This operation completely excises the diseased mucosa of the large intestine, and yet it preserves transanal defecation and reasonable fecal continence and avoids a permanent ileostomy. These results are achieved because the anal sphincters remain intact to provide fecal continence and because the ileal pouch provides a satisfactory reservoir for feces (1).

This newly devised operation, however, is accompanied by morphological changes in the mucosa of the ileal reservoir as it adapts to its new luminal environment. In addition, inflammatory changes may occur in the mucosa of the pouch and cause a condition now referred to as "pouchitis." In fact pouchitis, a condition first described by Kock, who noted it in patients with a continent ileostomy (2), has become the most frequent long-term complication of ileal-pouch/anal canal anastomosis.

This chapter will deal with the presentation, diagnosis, prevalence, cause, treatment, outcome, and prevention of pouchitis.

Presentation

Symptoms and Signs

Pouchitis is characterized mainly by diarrhea, sometimes containing blood. The diarrhea is usually watery and foul smelling. The onset of the diarrhea is often rapid and accompanied by a painful sensation in the deep pelvis, abdominal cramps, urgency, anal soiling, and incontinence. General malaise and low-grade fever may be present. When severe, the pouchitis can also be associated with weight loss and fever (3). In some cases, extraintestinal manifestations, such as arthritis, uveitis, erythema nodosum and pyoderma gangrenosum, can appear, even though the large intestine has been resected (4). The intensity of the extraintestinal manifestations often parallels that of the intestinal symptoms (5). Subjectively, patients are reminded of the symptoms they had when they had colitis.

On physical examination, the patient may be febrile and dehydrated. The anal canal and the distal portion of the ileal reservoir are painful on digital rectal examination which often reveals blood on the examining finger.

Endoscopic Findings

The healthy small intestinal mucosa shows a clearly visible vascular pattern at endoscopy. In ileal pouches, the vascular pattern often disappears once the diverting ileostomy is closed (4). With pouchitis, the endoscopic aspects are similar to those of an acute mucosal colitis. The mucosa becomes edematous, hyperemic, friable, and granular, with punctate ulcers present (Fig. 41.1). Occasionally, superficial, linear ulcers can be seen. The presence of rake-type ulcers, however, should raise the suspicion of Crohn's disease (6), although rake ulcers are sometimes seen in patients with severe pouchitis (7). The changes can be diffuse or patchy, and can extend into the ileum proximal to the pouch (8). Changes that resemble pseudomembranous enteritis with a whitish exudate on the

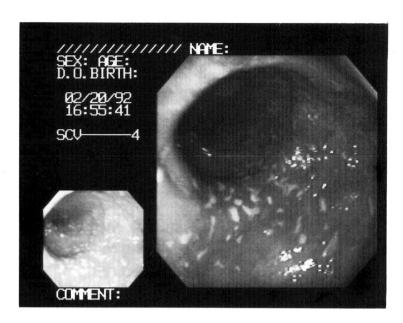

Fig. 41.1. Endoscopic appearance of ileal pouchitis.

surface of the mucosa also may be found. Thus, the endoscopic pattern of pouchitis is polymorphic.

Some patients with characteristic symptoms of pouchitis may have a normal appearing mucosa (9), although this is unusual. A correlation is usually present between the mucosal appearance, the mucosal histology and the symptoms. A linear relationship between the degree of acute inflammation present on pouch mucosal biopsy, the frequency of defecation, and the macroscopic evidence of inflammation within the pouch has been reported (10). Nonetheless, asymptomatic patients with normal endoscopy can show histological abnormalities, and vice versa (11).

Histologic Findings

Changes in the mucosa of the ileal pouch occur in response to the new luminal environment. The ileal mucosa assumes a colonic-like pattern that can be mistaken for colonic mucosa on biopsy. The villi atrophy, the crypts elongate, and the goblet cells enlarge (10,12). The goblet cells become distended with mucus. The mucus produced changes from that typical of ileum to a sulphomucin more typical of colon (13). Inflammatory cells, especially eosinophils, can be found in the lamina propria, although the colonic metaplasia can occur in the absence of inflammation (14). Paneth cells with atypical granules appear (15). Despite these changes, however, disaccharides characteristic of small intestinal mucosa are still produced by the mucosa (16). The changes

are usually well established by six months postoperatively (17). They are found in pouches of patients with ulcerative colitis and with familial adenomatous polyposis and are present in the absence of symptomatic pouchitis (14). Of interest is that similar changes have been described in the terminal ileum after a straight ileoanal anastomosis without a reservoir (18).

When symptoms of pouchitis appear, acute mucosal inflammation and ulceration are characteristically present in the pouch mucosa (Fig. 41.2). Crypt abscesses and goblet cell depletion also occur. The degree of acute inflammation can be mild, moderate or severe (10) (Table 41.1). Crypt cell proliferation is greater in pouches with pouchitis, compared to those without, and in pouches without pouchitis, compared to healthy ileum (19). The endoscopic changes of pouchitis can be patchy, so sampling errors can complicate the histological diagnosis. Biopsies should be obtained at a distance from the pouch/anal anastomosis and from pouch suture lines. The clinician should remember that acute inflammation can also occur in mucosal prolapse, mucosal ischemia, or infective enteritis (20).

The clinical syndrome of pouchitis usually correlates with the severity of the endoscopic and histologic features of acute inflammation (10). However, histologic inflammation does not correlate with the type of reservoir, the residual volume after evacuation and the compliance of the pouch (10). Also, no absolute correlation is present between the degree or severity of the clinical symptoms and the acute and chronic histologic changes, nor is a

Fig. 41.2. Histologic patterns: hematoxylin × eosin stain (× 44 magnification). (A) Villous pattern of healthy terminal ileum. (B) Adaptive changes. Villous atrophy, elongated ileal crypts and chronic inflammation in an ileal pouch. (C) Acute inflammation with predominance of neutrophils and ulceration in patients with ileal pouchitis.

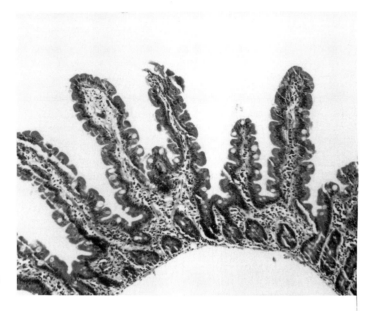

A

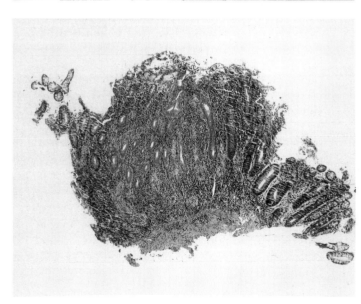

B

C

Table 41.1.   Histopathological criteria for severity of inflammation.*

	Score
Acute	
- polymorph infiltration	
mild	1
moderate + crypt abscess	2
severe + crypt abscess	3
- ulceration per low power field	
<25%	1
≥25%≤50%	2
>50%	3
- total possible	6
Chronic	
- chronic inflammatory cell infiltration	
mild	1
moderate	2
severe	3
- villous atrophy	
partial	1
subtotal	2
total	3
- total possible	6

*Data from Moskowitz et al. (10).

correlation present between the severity of inflammation and the preoperative duration of disease, the presence of cancer or dysplasia in the original operative specimen and the extraalimentary manifestations (21).

Radiologic Findings

Radiographic studies are usually not helpful in establishing the diagnosis of pouchitis. Fistulas, stenoses, and other abnormalities found on radiologic "pouchogram" prior to ileostomy closure indicate those patients at high risk of long-term complications following ileal-pouch/anal canal anastomosis (22), but no correlation has been established between such abnormalities and subsequent development of pouchitis. Pouchograms and computerized axial tomography (23) can detect peripouch inflammatory complications such as anastomotic dehiscence, phlegmon and abscess, but not pouchitis. Endoluminal transpouch ultrasonography (24) also can detect anastomotic dehiscences and peripouch sepsis, but again, not pouchitis.

In contrast, [111]Indium-labeled granulocyte scans are helpful in the diagnosis of pouchitis. In a group of patients with pouchitis, radioactive granulocytes localized to the pouch mucosa (25). The infiltration with granulocytes lessened after metronidazole therapy.

Other Laboratory Findings

Little information exists regarding other laboratory abnormalities in pouchitis. One paper did report increases in the sedimentation rate and a low serum iron in patients with pouchitis, perhaps the result of severe inflammation in the pouch (26). If mucosal friability and bloody diarrhea persist, however, a microcytic anemia can develop secondary to blood loss and iron deficiency, as observed in 30 percent of patients in one study (27).

Stool examination for parasites, enteric pathogens, and the toxin of clostridium difficile should be performed. These studies are usually negative. Elevated perinuclear antineutrophilic cytoplasmic antibodies (pANCA) levels occur more frequently in patients affected by chronic pouchitis (28) than in those without pouchitis.

Diagnosis

A diagnosis of pouchitis is made after other causes of postoperative diarrhea have been excluded. A careful evaluation should rule out partial small bowel obstruction either at the junction between the ileum and pouch or more proximally, a stenosis of the ileo-anal anastomosis or a peripouch inflammatory process. A deficiency in lactase should be excluded. Also, specific infections with enteric pathogens (*Salmonella, Clostridium Difficile, Yersinia,* and others) should be excluded by appropriate stool cultures and examinations. The diagnosis of Crohn's disease in an ileal pouch should be ruled out by reexamination of the original proctocolectomy specimen and by reevaluation of the remaining intestine and the pouch.

At the Mayo Clinic in Rochester, Minnesota, a diagnosis of pouchitis is made when the patients present a clinical syndrome consisting of frequent, watery, and often bloody stools associated with fecal urgency, incontinence, abdominal cramping, malaise, and fever. The symptoms must be present for more than two days, and they must respond promptly to metronidazole (29). At St. Mark's Hospital in London, a diagnosis of pouchitis is made when the patients have diarrhea, endoscopic features of inflammation in the pouch and histologic evidence of acute pouch inflammation (30).

A quantitative Pouchitis Disease Activity Index similar to that developed for Crohn's disease (29) has been proposed (Table 41.2). This index should facilitate comparisons between medical centers and quantification of the response to treatment.

Table 41.2. Pouchitis disease activity index.*

Criteria	Score
Clinical	
postoperative stool frequency	
- usual	0
- 1–2 stools/day more than usual	1
- 3 or more stools/day more than usual	2
rectal bleeding	
- none or rare	0
- present daily	1
fecal urgency/abdominal cramps	
- none	0
- occasional	1
- usual	2
fever (temperature > 100°F)	
- absent	0
- present	1
Endoscopic	
edema	1
granularity	1
friability	1
loss of vascular pattern	1
mucous exudate	1
ulceration	1
Acute histological	
polymorph infiltration	
- mild	1
- moderate + crypt abscess	2
- severe + crypt abscess	3
ulceration per lower power field (average)	
- <25%	1
- ≥25≤50%	2
- >50%	3

*Data from Sandborn (29).
Note: Pouchitis is defined as a total score ≥7.

Incidence and Prevalence

The incidence of pouchitis varies with the duration of follow-up, the definition of pouchitis, the number of patients followed, and the thoroughness of the evaluation (7). The first episode of pouchitis occurs within the first year after operation in 51% of patients (31) (Table 41.3), whereas the cumulative incidence increases over time. At the Mayo Clinic, the cumulative percent of colitis patients who had developed at least one episode of pouchitis over a mean period of 8 years after ileal-pouch/anal canal anastomosis was 32% (32). Of patients with pouchitis, 39% had a single acute episode that responded to treatment with antibiotics (5). The remaining 61% of patients had at least one recurrent episode, and 7% of these patients had pouchitis that recurred often enough to constitute a chronic problem (29).

Some have separated patients with pouchitis into three clinical groups according to frequency and severity of symptoms (31) (Table 41.4). Patients in group I (76%) will present with a single or a few mild episodes with various intervals between attacks. They respond promptly to treatment. Patients in group II (18%) develop frequent relapsing, mostly mild, short lasting episodes. Patients in group III (6%) have chronic, continuous troublesome symptoms from pouchitis.

Pouchitis is rare among patients who have had ileal-pouch/anal canal anastomosis for familial adenomatous polyposis compared to those who have the operation for ulcerative colitis (5). In our series, only 7% of patients with polyposis had had a bout of pouchitis by a mean of 36 months after operation, compared to 22% of patients with colitis (33). Pouchitis occurs more frequently in patients who had universal colitis prior to colectomy than in those with left-sided colitis (34). Patients with sclerosing cholangitis or other extraintestinal manifestations of colitis preoperatively are also at higher risk of pouchitis (5,35). Pouchitis occurs rarely before closure of a diverting ileostomy (8,12,36). The incidence of pouchitis is not influenced by the type of reservoir, the presence or absence of postoperative pelvic sepsis or by the age or

Table 41.3. Pouchitis: occurrence of first episode after operation.*

| Postoperative interval | No. (%) of patients with pouchitis | | |
	Continent ileostomy (n = 28)	Pelvic pouch (n = 45)	p-value
Within 6 months	16 (57%)	16 (36%)	NS
Within 1 year	18 (64%)	23 (51%)	NS
Within 2 years	24 (86%)	32 (71%)	NS
Within 4 years	28 (100%)	44 (98%)	NS
Within 5 years		45 (100%)	

*Data from Svaninger, et al. (31).

Table 41.4. Pouchitis: distribution among clinical groups.

| Patient category | No (%) of patients with pouchitis | |
	Continent ileostomy (n = 28)	Pelvic pouch (n = 45)
Group I	18 (64%)	34 (76%)
Group II	5 (18%)	8 (18%)
Group III	5 (18%)	3 (6%)

SOURCE: Data from Svaninger, et al. (31).
Group I = a single or few mild episodes of pouchitis with various intervals responding promptly to treatment.
Group II = frequently relapsing, mostly mild, short lasting episodes.
Group III = chronic, continuous severe symptoms from pouchitis.

sex of the patients. Pouchitis is not more common among patients who have backwash ileitis (37).

Etiology

The etiology of pouchitis remains unknown. Pouchitis may result from several abnormalities that merge to form a single clinical entity. In fact, it has been referred to as a "waste basket diagnosis" (38). Many etiologic factors are potentially at interplay in the pathogenesis of the condition. They include outflow obstruction of the pouch, persistence of diseased ileal or rectal mucosa, stasis in the pouch with overgrowth of bacteria, abnormal mucus, insufficient short-chain fatty acids in the pouch lumen, excessive release of inflammatory mediators, immunological or hormonal imbalances, pouch ischemia, and technical factors. Crohn's disease in the ileal pouch should also be considered. More recently, the complex interaction between the patient, who is genetically or immunologically susceptible to ulcerative colitis, and an ileal pouch that has undergone functional adaptation to a colon-like morphology in response to fecal stasis has been proposed as the predisposing condition for pouchitis (7).

Pouch Outflow Obstruction

After proctocolectomy and ileostomy, a type of prestomal ileitis that was relieved by stomal dilatation and lavage with a catheter was ascribed to stenosis at the outlet of the ileostomy (39,40). Indeed, Kock (41) believed that the inflammatory process observed in a continent ileal pouch was probably of bacterial origin and was similar to the nonspecific ileitis that sometimes complicates conventional ileostomies with an outflow obstruction. Also, a cor-

relation between the presence of an anastomotic stricture at a pouch-anal anastomosis that required intubation for pouch emptying and the development of pouchitis has been noted (42). However, in our experience, pouchitis can occur when patients have no significant anastomotic stricture, no outflow problem, and do not require intubation.

Persistent Diseased Rectal Mucosa

Ileal-pouch/distal rectal anastomosis has been proposed as an alternative to ileal-pouch/anal canal anastomosis to avoid anal "mucosectomy" and to facilitate the procedure from the technical standpoint. The distal rectal and proximal anal mucosa left behind, however, can be the site of inflammation and even dysplasia (43).

A subgroup of patients in whom inflammation of the reservoir is confined to the perianastomotic area and the area just distal to the anastomosis has been identified. The term "short strip pouchitis" has been used to describe the problem (38). These patients may have the same symptoms as patients with generalized inflammation of the pouch. The condition has even been described, surprisingly, among patients in whom the surgeon reported removing all diseased columnar mucosa down to the dentate line. Endoscopic and histologic examination of the area with simultaneous biopsy of ileal reservoir mucosa and anorectal mucosa is helpful in the identification of inflammation in residual rectal mucosa masquerading as pouchitis.

Whether persistent rectal mucosa is associated with a higher frequency of pouchitis is unknown. Large clinical series of patients have not documented an increased incidence of pouchitis in patients with retained rectal mucosa (44). In contrast, symptomatic inflammation in the retained mucosa was present in 15% of patients in one report (45).

Persistent Diseased Ileal Mucosa

The presence of backwash ileitis at the time of colectomy for ulcerative colitis does not predispose to subsequent pouchitis (37,38,46). A flare-up of Crohn's disease of the ileum in patients who have undergone proctocolectomy for presumed ulcerative colitis, is always a consideration when recurrent symptoms occur. Interestingly, no increased incidence of pouchitis has been observed in patients with histologically indeterminate colitis compared to patients with classic ulcerative colitis (46,47). Even in the presence of aphthous ulcers, serpiginous ulcers, ileitis proximal to the ileal reservoir and cobblestone mucosa, establishing a link between refractory pouchitis and underlying Crohn's disease is difficult (46). The endoscopic appearance, the precolectomy history, the colectomy specimen, and the postoperative histologic findings often are more compatible with a diagnosis of nonspecific pouchitis rather than Crohn's disease of the pouch.

The diagnosis of Crohn's disease in an ileal pouch should be made only when reexamination of the original proctocolectomy specimen and examination of the remaining gut are consistent with Crohn's disease. The diagnosis should not be made based solely on findings in the pouch (7,12). The role of the pathologist in the exact diagnosis of chronic ulcerative colitis versus Crohn's disease cannot be over emphasized (20).

Stasis

The term pouchitis, or nonspecific ileitis, was utilized early on by Kock in patients with continent ileostomy (48). Early reports suggested that the mucosal inflammation in these pouches and in pouches anastomosed to the anal canal was due to stasis and overgrowth of bacteria (11,40). The pouchitis in these patients was sometimes successfully treated by catheter drainage and sulphasalazine. However, if stasis were the main mechanism, a similar incidence of pouchitis would be expected in patients with ulcerative colitis as in patients with familial adenomatous polyposis. In fact, the incidence is far less in polyposis than in colitis. Also, patients who irrigate their continent ileostomy with saline after evacuation have a similar risk of pouchitis as the others (49).

Several methods which quantify pouch evacuation have been developed. A direct relationship was found between the efficiency of ileal pouch evacuation and the functional results (50), but ileal pouch evacuation was not different in patients with recurrent pouchitis as compared to patients with a good clinical outcome (51). These studies, however, have not been done prospectively. Others have shown using radiolabeled egg albumin (52) and methyl cellulose (53) that ileal pouch evacuation is less complete than rectal evacuation in healthy subjects. Thus, chronic stasis in pouches likely does exist.

Bacterial Overgrowth

That the clinical features of pouchitis respond to antibiotics such as metronidazole suggests a bacterial etiology (54). Pathogens such as *Clostridium difficile*, *Yersinia* spp., *Campylobacter* spp., *Salmonella*,

Shigella, *Vibrio*, and enterotoxigenic *Escherichia coli*, however, have not been consistently detected in stool cultures from patients with pouchitis (55). Nonetheless, the fecal flora of ileal pouches is altered compared to normal ileal effluent. The proportion of anaerobic bacteria to aerobic bacteria is increased in pouch patients (56,57). The degree of villous atrophy correlates with the number of bacteroides and with the concentration of butyrate in the stool (56). All patients irrespective of their clinical results have bacterial overgrowth in the ileal pouch (51). However, quantitative cultures of the fecal content of pouches does not reveal a greater number of anaerobes in patients with pouchitis compared to those without pouchitis (51,57). In one study (58), all patients with pouchitis had bacteria present in mucosal biopsy samples, all had facultative anaerobes in the biopsies and half had obligatory anaerobes. In some patients with poor functional outcome but without pouchitis, an overgrowth of bacteria in the proximal small bowel was associated with high stool volume (51). A similar finding was made with continent ileostomy patients (54). The role of gastric hypochlorhydria predisposing to bacterial proliferation has also been raised (59).

Quantitative bacteriology may vary with the duration of follow-up and the activity of pouchitis at the time of stool collection. In most reports, the number of patients with pouchitis is small. Drawing conclusions based on a small number of subjects is difficult and may explain contradictory results. In one study, the severity of histologically verified acute inflammation correlated with the number of aerobes, whereas the severity of chronic inflammation correlated with the number of anaerobes (60). In another study, the flora of patients with pouchitis had an increased number of aerobes and a higher pH (61). Bacteria are known to be potent producers of metabolites and toxins that can potentially damage the pouch mucosa. The protection of the pouch epithelium by the mucous layer may be overcome by the increased activity of bacteria and their products.

Abnormal Mucus

An important function of intestinal mucus is to protect the mucosal epithelial cells from mechanical injury, the action of antigens and toxins and the invasion of enteric bacteria (61). The recent histochemical finding that pouch mucin resembles colonic mucin rather than small bowel mucin is of interest (13). It is known that colonic mucin from patients with ulcerative colitis differs from that of normal subjects (62). Perhaps an abnormal pouch mucin in pouchitis allows bacteria and their toxins to diffuse from the bowel lumen into the mucosa, thus, resulting in inflammation (4).

A dual isotopic metabolic labeling technique has been used to follow mucin synthesis in ileal pouches (63). Further studies in this area may shed light on the role of mucus in the pathogenesis of pouchitis.

Free Fatty Acids and Mediators of Inflammation

Reduced concentrations of short-chain fatty acids in pouch effluent have been found. The low concentrations may correlate with villous atrophy and pouchitis (64). Short chain fatty acids may serve as a major energy source for the colonic-like epithelium of the pouch, just as they do for normal colonic epithelium. The lack of short chain fatty acids may make the pouch epithelial cells more susceptible to inflammation.

The role of platelet activating factor (PAF) as a local mediator of intestinal inflammation has been investigated (4). PAF was found not to be increased in pouchitis mucosa. However, increased cytokine expression does occur in both active ulcerative colitis and pouchitis (65).

Ischemia

Another hypothesis (66) proposes that pouchitis is caused by oxygen free radical injury to the mucosa of the ileal pouch. The process is initiated by transient ischemia of the pouch and subsequent reperfusion. Mucosal ischemia can occur by pouch distension or by inadequate perfusion of the reservoir by the ileal vessels. Frequently, some of the blood vessels supplying the reservoir must be divided to provide adequate length for a tension-free, pouch-anal anastomosis. Using intraoperative fluorescein flowmetry (67) or bidirectional laser Doppler, some studies have shown a reduction of blood flow to the ileal pouch (68). Nonetheless, treatment of pouchitis with an oxygen free radical scavenger does not clearly improve pouchitis compared to controls (69).

Immunological and Hormonal Imbalance

The presence of perinuclear antineutrophil cytoplasmic antibodies (pANCA) in patients with ulcerative colitis reinforces the likelihood of immunologic dysregulation in this disease (70). Perinuclear antineutrophil cytoplasmic antibodies is present in 60% of patients with ulcerative colitis and may be a marker for a genetically distinct subset of patients who develop chronic pouchitis after undergoing ileal-pouch/anal canal anastomosis. The frequency of pANCA positivity in patients with chronic pouchitis is 100% compared to only 50% in patients without pouchitis and to 70% in patients with a Brooke ileostomy (7).

RFD9+ macrophages and CD16 macrophages are abundant in the mucosa of patients with pouchitis just as in patients with ulcerative colitis (71). Their presence suggests that effector mechanisms similar to those triggering the original ulcerative colitis may also be operative in pouchitis.

Immunoreactive leukotriene B4 and prostaglandin E2 are present in greater amounts in inflamed pouch mucosa than in uninflamed mucosa (72). Inhibition of leukotriene synthesis or receptor antagonism merit therapeutic evaluation in pouchitis. Greenberg et al. (73) found that nerves immunoreactive to vasoactive intestinal peptide (VIP) were increased in number and coarsened in patients with pouchitis. Mucosal concentrations of VIP, however, were similar to those of controls.

Pouch Size

Fischer believes that the size of the pouch has a significant influence on the incidence of pouchitis; the larger the pouch, the greater the incidence of pouchitis. He states that a smaller pouch usually empties better than a larger pouch and so may be less susceptible to pouchitis (74). He advises making a smaller pouch.

Treatment

In the absence of a definite etiology for pouchitis, the treatment of pouchitis remains empirical (Table 41.5). Initial episodes of pouchitis are usually treated successfully by administration of metronidazole (250 mg po tid), ciprofloxacin (500 mg po bid) or other antibiotics with activity directed especially against anaerobic bacteria (54). Recur-

Table 41.5.   Therapies of pouchitis.

- Frequent catheter drainage and lavage of pouch	- Oxygen free radical scavengers
- Metronidazole and other antibiotics	- Kaopectate
- 5 amino-salicylic acid	- Lidocaine
- Steroids, including budesonide	- Immunosuppressants
- Glutamine	- Pouch excision
- Short chain fatty acids	- Diverting ileostomy

rent episodes have also been treated successfully with the same medications. In chronic, unremitting pouchitis, daily oral dosing with metronidazole has been shown to be superior to placebo in reducing the median number of stools per day (30). Topical applications of metronidazole also relieve symptoms of pouchitis (75) and are well tolerated as a long-term treatment. When daily oral metronidazole is not effective in chronic pouchitis, administration of daily oral ciprofloxacin may be tried with success.

Patients intractable to antibiotics require antiinflammatory therapy similar to that directed at ulcerative colitis. Topical administration of a 5-aminosalicylic acid (76) or enemas containing steroids have been used with some success. Because of its affinity for mucosal steroid receptors and its rapid hepatic conversion to metabolites without significant steroid activity, budesonide given per annum may have a superior systemic tolerance with a similar therapeutic efficacy for pouchitis when compared with other corticosteroids (77). Other avenues of medical therapy, including glutamine (78), short-chain fatty acids, oxygen free radical scavengers, kaopectate, lidocaine, and immunosuppressives, are currently under investigation.

Although response to medical therapy is generally prompt and effective, about 10% of patients with pouchitis do not have a satisfactory response to treatment. They regard their pouchitis as a medical, social, and occupational encumbrance (5,34). In these patients, operative therapy should be considered. Diversion of the fecal stream by a loop ileostomy placed proximal to the pouch or pouch excision with permanent end ileostomy are the two options most commonly employed. Both usually give immediate and long-lasting relief of symptoms.

Long-Term Outcome

The long-term consequences of an ileal-pouch/anal canal anastomosis are unknown. No serious oncologic, nutritional, or renal complications have been reported in the almost 30-year follow-up of patients with a continent ileostomy (26,79). These results are reassuring, but 30 years is still not a lifetime when studying the sequelae of chronic stasis and inflammation (26). Epithelial dysplasia associated with nuclear aneuploidy has been described in ileal pelvic pouches anastomosed to the anal canal (80). When subtotal or total villous atrophy accompanies severe pouchitis, the risk of dysplasia appears greater (81). The concern that malignant

transformation may occur in chronically inflamed pelvic pouches is still present.

The follow-up should include endoscopic and histologic surveillance of pouch mucosa (13,82). The presence of high-grade dysplasia may be an indication for excision of the pouch. Fortunately, in several large series of patients, pouchitis and high-grade dysplasia were rare long-term causes of pouch failure, occurring in only about two percent of patients to date (1,83).

Prevention

Patients at risk of developing chronic pouchitis can be identified on histological criteria within weeks of closure of the ileostomy (21). These patients may benefit from measures designed to prevent the development of pouchitis. For example, metronidazole has been administered prophylactically to patients after pouch construction in an attempt to prevent pouchitis (84). Because of the similarity between ulcerative colitis and pouchitis, measures known to prevent relapse of ulcerative colitis might also be helpful in the prevention of pouchitis.

Experimental and clinical studies are clearly needed to better define the pathophysiology of pouchitis and to develop a therapy that would prevent or cure this important clinical problem. A resolution of the problem of pouchitis might well lead to a resolution of the larger problem of chronic ulcerative colitis itself.

References

1. Pemberton JH, Kelly KA, Beart RW, Jr, et al. Ileal pouch anal anastomosis for chronic ulcerative colitis. Long-term results. Ann Surg 1987;206:504–13.
2. Kock NG, Darle N, Hulten L, et al. Ileostomy. Curr Probl Surg 1977;14:36–8.
3. Klein K, Stenzel P, Katon RM, Pouch ileitis: report of a case with severe systemic manifestations. J Clin Gastroenterol 1983;5:149–53.
4. Tytgat GNJ, van Deventer SJH. Pouchitis. Int J Colorectal Dis 1988;3:226–8.
5. Lohmuller JL, Pemberton JH, Dozois RR, et al. Pouchitis and extraintestinal manifestations of inflammatory bowel disease after ileal pouch-anal anastomosis. Ann Surg 1990;211:622–7.
6. Beart RW, Jr. Pouchitis: a clarification (letter). Gastroenterology 1995;109:1022–3.
7. Sandborn WJ. Pouchitis following ileal pouch-anal anastomosis: definition, pathogenesis, and treatment. Gastroenterology 1994;107:1856–60.
8. Di Febo G, Miglioli M, Lauri A, et al. Endoscopic assessment of acute inflammation of the ileal reservoir after restorative ileo-anal anastomosis. Gastrointest Endosc 1990;36:6–9.

9. Church JM, Fazio VW, Lavery IC. The role of fiberoptic endoscopy in the management of the continent ileostomy. Gastrointest Endosc 1987;33:203–9.

10. Moskowitz RL, Shepherd NA, Nicholls RJ. An assessment of inflammation in the reservoir after restorative proctocolectomy with ileo-anal ileal reservoir. Int J Colorectal Dis 1986;1:167–74.

11. Phillips B. Mucosal morphology, bacteriology, and absorption in intra-abdominal ileostomy reservoir. Scand J Gastroenterol 1975;10:145.

12. Shepherd NA, Hulten L, Tytgat GN, et al. Pouchitis. Int J Colorectal Dis 1989;4:205–29.

13. Shepherd NA, Jass JR, Duval I, et al. Restorative proctocolectomy with ileal reservoir: pathological and histochemical study of mucosal biopsy specimens. J Clin Pathol 1987;40:601–7.

14. Campbell AP, Merrett MN, Kettlewell M, et al. Expression of colonic antigens by goblet and columnar epithelial cells in ileal pouch mucosa: their association with inflammatory change and fecal stasis. J Clin Path 1994;47:834–8.

15. Lerch MM, Braun J, Harder M, et al. Postoperative adaptation of the small intestine after total colectomy and J-pouch-anal anastomosis. Dis Colon Rectum 1989;32:600–8.

16. de Silva HJ, Millard PR, Kettlewell M, et al. Mucosal characteristics of pelvic ileal pouches. Gut 1991;32:61–5.

17. Apel R, Cohen Z, Andrews CW, et al. Prospective evaluation of early morphological changes in pelvic ileal pouches. Gastroenterology 1994;107:435–43.

18. Heppell J, Kelly KA, Phillips SF, et al. Physiologic aspects of continence after colectomy, mucosal proctectomy and endorectal ileo-anal anastomosis. Ann Surg 1982;195:435–43.

19. de Silva HJ, Gatter KC, Millard PR, et al. Crypt cell proliferation and HLA-DR expression in pelvic ileal pouches. J Clin Pathol 1990;43:824–8.

20. Warren BF, Shepherd NA. The role of pathology in pelvic ileal reservoir surgery. Int J Colorectal Dis 1992;7:68–75.

21. Setti Carrato P, Talbot IC, Nicholls RJ. Longterm appraisal of the histological appearance of the ileal reservoir mucosa after restorative proctocolectomy for ulcerative colitis. Gut 1994;35:1721–17.

22. Tsao JI, Galandiuk S, Pemberton JH. Pouchogram: predictor of clinical outcomes following ileal-pouch anal anastomosis. Dis Colon Rectum 1992;35:547–51.

23. Hagen G, Kolmannskog F, Aesen S, et al. Radiology of the ileal J-pouch-anal anastomosis (IPAA). Acta Radiologica 1993;34:563–8.

24. Solomon MJ, McLeod RS, O'Connor BI, et al. Assessment of peripouch inflammation after ileoanal anastomosis using endoluminal ultrasonography. Dis Colon Rectum 1995;38:182–7.

25. Kmiot WA, Youngs DJ, Winslet MC, et al. Ileal adaptation following restorative proctocolectomy. Br J Surg 1989;76:625.

26. Hultén L. Pouchitis-incidence and characteristics in the continent ileostomy. Int J Colorectal Dis 1989;4:208–10.

27. Mortensen N. Restorative proctocolecotmy—the pouch operation: good or bad? Scand J Gastroenterol (Suppl) 1992;192:130–5.

28. Sandborn WJ, Landers CJ, Termaine WJ, et al. Antineutrophil cytoplasmic antibody correlates with chronic pouchitis after ileal pouch-anal anastomosis. Am J Gastroenterol 1995;90:740–7.

29. Sandborn WJ, Tremaine WJ, Batts KP, et al. Pouchitis after ileal pouch-anal anastomosis: a pouchitis disease activity index. Mayo Clin Proc 1994;69:409–15.

30. Madden MV, Farthing MJ, Nicholls RJ. Inflammation in ileal reservoirs: 'pouchitis'. Gut 1990;31:247–9.

31. Svaninger G, Nordgren S, Oresland T, et al. Incidence and characteristics of pouchitis in the Kock continent ileostomy and the pelvic pouch. Scand J Gastroenterol 1993;28:695–700.

32. Pena JP, Gemlo BT, Rothenberger DA. Ileal pouch-anal anastomosis: state of the art. Baillieres Clin Gastroenterol 1992;6:113–27.

33. Dozois RR, Kelly KA, Welling DR, et al. Ileal pouch-anal anastomosis: comparison of results in familial adenomatous polyposis and chronic ulcerative colitis. Ann Surg 1989;210:268–71.

34. Farrands P, Nicholls RJ. Paper presented at the Association of Surgeons of great Britain and Ireland, 1989 quoted by Madden MV, Farthing MJG, Nicholls RJ. Inflammation in ileal reservoirs: "pouchitis." Gut 1990;31:247–9.

35. Penna C, Dozois R, Tremaine W, et al. Pouchitis after ileal pouch-anal anastomosis for ulcerative colitis occurs with increased frequency in patients with associated primary sclerosing cholangitis. Gut 1996;38:234–9.

36. Trabucchi E, Doldi SB, Foschi D, et al. Pouch ileitis in excluded reservoir: an unusual complication of restorative proctocolectomy for ulcerative colitis. Int Surg 1988;73:187–9.

37. Gustavsson S, Weiland LH, Kelly KA. Relationship of backwash ileitis to ileal pouchitis after ileal pouch-anal anastomosis. Dis Colon Rectum 1987;30:25–8.

38. Rauh SM, Schoetz DJ Jr, Roberts PL, et al. Pouchitis—is it a wastebasket diagnosis? Dis Colon Rectum 1991;34:685–9.

39. Counsell B. Lesions of the ileum associated with ulcerative colitis. Br J Surg 1956;44:276.

40. Scott AD, Phillips RK. Ileitis and pouchitis after colectomy for ulcerative colitis. Br J Surg 1989;76:668–9.

41. Kock NG, Myrvold HE, Nilsson LO, et al. Continent ileostomy. An account of 314 patients. Acta Chir Scand 1981;147:67–72.

42. Fleshman JW, Cohen Z, McLeod RS, et al. The ileal reservoir and ileoanal anastomosis procedure. Factors affecting technical and functional outcome. Dis Colon Rectum 1988;31:10–6.

43. King DW, Lubowski DZ, Cook TA. Anal canal mucosa in restorative proctocolectomy for ulcerative colitis. Br J Surg 1989;76:970–2.

44. Fazio VW, Ziv Y, Church J-M, et al. Ileal pouch-anal anstomoses complications and function in 1005 patients. Ann Surg 1995;222:120–7.

45. Lavery IC, Sirimarco MT, Ziv Y, et al. Anal canal inflammation after ileal pouch-anal anastomosis. The need for treatment. Dis Colon Rectum 1995;38: 803–6.

46. Subramani K, Harpaz N, Bilotta J, et al. Refractory pouchitis: does it reflect underlying Crohn's disease. Gut 1993;34:1539–42.

47. Pezim ME, Pemberton JH, Beart RW, et al. Outcome of indeterminant colitis. Dis Colon Rectum 1989; 32:653–8.

48. Kock NG. Present status of continent ileostomy: surgical revision of the malfunctioning ileostomy. Dis Colon Rectum 1976;19:200–6.

49. Hultén L, Svaninger G. Facts about the Kock continent ileostomy. Dis Colon Rectum 1984;27:553–7.

50. Stryker SJ, Kelly KA, Phillips SF, et al. Anal and neorectal function after ileal pouch-anal anastomosis. Ann Surg 1986;203:55–61.

51. O'Connell PR, Rankin DR, Weiland LH, et al. Enteric bacteriology, absorption, morphology and emptying after ileal pouch-anal anastomosis. Br J Surg 1986;73:909–14.

52. Heppell J, Belliveau P, Taillefer R, et al. Quantitative assessment of pelvic ileal reservoir emptying with a semisolid radionuclide enema. A correlation with clinical outcome. Dis Colon Rectum 1987;30:81–5.

53. Nasmyth DG, Johnston D, Godwin PG, et al. Factors influencing bowel function after ileal pouch-anal anastomosis. Br J Surg 1986;73:469–73.

54. Kelly DG, Phillips SF, Kelly KA, et al. Dysfunction of the continent ileostomy: clinical features and bacteriology. Gut 1983;24:193–201.

55. Hill MJ, Fernandez F, Bacteriology II in Pouchitis (Workshop). Int J Colorectal Dis 1989;4:217–9.

56. Nasmyth DG, Godwin PG, Dixon MF, et al. Ileal ecology after pouch-anal anastomosis or ileostomy. A study of mucosal morphology, fecal bacteriology, fecal volatile fatty acids, and their interrelationship. Gastroenterology 1989;96:817–24.

57. Luukkonen P, Valtonen V, Sivonen A, et al. Fecal bacteriology and reservoir ileitis in patients operated on for ulcerative colitis. Dis Colon Rectum 1988; 31:864–7.

58. Onderdonk AB, Dvorak AM, Cisneros RL, et al. Microbiologic assessment of tissue biopsy samples from ileal pouch patients. J Clin Microbiol 1992;30:312–7.

59. Dube S, Heyen S. Pouchitis and gastric hyposecretion: cause or effect? Int J Colorectal Dis 1990;5: 142–3.

60. Santavirta J, Mattila J, Kokki M, et al. Mucosal morphology and faecal bacteriology after ileoanal anastomosis. Int J Colorectal Dis 1991;6:38–41.

61. Ruseler-van Embden JG, Schouten WR, van Lieshout LM. Pouchitis: result of microbial imbalance? Gut 1994;35:658–64.

62. Podolsky DK, Isselbacher KJ. Glycoprotein composition of colonic mucosa. Specific alterations in ulcerative colitis. Gastroenterol 1984;87:991–8.

63. Corfield AP, Warren BF, Bartolo DC, et al. Mucin changes in ileoanal pouches monitored by metabolic labelling and histochemistry. Br J Surg 1992;79: 1209–12.

64. Clausen MR, Tvede M, Mortensen PB. Short-chain fatty acids in pouch contents from patients with and without pouchitis after ileal pouch-anal anastomosis. Gastroenterology 1992;103:1144–53.

65. Patel RT, Bain I, Youngs D, et al. Cytokine production in pouchitis is similar to that in ulcerative colitis. Dis Colon Rectum 1995;38:831–7.

66. Levin KE, Pemberton JH, Phillips SF, et al. Role of oxygen free radicals in the etiology of pouchitis. Dis Colon Rectum 1992;35:452–6.

67. Perbeck L, Lindqvist K, Liljeqvist L. The mucosal blood flow in pelvic pouches in man: a methodologic study of fluorescein flowmetry. Dis Colon Rectum 1985;28:931–6.

68. Sakaguchi M, Hosie K, Tudor R, et al. Mucosal blood flow following restorative proctocolectomy: pouchitis is associated with mucosal ischemia. Br J Surg 1989;76:1331.

69. Levin KE, Pemberton JH, Phillips SF, et al. Role of oxygen free radicals in the etiology of pouchitis. Dis Colon Rectum 1991;34:P20.

70. Colombel JF, Reumaux D, Duthilleul P, et al. Antineutrophil cytoplasmic autoantibodies in inflammatory bowel disease. Gastroenterol Clin Biol 1992; 16:656–60.

71. de Silva HJ, Jones M, Prince C, et al. Lymphocytes and macrophage subpopulations in pelvic ileal pouches. Gut 1991;32:1160–5.

72. Gertner DJ, Rampton DS, Madden MV, et al. Increased leukotreine by release from ileal pouch mucosa in ulcerative colitis compared with familial adenomatous polyposis. Gut 1994;35:1429–32.

73. Greenberg GR, Buchan AM, McLeod RS, et al. Gut hormone response after reconstructive surgery for ulcerative colitis. Gut 1989;30:1721–30.

74. Fischer JE, Nussbaum MS, Martin CW, et al. The pull-through procedure: technical factors in influencing outcome, with emphasis on pouchitis. Surgery 1993;114:828–34.

75. Nygaard K, Bergan T, Bjornek-Lett A, et al. Topical metronidazole in treatment of pouchitis. Scand J Gastroenterol 1994;29:462–7.

76. Miglioli M, Barbara L, DiFetso G, et al. Topical administration of 5-amino salicylic: a therapeutic proposal for the treatment of pouchitis (letter). N Engl J Med 1989;320;257.

77. Brattsand R. Overview of newer glucocorticosteroid preparations for inflammatory bowel disease. Can J Gastroenterol 1990;4:407–14.

78. Wischmeyer PE, Tremaine WJ, Addad AC, et al. Fecal short chain fatty acids in patients with pouchitis after ileal pouch anal anastomosis (abstract). Gastroenterology 1991;100:848.

79. Ojerskog B, Kock NG, Nilsson LO, et al. Long-term follow-up of patients with continent ileostomies. Dis Colon Rectum 1990;33:184–9.

80. Lofberg R, Liljeqvist L, Lindqvist K, et al. Dysplasia and DNA aneuploidy in pelvic pouch. Report of a case. Dis Colon Rectum 1991;34:280–4.

81. Veress B, Reinholt FP, Lindqvist K, et al. Long-term histomorphological surveillance of the pelvic ileal pouch: dysplasia develops in a subgroup of patients. Gastroenterology 1995;109:1090–7.

82. Mignon M, Settler C, Phillips SF, Pouchitis—a poorly understood entity. Dis Colon Rectum 1995;38:100–3.

83. Gemlo BT, Wong WD, Rothenberger DA, et al. Ileal pouch-anal anastomosis. Patterns of failure. Arch Surg 1992;127:784–6; discussion 787.

84. Fonkalsrud EW. Update on clinical experience with different surgical techniques of the endorectal pull-through operation for colitis and polyposis. Surg Gynecol Obstetr 1987;165:309–16.

Index

ISBN 0-387-94966-6